Neurosurgical Intensive Care

NOTICE

Medicine is an ever-changing science. As new research and clinical experience broaden our knowledge, changes in treatment and drug therapy are required. The editors and the publisher of this work have checked with sources believed to be reliable in their efforts to provide information that is complete and generally in accord with the standards accepted at the time of publication. However, in view of the possibility of human error or changes in medical sciences, neither the editors nor the publisher nor any other party who has been involved in the preparation or publication of this work warrants that the information contained herein is in every respect accurate or complete, and they are not responsible for any errors or omissions or for the results obtained from use of such information. Readers are encouraged to confirm the information contained herein with other sources. For example and in particular, readers are advised to check the product information sheet included in the package of each drug they plan to administer to be certain that the information contained in this book is accurate and that changes have not been made in the recommended dose or in the contraindications for administration. This recommendation is of particular importance in connection with new or infrequently used drugs.

Neurosurgical Intensive Care

Editor
Brian T. Andrews, M.D.
Assistant Clinical Professor of Neurosurgery
Department of Neurosurgery
University of California
at San Francisco:
Attending Neurosurgeon,
the Neurosurgical Service
San Francisco General Hospital
San Francisco, California

This textbook has been endorsed by the Joint Section on Neurotrauma and Critical Care of the American Association of Neurological Surgeons and Congress of Neurological Surgeons. While the Joint Section considers this to be a useful source of information on neurosurgical intensive care, the opinions on specific management issues contained in this text are strictly those of the authors and do not necessarily reflect any official policy of the neurosurgical organizations or its officers.

McGRAW-HILL, INC.
Health Professions Division

New York St. Louis San Francisco Auckland
Bogotá Caracas Lisbon London Madrid Mexico
Milan Montreal New Delhi Paris San Juan
Singapore Sydney Tokyo Toronto

NEUROSURGICAL INTENSIVE CARE

1234567890 KGP KGP 9876543

ISBN 0-07-001849-9

This book was set in Times Roman by Digitype, Inc.
The editors were Jane Pennington and Susan Finn.
The production supervisor was Clare Stanley.
The cover was designed by Karen Quigley.
The index was prepared by Barbara Littlewood.
Arcata Graphics/Kingsport Press was the printer and binder.

INTERNATIONAL EDITION

When ordering this title, use ISBN 0-07-112535-3

Library of Congress Cataloging-in-Publication Data

Neurosurgical intensive care / editor, Brian T. Andrews.
p. cm.
Includes bibliographical references and index.
ISBN 0-07-001849-9
1. Neurological intensive care. 2. Surgical intensive care.
I. Andrews, Brian T.
[DNLM: 1. Intensive Care—methods. 2. Monitoring, Physiologic. 3. Neurosurgery. WL368 N4955]
RC350.N49N484 1993
617.4′8028—dc20
DLC
for Library of Congress 92-49880
CIP

Contents

Contributors*

Brian T. Andrews, M.D. [2,10,14,18]
Assistant Clinical Professor of Neurosurgery
Department of Neurosurgery
University of California
at San Francisco;
Attending Neurosurgeon, the Neurosurgical Service
San Francisco General Hospital
San Francisco, California

Stanley L. Barnwell, M.D., Ph.D. [16]
Associate Professor
Division of Neurosurgery
Department of Surgery
University of Oregon Health Sciences Center
Portland, Oregon

Daniel L. Barrow, M.D. [8]
Associate Professor
Department of Neurosurgery
The Emory University Hospital
Atlanta, Georgia

Gregory D. Cascino, M.D. [17]
Assistant Professor
Department of Neurology
The Mayo Clinic
Rochester, Minnesota

Joseph M. Darby, M.D. [6]
Associate Professor
Division of Critical Care Medicine
Department of Anesthesia
Presbyterian University Hospital
University of Pittsburgh, Pennsylvania

L. D. Dickenson, M.D. [9]
Resident in Neurosurgery
Section of Neurosurgery, Department of Surgery
University of Michigan
Ann Arbor, Michigan

*The numbers in brackets following the contributor name refer to chapter(s) authored or coauthored by the contributor.

Curtis A. Dickman, M.D. [11]
Attending Neurosurgeon
Department of Neurosurgery
Barrow Neurological Institute
St. Joseph's Hospital and Medical Center
Phoenix, Arizona

Grant E. Gauger, M.D. [21]
Clinical Professor of Neurosurgery
Department of Neurosurgery
University of California at San Francisco;
Chief of Neurosurgery
Highland General Hospital
Oakland, California

Philip H. Gutin, M.D. [18]
Professor of Neurosurgery
University of California at San Francisco
San Francisco, California

Gregory Hammer, M.D. [19]
Co-Director of the Pediatric Intensive Care Unit
Department of Pediatrics and Anesthesia
California Pacific Medical Center
San Francisco, California

Mark E. Harris, M.D. [5]
Resident in Neurosurgery
Department of Neurosurgery
The Emory University Medical Center
Atlanta, Georgia

J. T. Hoff, M.D. [9]
Professor and Chairman
Section of Neurosurgery, Department of Surgery
University of Michigan
Ann Arbor, Michigan

Patricia A. Hudgins, M.D. [5]
Assistant Professor of Radiology
Division of Neuroradiology
Department of Radiology
The Emory University Medical Center
Atlanta, Georgia

Rohit Khanna, M.D. [13]
Research Fellow
Cerebral Blood Flow Laboratory
Division of Neurosurgery
University of California at Los Angeles
Los Angeles, California

James N. Lindsay, M.D. [19]
Co-Director of the Pediatric Intensive Care Unit
Department of Pediatrics
California Pacific Medical Center
San Francisco, California

John M. Luce, M.D. [1,20]
Associate Director of Critical Care
San Francisco General Hospital;
Associate Professor of Medicine and Anesthesia
Departments of Medicine and Anesthesia
University of California at San Francisco
San Francisco, California

Neil A. Martin, M.D. [13]
Associate Professor
Head, Neurovascular Surgery Section
Director, Cerebral Blood Flow Laboratory
Division of Neurosurgery
University of California at Los Angeles
Los Angeles, California

Frederick B. Meyer, M.D. [15]
Associate Professor of Neurosurgery
Department of Neurosurgery
The Mayo Clinic
Rochester, Minnesota

Michon Morita, M.D. [18]
Senior Resident in Neurosurgery
Department of Neurosurgery
University of California at San Francisco
San Francisco, California

Paul B. Nelson, M.D. [6]
Associate Professor of Neurosurgery
Department of Neurosurgery
Presbyterian University Hospital
University of Pittsburgh
Pittsburgh, Pennsylvania

William G. Obana, M.D. [2,14]
Chief Resident
Department of Neurosurgery
University of California at San Francisco
San Francisco, California

Linda Ott, R.N. [7]
Division of Neurosurgery
Department of Surgery
University of Kentucky Medical Center
Lexington, Kentucky

Gerald Rodts, M.D. [13]
Senior Resident
Division of Neurosurgery
University of California at Los Angeles
Los Angeles, California

Michael J. Rosner, M.D. [4]
Associate Professor of Neurosurgery
Department of Neurosurgery
University of Alabama
Birmingham, Alabama

Volker K. H. Sonntag, M.D. [11]
Attending Neurosurgeon and Director of Spinal Surgery
Department of Neurosurgery
Barrow Neurological Institute
St. Joseph's Hospital and Medical Center
Phoenix, Arizona

Philip Villanueva, M.D. [3]
Associate Professor of Neurosurgery
Department of Neurosurgery
Director of the Neurosurgical Intensive Care Unit
University of Miami
Miami, Florida

David H. Wisner, M.D. [12]
Associate Professor of Surgery
Head, Section of Trauma Surgery
Department of General Surgery
University of California at Davis
Sacramento, California

Byron Young, M.D. [7]
Professor and Chief
Division of Neurosurgery
Department of Surgery
University of Kentucky Medical Center
Lexington, Kentucky

Preface

Neurosurgical management of patients with insults or injury to the central nervous system has long relied on the intensive care unit for monitoring of systemic vital signs and neurologic function and, on occasion, on specific techniques such as intracranial pressure monitoring.

Recently there have occurred a number of advances in ICU care that are of benefit to the neurosurgeon and supporting staff. First has been the development of specific *neurosurgical intensive care units* where the staff and support personnel treat such patients full time, with particular attention to newer methods of neurologic monitoring. Second is the training of physicians specializing in critical care, often coming out of the ranks of those in anesthesia or internal medicine, who are developing a more cooperative role with the neurosurgeon in the joint management of ICU patients. Finally, there has been rapid growth in methods for physiologic monitoring of the injured brain, such as intracranial pressure monitoring, measurement of cerebral bloodflow, perfusion and oxygen consumption, and monitoring of electrophysiologic function. I am pleased to say that the major research and development in these areas are coming from neurosurgical laboratories.

Whereas in years past the ICU was the setting for treatments that were primarily supportive, such as mechanical ventilation, control of vital signs, and treatment of infections, with the advent of more sophisticated monitoring we are now seeing wider and more effective attempts at therapies designed to reverse abnormalities of neurophysiology, such as hemodynamic therapies, and pharmacologic treatments to improve brain tolerance to injury.

The goal of this book is to provide neurosurgeons, critical care specialists, and all those who care for neurosurgical patients with an up-to-date reference. I offer heartfelt thanks to the chapter authors and know that the reader will benefit from their thoughtful contributions.

CHAPTER 1

Cardiopulmonary Physiology and Management in Neurosurgical Intensive Care

John M. Luce

CARDIOPULMONARY PROBLEMS IN NEUROSURGICAL PATIENTS

Underlying Medical Diseases

Depending on age and other factors, neurosurgical patients may suffer from chronic cardiac conditions such as ischemic heart disease (IHD). Asthma, chronic obstructive pulmonary disease (COPD), and other respiratory problems may occur in the same patients. At the same time, preexisting nervous system disorders such as epilepsy and neuromuscular disease may be present. All of these conditions may be exacerbated by the stress of neurosurgical illnesses and may complicate its management.

Perioperative Complications

Operative intervention may worsen preexisting medical conditions. For example, hyperventilation therapy used to reduce cerebral blood flow at the time of surgery may precipitate arrhythmias due to the effects of alkalemia and electrolyte shifts on the heart. Similarly, hyperosmolar therapy and the use of diuretics may severely compromise cardiac output in patients with inadequate intravascular volume, with myocardial infarction and cardiorespiratory arrest as potential perioperative complications in patients with IHD.

Complications of Intensive Care

Although intensive care units (ICUs) were created to improve and prolong life, they frequently are the setting for complications that increase morbidity and mortality. Such complications may result from pulmonary artery catheter placement that may cause vascular rupture, or from mechanical ventilators that may produce barotrauma and "volutrauma." Nosocomial pneumonia is all too common among neurosurgical patients receiving intensive care, and complications such as adult respiratory distress syndrome (ARDS) and multiple organ system failure (MOSF) also may occur.

Importance of Understanding Cardiopulmonary Function and Failure

Neurosurgical patients are managed in ICUs because they are expected to benefit from the monitoring techniques and therapeutic devices available there despite the possibility of complications. To minimize complications and to maximize patient benefit, clinicians who practice in the units must understand cardiopulmonary function and failure. This applies both to neurosurgeons and to critical care practitioners.

MONITORING OF CARDIOVASCULAR AND RESPIRATORY FUNCTION

Cardiovascular Monitoring

The adequacy of cardiac output ($\dot{Q}_T$) and tissue perfusion can be inferred from the strength of peripheral pulses, the warmth and color of the hands or feet, and the time required to refill superficial capillaries after they have been blanched; normally, 2 to 3 s are required. Most ICUs also have the capacity to monitor heart rate (HR), rhythm, and systemic arterial pressure (P_{SA}).[1]

Systemic Arterial Pressure Monitoring HR and P_{SA} may be determined in an on-line fashion with indwelling systemic arterial catheters that also may be used to obtain samples for systemic arterial blood gas analysis. These catheters are usually placed in the radial or femoral arteries. Complications such as local hematoma formation, ischemia distal to the site of insertion, or local infection may be minimized by using pressure dressings, devices that continually flush the catheters with dilute solutions containing heparin, and sterile catheter insertion and maintenance techniques.

Although HR is easy to measure, stroke volume (SV) is difficult to estimate and requires radionuclide or ultrasonographic studies that cannot routinely be performed at the bedside. Because of this, clinicians commonly must infer SV by estimating preload, one of its three determinants. Preload cannot be measured directly but is equivalent to ventricular end-diastolic volume, which is similar to—but not always the same as—ventricular end-diastolic pressure.

Central Venous Pressure Monitoring Right ventricular end-diastolic pressure may be obtained by passing a catheter into the superior vena cava and measuring mean right atrial pressure ($\bar{P}_{RA}$) when the tricuspid valve is open. Central venous pressure (CVP) monitoring carries the risk of perforating a major vein or the right atrium and providing a nidus for infection, especially if the catheter is inserted in unsterile fashion or left in place too long. Nevertheless, the pressure measurement provides an approximation of right ventricular preload if ventricular compliance is normal, as it usually is in young patients with neurosurgical disease.

Central venous pressure measurement also may be used to estimate left ventricular end-diastolic pressure and volume if one assumes that right and left ventricular pressures are similar in diastole. The $\bar{P}_{RA}$ is particularly helpful when it is less than its normal level of approximately 5 mmHg as pressure in the right ventricle is seldom much higher than that in the left; thus, a low $\bar{P}_{RA}$ suggests decreased intravascular volume. However, the $\bar{P}_{RA}$ may be increased due to elevated pressure in pulmonary circulation when left ventricular pressure is normal, just as left ventricular pressure may be elevated when right ventricular pressure is normal. Therefore, it may be preferable to assess left ventricular pressure more directly, especially in older patients.

Pulmonary Artery Pressure Monitoring Left ventricular end-diastolic pressure may be estimated by passing a balloon-tipped catheter into the central venous circulation. With the balloon inflated, the catheter travels with venous blood through the right atrium, right ventricle, and main pulmonary artery. The catheter then floats into a branch of the pulmonary artery and occludes it by "wedging" there. Blood flow distal to the balloon ceases, and the pulmonary artery occlusion pressure (P_{PAO}) measured at the catheter tip just distal to the balloon reflects the downstream pressure. This pressure is usually equal to left atrial pressure (P_{LA}), which is the same as left ventricular end-diastolic pressure when the mitral value is open, assuming that pulmonary venous pressure is not higher. The left ventricular end-diastolic pressure is assumed to be an approximation of left ventricular end-diastolic volume, that is, preload. In addition to estimating preload, the pulmonary artery catheter with an incorporated thermister may be used to measure $\dot{Q}_T$.[2]

The indications for pulmonary artery catheterization include estimation of intravascular volume in patients whose volume status is uncertain, determination of $\dot{Q}_T$, and measurement of intracardiac pressures to help diagnose disorders such as pulmonary hypertension and cardiac tamponade. The contraindications include lack of vascular access, untreatable bleeding disorders, and patient instability that does not allow time for the procedure.

The complications of pulmonary artery catheterization include vascular laceration during insertion and infection, as with central venous catheterization. In addition, because the catheter is passed through the heart, it may cause arrhythmias and heart block. For this reason, pulmonary artery catheterization should be performed under electrocardiographic monitoring with resuscitation equipment and intravenous lidocaine available.

Once the catheter is in the pulmonary artery, it may cause vessel rupture or infarction if it migrates into a distal vessel. These complications may be avoided by determining the position of the catheter tip on the chest radiograph, monitoring the pulmonary artery pressure (P_{PA}) waveform to be certain that the P_{PAO} tracing is not present when the balloon is deflated, and making certain that a P_{PAO} tracing can be obtained only by inflating the balloon with at least 1 mL of air.

Proper interpretation of measurements made with central venous and pulmonary artery catheters requires that intravascular pressures be referenced to the extravascular pressures around them. Thus, the P_{PAO} will actually be lower than the true ventricular filling pressure if it is measured in a spontaneously breathing patient during inspiration when pleural pressure may be greatly negative. On the other hand, the P_{PAO} will be higher than the true filling pressure if it is measured in a mechanically ventilated patient during an inspiration with positive pressure. To avoid erroneous interpretation, the P_{PAO} should be measured in end expiration. If patients are receiving positive end-expiratory pressure (PEEP) at levels above 10 cmH_2O from the ventilator, approximately one quarter of the PEEP should be subtracted from the measured P_{PAO} to approximate the true P_{PAO}. It is less important to subtract an exact amount than it is to recognize that the P_{PAO} is at best an approximation of left ventricular end-diastolic pressure, which is only an approximation of left ventricular end-diastolic volume.[3]

The combination of systemic and pulmonary artery catheterization also facilitates measurement of the pressure across the systemic ($\overline{P_{SA}}$ minus $\overline{P_{RA}}$) and pulmonary (mean $\overline{P_{PA}}$ minus $\overline{P_{LA}}$ or $\overline{P_{PAO}}$) circulations. In concert with $\dot{Q}_T$, these data allow determination of the systemic and pulmonary vascular resistances (SVR, PVR). Pulmonary artery catheterization also provides information about mixed venous blood gas values.

Respiratory Monitoring

Breathing Patterns Physical examination may be very helpful in assessing respiratory function. For example, rapid breathing and intercostal muscle retraction may reflect respiratory distress. Abdominal paradox, an inward movement of the abdominal wall during inspiration, signifies that the diaphragms are not contracting normally; this may be seen in patients with high cervical spinal cord injury above or involving the phrenic nerve nuclei (level C_3 through C_5) (Fig. 1-1). Patients with low cervical spinal cord lesions do not manifest abdominal paradox (Fig. 1-2).[4]

Six breathing patterns have been said to result from head trauma and other insults to the central nervous system: (1) eupneic or normal respiration, which may occur in the presence of small lesions; (2) Cheyne-Stokes asthma or periodic respiration, which is associated with bilateral hemispheric disease; (3) central neurogenic hyperventilation, which may be due to lesions at the pontine level; (4) apneustic respiration, which also may reflect damage to the pons; (5) ataxic respiration related to injury in the medulla; and (6) apnea caused by overwhelming damage to the medullary respiratory control center.[5] However, precise localization of lesions based on respiratory pattern is not

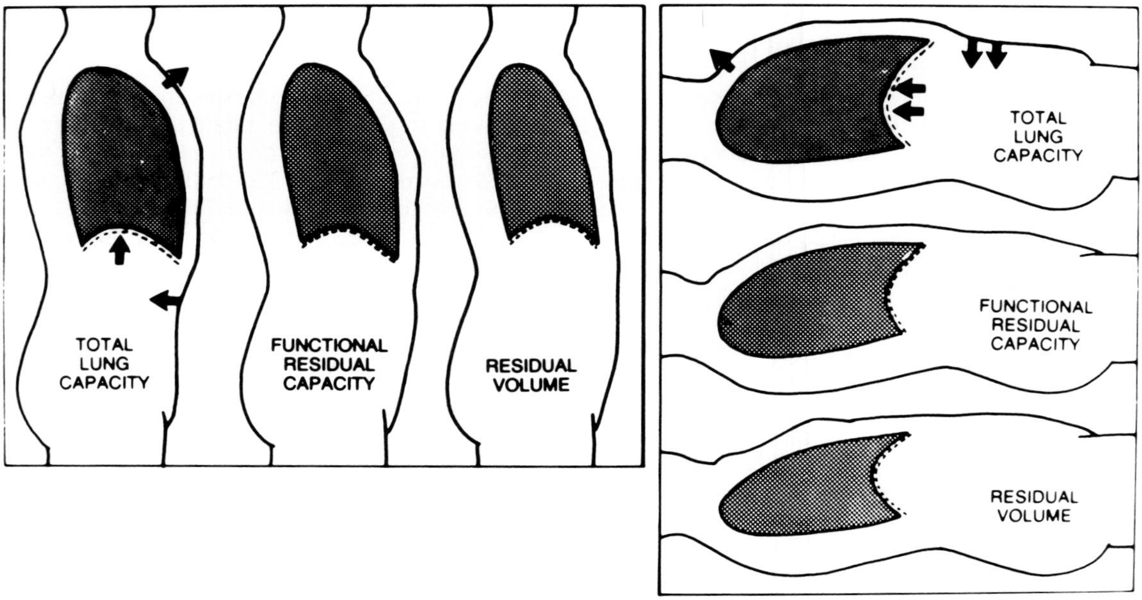

Figure 1-1 Breathing patterns in the upright and supine positions in patients with high cervical spinal cord lesions. Because the phrenic and intercostal nerves do not function, patients inspire from functional residual capacity to total lung capacity only with their accessory respiratory muscles, and only their upper rib cage moves outward (arrows). Their abdominal wall actually moves inward during inspiration, a sign called abdominal paradox. Inspiration is worsened in the supine position because the abdominal contents force the flaccid diaphragms further cephalad. Because the intercostal and abdominal nerves do not function, expiration to residual volume is compromised. (Adapted, with permission, from Luce JM, Tyler ML, Pierson DJ: *Intensive Respiratory Care*. Philadelphia, Saunders, 1984, p 69.)

always possible.[6] Furthermore, although respiratory patterns may provide a rough approximation of the level of the lesion, they cannot substitute for arterial blood gas analysis in the detection and evaluation of respiratory failure.

Assessment of Ventilation Samples of systemic arterial blood for measurement of partial arterial pressures of carbon dioxide (Pa_{CO_2}), oxygen (Pa_{O_2}), pH, and the bicarbonate concentration ($[HCO_3^-]$) may be obtained from either repeated percutaneous arterial punctures or indwelling arterial catheters. The Pa_{CO_2} is used to assess the adequacy of ventilation and diagnose hypercapneic respiratory failure, which is also called ventilatory failure. Similarly, the pH and $[HCO_3^-]$ measurements can be used to determine whether hypercapnia is acute or chronic.

An approximation of Pa_{CO_2} may be made by measuring the end-tidal CO_2 tension (PET_{CO_2}) in expired gas. This is most conveniently measured in mechanically ventilated patients. If the PET_{CO_2} is to substitute for Pa_{CO_2}, the two values should be correlated using several paired measurements. The PET_{CO_2} usually is slightly less than the Pa_{CO_2}. Measurement of PET_{CO_2} is particularly helpful in patients with head trauma and other conditions who are being hyperventilated and in whom PET_{CO_2} and Pa_{CO_2} are well correlated if there is no concurrent lung disease.

Ventilatory variables such as respiratory rate (F) and tidal volume (V_T) and their product, the minute ventilation ($\dot{V}_E$), may be accurately measured by a technique called respiratory inductance plethysmography, which uses wire coils imbedded in bands that fit around the chest and abdomen to

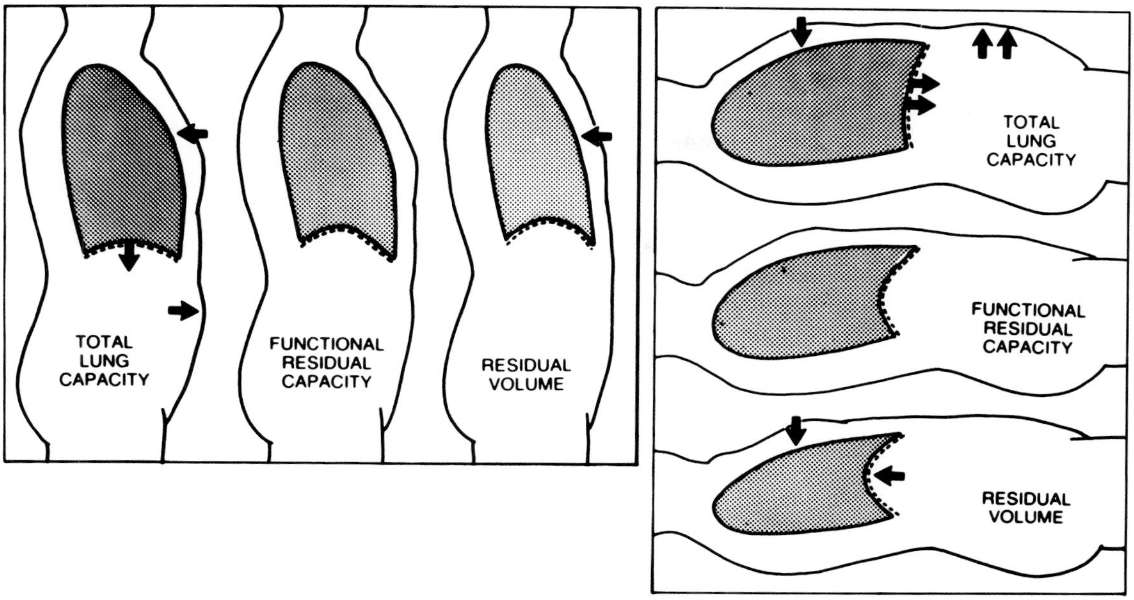

Figure 1-2 Breathing patterns in the upright and supine positions in patients with low cervical spinal cord lesions. Because the phrenic nerves function, patients inspire reasonably well from functional residual capacity and do not manifest abdominal paradox (arrows). Therefore, they achieve a total lung capacity that is near normal and is limited only by a lack of intercostal and abdominal muscle contraction. Inspiration is aided in the supine position, when the abdominal contents force the diaphragms into a domed position from which they contract more effectively. Expiration to residual volume is limited by intercostal and abdominal muscle dysfunction, although patients learn to aid expiration by contracting their pectoralis major muscles. (Reproduced, with permission, from Luce JM, Tyler ML, Pierson DJ: *Intensive Respiratory Care*. Philadelphia, Saunders, 1984, p 67.)

detect movements of these areas. These variables also may be measured by a pneumotachygraph or other types of spirometers in patients who are breathing through endotracheal tubes. Neither alveolar ventilation ($\dot{V}_A$) nor dead-space ventilation ($\dot{V}_D$) can be directly measured, although the value of $\dot{V}_A$ may be inferred if $\dot{V}_E$ and $\dot{V}_D$ are known. The ratio of V_D to V_T per breath can be calculated in patients whose Pa_{CO_2} and PET_{CO_2} are known, using the modified Bohr equation:

$$V_D/V_T = \frac{Pa_{CO_2} - PET_{CO_2}}{Pa_{CO_2}} \qquad (1)$$

The V_D/V_T is usually 0.30 to 0.35 in healthy persons breathing spontaneously. In patients with normal lungs being mechanically ventilated the V_D/V_T is approximately 0.50.[1]

Carbon dioxide production ($\dot{V}_{CO_2}$) may be measured by closed systems in patients breathing spontaneously or receiving mechanical ventilation. Once $\dot{V}_{CO_2}$ is measured, V_D/V_T is calculated from Eqs. 1 and $\dot{V}_A$ is inferred, one can determine which abnormality in the alveolar ventilation relationship (Eqs. 2 and 3) is responsible for ventilatory failure.

Three other variables that reflect ventilatory capability are the maximum inspiratory pressure (MIP), the vital capacity (VC), and the ratio of the forced expiratory volume in 1 s (FEV_1) to the forced VC. In the MIP maneuver, a manometer is used to measure the negative pressure patients can generate when inspiring from a low lung volume. An MIP that is less negative than -20 cmH_2O, as might be seen in patients with neuromuscular disease, suggests the need for ventilatory support. On the other hand, an MIP that is more negative than -20 cmH_2O correlates with successful weaning from mechanical ventilation.[7]

The VC, the greatest amount of gas that can be inhaled or exhaled in a single breath, can be measured with any of a variety of spirometers. The normal VC is approximately 50 mL/kg of body weight. A VC of less than 10 mL/kg, which also may be seen in patients with neuromuscular disease, usually indicates the need for institution or continuation of mechanical ventilation. The FEV_1 also can be measured by spirometry. Normally the FEV_1 is approximately 75 to 80 percent of the forced VC; reductions in this ratio may occur in patients with airway obstruction due to asthma or COPD.

Assessment of Auto-PEEP Another measurement that may be made on mechanically ventilated patients is intrinsic or auto-PEEP. Auto-PEEP occurs primarily in patients with airway obstruction due to asthma or COPD who fail to complete expiration either during spontaneous breathing or before they receive the next breath from a mechanical ventilator. This results in air trapping that produces positive pressure at end expiration. The auto-PEEP effect can reduce cardiac filling pressures and $\dot{Q}_T$ and elevate P_{PAO} readings unless it, like intentionally administered PEEP, is accounted for. Auto-PEEP can be measured in mechanically ventilated patients by stopping airflow at end expiration just before the next breath, allowing the pressure in the airways and the ventilator tubing to equilibrate, and reading the pressure from the ventilator manometer.[8]

Assessment of Arterial Oxygenation Just as measurement of Pa_{CO_2} is the means by which ventilatory failure is diagnosed, failure of arterial oxygenation can be diagnosed only by determining the Pa_{O_2}. Introducing the values for Pa_{CO_2} and the partial pressure of oxygen in inspired gas (PI_{O_2}) into the alveolar gas equation (Eq. 4) enables determination of the alveolar to arterial oxygen pressure difference [$P(A\text{-}a)_{O_2}$]. This in turn provides insight into the probable cause of hypoxemia in a given patient.

Because systemic arterial blood sampling may be associated with complications, a less invasive approximation of the state of arterial oxygenation often is desirable. This may be accomplished through pulse oximetry in which the differential absorption of certain wavelengths of light passed through a finger or other appendage is used to calculate the systemic arterial oxygen saturation (Sa_{O_2}). This technique accurately measures Sa_{O_2} above levels of 80 percent in patients with adequate peripheral blood flow. It is particularly helpful as a continuous measurement in patients who are relatively stable and in whom a normal oxyhemoglobin saturation curve enables good correlation between Sa_{O_2} and Pa_{O_2}. The Sa_{O_2} measured by oximetry does not account for hemoglobin that is saturated by substances other than oxygen, such as carbon monoxide.[9]

The Sa_{O_2} also may be derived from the Pa_{O_2}. The Sa_{O_2}, hemoglobin (Hb) concentration, and Pa_{O_2} are the determinants of the systemic arterial oxygen content (Ca_{O_2}) (Eq. 2). Once Ca_{O_2} is known, it can be multiplied by the $\dot{Q}_T$ to determine oxygen transport ($\dot{T}_{O_2}$). Thus, systemic arterial blood gas analysis helps diagnose failure of oxygen transport, determine the abnormalities responsible for such failure, and assess its severity.

Pulmonary arterial blood gas analysis provides information about the partial pressure, saturation, and content of oxygen in mixed venous blood ($P\bar{v}_{O_2}$, $S\bar{v}_{O_2}$, $C\bar{v}_{O_2}$). In addition, $S\bar{v}_{O_2}$ may be measured continuously with oxymetric pulmonary artery catheters. Combined with values for $\dot{Q}_T$ and Ca_{O_2} obtained by systemic arterial blood gas analysis, the $C\bar{v}_{O_2}$ may be inserted into Eq. 7 to calculate the oxygen consumption ($\dot{V}_{O_2}$). Alternatively, $\dot{V}_{O_2}$ may be determined directly by measuring concentrations of oxygen in inspired and expired gas and the inspired and expired volumes. Even if $\dot{V}_{O_2}$ is not calculated or precisely known, the decrease in $P\bar{v}_{O_2}$, $S\bar{v}_{O_2}$, and $C\bar{v}_{O_2}$ and the increase in the arterial to mixed venous content difference ($C[a\text{-}\dot{v}]_{O_2}$) that characterize adequate oxygen transport can be assessed by analysis of systemic and pulmonary artery blood gas samples, as can the increase in $P\bar{v}_{O_2}$, $S\bar{v}_{O_2}$, and $C\bar{v}_{O_2}$, and the decrease in $C(a\text{-}\dot{v})_{O_2}$ that characterize inadequate oxygen extraction.

Assessment of Tissue Oxygenation As suggested by the previous discussion, the data obtained from combined systemic and pulmonary artery blood gas analysis may be very helpful in managing critically ill patients. Nevertheless, not all such patients require such sophisticated monitoring techniques, and the techniques still cannot provide an ideal assessment of oxygenation at a tissue level. The same can be said for serial measurement of serum lactate levels, which some physicians use as a monitoring tool. Despite these and other technological advances in critical care monitoring, assessment of tissue oxygenation probably is best performed by analyzing individual organ system function by simple biochemical tests, such as renal and hepatic indices, measuring urine output, and observing mental status.

PATHOPHYSIOLOGY OF CIRCULATORY AND RESPIRATORY FAILURE

Aerobic Metabolism

Aerobic metabolism in man is made possible by four processes that involve the cardiovascular and respiratory systems. These processes include (1) ventilation, in which O_2 is inhaled from the atmosphere and CO_2 is excreted into it; (2) arterial oxygenation, in which O_2 is transferred from the alveoli into mixed venous blood in the pulmonary capillaries in exchange for CO_2; (3) O_2 transport, in which O_2 is carried in systemic arterial blood to the tissues; and (4) O_2 extraction and utilization, in which the tissues take up O_2 from the blood and give up CO_2, which is transported in mixed venous blood to the lungs.[1]

Ventilation

The adequacy of ventilation is determined by measurement of the Pa_{CO_2} in systemic arterial blood. At sea level, the normal Pa_{CO_2} is approximately 40 mmHg. Hypoventilation and hypercapnia exist when the Pa_{CO_2} exceeds this level, and hypercapneic respiratory failure is diagnosed when the Pa_{CO_2} is 50 mmHg or greater at sea level unless this is a compensation for metabolic alkalosis. Hypercapneic respiratory failure is also called ventilatory failure.[10]

The pathophysiology of ventilatory failure is explained by examining the factors that determine the Pa_{CO_2}. The Pa_{CO_2} is directly related to the body's carbon dioxide production per minute ($\dot{V}_{CO_2}$) and inversely proportional to $\dot{V}_A$. Thus,

$$Pa_{CO_2} \approx \frac{\dot{V}_{CO_2}}{\dot{V}_A} \tag{2}$$

The normal $\dot{V}_{CO_2}$ of a healthy young person is approximately 200 mL/min and $\dot{V}_A$ is approximately 5 L.

Alveolar ventilation is equal to the $\dot{V}_E$, which is the amount of gas that enters the upper respiratory tract each minute, minus the $\dot{V}_D$, which is the inhaled gas that does not participate in gas exchange either because it remains in the upper airways or because it enters areas of the lung where blood flow is insufficient for the matching of ventilation and perfusion. The $\dot{V}_E$ is the product of V_T, which is normally 450 mL and F, which is normally 12 to 22/min. Thus,

$$Pa_{CO_2} \approx \frac{\dot{V}_{CO_2}}{(V_T \times F) - \dot{V}_D} \tag{3}$$

From Eqs. 2 and 3, it follows that hypercapnia can occur if $\dot{V}_{CO_2}$ increases and $\dot{V}_A$ does not, if $\dot{V}_A$ decreases and $\dot{V}_{CO_2}$ does not, or if $\dot{V}_D$ increases out of proportion to $\dot{V}_E$. The example of the first situation might be a patient who becomes febrile due to infection and thereby increases $\dot{V}_{CO_2}$ but cannot increase $\dot{V}_A$ because of respiratory muscle weakness. Patients with severe asthma and COPD may have ventilatory failure because $\dot{V}_A$ is reduced due to airway obstruction, especially when $\dot{V}_{CO_2}$ is increased. A primary reduction in $\dot{V}_A$ is also seen in narcotic or sedative drug overdosage. In conditions such as ARDS, $\dot{V}_D$ may increase due to vascular obstruction and can cause ventilatory failure if patients cannot increase $\dot{V}_E$ due, for example, to oversedation.

The physiologic consequences of hypercapnia depend largely on the rate of increase in Pa_{CO_2} and the level it reaches. An increased Pa_{CO_2} dilates cerebral blood vessels, increases cerebral blood flow, and may increase intracranial pressure (ICP), especially if ICP is increased to begin with.[11] In addition, every 1 mmHg rise in Pa_{CO_2} causes the pH in systemic arterial blood to fall by 0.0075 units. The acute respiratory acidosis that results may depress the function of the heart and other organs until the serum [HCO_3^-] rises and buffers the fall in pH. Thus, gradual increases in Pa_{CO_2} are compensated for by an increasing [HCO_3^-]. Chronic metabolic alkalosis of this sort is of little physiologic consequence. However, an increase in Pa_{CO_2} will result in a reduction of the partial pressure of oxygen in alveolar gas and thus a decrease in the partial pressure of oxygen in systemic arterial blood unless supplemental O_2 is administered.

Arterial Oxygenation

The adequacy of arterial oxygenation is determined by the Pa_{O_2}, which in healthy young persons is approximately 95 mmHg at sea level. Hypoxemia exists when the Pa_{O_2} is below this value, and hypoxemic respiratory failure is diagnosed if the Pa_{O_2} is less than 50 to 60 mmHg at sea level. Hypoxemic respiratory failure is also called failure of arterial oxygenation.[10]

The alveolar gas equation states that PA_{O_2} is equal to the partial pressure of oxygen in inspired air (PI_{O_2}) minus the partial pressure of carbon dioxide in alveolar gas (PA_{CO_2}), divided by the respiratory quotient (RQ). Thus,

$$PA_{O_2} = PI_{O_2} - \frac{PA_{CO_2}}{RQ} \tag{4}$$

The PI_{O_2} is equal to the fraction of inspired oxygen (FI_{O_2}) which is normally 0.21 times the barometric pressure corrected for water vapor (PB − 47 mmHg) and is approximately 150 mmHg at sea level. The PA_{CO_2} is equal to the Pa_{CO_2} and, therefore, is normally 40 mmHg. The RQ is the ratio of $\dot{V}_{CO_2}$ to $\dot{V}_{O_2}$ and usually is assumed to be 0.8. Substituting these values in Eq. 4, the PA_{O_2} should equal approximately 100 mmHg in healthy young persons breathing ambient air at sea level. With an FI_{O_2} of 0.21, the difference between PA_{O_2} and Pa_{O_2}, the $P(A\text{-}a)_{O_2}$ is less than 10 mmHg.

From Eq. 4 and the normal value for $P(A\text{-}a)_{O_2}$ just derived, it follows that a fall in the Pa_{O_2} to below 50 to 60 mmHg can occur if PI_{O_2} decreases, if Pa_{CO_2} increases, or if $P(A\text{-}a)_{O_2}$ increases. A marked decrease in PI_{O_2} might occur while breathing air at high altitude where PB is reduced or during a fire because it consumes oxygen. In the latter case, FI_{O_2} will be less than 0.21. An increase in Pa_{CO_2} above 40 mmHg is ventilatory failure by definition. Ventilatory failure may cause failure of arterial oxygenation unless the PI_{O_2} is increased by the administration of supplemental oxygen to offset the fall in PA_{O_2}. An increased $P(A\text{-}a)_{O_2}$ is primarily the result of ventilation-perfusion mismatching and shunting of mixed venous blood either within the heart or past unventilated areas of the lung. The latter is actually an extreme form of ventilation-perfusion mismatching. The hypoxemia associated with asthma and COPD are largely attributable to ventilation-perfusion mismatching, whereas the hypoxemia associated with ARDS is attributable to intrapulmonary shunting.[1]

The physiologic consequences of hypoxemia depend on the rate of decline of Pa_{O_2} and its severity and duration. Some persons who are born at high altitude or who have congenital cyanotic heart disease live normally with a Pa_{O_2} less than 50 mmHg. However, failure of arterial oxygenation usually leads to some mental impairment and reduced exercise performance regardless of its chronicity, and it is likely to be catastrophic in depressing organ function in patients unaccustomed to hypoxemia.

Oxygen Transport

The amount of oxygen transported ($\dot{T}_{O_2}$) to the tissues is the product of the cardiac output $\dot{Q}T$ and the Ca_{O_2}. Thus,

$$\dot{T}_{O_2} = (\dot{Q}T)\,(Ca_{O_2}) \tag{5}$$

The Ca_{O_2} is the oxygen that is bound to Hb plus the small amount that is dissolved in plasma. This is described by the following equation:

$$Ca_{O_2} = (1.39)\,(Hb)\,(Sa_{O_2}) + (0.003)\,(Pa_{O_2}) \tag{6}$$

where 1.39 is the oxygen carrying capacity of Hb in milliliters per gram and 0.003 is the solubility of oxygen in plasma at 37°C in mL O_2/mL blood. If arterial blood has a Hb concentration of 15 g/mL and the Hb is 98 percent saturated, the Hb carries 19.7 mL O_2/dL blood. The amount of oxygen in solution at a Pa_{O_2} of 95 mmHg is 0.3 mL/dL blood. Thus, the Ca_{O_2} normally is 20 mL O_2/dL blood or 200 mL O_2/L. Multiplying by the normal $\dot{Q}T$ of 5 L/min, $\dot{T}_{O_2}$ is approximately 1 L/min.

The relationship between Pa_{O_2}, Sa_{O_2}, and Ca_{O_2} is described by the oxyhemoglobin dissociation curve (Fig. 1-3). Some laboratories use an idealized version of this curve to calculate the Sa_{O_2} and Ca_{O_2} from the measured Pa_{O_2}. However, the idealized curve assumes that Hb and metabolic status are normal. In patients the oxyhemoglobin dissociation curve frequently is shifted to the left due to alkalosis, Hb with a high affinity for O_2, and CO poisoning in which Hb also binds more avidly than O_2, causing a functional anemia. As a result of this left shift, the Sa_{O_2} is higher at a given Pa_{O_2}, so less O_2 is extracted by the tissues. By contrast, the curve is shifted to the right by acidosis, Hb with a weak affinity for O_2, and 2, 3-diphosphoglycerate, which is produced in increased amounts in response to hypoxia. This right shift results in a lower Sa_{O_2} for a given Pa_{O_2}, so that more O_2 is extracted by the tissues. The true Sa_{O_2} can be known only by oximetric analysis of arterial blood, a fact that is of particular relevance in evaluating patients with CO poisoning.[1]

Inspection of the oxyhemoglobin dissociation curve reveals other important aspects of $\dot{T}_{O_2}$. One is that with a normal Hb concentration the Ca_{O_2} remains near 20 mL/dL blood above a Pa_{O_2} of 60 mmHg and Sa_{O_2} of 90 percent, but that the Ca_{O_2} diminishes rapidly below these levels. Because of this, the physiologic consequences of hypoxemia usually begin to occur at a Pa_{O_2} of approximately 60 mmHg and can be avoided if the Pa_{O_2} is raised above this level. Note also that the Ca_{O_2} can be increased only slightly by raising the Pa_{O_2} above the normal level of 95 mmHg. This is because the Hb

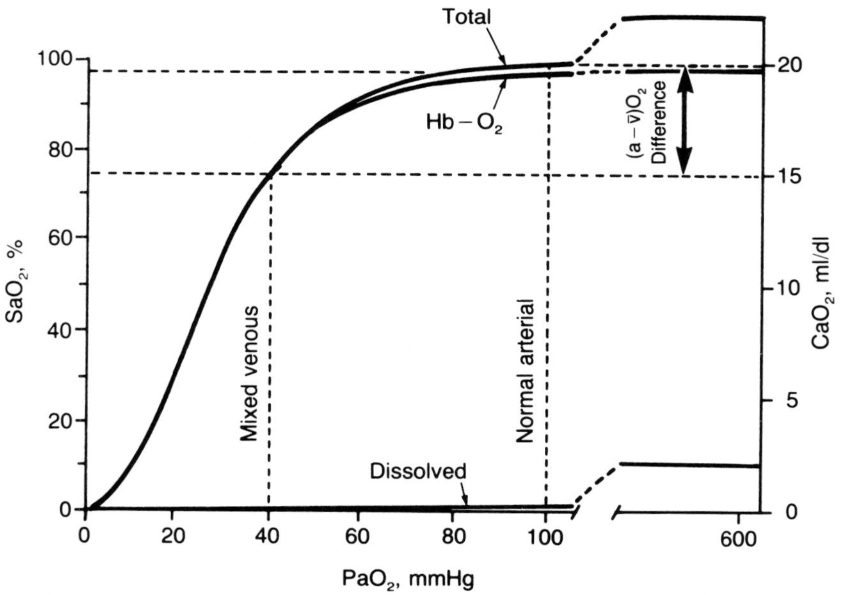

Figure 1-3 The oxyhemoglobin dissociation curve relating the partial pressure of oxygen in systemic arterial blood (Pa_{O_2}) to arterial O_2 saturation (Sa_{O_2}) and to the O_2 content of arterial blood (Ca_{O_2}) and assuming a normal hemoglobin (Hb) concentration. The curve descends steeply below Pa_{O_2} values of 60 mmHg, indicating severely reduced O_2-carrying capacity of Hb below this Pa_{O_2}. The lower line represents O_2 in solution in the blood; the middle line depicts O_2 bound to Hb at that Pa_{O_2}; the upper line shows O_2 bound to Hb plus O_2 dissolved. Note that dissolved O_2 contributes little to Ca_{O_2} at a Pa_{O_2} in the normal range. (Reproduced, with permission, from Luce JM, Tyler ML, Pierson DJ: *Intensive Respiratory Care*. Philadelphia, Saunders, 1984, p 26.)

is fully saturated at this level and only a little more O_2 can be dissolved in blood.

The oxyhemoglobin dissociation curve also gives information regarding the $P\bar{v}_{O_2}$, $S\bar{v}_{O_2}$, and $C\bar{v}_{O_2}$. The relationship between these values and their counterparts in systemic arterial blood is described by the Fick equation, which holds that the $\dot{V}_{O_2}$ is the difference between the $\dot{T}_{O_2}$, and the O_2 returned from the tissues in mixed venous blood to the right side of the heart, which is the product of $\dot{Q}_T$ and the $C\bar{v}_{O_2}$. By combining terms, the Fick equation can be expressed as

$$\dot{V}_{O_2} = \dot{Q}_T[C(a\text{-}\bar{v})_{O_2}] \tag{7}$$

Figure 1-3 shows that the $P\bar{v}_{O_2}$ normally is approximately 40 mmHg, the $S\bar{v}_{O_2}$ is 75 mmHg, the $C\bar{v}_{O_2}$ is 15 mL/dL blood, and the $C(a\text{-}\bar{v})_{O_2}$ is 5 mL/dL blood; given a $\dot{Q}_T$ of 5 L/min, $\dot{V}_{O_2}$ is approximately 250 mL O_2/min. These values indicate that normally only 25 percent of the O_2 in systemic arterial blood is extracted by the tissues, leaving a large O_2 reserve. Patients characteristically call upon this reserve when $\dot{V}_{O_2}$ increases or when $\dot{T}_{O_2}$ decreases due to a fall in $\dot{Q}_T$, Ca_{O_2}, or both. This in turn causes a decrease in the $P\bar{v}_{O_2}$, $S\bar{v}_{O_2}$, Cv_{O_2} and an increase in the $C(a\text{-}\bar{v})_{O_2}$.

A shift from aerobic to anaerobic metabolism and an increased production of lactic acid may be observed in conditions such as severe anemia, CO poisoning; hypovolemic, obstructive, and cardiogenic shock; and cardiorespiratory arrest. These findings are associated with decreases in $P\bar{v}_{O_2}$ below 30 mmHg, the $S\bar{v}_{O_2}$ below 60 percent, and the $C\bar{v}_{O_2}$ below 10 mL O_2/dL blood, and an increase in the $C(a\text{-}\bar{v})_{O_2}$ above 10 mL/dL. Such values are indicative of failure of oxygen transport.[10]

From Eq. 5, it can be seen that inadequate $\dot{T}_{O_2}$ can result from a decrease in either Ca_{O_2} or $\dot{Q}_T$. Cardiac output itself is the product of HR and SV. Thus,

$$\dot{Q}_T = (HR)\,(SV) \tag{8}$$

Heart rate, which normally averages 70 beats/min, is determined by autonomic influences on the intrinsic cardiac pacemakers. SV, which averages 70 mL/beat, is determined by three factors: (1) preload is the length of cardiac muscle fibers at the start of contraction and is equal to ventricular end-diastolic volume and is approximated as end-diastolic pressure; (2) afterload is the tension the heart muscle develops during systole, which is usually equated with the blood pressure or vascular resistance the ventricle must overcome to pump blood into either the pulmonary or systemic circulation; and (3) contractility is the inotropic state of the muscle, which may be expressed as the velocity of muscle shortening.

Cardiac output is also equal to the perfusion pressure (P_{circ}) across the circulation into which the ventricle is pumping, which is the difference between arterial inflow and venous outflow pressures, divided by the resistance of that circulation (R_{circ}). Thus,

$$R_{circ} = P_{circ}/\dot{Q}_T \tag{9}$$

Pulmonary vascular resistance is equal to $\overline{P_{PA}}$ minus $\overline{P_{LA}}$ divided by $\dot{Q}_T$. Normally, $\overline{P_{PA}}$=approximately 15 mmHg, $\overline{P_{LA}}$ = 10 mmHg, and $\dot{Q}_T$ = 5 L/min, so PVR = 1 mmHg/L/min; this usually is multiplied by 80 and expressed as 80 dyne·s/cm^5. On the other hand, SVR is equal to $\overline{P_{SA}}$ minus $\overline{P_{RA}}$, divided by the $\dot{Q}_T$. Normally, $\overline{P_{SA}}$ = approximately 85 mmHg, $\overline{P_{RA}}$ = 5 mmHg and $\dot{Q}_T$ = 5 L/min, so SVR = 16 mmHg/L/min, or 1280 dyne·s/cm^5.[1]

Oxygen Extraction

Some critically ill patients shift from aerobic to anaerobic metabolism and develop lactic acidosis despite what appears to be a normal or even increased $\dot{Q}_T$ and Ca_{O_2}. Such patients have what may be called failure of O_2 extraction. They characteristically have a $P\bar{v}_{O_2}$ of greater than 60 mmHg, a $S\bar{v}_{O_2}$ of greater than 80 percent, a $C\bar{v}_{O_2}$ of greater than 18 mL O_2/mL, and a $C(a\text{-}\bar{v})_{O_2}$ of less than 5 mL O_2/mL blood. Failure of O_2 extraction is characterized by a reduction in $\dot{V}_{O_2}$ (Eq. 7). Such a reduction occurs in cyanide poisoning because the cyanide ion interrupts intracellular mitochondrial O_2 transport. More common examples are distributive shock, ARDS, and the MOSF.[10]

GENERAL MANAGEMENT OF CIRCULATORY AND RESPIRATORY FAILURE

Therapy to Improve Ventilation

The Pa_{CO_2} may be improved by manipulating the variables that affect it: $\dot{V}_{CO_2}$ and $\dot{V}_A$ ($\dot{V}_A$ is equal to $\dot{V}_E - \dot{V}_D$).[12] Manipulation of $\dot{V}_A$ may involve any or all components of the respiratory system. These include the respiratory control centers in the brainstem that regulate $\dot{V}_A$, the nerves that transmit messages from the control centers to the respiratory muscles, the muscles themselves, the chest wall to which the muscles are attached, the pleura that lines the lungs, the lung parenchyma, and the upper and lower airways.

Ventilation may be improved in patients who have overdosed on narcotics by the administration of intravenous naloxone in 0.4 mg doses as required. At the very least, narcotics and sedatives should be administered cautiously to patients at risk of ventilatory failure. This is particularly true of neurosurgical patients whose consciousness already is depressed.

Disorders of the chest wall such as massive obesity and kyphoscoliosis usually are not amenable to specific treatment. However, this is not true of neuromuscular diseases that cause respiratory muscle weakness or paralysis. Beyond therapies for neuromuscular diseases, there are few measures that improve respiratory muscle weakness. Theophylline has been shown to increase ventilatory capacity in some, but not all, patients with COPD.[13] Nutrition also improves respiratory muscle function to a limited extent, but it also increases $\dot{V}_{CO_2}$, which may offset any increase in $\dot{V}_E$.

Pleural and parenchymal diseases limit $\dot{V}_A$ by restricting lung expansion and by increasing $\dot{V}_D$. These disorders also increase the work of breathing, which increases $\dot{V}_{CO_2}$ and may fatigue the respiratory muscles. Evacuation of the pleural space, usually by means of tube thoracostomy, is called for in patients compromised by pneumothorax, hemothorax, or pleural empyema.[14]

Anatomic obstruction of the upper airways should be removed or bypassed when it causes or could cause hypercapnia. This applies to excessive soft tissue as well as to aspirated material. Inspissated secretions frequently cause or contribute to ventilatory failure in a variety of patients, including those with neurosurgical disorders. Secretion removal may be facilitated by chest physiotherapy, gentle endotracheal suctioning, and, if necessary, fiber-optic bronchoscopy.

The $\dot{V}_{CO_2}$ may be reduced by lowering the metabolic rate and thereby the need for increased ventilation. For example, seizures may respond to phenytoin administration at 50 mg/min intravenously up to a loading dose of 1000 mg, followed by 300 mg/day. Shivering may be prevented by chloropromazine doses of 25 to 75 mg intramuscularly. Fever may be reduced by the administration of antipyretics such as aspirin or acetaminophen, which are more effective than cooling blankets or sponge baths in decreasing core temperature.

Therapy to Improve Arterial Oxygenation

The Pa_{O_2} may be improved by manipulating the variables that affect it: Pa_{CO_2}, PI_{O_2}, and $P(A\text{-}a)_{O_2}$.[15] Thus, if hypoventilation is the sole cause of hypoxemia, as might be the case in a narcotic overdosage, the Pa_{O_2} increases as the Pa_{CO_2} decreases in response to naloxone. Similarly, if the PI_{O_2} is reduced by the combustion of O_2 in a fire or by high altitude residence, the Pa_{O_2} should improve if the patient breathes atmospheric air with an inspired fraction of O_2 (FI_{O_2}) at the same PB as at sea level. Patients whose $P(A\text{-}a)_{O_2}$ is increased require therapy for the underlying cause of their hypoxemia as well as supplemental O_2.

Positioning Alveolar collapse, or atelectasis, commonly occurs in dependent regions of the lung. Atelectasis is particularly problematic in supine patients whose lung expansion is limited by obesity, pain on deep breathing, or the presence of restricting bandages over the abdomen or chest. Neurosurgical patients who are obtunded or comatose may not reposition themselves in bed spontaneously and therefore may develop atelectasis. Positioning such patients upright from time to time and turning them from side to side may greatly improve the Pa_{O_2}, although such maneuvers may not be possible due to conditions such as cervical spinal cord injury. Bronchoscopy is rarely effective in permanently relieving atelectasis because the condition rarely is due primarily to impaired secretion clearance.[16]

Adults with unilateral parenchymal lung disorders such as pneumonia may become more hypoxemic when their diseased lung is dependent. The Pa_{O_2} of these patients may improve when they lie on the side of the nondiseased lung. Pulmonary edema tends to occur in dependent lung regions because the intravascular hydrostatic pressure is greatest there. For this reason, the Pa_{O_2} of patients with pulmonary edema may improve, at least temporarily, if they are moved from the supine to the prone position. Unfortunately, such positioning may complicate nursing care and is impossible in patients with many types of neurosurgical diseases.

Oxygen Delivery Systems Hypoxemia usually responds to increasing the FI_{O_2} and thereby the PI_{O_2}. Hypoxemia associated with disorders such as asthma and COPD that are characterized by ventilation-perfusion mismatching but not by intrapulmonary shunt are usually relieved by supplementing O_2 at a low FI_{O_2}. An FI_{O_2} of 0.24 to 0.35 can usually be achieved by delivering O_2 through nasal prongs at flow rates of 5 to 6 L/min; higher flow rates dry the nasal mucosa and do not further increase the FI_{O_2} because patients dilute the O_2 with ambient air. Open face masks provide a higher flow of humidified, premixed air and O_2 at an FI_{O_2} of up to 0.5.[1]

Tightly fitting face masks with a nonbreathing valve and reservoir bag can be used to provide even higher concentrations of O_2 in patients whose hypoxemia is caused by shunting associated with disorders such as severe pneumonia and ARDS. However, tightly fitting face masks are uncomfortable and may cause nasal necrosis if left in place for several days.

Endotracheal Intubation

Indications for Intubation Humidified O_2 at an FI_{O_2} higher than 0.50 is most reliably delivered through the closed system provided by an endotracheal tube. Intubation also is commonly indicated to protect the airway and lungs from aspiration of gastric contents, to prevent asphyxia due to upper airway obstruction, and to provide a route for tracheobronchial toilet.

Kinds of Intubation Endotracheal intubation may be performed either translaryngeally through the nose or mouth, or via a tracheostomy. Tracheostomy tubes once were used routinely in patients requiring intubation for longer than 1 or 2 days, including neurosurgical patients. However, the development of low-pressure and high-compliance cuffs that limit tracheal damage from nasal or oral tubes, the demonstration that such tubes can be left in place for weeks and even months without severe sequellae, and the documentation of complications after tracheostomy have led to a preference for nasotracheal or orotracheal intubation over tracheostomy in all but a few patients. Such patients include those with laryngeal fractures; those who require intubation for longer than a month or so, such as patients with cervical spinal cord injury; and those in whom rapid airway access may be desirable in the future. Tracheostomy tubes generally are more comfortable than translaryngeal tubes. Tracheostomy tubes are also easier to suction through, and talking may be made possible by fitting the tubes with a device that directs a stream of retrograde air through the larynx above the cuff site.

Nasal intubation provides good support for the endotracheal tube and often allows patients to swallow their secretions better than when the tube passes orally. Oral intubation may allow passage of a tube with a larger diameter (8 mm or more) than that which the nostril will accommodate, and usually is the preferred method for emergency intubations. Whichever route is chosen, the tube diameter should be sufficient to seal the trachea without cuff pressures in excess of 20 to 25 mmHg. These pressures should be monitored regularly. Tube position should be determined by chest radiograph immediately following insertion and on a regular basis thereafter. Intubation of the right mainstem bronchus, which extends from the trachea at less of an angle than the left mainstem bronchus, should be looked for in particular.

Complications of Intubation Excessive cuff pressure requirements, self-extubation, and inability to seal the airway are the most common complications with nasotracheal and orotracheal tubes. Problems associated with tracheostomy include stomal hemorrhage, excessive cuff pressure requirements, and subcutaneous emphysema. Tracheal stenosis is more common with tracheostomies than with translaryngeal intubation, although laryngeal complications are more common with the latter.[17]

Extubation In general, endotracheal tubes may be removed when the original indications for insertion are no longer present. For example, extubation frequently follows the return of consciousness and an adequate gag reflex in previously comatose patients or the restoration of adequate ventilation and arterial oxygenation in patients with respiratory failure. If an endotracheal tube has been in place only briefly, it may be removed after secretions have been suctioned from above the cuff site and the patient has been seated upright. Depending on physical and mental status, a patient with a tracheostomy may be progressed from a cuffed to a noncuffed or fenestrated tube, and then may be extubated.

Mechanical Ventilation

Indications for Mechanical Ventilation Mechanical ventilation may be necessary in patients who have inadequate ventilation, inadequate arterial oxygenation, or both. Furthermore, severe airway obstruction caused by asthma and COPD or parenchymal disease caused by disorders such as ARDS may increase the work of breathing to levels that cannot be maintained by spontaneous breathing. Finally, mechanical ventilation may be required in clinically unstable patients such as those in shock and those who require hyperventilation to decrease cerebral blood flow and ICP.

Devices to Assist Ventilation Ventilation may be assisted by devices that substitute for the functions of the diaphragm. One such device is the rocking bed, which swings the patient in a 60 degree arc, forcing the weak or paralyzed diaphragm into inspiratory and expiratory positions by gravity. The rocking bed was commonly used in patients with diaphragmatic paralysis due to neuromuscular disease.

Negative-Pressure Ventilation Ventilation can also be supported by devices that generate a negative pressure around the chest during inspiration to substitute for the negative pleural and airway pressures normally created by contraction of the respiratory muscles. Negative-pressure ventilation can be achieved by including the entire body except the head and neck in an "iron lung," by encompassing the thorax in a garment wrap, or by fitting a cuirass to the anterior chest. As with machines that substitute for the diaphragm, negative-pressure ventilators are best suited to stable patients with neuromuscular diseases whose lungs are normal and who do not require endotracheal intubation for delivery of O_2 at a high FI_{O_2}.

Positive-Pressure Ventilation Due to the limitations of the aforementioned devices, positive-pressure ventilation (PPV) is the kind of mechanical ventilation most widely used today. With PPV, gas is delivered under positive pressure, usually through an endotracheal tube into the airways and the lungs. In contrast to negative-pressure ventilation, PPV produces a positive airway pressure during inspiration. This inflates the alveoli, providing both ventilation and arterial oxygenation while reducing the work of breathing.[1]

Most positive-pressure ventilators may be used to deliver gas up to a preset pressure or volume. The first approach allows limits to be established on the peak pressure (P_{max}) used for lung inflation but allows V_T and $\dot{V}_E$ to vary depending on respiratory system compliance. Alternatively, the ventilators may deliver a preset V_T at whatever P_{max} is required for lung inflation, which guarantees $\dot{V}_E$ but may increase P_{max} and pressure in the alveoli. Cycling of standard ventilators occurs whenever a certain pressure or volume is reached or at preset time intervals. Time cycled ventilation is used primarily in infants or adults who are ventilated at a high F that precludes pressure or volume cycling.

Modes of Positive-Pressure Ventilation Perhaps the simplest mode of PPV is controlled mechanical ventilation (CMV), in which the ventilator delivers gas at a preset F and either a preset P_{max} or V_T. Volume cycled CMV most often is used in patients who are unconscious due to illness or drugs, who are being intentionally hyperventilated, or who are recovering from anesthesia. Patients whose ventilatory drives are intact must often be hyperventilated or given sedatives to diminish their tendency to breathe asynchronously with the ventilator while receiving CMV. As with most other modes of PPV, an inspiratory to expiratory (I:E) ratio of 1:3 or less is generally used with CMV to allow adequate time for expiration and thereby avoid auto-PEEP. Because patients receiving CMV cannot increase their V̇E voluntarily, their ventilatory status must be followed closely. Thus, the advantage of CMV, complete control of ventilating function, is also its major limitation.

Assisted mechanical ventilation (AMV) is a PPV mode in which the patient triggers the ventilator to deliver a preset VT. Triggering is accomplished by generating an airway pressure less than that in the ventilator and tubing. If the ventilator is sensitive to this pressure it will increase F and V̇E in response to patient demands. The machine will not trigger if it is insensitive, however, and if unduly sensitive, it will trigger in response to small fluctuations in airway pressure in addition to attempts to breathe. The latter problem may be circumvented by establishing a proper sensitivity or, if this is not possible, by sedating the patient. Because sedation or neurologic changes may prevent patients from adjusting V̇E, an obligatory backup (or CMV) rate that will provide the minimum allowable V̇E should be used with AMV. The combination of AMV and CMV, which is called the assist/control mode, offers the great advantage of responding to changes in patient status without the close monitoring required of CMV.

A third mode of PPV is intermittent mandatory ventilation (IMV), in which the ventilation delivers a preset VT at specific intervals while also providing a flow of gas for spontaneous breathing. The form of IMV most often used today is synchronized IMV (SIMV), in which ventilator breaths are delivered only after the end of a spontaneous expiration so that patients are not hyperinflated by receiving spontaneous and machine-delivered inspirations simultaneously. With SIMV, the ventilator F may be initially set high enough to provide most, if not all, of the patient's V̇E. F then may be lowered as the patient improves. The potential benefits of SIMV include less asynchronous breathing, lowered sedation requirements, reduced mean airway pressure by combining spontaneous and machine breaths, and improved respiratory muscle function by allowing patients to breathe spontaneously. Disadvantages include the lack of a backup to guarantee V̇E in unstable patients and the possibility of causing respiratory muscle fatigue in patients who receive SIMV at a low ventilator F.

Pressure support ventilation (PSV), a fourth mode of PPV, augments spontaneous ventilatory efforts with a level of positive airway pressure that is preset to achieve a desired VT. This mode of ventilation allows patients to set their own F and timing of breaths, which may be more comfortable than other modes of PPV. PSV is also useful in overcoming the work of breathing through an endotracheal tube. Inasmuch as patients must initiate breaths with PSV, it should not be used in unstable patients and is most applicable during weaning.[18]

A fifth PPV mode is pressure control ventilation (PCV). With this mode, gas is not delivered at a constant VT. Instead, it is delivered until a preset P_{max} is reached, and the patient's V̇E is determined by the preset P_{max}, ventilator F, and inspiratory time. In contrast to the square wave gas flow pattern used with CMV and AMV, inspiratory flow with PCV decelerates when the P_{max} is reached. Advocates of this mode state that complications are reduced with PCV because P_{max} is limited. In addition, the decelerating waveform is thought to provide ventilation of more alveoli. This might be particularly helpful in patients with ARDS, although PCV may not provide a V̇E that is sufficient to prevent hypoventilation.[19]

Complications of Positive-Pressure Ventilation One possible result of PPV is that inflation at high pressure may damage the lung. Such damage has been described traditionally as barotrauma, implying that it is the consequence of pressure changes. However, because alveolar distension occurs as a result of changes in pressure, "volutrauma" may be an equally accurate term. Pneumothorax is a common kind of barotrauma, but subcutaneous and mediastinal emphysema, parenchymal lung cysts, and systemic air embolism also may occur. Some investigators believe that PPV at high pressures and volumes also cause bronchopulmonary dysplasia and diffuse alveolar damage that is identical to ARDS and may cause or perpetuate the syndrome.[20]

In addition to these respiratory effects, PPV may also compromise the cardiovascular system because the positive airway pressure during inspiration reduces venous return to the chest and may depress $\dot{Q}_T$. This effect may be increased if auto-PEEP is produced by PPV. On the other hand, it may be decreased if adequate time is allowed for airway and alveolar pressure to return to ambient levels during exhalation.[21]

Weaning from Positive-Pressure Ventilation Mechanical ventilatory support can generally be withdrawn when the reasons for its initiation no longer are present. This generally means complete or near-complete resolution of the patient's disease process whether or not it involves the lungs. Such resolution should be reflected in clinical stability, a return of $\dot{V}_E$ to below 10 L/min, spontaneous V_T to between 10 and 15 mL/kg, MIP to more negative than -20 cmH_2O, V_D/V_T to below 0.6, Pa_{O_2} to above 50 to 100 mmHg on an FI_{O_2} of 0.4, and $P(A\text{-}a)_{O_2}$ to less than 300 mmHg on an FO_{O_2} of 1.0.[7]

Weaning from AMV and other modes of PPV may be accomplished by connecting the endotracheal tube to a piece of tubing, called a T-piece, that is connected to a source of O_2 diluted with air to create the desired FI_{O_2}. The patients may then breathe spontaneously through the T-piece at their own F and V_T until they meet some or all of the weaning criteria. Otherwise healthy persons recovering from anesthesia or drug overdosages may be put on a T-piece when they wake up and may be intubated after a 15 to 30 min period. Chronically ventilated patients may be put on a T-piece for a few minutes each hour or a few hours each day. When their respiratory muscles are less fatigued and they can tolerate longer periods on a T-piece, discontinuation of the ventilator may be appropriate.

Weaning from SIMV may be accomplished by progressively reducing the ventilator F until the patient can maintain an adequate $\dot{V}_E$ by breathing spontaneously. Patients initially receiving AMV or other PPV modes can be weaned with SIMV without ever using a T-piece. Finally, SIMV and PSV may be combined to facilitate weaning. The PSV level is reduced so long as the patient's V_T remains adequate and SIMV is begun at an intermediate rate and reduced to an F of 2 or so to periodically inflate the lungs and limit atelectasis.

Positive End-Expiratory Pressure

Positive end-expiratory pressure improves arterial oxygenation by increasing lung volume. This has the effect of preventing or reversing atelectasis and redistributing intraalveolar edema into a thinner meniscus within the alveoli or out of the alveoli into the interstitium of the lung. The end result is recruitment of alveoli for better O_2 exchange. It should be noted that PEEP does not improve ventilation. In fact, the Pa_{CO_2} may increase because PEEP increases V_D/V_T by distending the airways and alveoli.[22]

Indications for Positive End-Expiratory Pressure One indication for PEEP is to prevent or reverse atelectasis. For example, low levels such as 5 cmH_2O of PEEP commonly are administered to supine intubated patients. Some investigators believe that low levels of PEEP facilitate weaning from mechanical ventilation by maintaining higher lung volumes while patients breathe through an endotracheal tube. They therefore continue PEEP during T-piece trials and when patients are receiving SIMV at a low ventilator F, with or without PSV.

The other major indication for PEEP is to improve arterial oxygenation in patients with diffuse parenchymal lung disorders such as ARDS. Because their hypoxemia is primarily due to interpulmonary shunt, such patients often cannot be oxygenated adequately even at an FI_{O_2} of 1.0. Administered in levels in excess of 5 cmH_2O, PEEP usually improves the Pa_{O_2} of these patients. It also allows the FI_{O_2} to be reduced to levels of 0.6 or less, thereby minimizing the risk of oxygen toxicity.

Modes of Positive End-Expiratory Pressure Positive end-expiratory pressure may be administered to spontaneously breathing patients either through a tightly fitting face mask or an endotracheal tube, in which case it is called continuous positive airway pressure (CPAP). It also may be combined with CMV, AMV, IMV, or PCV in mechanically ventilated patients to create what is called continuous positive pressure ventilation (CPPV). CPAP patients who merely have atelectasis, including neurosurgical patients who cannot be positioned readily in bed, often may be managed solely with CPAP. However, because they also have edema and because their ventilatory needs are greater, patients with diffuse parenchymal lung disease generally receive PEEP with mechanical ventilation.[22]

Complications of Positive End-Expiratory Pressure As with its benefits, the complications of PEEP are related to lung volume and airway pressure. The delivery of gas at high pressure to achieve an increase in lung volume throughout the ventilatory cycle is more likely to cause barotrauma or "volutrauma" than is the delivery of pressurized gas solely during inspiration. It is also more likely to decrease venous return to the chest and thereby depress PSA and $\dot{Q}_T$. Although the incidence of complications due to PEEP has not been well-studied, these complications appear to be significant if high levels are used.[21]

Weaning from Positive End-Expiratory Pressure Patients who are receiving low levels of PEEP for atelectasis can usually be weaned from PEEP without difficulty. However, premature withdrawal or reduction of PEEP from patients with diffuse parenchymal lung disorders can worsen oxygenation and cause clinical deterioration that requires hours or days of therapy to reverse. For this reason, PEEP should be withdrawn slowly, in small (2 to 5 cmH_2O) increments, with close monitoring of Pa_{O_2} or Sa_{O_2} in such patients. Premature reduction of PEEP can be avoided if the disease process for which PEEP was initiated has resolved or is substantially improved, if the Pa_{O_2} is 80 mmHg or greater on an FI_{O_2} of 0.4 or less, and if these conditions have been present for several hours.

Therapy to Improve Oxygen Transport

Oxygen transport may be improved by manipulating the variables that affect it—Ca_{O_2} and $\dot{Q}_T$. The major determinants of Ca_{O_2} are the Hb concentration and Sa_{O_2}. Most physicians are familiar with the need to optimize Sa_{O_2} by the methods discussed earlier, but many forget that $\dot{T}_{O_2}$ often can be improved by restoring the Hb concentration to normal (Fig. 1-4).

CO poisoning causes a functional anemia that may impair $\dot{T}_{O_2}$. The oxyhemoglobin dissociation curve is shifted to the left in patients with CO poisoning, which results in less O_2 being available to the tissues. However, because the Pa_{O_2} is normal, the possibility of CO poisoning may be overlooked unless the Sa_{O_2} or the Ca_{O_2} is measured directly. CO poisoning is treated with supplemental O_2 at an FI_{O_2} of 1.0 and occasionally with hyperbaric oxygenation. Both of these maneuvers improve $\dot{T}_{O_2}$ by dissolving O_2 in plasma and displacing CO from Hb.

Manipulation of $\dot{Q}_T$ in patients with failure of $\dot{T}_{O_2}$ often involves administration of drugs to alter HR, SV, and vascular pressures and resistances. Alteration of HR includes measures to reverse bradyarrhythmias or tachyarrhythmias if they are present. In general, sinus bradycardia severe enough to compromise $\dot{Q}_T$ and PSA may be treated with parasympatholytic drugs such as atropine (0.5 to 1.0 mg intravenously), beta- and $beta_2$-adrenergic agonists such as isoproterenol (1 to 2 mg in 500 mL dextrose and water given at 2 to 20 μg/min), or by cardiac pacing. Sinus tachycardia may be treated by reversing its underlying causes, which include hypovolemia, pain, and hyperthyroidism.[1]

Supraventricular tachycardia may respond to vagal maneuvers such as carotid sinus massage, $beta_1$ and $beta_2$ antagonists such as esmolol (5 g in 500 mL dextrose and water given as a loading dose of 500 μg/kg over 1 min followed by an infusion of 50 μg/min for 4 min), and calcium channel blockers such as verapamil (5 to 10 mg intravenously as needed). Ventricular tachycardia is treated with lidocaine or bretylium; ventricular fibrillation is treated with electrical defibrillation.

Manipulation of SV requires alterations of its three determinants: preload, afterload, and contractility. For example, preload should be restored with crystalloid, colloid, or red blood cell transfusions when it is decreased sufficiently to cause hemodynamic compromise. When preload is increased, especially when pulmonary edema is

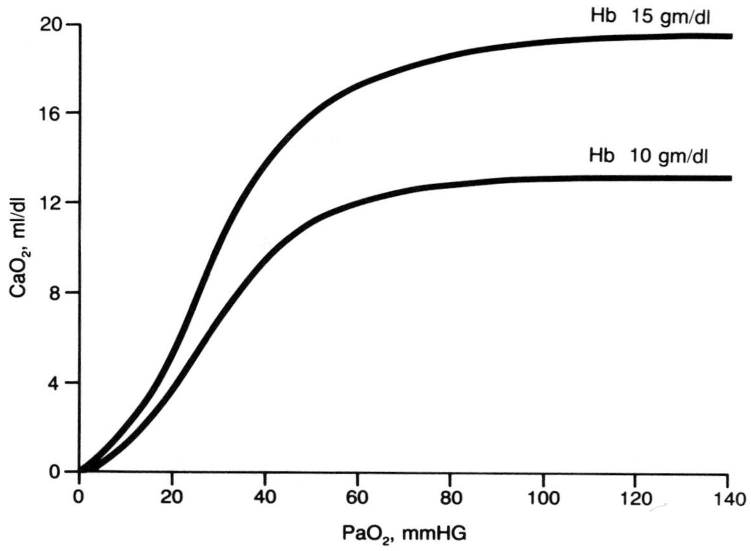

Figure 1-4 Difference in arterial oxygen content (Ca_{O_2}) attainable at partial oxygen pressure (Pa_{O_2}) values of up to 140 mmHg, with blood hemoglobin (Hb) values of 10 vs. 15 g/dL. (Reproduced, with permission, from Luce JM, Tyler ML, Pierson DJ: *Intensive Respiratory Care*. Philadelphia, Saunders, 1984, p 225.)

present, it may be reduced with diuretics such as furosemide (40 mg intravenously as needed), or with nitroglycerin (given transcutaneously, sublingually, orally, or intravenously; the intravenous dose is 10 μg/min titrated as high as 200 to 300 μg/min), or other agents that cause venodilation. Left ventricular afterload may be reduced by agents that cause arterial dilation and thereby reduce SVR, such as nitroprusside (10 μg/min intravenously titrated as high as 300 to 400 μg/min).

Normally, arterial inflow pressures ($\overline{\text{PPA}}$, $\overline{\text{PSA}}$) must be sufficiently high and venous outflow pressures ($\overline{\text{PLA}}$, $\overline{\text{PRA}}$) must be sufficiently low to provide adequate perfusion across the pulmonary and systemic circulations. At the same time, perfusion pressure must be balanced by circulatory resistances (PVR, SVR) to maintain an adequate $\dot{Q}$T. Systemic arterial pressure may be increased by $alpha_1$ agonists such as phenylephrine (50 to 100 μg/min bolus, titrated thereafter), norepinephrine (4 to 8 mg in 500 mL dextrose and water given at 4 to 12 μg/min), or high-dose dopamine. Left atrial pressure and PRA may be reduced by nitrates and other agents that decrease preload. Similarly, SVR may be increased by $alpha_1$ agonists and decreased by drugs such as nitroprusside.

The drugs most commonly used to improve $\dot{Q}$T in critically ill patients are dopamine and dobutamine. Dopamine may be given in low doses (usually 2.0 to 5.0 μg/min) to enhance renal and mesenteric perfusion through its dopaminergic effects. Intermediate doses of 5.0 to 10.0 μg/min of dopamine improves $\dot{Q}$T through its $beta_1$ effects, whereas high doses of (>10.0 μg/min) dopamine increase PSA through its $alpha_1$ properties. The pharmacological effects of dopamine are not always predictable in all patients, and the drug must be carefully titrated to achieve its desired effects.

Unlike dopamine, dobutamine does not selectively enhance renal and mesenteric perfusion because it lacks dopaminergic properties. It also does not generally increase PSA or PAO because its $alpha_1$ properties are balanced by its $beta_1$ properties; in fact, dobutamine may reduce PSA and PAO in some labile patients when its $beta_2$ properties predominate. However, dobutamine improves $\dot{Q}$T through its $beta_1$ properties. If PSA is reduced, dobutamine may be combined with high-dose dopamine or other $alpha_1$ agonists. The usual dose of dobutamine is 2.5 to 10 μg/min up to a maximum dose of 30 μg/min.

Therapy to Improve Oxygen Extraction

Oxygen extraction may be improved by increasing $\dot{V}_{O_2}$. In patients with cyanide poisoning, this traditionally has involved the administration of amyl nitrate by inhalation and sodium nitrite intravenously. These drugs produce methemoglobin, which binds free cyanide ions. Intravenous sodium thiosulfate is then given to enhance conversion of cyanide to thiosulfate, which is less toxic and is readily excreted. Vitamin $B_{12}A$ will soon be available for treating cyanide poisoning in the United States.[1]

PATHOPHYSIOLOGY, MONITORING, AND MANAGEMENT OF COMMON CAUSES OF CIRCULATORY AND RESPIRATORY FAILURE

Neuromuscular Diseases Causing Respiratory Failure

A wide variety of neuromuscular diseases cause weakness or paralysis that may lead to hypercapneic respiratory failure. These disorders may involve the upper motor neurons (e.g., cervical spinal cord injury), lower motor neurons (e.g., amyotrophic lateral sclerosis), peripheral nerves (e.g., Guillian Barré syndrome), myoneural junction (myasthenia gravis), or the muscles themselves (e.g, muscular dystrophies). The overall approach to patients with these conditions is to diagnose and treat specific neuromuscular disease if possible, diagnose precipitating factors prompting ICU admission, evaluate the need for respiratory support, provide support on an acute basis, and consider chronic support when required.[23]

Once weakness or paralysis is appreciated, most neuromuscular diseases causing these symptoms can be differentiated by means of clinical characteristics, cerebrospinal fluid analysis, provocative tests such as the administration of cholinergic drugs, nerve conduction studies and electromyography, and occasionally muscle biopsy. Determination of the location and completeness of the lesion is essential in patients with acute cervical spinal cord injury. Severe damage to or above cord segments C_3 to C_5 involves the phrenic nerve nuclei and causes bilateral diaphragmatic paralysis, whereas damage to segments below this level customarily leaves diaphragmatic function intact.[4]

In terms of specific therapy, methylprednisolone is given to patients with acute cervical spinal cord injury, and plasmapheresis is used for patients with the Guillain Barré syndrome.[24] Myasthenia gravis is treated with relatively long-acting anticholinesterase agents such as pyridostigmine; and with plasmapheresis, corticosteroids, and thymectomy. Specific therapy for botulism involves elimination of malabsorbed neurotoxin from the gut by means of enemas and gastric lavage, administration of trivalent antitoxin, the administration of high-dose penicillin, and surgical debridement of contaminated wounds.

Although some patients with neuromuscular disease need critical care solely because of progressive muscle dysfunction, admission often is precipitated by other factors. For example, patients with bulbar involvement may aspirate or develop upper airway obstruction, whereas atelectasis and pneumonia are more common in patients with generalized weakness. Pulmonary hypertension and right heart failure should be anticipated in chronically hypoxemic patients, including those whose muscle weakness is compounded by kyphoscoliosis. Intercurrent illnesses, such as urinary tract infection and pulmonary thromboembolism, also may occur.[23]

The need for respiratory support in patients with neuromuscular disease can be assessed by the MIP and VC maneuvers. As noted earlier, intubation and mechanical ventilation generally are required if the MIP is less negative than -20 cmH_2O and the VC is approximately 10 mL/kg. It should be noted that impaired secretion clearance may occur at a VC that is less than 30 mL/kg and may require intubation but not mechanical ventilation.[25]

Hypoxemic respiratory failure in patients with neuromuscular disease can usually be treated adequately with supplemental O_2 delivered through nasal prongs or a face mask, coupled with frequent positioning and the delivery of CPAP via a tightly fitting face mask to treat atelectasis. However, intubation and mechanical ventilation are usually called for if muscle strength and lung volumes have declined to the level mentioned previously and always are necessary if hypercapnia is acute and severe. Patients with rapidly reversible muscle weakness or paralysis should be intubated by the translaryngeal route in most instances, but tracheostomy is indicated if patients require intubation for longer than a month or so.

No particular kind of ventilatory support has been demonstrated to be superior in patients with neuromuscular disease, although PPV is preferred over negative-pressure ventilation in the ICU, especially if admission has been prompted by pneumonia or some other intermittent illness that requires supplemental O_2 at a high $F_{I_{O_2}}$. The value of various modes of PPV is open to debate. Nevertheless, because SIMV can be used only in those patients who can generate substantial inspiratory pressures, patients with severe weakness or paralysis are ventilated at least initially with CMV or AMV. In patients who are improving, SIMV may be used if it does not cause fatigue. Weaning by SIMV, T-piece, or PSV should be attempted only when patients demonstrate improvement in the MIP and VC.

Oxygen transport is usually adequate in patients with neuromuscular disease who are not hypoxemic or anemic and do not have concurrent IHD. Nevertheless, autonomic dysfunction in patients with Guillain Barré syndrome and other disorders may take the form of over- or underactivity of the sympathetic nervous system. Hypertension, diaphoresis, and tachycardia may be treated with titratable agents such as esmolol to prevent overswings in HR and PSA. The hypotension that often accompanies cervical spinal cord injury and other conditions may be treated with intravenous fluids or $alpha_1$ agonists such as phenylephrine or high-dose dopamine. Bradycardia is treated with atropine. Patients with profound vagal tone in whom bradycardia progresses to asystole may be candidates for cardiac pacing.

Asthma and Chronic Obstructive Pulmonary Disease

The primary pathophysiologic abnormalities in asthma and COPD is an increased resistance in airflow resulting from narrowing of the airways by bronchospasm, inflammation, mucous, or loss of airway tethering forces by parenchymal lung destruction. The airflow resistance causes air trapping and an abnormal increase in lung volume. Patients also have hypoxemia caused by mismatching of ventilation, perfusion and hypercapnia caused by the airway obstruction itself, plus fatigue of the respiratory muscles.

In patients with asthma and COPD, Pa_{CO_2} usually begins to increase when the FEV_1 is reduced to approximately 750 mL, or 25 percent of the predicted value. This reduction may result from a gradually progressive disease but more often occurs in the setting of acute exacerbations of obstruction due, for example, to acute bronchitis. An increase in Pa_{CO_2} without a deterioration in FEV_1 may be the result of decreased ventilatory drive due to narcotic or sedative drugs or the inhalation of oxygen at a high $F_{I_{O_2}}$. Alternatively, it may result from increased $\dot{V}_{CO_2}$ in a patient with a limited ability to increase $\dot{V}_A$. As previously described, the distinction between acute and chronic respiratory acidosis can be determined by analyzing the relationships among Pa_{CO_2}, pH, and $[HCO_3^-]$. Acute hypoventilation obviously dictates a more prompt response than chronic, partially compensated respiratory acidosis, as does neuromuscular disease.

Metabolic acidosis is a more ominous finding than pure respiratory acidosis in the setting of airway obstruction. It implies a failure of oxygen transport to meet the demands imposed by the increased work of breathing. This failure may result from a decrease in Ca_{O_2} due to processes such as hypoxemia or anemia or a decrease in $\dot{Q}_T$ due to concurrent ischemic heart disease, inadequate intravascular volume, or auto-PEEP caused by air trapping. Unless patients with inadequate oxygen transport improve, their condition will rapidly deteriorate.

Patients with asthma and COPD may be treated with $beta_2$-adrenergic agonists, theophylline, anticholinergic agents, and corticosteroids. $Beta_2$ agonists such as metaproterenol and albuterol relax bronchial smooth muscle through their action on $beta_2$ receptors in the airways and have little effect on $beta_1$ receptors in skeletal muscles, systemic vessels, and the heart. Therefore, they are preferred to agents such as epinephrine and isoproterenol that have mixed $beta_1$ and $beta_2$ properties. The mild tachycardia, tremulousness, and other cardiovascular side effects of $beta_2$ agonists can be minimized if the drugs are taken in aerosol form. Average doses of aerosolized metaproterenol and albuterol are 15 and 2.5 mg, respectively, given every 2 to 4 h.[1]

Theophylline has fallen into disfavor because of its limited bronchodilating properties and its potential for toxicity. Theophylline may be administered as aminophylline in a loading dose of 5 to 6 mg/kg intravenously followed by an infusion of 0.4 to 0.9 mg/kg/n to achieve a mean serum level of approximately 10.0 μg/mL. Serum levels should be followed regularly in patients receiving intravenous theophylline.

Aerosolized anticholinergic agents such as ipratropium bromide, which may be given via an inhaler at a dose of 0.04 mg every 2 to 4 h, are both effective and safe due to their lack of systemic side effects.[26] Corticosteroids suppress inflammation and increase responsiveness to beta$_2$ stimulation. These agents are available in aerosol, oral, or intravenous forms. Intravenous methylprednisolone commonly is administered to the critically ill with asthma and COPD in the range of 0.5 to 1.0 mg/kg four times daily.[27]

Although hypoxemia invariably is present in patients with severe airway obstruction, the degree of reduction in Pa_{O_2} generally is not sufficient to require respiratory support other than supplemental O_2 delivered with external devices. Hypoxemia should usually be corrected only to a Pa_{O_2} of approximately 60 mmHg using as low an FI_{O_2} as possible to avoid ventilatory depression. This will significantly improve the Sa_{O_2} and Ca_{O_2} (Fig. 1-5). If a high FI_{O_2} must be used in patients with intercurrent illnesses such as pneumonia, endotracheal intubation and mechanical ventilation may be required.

One cannot definitely state criteria for intubating and ventilating patients with severe airway obstruction. Arterial blood gas and pH values at a single point in time showing marked acute respiratory acidosis with or without metabolic acidosis may be sufficient information on which to base the decision to provide mechanical ventilation. More commonly, however, it is necessary to evaluate the patient during a period of time while drugs are being administered and to evaluate the response to therapy. If blood gas values are worsening or not

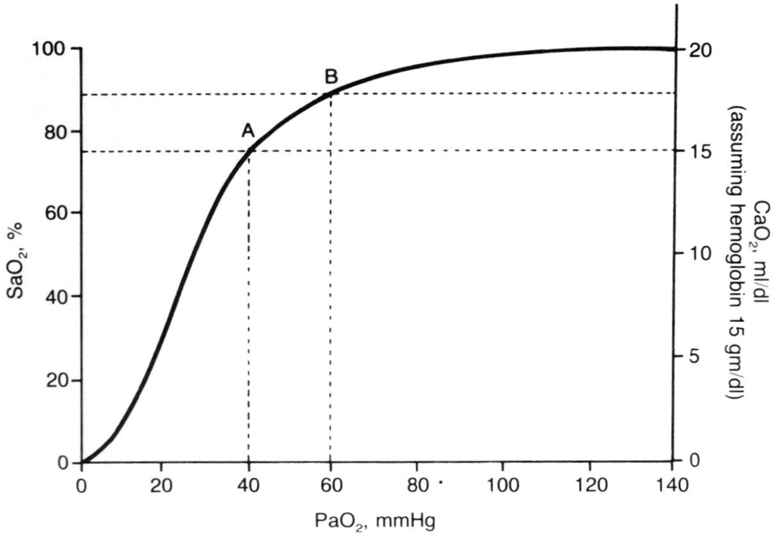

Figure 1-5 Raising the partial pressure of oxygen in systemic arterial blood (Pa_{O_2}) from 40 mmHg (point A) to 60 mmHg (point B) increases arterial O_2 saturation (Sa_{O_2}) from about 75 to about 90 percent and arterial O_2 content (Ca_{O_2}) from 15 to 18 mL/dL. This corrects hypoxemia of a life-threatening degree and is especially useful in patients with chronic obstructive pulmonary disease whose respiratory drives may be depressed. (Reproduced, with permission, from Luce JM, Tyler MT, Pierson DJ: *Intensive Respiratory Care*. Philadelphia, Saunders, 1984, p 211.)

improving in spite of maximal treatment, mechanical ventilation is the next logical step. In addition to the objective evaluation provided by arterial blood gas and pH measurements, subjective assessments are of value. Patients who are confused, somnolent, or uncooperative may require ventilatory support because their mental status may indicate inadequate oxygen transport and because they cannot cooperate with conservative management.

Severe airway obstruction presents a difficult situation in which to apply PPV. There is need to allow adequate expiratory time to avoid auto-PEEP, but also slow inspiratory flows are desirable to optimize the distribution of ventilation and to minimize the airway pressure required to deliver a preset VT. To accomplish these goals, at least early in the course of mechanical ventilation, it often is necessary to sedate the patient receiving CMV or AMV in order to provide a slow ventilator F, which allows a small I : E ratio to be used. Some patients will benefit from SIMV in this situation. The VT should be between 7 to 10 mL/kg and the FI_{O_2} adjusted to provide an adequate Pa_{O_2}. The Pa_{CO_2} may rise due to the relatively low F and VT, but severe drops in pH can be treated with HCO_3^- if necessary. If the Pa_{CO_2} remains elevated, or if the patient already has chronic hypoventilation, it is important not to reduce the Pa_{CO_2} rapidly because doing so will result in uncompensated metabolic alkalosis.[1]

Positive end-expiratory pressure would appear to be contraindicated in patients with asthma and COPD whose lung volumes already are increased above normal. Certainly, high levels of PEEP are potentially dangerous and are unnecessary because these patients do not have failure of arterial oxygenation due to diffuse parenchymal lung disease. Nevertheless, recent studies have suggested that PEEP in levels of approximately 5 cmH_2O does not commonly cause hyperinflation in patients with airway obstruction. Indeed, low levels of PEEP may reduce the work or breathing of some obstructed patients, including those receiving mechanical ventilation.[28]

The adequacy of oxygen transport in patients with asthma and COPD generally can be assessed by physical examination, measurement of urine output, and monitoring of PSA. Central venous and pulmonary artery catheterization rarely are required but may be helpful in evaluating patients whose $\dot{Q}$T is known or suspected to be depressed and in evaluating their response to fluids and agents such as dopamine or dobutamine. The elevation of PPAO by auto-PEEP should be taken into account when estimating intravascular volume.

In patients with airway obstruction, weaning from mechanical ventilation also may present difficulties. Patients with asthma usually may be weaned and extubated quickly after they have responded to treatment. However, patients with COPD may at best have marginal lung function with persistent retention of CO_2. In general, the arterial blood gas pattern that exists when the patient is "well" should be approximated while mechanical ventilation is still being used. Ideally, weaning with SIMV or a simple T-piece with or without PSV and small amounts of PEEP then can proceed using previously described criteria.

In some instances, patients with COPD never meet the objective criteria for weaning and extubation. When this occurs, the decisions regarding weaning and extubation are based on subjective criteria, such as level of alertness, patient cooperation, and prognosis. These factors obviously cannot be quantitated. Once the patient has demonstrated the ability to maintain a desired $\dot{V}$E spontaneously for 30 to 60 min, the endotracheal tube should be removed.[1]

Infectious Pneumonia

The terms pneumonia and pneumonitis refer to inflammation that is located in the lung interstitium, which normally contains capillaries, connective tissue, and a variety of cellular components; the alveolar space, which normally contains air and a small amount of water, surfactant, and cells such as macrophages; and a combination of the two. Infectious pneumonia may be caused by a variety of microorganisms including viruses, bacteria, fungi, rickettsiae, and protozoa. Infectious pneumonia characteristically involves the alveoli.

Infectious pneumonias may be divided epidemiologically into the community-acquired type, implying that the pathogens were acquired in the patient's normal environment, and the nosocomial, or hospital-acquired type. Another approach, which is based on the characteristics of the human host, is to describe infectious pneumonia as either routine, in that it occurs in an immunocompetent patient, or opportunistic, in that the patient is immunocompromised by, for example, cancer or infection with the human immunodeficiency virus (HIV).[29]

Microorganisms reach the lungs either by direct inhalation from air or from respiratory therapy devices, aspiration of secretions from the mouth and nasopharynx, hematogenous spread from other body sites, or direct penetration of the chest wall. Usually the mouth and nasopharynx are populated predominantly by anaerobic bacteria that are kept out of the lungs due to intact gag and cough reflexes and the mucocilliary clearance mechanisms of the trachea and bronchi. However, this resident flora is rapidly replaced by aerobic bacilli, including those found in ICUs, when illness supervenes.[30] Approximately one-fourth of patients who become colonized in this fashion go on to develop either bacterial tracheobronchitis or pneumonia, in large part because their gag and cough reflexes and mucocilliary clearance mechanisms are depressed by disease, medications, or the presence of an endotracheal tube.[31]

Bacteria that proliferate in the alveoli generally elicit an inflammatory response characterized by complement activation and phagocytosis by alveolar macrophages and neutrophils that are attracted to the lung. This is accompanied by an increase in permeability of the endothelium of the pulmonary capillaries and the epithelium of the alveolar wall. The increased permeability allows water and proteins to leak from the vessels into the air spaces even though the hydrostatic pressure within the capillaries is normal. As the lung tissues become consolidated, local pulmonary compliance diminishes, and hypoxemia results from mismatching of ventilation and perfusion in the lung.

Bacterial pneumonia may be diagnosed by the constellation of fever, neutrophilia or neutropenia, hypoxemia, the finding of focal consolidation on physical examination of the chest, focal infiltrates on the chest radiograph, and the presence of purulent sputum. Some of these findings may be insensitive and nonspecific in critically ill patients but radiographic infiltrates and sputum should be required for the diagnosis. If infiltrates are not present but purulent sputum is, the diagnosis most likely is tracheobronchitis and not pneumonia.

Spontaneously produced sputum or secretions that have been suctioned from the tracheobronchial tree should be Gram stained and examined for abundant neutrophils as a reflection of purulence and for potentially pathogenic bacteria. Several types of bacteria may be seen in critically ill patients, especially those who are intubated, if their pneumonia is due to more than one microorganism. Sputum and tracheobronchial secretions also should be cultured to determine which microorganisms are predominant. However, it should be noted that the presence of positive cultures does not confirm the diagnosis of either tracheobronchitis or pneumonia, in that critically ill patients without these disorders may have positive cultures due to airway colonization.

Some clinicians treat any respiratory infection in hospitalized patients, reasoning that if tracheobronchitis is present, pneumonia cannot be far behind. Most, however, prefer not to give antibiotics for mild-to-moderate cases and wait until tracheobronchitis is severe or, more often, until pneumonia is documented by chest radiograph. Antibiotic therapy may be empiric or based on the results of Gram stain, culture, or both. Therapeutic recommendations are included in Table 1-1.

Most bacterial pneumonias respond to antibiotic treatment and maneuvers to aid secretion clearance, so that radiographic infiltrates should begin to clear after several days. This may not be the case in critically ill patients, however, because their infiltrates are due to some other cause such as atelectasis, they cannot ward off an identified pathogen due to its virulence or their depressed host defenses, the pathogen is insensitive to the antibiotics begin given, or the patients are infected with an undiagnosed and perhaps opportunistic, nonbacterial microorganism. Because of the last possibility, patients who do not improve with treatment may be subjected to diagnostic tests more invasive than sputum analysis, such as bronchoscopy with protected brush catheterization of the lower airways, or bronchoalveolar lavage.

Table 1-1 Infectious Pneumonias

Kind of patient	Likely offending microorganisms	Initial antimicrobial therapy (pending sensitivities)	Average dose	Route	Interval
Normal young host with community-acquired pneumonia	Mycoplasma				
	Mycoplasma pneumoniae	Erythromycin or	0.5 g	PO	qid
		tetracycline	0.5 g	PO	qid
	Gram-positive aerobic bacteria				
	Streptococcus pneumoniae	Penicillin G or	600,000 units	PO, IM, IV	bid
		erythromycin	0.5 g	PO, IM, IV	qid
	Viruses				
	Influenza A	No therapy or			
	Adenovirus	amantadine	0.2 g	PO	qid
	Fungi (in endemic areas) *Coccidioides immitis* *Histoplasma capsulatum*	Usually untreated unless dissemination occurs or pulmonary infection becomes chronic. Then use amphotericin B as below.			
Elderly host, heavy smoker, or alcoholic individual with nosocomial pneumonia	Gram-positive aerobic bacteria				
	Streptococcus pneumonia	Penicillin G or	600,000 units	IM, IV	bid
		erythromycin	0.5 g	IM, IV	qid
	Staphylococcus aureus	Nafcillin or	1–2 g	IV	q4h
		vancomycin	1 g	IV	q12h
	Gram-negative aerobic bacteria				
	Hemophilus influenzae	Ampicillin or	0.5–1 g	IV, PO	qid
		cefuroxime	1.0 g	IV	q8h
				IV	q8h
	Klebsiella pneumoniae	Cefazolin and gentamycin or tobramycin	1.5 mg/kg	IV	q8h
	Legionella pneumophilia	Erythromycin	0.5–1 g	IV	qid
	Anaerobic bacteria				
	Bacteroides fragilis	Metronidazole or	500 mg	IV	q8h
		clindamycin	0.3 g	IV, PO	qid
	Mycobacteria				
	Mycobacterium tuberculosis	Isoniazid and rifampin	300 mg	PO	qd
			600 mg	PO	qd
	Viruses and fungi (as in young hosts)	As above			
Normal young or elderly host with nosocomial pneumonia	Gram-positive aerobic bacteria				
	Staphylococcus aureus	Nafcillin or	1–2 g	IV	q4h
		vancomycin	1 g	IV	qid

continued

Table 1-1 Infectious Pneumonias (Continued)

Kind of patient	Likely offending microorganisms	Initial antimicrobial therapy (pending sensitivities)	Average dose	Route	Interval
	Streptococcus fecalis (nonendocarditis)	Ampicillin and	1 g	IV	q8h
		gentamycin or tobramycin	1.5 mg/kg	IV	qid
	Gram-negative aerobic bacteria				
	Escherichia coli	Ampicillin alone or	1 g	IV	qid
		gentamycin or tobramycin and	1.5 mg/kg	IV	qid
		carbenicillin or ticarcillin	3–6 g	IV	q4h
	Pseudomonas aeruginosa	Carbenicillin or ticarcillin	3–6 g	IV	q4h
		and gentamycin or tobramycin	1.5 mg/kg	IV	qid
	Proteus mirabilis	Ampicillin or	1 g	IV	qid
		ticarcillin	3–6 g	IV	q4h
	Klebsiella pneumoniae	Cefazolin and	1–2 g	IV	q8h
		gentamycin or tobramycin	1.5 mg/kg	IV	qid
	Enterobacter species	Cefamandole and	2 g	IV	qid
		gentamycin or tobramycin	1.5 mg/kg	IV	qid
Immunocompromised host with community- or hospital-acquired pneumonia	Gram-negative aerobic bacteria, as above	As above; prefer combination			
	Viruses				
	Cytomegalovirus	Gancyclovir			
	Varicella-zoster	Acyclovir			
	Herpes simplex	Acyclovir			
	Fungi				
	Candida albicans	Amphotericin B	0.025–0.1 g	IV	qd
	Aspergillus fumigatus	Amphotericin B	0.025–0.1 g	IV	qd
	Cryptococcus neoformans	Amphotericin B	0.025–0.1 g	IV	qd
	Protozoa				
	Pneumocystis carinii	Trimethoprimsulfamethoxazole or	20 mg/kg	IV, PO	qid
		pentamidine isethionate	4 mg/kg	IV	qd

(Adapted, with permission, from Luce JM, Tyler ML, Pierson DJ: *Intensive Respiratory Care*. Philadelphia, Saunders, 1984, pp 306–308.)

Adult Respiratory Distress Syndrome and Multiple Organ System Failure

A constellation of clinical, radiographic, and pathophysiologic findings that result from diffuse injury to the lung parenchyma define ARDS. The characteristics of this syndrome are severe hypoxemia due to intrapulmonary shunting of blood, the presence of diffuse infiltrates on the chest radiograph, and noncardiogenic pulmonary edema related to increased permeability of the capillary endothelium and the alveolar epithelium. The syndrome is associated with a variety of clinical conditions including lung contusion, multiple transfusions, overwhelming pneumonia, pancreatitis, aspiration of gastric contents, and especially, the sepsis syndrome.

Regardless of the type of mechanism of injury, the damage to the lungs of patients with ARDS is diffuse compared with diseases such as focal pneumonia. However, the damage is nonhomogeneous, and some areas of lung parenchyma may be spared. In damaged areas, the lung is atelectatic, edematous, and hemorrhagic. Microscopic examination reveals intraalveolar collections of proteinaceous fluid, red blood cells, and inflammatory cells. Microthrombi or white cell aggregates may be seen in small vessels. After 24 to 48 h, hyaline membranes formed by fibrin that have escaped through the capillaries line the alveoli. Subsequently, as repair of the injury occurs, fibrosis may ensue.[1]

The major and most frequent gas exchange abnormality in ARDS is hypoxemia caused by the loss of functional alveoli. In severe forms of ARDS, as the process evolves from injury to repair, gas exchange abnormalities also evolve. Lung fibrosis may result in obliteration of capillaries and coalescence of alveoli to produce an increased V_D/V_T. Unless $\dot{V}_E$ can be increased, which may be difficult, hypercapnia will result.

Some, but not all patients with ARDS develop dysfunction or failure of one or more organ systems sequentially or simultaneously. By contrast, other patients develop MOSF without having ARDS, although they may have less severe degrees of parenchymal lung injury. MOSF is associated with the same clinical conditions as ARDS. Furthermore, as with ARDS, it is most commonly associated with sepsis syndrome. This suggests that ARDS is a respiratory manifestation of MOSF, just as distributive shock is a cardiovascular manifestation. Alternatively, ARDS and MSOF may be aspects of sepsis syndrome. Some investigators have broadened the use of the term sepsis syndrome to include any generalized inflammatory process that may cause or contribute to widespread organ dysfunction.[32]

This generalized inflammatory process may be mediated by a variety of circulating substances with vasoactive, inflammatory, and tissue damaging properties. These substances, which may include endotoxin, histamine, arachidonic acid metabolitis, complement, myocardial depressant factor, and tumor necrosis factor, may cause systemic vasodilation, microvascular vasoconstriction, altered myocardial contractility, capillary microembolization, and endothelial cell disruption. The end result is increased capillary permeability with intravascular fluid loss, interstitial fluid accumulation, impaired microcirculatory blood flow, and inadequate tissue oxygenation in the lungs and other organs. Patients may die of refractory hypotension, hypoxemia attributable to ARDS, or other manifestations of MOSF such as disseminated intravascular coagulation.[33]

It is not clear whether the term sepsis syndrome should be applied to patients with ARDS and MOSF who are not truly infected. Nevertheless, such patients probably should be assumed to be infected unless there is another explanation for their condition. If bacterial infection is suspected or known to exist, broad spectrum antibiotics such as ampicillin, metronidazole, and gentamycin should be given intravenously to cover gram-positive and gram-negative pathogens and then tailored to culture results. Suspected or documented infections with other organisms should be treated appropriately. In addition, abcesses should be searched for by computed tomography and other techniques when appropriate. If detected, they should be drained percutaneously or at surgery.[34]

The unusual patient with MOSF who does not have severe parenchymal lung disease may benefit from endotracheal intubation and mechanical ventilation merely because of hemodynamic instability. Vital organ perfusion may also be enhanced if the work of breathing is reduced by mechanical ventilation. Patients with ARDS, however, invariably require both PPV and PEEP to improve arterial oxygenation. The need for such support may be evaluated by monitoring the Pa_{O_2} and $P(A\text{-}a)_{O_2}$. Respiratory or metabolic acidosis is ominous in this setting. Because patients with ARDS, MOSF, or both may deteriorate rapidly, it generally is better to provide intubation and mechanical ventilation earlier rather than later.

The use of PPV in patients with ARDS and MOSF varies. Most physicians probably administer CMV, AMV, or IMV with a VT of 10 to 15 mL/kg, an I:E ratio of 1:3 or greater, and a P_{max} as required to deliver a VT in the aforementioned range. Positive end-expiratory pressure is used at levels necessary to reduce the FI_{O_2} to 0.6 or less. However, increasing concern over the possible effects of high alveolar pressures and volumes in causing barotrauma or "volutrauma" has led some investigators to advocate the use of PCV and a larger I:E ratio of approximately 1:1, despite the fact that this approach has not been demonstrated to be more effective than other methods shown to be superior to older ones. It is argued that when older modes of PPV are employed, VT should be as low as 5 to 7 mL/kg, ventilators should be pressure cycled, and high levels of PEEP should be avoided if possible, even if the FI_{O_2} exceeds 0.6 in the process.

Appropriate use of intravenous fluid is an essential component of the management of ARDS and MOSF. Because pulmonary capillary permeability is increased, administration of fluid, which increases the capillary hydrostatic pressure, tends to increase the amount of lung water. On the other hand, adequate pulmonary perfusion may be important in preventing or ameliorating lung damage, and systemic perfusion clearly is essential in maintaining renal, cardiac, and CNS function. Thus, the effects of crystalloid, colloid, or red blood cell administration should be carefully monitored with clear endpoints in mind. In addition to measuring PSA and other variables, indices of end-organ perfusion such as urine output and mental status should be followed.

Pulmonary artery catheterization may be extremely helpful in assessing hemodynamic status, at least early in the course of ARDS and MOSF. Although the correlation between PPAO and the outcome of these disorders has not been determined, it appears reasonable to maintain the PPAO at a normal or slightly below normal level so long as perfusion of vital organs is maintained. If perfusion is inadequate or if $\dot{Q}T$ is depressed by the patient's underlying disease or its treatment, the circulation can be supported with dopamine or dobutamine.

Ideally, the combination of specific therapy for associated conditions such as sepsis syndrome and appropriate cardiovascular and respiratory system support should improve $\dot{T}_{O_2}$ in patients with ARDS and MOSF. It is important to keep this goal in mind for at least three reasons. First, $\dot{T}_{O_2}$ and its components (Ca_{O_2} and $\dot{Q}T$) can be quantified, and therapies that increase one component at the expense of the other may be modified. Second, there is no specific antidote for the inadequate O_2 extraction that so often characterizes ARDS and MOSF. Therapies to improve $\dot{T}_{O_2}$ are the only ones available. A third reason to improve $\dot{T}_{O_2}$ is that the apparent failure of O_2 extraction in patients with ARDS and MOSF may actually be a complicated form of $\dot{T}_{O_2}$ failure. This is supported by the demonstration that $\dot{V}_{O_2}$ appears to be dependent upon $\dot{T}_{O_2}$ at some critical level of $\dot{T}_{O_2}$ in these conditions.[35] It is also supported by the finding that some patients with ARDS and MOSF increase $\dot{V}_{O_2}$ and resolve their lactic acidosis with increases in $\dot{T}_{O_2}$.[36] Given this finding, some investigators advocate fluid loading, hypertransfusion with red blood cells, or the administration of dobutamine to patients with ARDS and MOSF to increase Ca_{O_2} and $\dot{Q}T$ to arbitrarily high levels.[37] The general benefit of this approach has not been determined, however, and it cannot be recommended at the present time.[1]

Shock

The concepts in Eqs. 8 and 9 help to explain the various kinds of shock that produce inadequate O_2 transport and O_2 extraction. For example, hypovolemic shock, in which $\dot{Q}T$ is depressed because SV is inadequate, is associated with hemorrhage or other intravascular fluid losses. Obstructive shock may result from pulmonary thromboembolism, in which right ventricular output falls because PPA and PVR increase; or from cardiac tamponade, in which an accumulation of pericardial fluid interferes with ventricular filling and SV.[1]

Cardiogenic shock usually results from left ventricular dysfunction following massive myocardial infarction in patients with IHD; right ventricular infarction rarely causes cardiogenic shock. Left ventricular dysfunction leads to a fall in SV and an increase in SVR as the body attempts to maintain PSA and coronary perfusion. Left ventricular pressure, PLA and pulmonary capillary pressure also may increase, and fluid may transudate into the pulmonary interstitial space and ultimately the alveoli, causing pulmonary edema and reducing Pa_{O_2}. With either left or right ventricular infarction, PRA may increase, and peripheral edema may result from increased systemic venous pressure. Both forms of infarction may be complicated by bradyarrhythmias, in which $\dot{Q}T$ is further reduced by a fall in HR and by tachyarrhythmias, which reduces SV by decreasing the duration of diastole and thereby compromising ventricular filling.

Distributive shock is characterized by a fall in SVR and a rise in $\dot{Q}T$ as left ventricular afterload is reduced. Despite this increase in $\dot{Q}T$, however, organ perfusion is often inadequate because of abnormalities in regional blood flow. Distributive shock is seen mostly in patients with sepsis syndrome due to a variety of organisms. Patients with pancreatitis, anaphylaxis, overdosage of drugs such as aspirin, and severe liver failure also may have distributive shock.

Spinal or neurogenic shock is a form of distributive shock seen primarily in patients with cervical spinal cord injury. The primary pathogenic mechanism of spinal shock is an interruption of sympathetic tone below the level of the cord lesion that causes vasodilation and a pooling of blood in the extremities. This may be accompanied by unopposed vagal influences on the heart, so that bradycardia develops. Cardiac output may be depressed due to the bradycardia, and spinal cord perfusion may decrease due to the fall in PSA.

Treatment of the various kinds of shock is based on their underlying pathophysiology. For example, hypovolemic shock is best treated with intravascular fluids including blood that restore preload. $Alpha_1$ agonists such as phenylephrine or high-dose dopamine that increase P_{circ} and R_{circ} should be used only temporarily to support PSA in patients with hypovolemic shock because they do not affect the underlying volume loss. Similarly, obstructive shock should be treated with measures that relieve the obstruction. Thus, the abnormal rise in PPA and PVR that accompanies pulmonary thromboembolism may be ameliorated by thrombolytic agents. Oxygen also should be administered to prevent increases in PVR caused by alveolar hypoxia. At the same time, SV may be restored in patients with cardiac tamponade by removing pericardial fluid. The circulation can be supported in patients with these conditions with volume infusion and dobutamine to increase $\dot{Q}T$, given in concert with $alpha_1$ agonists if necessary to maintain PSA and perfusion of the coronary circulation.

The treatment of cardiogenic shock following left ventricular infarction depends on the patient's PLA as approximated by PPAO. If the PPAO is decreased, $\dot{Q}T$ may be increased by improving preload. Conversely, if PPAO is increased, it may be decreased by agents that reduce preload, left ventricular afterload, or both variables. Morphine at doses of 1 to 10 mg or more intravenously is a potent venodilator that reduces preload. This agent also relieves pain and reduces the liberation of endogenous catecholamines that increase SVR during infarction. Nitroglycerin also reduces preload by its effects on the venous circulation and limits ischemia through coronary vasodilation. Nitroprusside is preferred in reducing afterload because its effects are more pronounced on the arterial circulation. It should be noted that decreasing PPAO by reducing preload or afterload will in turn reduce pulmonary capillary pressure and edema formation as well as PRA. If right ventricular infarction has occurred, the output of that ventricle may be improved by either volume infusion or dobutamine. In patients with infarction of either ventricle, PSA may be supported with $alpha_1$-agonists to insure adequate coronary perfusion if necessary.

The general approach to patients with distributive shock is to insure adequate preload, add $alpha_1$ agonists to increase PSA and SVR if necessary, and administer dopamine in low doses to maintain renal and mesenteric blood flow. Dopamine also may be used in $beta_1$- and $alpha_1$-range doses in patients with sepsis syndrome, pancreatitis, and severe liver failure. Epinephrine, which also has $alpha_1$ and both $beta_1$ and $beta_2$ properties, traditionally has been given to patients with anaphylaxis at doses of 0.5 to 1 mg or 5 to 10 mL of a 1:10,000 solution. Although dobutamine may be useful in increasing $\dot{Q}T$ in patients with distributive shock, it may cause hypotension and require the simultaneous administration of $alpha_1$ agonists. Isoproterenol probably should be avoided because it is a $beta_1$ and $beta_2$ agonist without alpha$_1$ effects, and therefore has unopposed vasodilating properties. Alpha$_1$ agonists usually are given in conjunction with atropine to patients with spinal shock.

Cardiorespiratory Arrest

Cardiorespiratory arrest is the most profound form of cardiogenic shock and also the most extreme example of T_{O_2} failure. Cessation of effective $\dot{Q}T$ may be the culmination of a variety of shock states but most commonly is the result of ventricular fibrillation occurring either primarily or in the course of left ventricular infarction. As $\dot{Q}T$ abruptly falls, release of catecholamines results in peripheral vasoconstriction in an attempt to preserve blood flow to the brain, heart, and respiratory muscles at the expense of other organs, just as occurs in less severe shock. Lactic acid production increases unless $\dot{Q}T$ is restored, and the effectiveness of catecholamines is diminished. This results in generalized vasodilation that reduces the distribution of blood flow to vital organs.

Cardiorespiratory arrest is treated with CPR. This technique is based on the goal of augmenting both Ca_{O_2} and $\dot{Q}T$ by a series of basic life support maneuvers until advanced cardiac life support can be applied. An important determinant of CPR success is the provision of adequate $\dot{V}A$ to normalize Pa_{CO_2} and pH. When cardiac arrest occurs in nonintubated patients, the first step is to open the airway and assure its patency. The most common cause of obstruction is the tongue. This may be corrected simply by tilting the head backward and lifting the chin or lower jaw forward. Mouth-to-mouth ventilation then has to be applied unless a foreign body is obstructing the airway. Two quick breaths sufficient to make the chest wall rise should be given in single-rescuer CPR.[1]

A resuscitator's exhaled air may provide an FI_{O_2} of approximately 0.17 during mouth-to-mouth ventilation, and CO_2 will be eliminated because of passive lung deflation. This should alleviate the need for HCO_3^-, which is no longer recommended to reverse metabolic acidosis because it adds CO_2 to the body and may cause respiratory acidosis. Commonly, however, O_2 exchange within the lungs is not normal and significant hypoxemia develops. For this reason, supplemental O_2 should be administered as soon as it is available. Both oxygenation and ventilation can be accomplished via a tightly fitting face mask and ventilation bag, preferably one capable of delivering an FI_{O_2} of 1. Endotracheal intubation provides the most reliable closed system for oxygenation and ventilation, and also protects the airway against the aspiration of gastric contents.

Closed chest compression should be administered to patients who do not have a palpable pulse. The patient should be supine and on a firm surface. Sufficient pressure should be applied to the lower half of the sternum to depress it 4 to 5 cm in most adults and 2 cm in children in order to increase PSA. The pressure should be relaxed after each compression, allowing the sternum to return to its relaxed position, which will reduce PRA and enhance coronary perfusion. The recommended compression-to-relaxation ratio is 1:1, and the rate of compressions should be between 80 and 100/min. The adequacy of closed chest compression should be determined by attempting to palpate a carotid or femoral pulse produced by the compression.

The arrival of persons with additional training or equipment marks the start of advanced cardiac life support. Electrocardiographic monitoring enables proper application of direct current countershock for defibrillation or conversion of ventricular tachycardia. A current of 200 to 360 J should be used for ventricular fibrillation. The current given should be increased if there is no response to the initial shock. In patients with ventricular fibrillation, epinephrine should be routinely administered in doses of 1 mg or 10 mL of a 1:10,000 dilution intravenously (preferably via a central venous catheter), or via an endotracheal tube before countershock is applied. Epinephrine constricts peripheral vessels through its alpha$_1$ effects and enhances myocardial contractility through its beta$_1$ effects. This combination improves cerebral and cardiac perfusion. Intravenous lidocaine in a bolus of 1 mg/kg followed by additional boluses and a continuous infusion of 1 to 4 mg/min may also be helpful in treating ventricular ectopy, as may bretylium in an initial intravenous bolus of 5 to 10 mg/kg followed by an infusion of 1 to 2 mg/min. Calcium chloride is no longer recommended in the treatment of cardiorespiratory arrest because it has been shown to be ineffective and may contribute to ischemic injury.[38]

The major determinant of return of brain function is the adequacy of cerebral perfusion during the period of cardiac arrest. After recovery of cardiac function, all factors that influence O_2 delivery to the brain should be evaluated and made normal where possible. Measures to prevent possible elevations in ICP, such as head elevation, controlling arterial pH and Pa_{CO_2}, and treating seizures and agitation, should be undertaken. Neither barbiturates nor calcium channel-blocking agents have been demonstrated to minimize brain damage.[39,40]

REFERENCES

1. Luce JM, Hopewell PC: Critical care medicine. In: Wyngaarden JB, Smith LH, Bennett JC, Plum F (eds): *Cecil Textbook of Medicine*, 19th ed. Philadelphia, Saunders, 1992, pp 459–476.
2. Luce JM: Hemodynamic and respiratory monitoring in critical care medicine. In: Kelly WN (ed): *Textbook of Internal Medicine*, 2d ed. Philadelphia, Lippincott, 1992, pp 1845–1849.
3. O'Quin R, Marini JJ: Pulmonary artery occlusion pressure: Clinical physiology, measurement and interpretation. *Am Rev Respir Dis* 128:319, 1983.
4. Luce JM: Medical management of spinal cord injury. *Crit Care Med* 13:126, 1985.
5. Plum F, Posner JB: *The Diagnosis of Stupor and Coma*, 2d ed. Philadelphia, F.A. Davis, 1972, pp 13–65.
6. North JB, Jennett S: Abnormal breathing patterns associated with acute brain damage. *Arch Neurol* 31:338, 1974.
7. Sahn SA, Lakshiminarayan S, Petty JL: Weaning from mechanical ventilation. *JAMA* 235:2208, 1976.
8. Pepe PE, Marini JJ: Occult positive end-expiratory pressure in mechanically ventilated patients: The auto-PEEP effect. *Am Rev Respir Dis* 126:166, 1982.
9. Schnapp LM, Cohen NH: Pulse oximetry: Uses and abuses. *Chest* 98:1244, 1990.
10. Luce JM, Tyler ML, Pierson DJ: *Intensive Respiratory Care*. Philadelphia, Saunders, 1984, pp 93–110.
11. Luce JM: Neurologic monitoring. *Respir Care* 30:471, 1985.
12. Luce JM, Tyler ML, Pierson DJ: *Intensive Respiratory Care*. Philadelphia, Saunders, 1984, pp 190–206.
13. Murciano D, Aubuir M, Lecocquic Y, Poriente R: Effects of theophylline on diaphragmatic strength and fatigue in patients with chronic obstructive pulmonary disease. *N Engl J Med* 311:349, 1984.
14. Luce JM, Tyler ML, Pierson DJ: *Intensive Respiratory Care*. Philadelphia, Saunders, 1984, pp 156–173.
15. Luce JM, Tyler ML, Pierson DJ: *Intensive Respiratory Care*. Philadelphia, Saunders, 1984, pp 207–226.
16. Marini JJ, Pierson DJ, Hudson LD: Acute lobar atelectasis: A prospective comparison of fiberoptic bronchoscopy and respiratory therapy. *Am Rev Respir Dis* 119:971, 1979.
17. Stauffer JL, Olson DE, Petty TL: Complications and consequences of endotracheal intubation and tracheotomy. *Am J Med* 70:65, 1981.
18. MacIntyre NR: Respiratory function during pressure support ventilation. *Chest* 89:677, 1986.
19. Lain DC, DiBenedetto R, Morris SL, et al: Pressure control inverse ratio ventilation as a method to reduce peak inspiratory pressure and provide adequate ventilation and oxygenation. *Chest* 95:1081, 1989.
20. Dreyfus D, Basset G, Soler P: Intermittent positive-pressure hyperventilation with high inflation pressures produces pulmonary microvascular injury in rats. *Am Rev Respir Dis* 132:880, 1985.
21. Luce JM: The cardiovascular efforts of mechanical ventilation and positive end-expiratory pressure. *JAMA* 252:807, 1984.
22. Pierson DJ: Positive end-expiratory pressure. In: Luce JM, Pierson DJ (eds): *Critical Care Medicine*. Philadelphia, Saunders, 1988, pp 227–232.
23. Kelly BJ, Luce JM: The diagnosis and management of neuromuscular diseases causing respiratory failure. *Chest* 99:1485, 1991.
24. Brachen ME, Shepard MJ, Collins WF, et al: A randomized, controlled trial of methylprednisolone or naloxone in the treatment of acute spinal-cord injury. *N Engl J Med* 322:1405, 1990.
25. O'Donohue WJ, Baker JT, Bell GM, et al: Respiratory failure in neuromuscular disease. *JAMA* 235:773, 1976.
26. Rebuck AS, Chapman KR, Abboud R: Nebulized anticholinergic and sympathomimetic treatment of asthma and chronic obstructive pulmonary disease in the emergency room. *Am J Med* 82:59, 1987.
27. Albert RK, Martin TR, Lewis SW: Controlled clinical trial of methylprednisolone in patients with chronic bronchitis and acute respiratory failure. *Ann Intern Med* 92:753, 1980.
28. Tobin MJ: Mechanical ventilation. *Crit Care Clin* 6:489, 1990.
29. Luce JM, Tyler ML, Pierson DJ: *Intensive Respiratory Care*. Philadelphia, Saunders, 1984, pp 302–314.
30. Niederman MS, Rafferty TD, Sasaki CT, et al: Comparison of bacterial adherence to ciliated and squamous epithelial cells obtained from the human respiratory tract. *Am Rev Respir Dis* 119:971, 1979.
31. Pierce AK, Sanford JP: Aerobic gram-negative basillary pneumonias. *Am Rev Respir Dis* 110:647, 1974.
32. Dorinsky PM, Gadek JE: Mechanisms of multiple non-pulmonary organ failure in ARDS. *Chest* 96:855, 1989.
33. Knaus WA, Wagner DP: Multiple systems organ failure: Epidemiology and prognosis. *Crit Care Clin* 5:221, 1989.

34. Macho JR, Luce JM: Rational approach to the management of multiple systems organ failure. *Crit Care Clin* 5:379, 1989.
35. Danek SJ, Lynch JP, Weg JG, Dantzker DR: The dependence of oxygen uptake on oxygen delivery in the adult respiratory distress syndrome. *Am Rev Respir Dis* 122:387, 1980.
36. Gilbert EM, Haupt MT, Mandanas RY, et al: The effect of fluid loading, blood transfusion, and catecholamine infusion on oxygen delivery and consumption in patients with sepsis. *Am Rev Respir Dis* 134:873, 1986.
37. Shoemaker WC, Kram HB, Appel PL: Therapy of shock based on pathophysiology, monitoring, and outcome prediction. *Crit Care Med* 18:S19, 1990.
38. *Textbook of Advanced Cardiac Life Support*. Dallas, American Heart Association, 1987.
39. Brain Resuscitation Clinical Trial I Study Group: Randomized clinical study of thiopental broadening in comatose survivors of cardiac arrest. *N Engl J Med* 314:397, 1986.
40. Brain Resuscitation Clinical Trial II Study Group: A randomized clinical study of a calcium-entry blocker (lidoflazine) in the treatment of comatose survivors of cardiac arrest. *N Engl J Med* 324:1225, 1991.

CHAPTER 2

The Neurologic Examination and Neurologic Monitoring in the Intensive Care Unit

William G. Obana
Brian T. Andrews

The neurologic examination is perhaps the single most important method of assessing patients in the neurosurgical intensive care unit (ICU). The initial neurologic examination includes a complete medical history, vital signs, a physical examination, and assessment of neurologic function, including the use of intracranial pressure (ICP) monitors, if available. It is imperative to assess neurologic function on admission to the hospital or ICU and at regular intervals throughout the hospital course. Serial examinations and accurate documentation of the findings are essential, because the change or lack of change in neurologic findings over time is the most sensitive method of detecting early neurologic deterioration. It is when such observations are made that further workup is necessary. Using a systematic approach to the examination helps avoid significant omissions.

HISTORY

Knowledge of the history of the present illness, past medical history, and recent hospital or prehospital course provides valuable information for understanding a patient's neurologic condition. This information enables one to better direct the initial management, anticipate potential problems, and focus on certain aspects of the neurologic examination.

Aggressive efforts should be made to obtain a comprehensive history from all patients admitted to an ICU. In patients with depressed mental status due to subarachnoid or spontaneous intraparenchymal hemorrhage, brain tumors, or brain abscesses, this information should be sought from relatives and friends of the patient and from the referring physician.

In cases of traumatic head injury, it is essential

that some attempt be made to determine the circumstances surrounding the accident. Paramedics, witnesses, or family members may be able to provide valuable information for guiding management. The sudden onset of headache, seizure, loss of consciousness, or chest pain before an accident may indicate an underlying intracranial abnormality or cardiopulmonary insult. The type of accident should also alert one to the possibility of other injuries, such as spinal cord injury after a fall or leap from a high place, or an intrathoracic or intraabdominal injury after major blunt trauma (e.g., a pedestrian struck by a motor vehicle). The time of the injury may also be significant, as prolonged subsequent hypoxia or hypotension adversely affects neurologic function in head-injured patients.[1-5] All of this information should enable more directed care during the initial intensive care period.

Knowledge of the disease may allow the neurosurgeon to focus on particular aspects of the neurologic examination. Patients with traumatic head injury should be monitored for cerebrospinal fluid leakage and signs and symptoms of increased ICP due to hemorrhage, diffuse brain swelling, or cerebral edema. Patients with aneurysmal subarachnoid hemorrhage should be observed for evidence of rehemorrhage, vasospasm, and hydrocephalus. Resection of supratentorial parenchymal brain tumors increases the risk of elevated ICP due to cerebral edema or postoperative hemorrhage; infratentorial procedures increase the risk of obstructive hydrocephalus as well. Surgery in the region of the hypothalamus or pituitary gland may lead to metabolic changes such as dehydration, hyper- or hyponatremia, which may result in altered mental status.

It is helpful to know the duration of the neurologic signs or symptoms and the neurologic status at the initial evaluation by paramedics, at the time of admission to the hospital, or at surgery. The initial neurologic findings provide the baseline against which subsequent findings will be compared. It is also important to know of any preexisting neurologic deficits. Orthopedic problems or arthritis often make neurologic assessment more difficult. A thorough review of underlying medical illnesses is necessary, not only for the general medical management of the patient but also for evaluating neurologic problems.

VITAL SIGNS

Core body temperature, blood pressure, pulse, and respiratory rate and pattern are important aspects of the general neurologic examination.

Core Body Temperature

Hypothermia, defined as a core body temperature below 32.2°C, can significantly alter the neurologic findings.[6] Care must be taken to maintain normothermia, especially in the immediate postoperative period. Although hypothermia is most frequently observed in alcoholics, drug-intoxicated patients (phenothiazine or barbiturate), those overexposed to cold, and, less frequently, those with adrenal insufficiency, hypothalamic disorders, hypopituitarism, or hypoglycemia, it can have a profound effect on the neurologic findings in neurosurgical patients. Patients with a core body temperature above 32.2°C are usually conscious unless there is another reason for stupor or coma.[6] Patients with core body temperatures less than 32.2°C, however, may appear to be comatose or even brain dead.[6] In neurosurgical patients who have underlying cerebral dysfunction, neurologic deficits due to hypothermia may occur earlier or at higher temperatures. Dehydration, lactic acidosis, and cardiac arrhythmias are the main complications of severe hypothermia. Slow, progressive rewarming, for example with blankets, heating blankets, and increased room temperature, is necessary.

A core body temperature greater than 42°C, also has been known to cause coma.[6] Lesser temperature elevations are commonly associated with delirium. In neurosurgical patients, modest temperature elevations combined with other neurologic insults can alter mental status significantly. Although hyperthermia in the general population is usually associated with heat stroke, neurosurgeons most often see such temperature elevations in patients with hypothalamic dysfunction or infections. Hyperthermic patients without infections are often diagnosed with a "central fever," which, unlike the waxing and waning fever typical of infection, persists for several days in a steady fashion. Central fevers may be quite high, often approaching 40°C. In patients with acute brain injury, large fluctuations in temperature can be a grave prognostic sign, indicating severe hypothalamic damage.

It is imperative that every effort be made to keep the core temperature below 38.5°C. Fever increases not only cerebral blood flow and ICP, but also CO_2 production and Pa_{CO_2}, further exacerbating intracranial hypertension. Fans, cooling blankets, and antipyretics should be used as needed. When the core body temperature has normalized, neurologic dysfunction due to fever should resolve, except in cases of severe hyperthermia (>42°C), in which permanent neurologic sequelae such as cerebellar ataxia, dementia, and hemiparesis are not infrequent.[6]

Blood Pressure

Blood pressure measurements can provide important diagnostic information. Extreme variations can significantly reduce the reliability of the neurologic examination. Continuous monitoring of blood pressure may provide an early indicator of ICP elevation or direct brainstem compression.

Hypertension and bradycardia in a neurosurgical patient with cerebral injury should alert one to the likelihood of an expanding mass lesion and increased ICP. As ICP rises, there is a compensatory vasomotor response manifested by an increase in mean arterial pressure and usually bradycardia. In 1902, Cushing reported that this response was graded and occurred when ICP exceeded systolic blood pressure (SBP); he postulated that it was stimulated by brainstem ischemia.[7] This vasomotor response became known as the Cushing reflex. In classic feline experimental studies aimed at localizing the receptive areas that mediate the Cushing reflex, Hoff and Reis found that the pressor response was due to stimulation of pressure-sensitive regions in the dorsal brainstem extending paramedially along the floor of the fourth ventricle from the obex and rostrally to the level of the facial colliculus. Pressor responses were also elicited in the cervicothoracic spinal cord. Pressure on or stretching of neural tissue appeared to be an adequate stimulus.

In our experience, ICU patients with progressive increases in ICP may have both hypertension and bradycardia, but often have only blood pressure elevation without a change in heart rate; a few patients have bradycardia without hypertension. In deeply comatose patients, these clinical signs often precede further neurologic deterioration due to elevated ICP. The presence of hypertension or bradycardia should prompt a careful assessment of the patient and repeated computed tomography (CT) scanning or institution of ICP monitoring.

SBP less than 60 mmHg or cardiac arrest of any duration has been shown to nullify the neurologic examination in severely head-injured patients.[1,9] In their series of 100 head-injured patients with brainstem dysfunction, Andrews et al.[10] reported that 38 percent of patients were in cardiac arrest or had systemic hypotension with SBP < 90 mmHg on admission. They subsequently reviewed 36 head-injured patients who presented with brainstem dysfunction and cardiac arrest, a SBP less than 60 mmHg, or an SBP of 60 to 90 mmHg.[1,9] In patients with cardiac arrest or SBP less than 60 mmHg, the neurologic findings of brainstem dysfunction did not reliably indicate mechanical brainstem compression from a mass lesion but rather diffuse brain ischemia, whereas in those with an initial SBP greater than 60 mmHg, such findings accurately reflected brainstem compression.

If SBP remains above 60 mmHg, cerebral autoregulation maintains adequate cerebral blood flow.[1] Below this level, cerebral ischemia occurs as blood flow to the brain decreases linearly with decreasing blood pressure.[11,12] Cerebral ischemia due to compressive lesions or increased ICP is exacerbated by systemic hypotension, which decreases cerebral perfusion pressure. The result is worsening neurologic function and increased morbidity.[1,2,4,5,13]

In patients with severe head injury, cerebral autoregulation may fail at less severe levels of hypotension. The most common cause of hypotension in head-injured patients is hemorrhagic shock soon after injury; hypotension may also occur due to dehydration from the use of diuretics or from diabetes insipidus. Systemic hypotension and high fevers may also be seen in patients with sepsis. Thus, great care must be taken to avoid systemic hypotension in neurosurgical patients. In patients with SBP less than 60 mmHg, the neurologic examination may be both extremely abnormal and misleading.[1,9]

Heart Rate

Heart rate monitoring, combined with other cardiopulmonary findings, provides useful information about CNS status. Sinus tachycardia may indicate sympathetic stimulation, such as pain, fever, or early hemorrhagic shock, even if hypotension is not yet present. Bradycardia, when associated with increased SBP and decreasing mental status, suggests severely increased ICP (Cushing reflex). In contrast, the presence of bradycardia and hypotension in a trauma patient should quickly alert one to the possibility of a cervical or upper thoracic spinal cord injury. It is crucial to realize that this cardiovascular compromise is due to decreased sympathetic tone and should be treated with atropine and/or alpha agonists rather than with large amounts of volume expanders, unless there has also been significant blood loss. In patients with spinal cord injuries, close monitoring of heart rate and blood pressure is critical.

Respirations

The rate and pattern of respirations can be important indicators of underlying neurologic dysfunction. Patients in stupor or coma and those with upper cervical cord injuries or airway compromise commonly require ventilatory support, but most patients in a neurosurgical ICU are not intubated. Therefore, it is important to understand the implications of, and promptly identify, abnormal breathing patterns, especially posthyperventilation apnea, Cheyne-Stokes respirations, apneustic breathing, and ataxic breathing.

Posthyperventilation apnea, or respirations that stop when deep breathing has lowered Pa_{CO_2} below its usual resting level, is seen in patients with bihemispheric lesions.[6] Rhythmic breathing resumes when endogenous CO_2 production raises Pa_{CO_2} to normal.[6] Care must be taken to monitor patients with Cheyne-Stokes respiration for prolonged apnea. Normal persons whose Pa_{CO_2} is lowered by hyperventilation continue to breath regularly with a reduced tidal volume until the Pa_{CO_2} returns to normal.

Cheyne-Stokes respirations are characterized by escalating hyperventilation followed by decremental hypoventilation and, finally, apnea.[14] Hyperpnea alternates smoothly and regularly with apnea.[6] Arterial blood gases show a rise in pH and a falling Pa_{CO_2}, which becomes maximal when breathing ceases and never returns to normal.[14] This breathing pattern is usually caused by deep bilateral cerebral or diencephalic dysfunction resulting from intracranial lesions.[15,16] It is also seen in patients with metabolic disorders, bilateral cerebral infarcts, and hypertensive encephalopathy.[6,15] Although Cheyne-Stokes respirations may occur in normal people during sleep,[17] in patients with intracranial disease they indicate serious neurologic and/or circulatory abnormalities.[6,15] Patients with Cheyne-Stokes respirations have an abnormally increased ventilatory response to CO_2 stimulation, which causes hyperpnea, and an abnormally decreased forebrain ventilatory stimulus, which allows apnea.[6,15] This breathing pattern has been reported to be a valuable sign of incipient transtentorial herniation.[6] The level of consciousness, pupillary size, muscle tone, and cardiac rhythms may change cyclically in patients with Cheyne-Stokes respirations.[18]

Apneustic respirations are characterized by prolonged end-inspiratory pauses.[6,14] This rare breathing pattern is defined operationally as a failure of normal inspiratory off-switching[14] and reflects dysfunction of the pneumotaxic centers, which are located in the middle or lower pons at or below the level of the nucleus parabrachialis.[6,19,20] Brainstem lesions are usually located in the dorsolateral tegmentum. Apneustic respirations are common in patients with pontine infarctions due to basilar artery occlusion[21] and occasionally occur in patients with transtentorial herniation.

Ataxic breathing is completely irregular; it is characterized by deep and shallow breaths, random pauses, and occasionally apnea.[6] This breathing pattern reflects dysfunction in the region of the reticular formation, which is located in the dorsolateral medulla and extends down to the obex, which is the area responsible for respiratory rhythm.[6] In patients with ataxic breathing, the respiratory center is hypersensitive to depressant drugs, and even mild sedation can cause apnea. Ataxic breathing may indicate an expanding mass in the posterior fossa, which can rapidly lead to respiratory arrest.

PHYSICAL EXAMINATION

A general physical examination should be performed on admission and at regular intervals throughout the hospital course. The development of medical illnesses, including infections, cardiopulmonary compromise, hematologic abnormalities, gastrointestinal disorders, and renal disease, can significantly alter the neurologic status.

NEUROLOGIC EXAMINATION

To be useful in a critical care setting, the neurologic examination must be performed frequently and without variation. In head-injured patients, the Glasgow Coma Scale (Table 2-1) is used to assess hemispheric function on admission and repeatedly thereafter.[22] At San Francisco General Hospital Medical Center, a standard admission form is completed for all head-injured patients (Fig. 2-1). This form facilitates rapid and complete neurologic evaluation, documents the findings, and enables comparisons to be made with subsequent examinations.

Similarly, to minimize variations in the hourly neurologic assessment, which is usually performed by nurses, a standard neurologic flow sheet is used to evaluate the level of consciousness, brainstem function, and motor response (Fig. 2-2). A sensory examination is usually performed only in patients with spinal cord injuries. Using the flow sheet maximizes the objective portions of the neurologic examination and minimizes the subjective aspects.

Table 2-1 Glasgow Coma Scale

Category	Response	Score
Eye opening	None	1
	To pain	2
	To voice	3
	Spontaneously	4
Verbal	None	1
	Incomprehensible	2
	Garbled words	3
	Confused speech	4
	Oriented speech	5
Motor	Flaccid	1
	Abnormal extension	2
	Abnormal flexion	3
	Normal flexion	4
	Localizing pain	5
	Follows commands	6

Level of Consciousness and Mental Status

A change in the level of consciousness or mental status may be the first indication of neurologic deterioration. The standard terms used to describe the level of consciousness are awake and alert, lethargic, stuporous, obtunded, and comatose. The level of consciousness reflects both the level of arousal and the presence of cognition or conscious behavior. Arousal is dependent upon proper function of the reticular activating system (RAS), whereas conscious behavior is dependent on proper function of the cerebral hemispheres.[1,6]

The RAS is a diffuse network of neurons in the brainstem. It is located predominantly in the midbrain, where it forms part of the tegmentum,[1,6] and extends into the thalamus and subthalamus in the diencephalon. The neurons of the RAS are extensively interconnected and receive collateral input from every major somatic and special sensory pathway. Numerous axons ascend from the RAS through the central tegmental fasciculus of the midbrain and extend into the thalamus, hypothalamus, basal forebrain structures, including the limbic system, and diffusely into the neocortex.

Stimulation of the RAS produces generalized, nonspecific activation of the cerebral cortex.[1,6] This activity appears to occur in part through abolition of the tonically inhibitory influence of the thalamic reticular nucleus and through modulation of the limbic system by the hypothalamus. An injury that interrupts or reduces rostral input from the RAS in the mesencephalon and diencephalon decreases alertness and cortical arousal.

Conscious behavior is dependent upon arousal of the cerebral cortex in many localized areas that participate in specific cognitive functions.[1,6] Of

DATE TIME	PROBLEM NUMBER	FORMAT: PROBLEM NUMBER AND TITLE: S—Subjective A—Analysis O—Objective P—Plans
		NEUROSURGICAL HEAD INJURY ADMITTING SHEET
		Sex: ☐ Male / ☐ Female Age: Handedness: ☐ Left / ☐ Right
		Cause of Injury:
		Time from: Injury → Coma Injury → MEH Injury → Neuro Consult
	Physical Exam	Vital Signs BP HR TEMP

COMA SCORE	GROUP A	GROUP B	GROUP C	GROUP D
Eye Opening	None		To Pain	To Voice Spontaneously
Verbal Response	None	Sounds	Words	Confused Oriented
Motor Response	None Abnl. Extens. Abnl. Flexs.	Withdraws Localizes Pain		Follows Commands
	ALL circles here = A	HIGHEST circle here = B	ANY circle here = C	ALL circles must be here to = D

MOTOR EXAM:

	R	L
arms		
legs		

1 = no response
2 = abnormal extension
3 = abnormal flexion
4 = weakness
5 = normal

Spontaneous spasms (posturing)? ☐ Yes / ☐ No

PUPILS:	Ⓡ Size____mm Reaction + / - Ⓛ Size____mm Reaction + / -
EOMs:	III nerve palsy? ☐ Right ☐ Left ☐ Neither ☐ Both
	Spontaneous eye movements? Describe:
	Doll's eyes: ☐ Absent ☐ Sluggish ☐ Brisk ☐ Normal (awake)
	Calorics: ☐ None ☐ Dysconj. ☐ Conj. ☐ Nystagmus (BEST RESPONSE EITHER EAR)
CORNEALS:	Right + / - Left + / -
RESPIRATIONS:	☐ Regular ☐ Ataxic ☐ Periodic (Cheyne-Stokes)
	Apneic? ☐ Yes ☐ No Resp. Rate:
	Cough? ☐ Yes ☐ No Gag? ☐ Yes ☐ No

F 726N Rev 8/87

Figure 2-1 Standard admission form used for all head-injured patients at the San Francisco General Hospital Medical Center.

special importance are sensory and sensory association areas and regions important for motivation. Cortical lesions of increasing size cause a progressive decrease in alertness and cognitive function, regardless of their location, although earlier and more prominent findings may be noted if the left cerebral hemisphere is involved. When cortical function ceases, the patient loses all alertness, even if the RAS remains intact. Damage to connections between cortical regions probably explains the influence of a lesion on uninjured areas. Intact cognitive function may require continuous afferent stimulation from all other parts of the neocortex through both corticothalamic and direct cortical connections.

Orientation and mentation are assessed as a part of the routine neurologic evaluation. Changes in conscious behavior may signify a change in or the

Neuro Flowsheet

Glasgow Coma Scale

Pupil Scale (m.m.)

1 2 3 4 5 6 7 8

		Date																								
		Time	07	08	09	10	11	12	13	14	15	16	17	18	19	20	21	22	23	24	01	02	03	04	05	06
PUPILS	right	Size																								
		Reaction																								
	left	Size																								
		Reaction																								
COMA SCALE	Eyes Open	4 Spontaneously																								
		3 To speech																								
		2 To pain																								
		1 To none																								
	Best Motor Response	6 Obey commands																								
		5 Localize pain																								
		4 Flexion withdrawl																								
		3 Flexion normal																								
		2 Extension																								
		1 None																								
	Best Response to Auditory/ Visual Stimulus	ADULT																								
		5 Orientation																								
		4 Confused																								
		3 Inappropriate words																								
		2 Incomprehensible words																								
		1 None																								
		T= Endotracheal Tube or Tracheostomy																								
		L= Language Barrier																								
	COMA SCALE TOTALS																									
LIMB MOVEMENT			R/L	R/L	R/L	R/L	R/L	R/L	R/L	R/L	R/L	R/L	R/L	R/L	R/L	R/L	R/L	R/L	R/L	R/L	R/L	R/L	R/L	R/L	R/L	R/L
	ARMS	Voluntary motor (0-5)																								
		Flexion withdrawl																								
		Flexion Abnormal																								
		Extension																								
		No Response																								
	LEGS	Voluntary motor (0-5)																								
		Flexion																								
		Extension																								
		No Response																								
		MAP																								
		ICP																								

++ = brisk
+ = sluggish
- = no reaction
C = eye closed by swelling

Eyes closed by swelling = C

+ = Present
- = Absent
NT = Not Tested
0 = No Movement
1 = Trace Movement
2 = Movement, but not against gravity
3 = Movement against gravity, but not against resistance
4 = Movement against gravity and some resistance
5 = Full Power

Figure 2-2 Standard neurologic flow sheets used for all neurosurgical intensive care unit patients at the hospitals associated with the University of California, San Francisco.

development of an intracranial lesion. However, it is also important to check for other abnormalities that may contribute to or be responsible for a change in the level of consciousness. These include seizures, fever, hypothermia, hypotension, hypertension related to encephalopathy, hypoxia, hypercapnia, infection, metabolic changes, and sedatives or other pharmacologic agents.

Brainstem

Brainstem function should be evaluated systematically, beginning from the midbrain and extending down to the medulla. Olfaction and vision or visual fields are often difficult to test in ICU patients. Therefore, the brainstem reflexes must be tested to evaluate brainstem function.

Afferent defects in the optic nerve can be detected by evaluating the consensual pupillary response to light. For example, in the Marcus Gunn pupil test, when a light is swung from a normal eye to an impaired eye at 3-s intervals, both pupils will dilate when the light is directed toward the eye with an optic nerve defect. In such instances, the direct light stimulus is no longer sufficient to maintain the previously evoked consensual pupillary constriction. This test may be helpful in detecting changes in lesions in the region of the optic nerves.

Pupillary symmetry and reactivity are the most important part of the brainstem examination in patients at risk for expanding intracranial mass lesions. Unilateral pupillary dilatation most likely indicates transtentorial herniation.[1] The pupillary response to direct light reflects the integrity of the midbrain, including the third nerve nuclei and superior colliculi and the exiting third cranial nerves. Pupillary size is determined by the balance between the effects of the sympathetic and parasympathetic nervous system on the pupils.

Sympathetic innervation arises from the hypothalamus and brainstem and passes through the cervical spinal cord to synapses in the intermediolateral tract of the upper three thoracic spinal segments.[1] Preganglionic fibers pass through the ventral roots of the cervical spinal cord and through the inferior and middle cervical sympathetic ganglia to synapses in the superior cervical sympathetic ganglion. Postganglionic fibers pass through the internal carotid plexus along the internal carotid artery, enter the orbit through the superior orbital fissure with the nasociliary nerve, and then enter the globe as the long ciliary nerve. Sympathetic discharges innervate the dilator pupillae muscle, resulting in dilatation of the pupil.

Parasympathetic innervation arises from the Edinger-Westphal nucleus, dorsal to the third nerve nucleus in the mesencephalon.[1] The preganglionic fibers travel with the oculomotor nerve as it passes forward from the interpeduncular fossa and penetrates the dural edge of the incisura to enter the lateral wall of the cavernous sinus. The parasympathetic fibers lie peripherally in the nerve and are exquisitely sensitive to compression. When the oculomotor nerve enters the superior orbital fissure, the parasympathetic fibers travel to the ciliary ganglion and synapse. The postganglionic fibers form the short ciliary nerve, which enters the sclera and innervates the smooth muscle that constricts the pupil.

Transtentorial herniation causes compression of the ipsilateral oculomotor nerve or the ipsilateral third nerve nucleus and the Edinger-Westphal nucleus.[1] Initially, parasympathetic tone is disrupted, but sympathetic tone remains intact, causing pupillary dilatation or irregularity. The oval or irregular pupil is thought to result from centrally determined differences in parasympathetic tone to some segments of the pupillary sphincters.[23,24] As transtentorial herniation progresses, the midbrain becomes ischemic, and both parasympathetic and sympathetic tone are lost, resulting in fixed, midposition pupils of 4 to 5 mm. If transtentorial herniation persists and the more central fibers of the oculomotor nerve supplying the extraocular muscles are affected, ipsilateral extraocular movements mediated by the third nerve may be lost. Pupillary asymmetry in a patient with an intracranial mass lesion and a depressed level of consciousness signifies transtentorial herniation, which requires prompt neurosurgical attention.[1,6,9,10,23,25–30]

Unilateral pupillary dilatation does not always signify a mass lesion compressing the Edinger-Westphal nucleus or oculomotor nerve and/or nuclei. A patient who has undergone clipping of a basilar artery aneurysm or who has suffered eye trauma often has oculomotor nerve palsies from focal injury or surgical manipulation. In such cases, the possibility of an expanding intracranial mass lesion should not be easily dismissed. Other methods of assessment, such as ICP measurements and imaging studies, should be used.

With tegmental lesions, the pupils are usually midposition and unreactive. Pontine lesions most often cause pinpoint and unreactive pupils. Small reactive pupils are most commonly seen with hemorrhage into and around the third ventricle.

Many pharmacologic agents can affect pupillary function. Barbiturates and atropine are commonly used in a critical care setting. Barbiturates at lower doses usually cause pupillary constriction and in high doses may result in loss of pupillary reactivity.[30] Atropine, a parasympathetic antagonist most commonly used to treat bradycardia, also results in pupillary dilatation. Any pupillary asymmetry in patients receiving barbiturates or atropine should be presumed to be due to an intracranial mass until proven otherwise.

The corneal reflexes reflect the integrity of the fifth afferent and seventh efferent cranial nerves and their interconnections in the pons. Absence of the corneal reflex indicates probable pontine dysfunction.

If there is no cervical spinal injury or contraindication for cervical spinal manipulation, the oculocephalic reflex should be tested by the doll's eye maneuver to evaluate the midbrain and pons, specifically the integrity of the prepontine gaze centers, third and sixth nerve nuclei, and their interconnections via the medial longitudinal fasciculus. If cervical movement is contraindicated, the oculovestibular reflex can be evaluated by ice water calorics — instilling 100 mL ice water onto the tympanic membrane. If the reflex is intact, this maneuver produces a tonic deviation of both eyes toward the tested side. This test is contraindicated in patients with hemotympanum, tympanic membrane perforation, otorrhea, or basilar skull fractures.

The gag response evaluates the functioning of the ninth afferent and tenth efferent cranial nerves, the nuclei of which are located in the medulla. The respiratory status may need to be evaluated to assess the pontomedullary respiratory centers, especially when the determination of brain death is being made.

Motor Function

Asymmetric motor findings suggest increasing mass effect on the motor cortex or descending fibers in the corticospinal tracts. In patients with a depressed level of consciousness and unilateral pupillary dilatation, a contralateral hemiparesis completes the clinical triad for diagnosing transtentorial herniation.[1,10,26,28,29] However, in up to 25 percent of patients with transtentorial herniation, the hemiparesis is ipsilateral to the dilated pupil[28] because the brainstem is displaced away from the side of the mass, compressing the contralateral cerebral peduncle against the opposite dural edge of the incisura, a condition called Kernohan's notch phenomenon.[31]

In awake patients, the motor function of each extremity can be graded from 0 to 5 with 5/5 as normal strength, 4/5 as decreased strength to resistance, 3/5 as able to lift extremity against gravity, 2/5 as able to move an extremity with gravity eliminated, 1/5 as muscle contraction, and 0/5 as no visible movement. The notations "+" and "−" can be used to further convey more subtle changes.

In patients with a depressed level of consciousness, motor function is evaluated by testing the best motor response to voice or, if necessary, to deep pain. These movements can be recorded as normal, abnormal, or absent. Normal motor function is characterized by the ability to follow commands, purposeful spontaneous movements, brisk localization of supraorbital pain (lifting the hand above the chin), or brisk withdrawal of an extremity to deep peripheral pain (tested with a pencil across the fingernail while applying increasingly firm pressure). Abnormal motor function is characterized by flexor or extensor posturing. Absent movement or flaccidity is characterized by no response to painful stimulation. Abnormal flexor and extensor posturing can be produced experimentally in animals by lesions in several different locations in the brain. Therefore, the terms decorticate and decerebrate are probably misleading.[6] In humans, these anatomic and physiologic associations are even less clear.

Flexor posturing, or abnormal flexor response in the arm and extension of the leg, consists of a relatively slow flexion of the arm, wrist, and fingers with adduction in the upper extremity and extension, internal rotation, and plantar flexion in the lower extremity.[6] The extent of this response varies. The large size of fatal lesions in humans often precludes the use of autopsy material to localize these responses. Clinically, patients with these abnormal movements usually have hemispheric lesions rather than deeper lesions. Bricolo et al.[32] reported that 90 percent of their head-injured patients with "decorticate rigidity" had no neuroophthalmologic evidence of brainstem injury.

Extensor posturing, or abnormal extensor response in the arm and leg, consists of opisthotonos; clenching of the teeth; and extension, adduction, and hyperpronation of the upper extremity; which are accompanied by extension of the lower extremity and plantar flexion of the foot.[6] Clinically, these features are seen in patients with massive bilateral forebrain lesions, transtentorial herniation, expanding posterior fossa lesions causing midbrain and rostral pontine dysfunction, or severe metabolic disorders.[6]

Flaccidity is characterized by the absence of elicitable motor responses. It can be caused by peripheral denervation or dysfunction of central motor mechanisms in the medullopontine reticular formation.[6] Bilateral flaccidity is an ominous sign in patients with intracranial mass lesions. Flaccidity due to spinal shock can be an early consequence of spinal cord injury.

Myoclonus is common after hypoxic insults or cardiac arrest. Asterixis or tremors suggest other metabolic abnormalities.

OTHER FACTORS ASSOCIATED WITH THE NEUROLOGIC EXAMINATION AND NEUROLOGIC MONITORING

Arterial Blood Gases

In neurosurgical patients, the most common abnormalities in arterial blood gases are those reflecting respiratory failure. A Pa_{O_2} less than 60 mmHg or a Pa_{CO_2} greater than 50 mmHg unequivocally defines respiratory failure.[33] Patients with neurologic disease rarely complain of dyspnea. The more common premonitory neurologic signs of respiratory failure are confusion, restlessness, and headache.[33] As ventilation is further compromised, pupillary constriction, asterixis or tremors, papilledema, and coma ensue. In such patients, it is therefore important to avoid systemic hypoxia and hypercapnia and to interpret the neurologic findings with caution.

The effect of systemic hypoxia on the neurologic examination has been most often evaluated clinically in cases of acute airway obstruction, drowning, or suffocation. Systemic hypotension is often associated with acute hypoxia due to a centrally induced reflex depression of cardiac function.[34] Consequently, the adverse effects of acute hypoxia on the brain are partly due to hypoperfusion.[14] Cerebral ischemia may result from both systemic hypoxia and hypoperfusion.

If systemic hypotension is adequately treated, humans can tolerate extremely low Pa_{O_2} without obvious neurologic sequelae. In a series of 22 patients with a Pa_{O_2} less than 20 mmHg, Gray and Horner[35] reported that eight were alert, seven were somnolent, and seven were comatose. When systemic hypoxia ($Pa_{O_2} < 20$ mmHg) is combined with hypercapnia, however, neurologic function is poor and recovery infrequent.[36]

Severe hypoxia may cause clinical signs of a metabolic encephalopathy, including progressive alterations in the level of consciousness leading to coma; changes in respiratory patterns; and tremors, asterixis, myoclonus, and flexor or extensor posturing.[6,16] Brainstem reflexes usually remain intact until the anoxia becomes profound, at which time pupillary dilatation and loss of oculocephalic reflexes may occur.[6] Experimentally, acute anoxia has been shown to produce pupillary constriction until cardiac output has decreased by 70 percent.[37] The pupils then dilate and remain dilated until several minutes after death, when they return to the midposition. The pupils may, however, remain small until the time of death.[1]

Systemic hypoxia is a frequent complication of severe head injury. In a series of patients in coma after head injury, Katsurada et al.[38] found that 43 percent had a Pa_{O_2} less than 70 mmHg, 51 percent had an alveolar-arterial O_2 tension difference greater than 30 mmHg, 14 percent had Pa_{CO_2} greater than 45 mmHg, and 20 percent had an arterial pH less than 7.35. Similarly, Miller et al.[4] observed that 30 percent of severely head-injured patients had an initial Pa_{O_2} less than 65 mmHg. Systemic hypoxia in such instances may result from the immediate onset of apnea after head injury,[3] subsequent abnormal breathing patterns,[39] hypoventilation due to associated spinal cord injury causing paralysis of the thoracic musculature, airway obstruction due to facial or neck injuries, direct injury to the chest wall or lungs, or fat emboli in the pulmonary circulation.[40,41] In patients with systemic hypoxia, the neurologic findings should not be the sole basis for neurosurgical treatment decisions. The neurologic evaluation should be repeated as the respiratory and metabolic abnormalities are corrected, and other clinical findings, such as vital signs or ICP, should be taken into consideration.

Hypercapnia, or respiratory acidosis ($Pa_{CO_2} >$ 55 mmHg), is usually accompanied by systemic hypoxia and elevated cerebrospinal fluid pressure.[14] It is usually caused by severe neuromuscular or pulmonary disease or by depression of the respiratory centers. Neurologic dysfunction appears to be somewhat dependent on the rate of increase in Pa_{CO_2}; a rapid elevation may be more detrimental than a slow elevation.[14] Neff and Petty[42] reported 10 patients with slow increases in Pa_{CO_2} ranging from 75 to 110 mmHg who had no neurologic symptoms. In such patients, neurologic deterioration may be caused by respiratory failure or, conversely, the respiratory failure may be due to the underlying neurologic process. In a patient with an intracranial mass lesion, any elevation in Pa_{CO_2} may cause a rapid rise in ICP, a decrease in cerebral perfusion, and an abrupt or progressive decline in neurologic function.

Intracranial Pressure Monitoring

In patients at risk for increasing mass effect from an intracranial lesion, ICP monitors can provide valuable information that cannot be obtained from the standard neurologic examination.[1,25,27–29,43–45] This is especially true in comatose or sedated patients in whom clinical neurologic changes are less apparent. We routinely monitor ICP for a minimum of 24 h after clipping of a ruptured aneurysm, removal of most intraparenchymal lesions, or severe head injury.

Although ICP monitoring can help identify expanding mass lesions, its limitations must be recognized. Bullock et al.[40] analyzed 59 patients with recurrent hematomas after craniotomy for traumatic intracranial hemorrhage. ICP was monitored in 39 of these patients and allowed earlier detection of the hematoma in 22 (56 percent). However, in 17 patients (44 percent), ICP did not increase despite clinical deterioration. The delay in diagnosing recurrent hemorrhage in these patients significantly worsened their outcomes. Thus, one must continue to follow the neurologic examination carefully to rule out an expanding mass lesion in all patients with neurologic deterioration despite normal ICP readings.

Electrocardiogram

Neurogenic cardiac arrhythmias, including supraventricular and ventricular tachycardias, are common after head injury or acute intracranial hemorrhage. Most patients with subarachnoid hemorrhage have an abnormal electrocardiogram (ECG), reflecting arrhythmias or myocardial ischemia. Such changes have been attributed to the combination of intense parasympathetic-sympathetic stimulation and elevated levels of circulating catecholamines. Continuous ECG monitoring is an important element of intensive care monitoring, all ECG abnormalities should be thoroughly investigated to rule out new neurologic or myocardial insults.

ACKNOWLEDGMENTS
The authors thank Cheryl Christensen for manuscript preparation and Stephen Ordway for editorial assistance.

REFERENCES

1. Andrews BT, Pitts LH: *Traumatic Transtentorial Herniation.* New York, Futura, 1991.
2. Eisenberg HM: Outcome after head injury: General considerations and neurobehavioral recovery. In: Becker DP, Povlishock JT (eds): *Central Nervous System Trauma Status Report.* National Institutes of Neurological and Communicative Diseases and Stroke, Washington, DC, 1985, pp 271–280.
3. Miller JD: Head injury and brain ischaemia-implications for therapy. *Br J Anaesth* 547:120, 1985.
4. Miller JD, Sweet RC, Narayan R, et al: Early insults to the injured brain. *JAMA* 240:439, 1978.
5. Newfield P, Pitts LH, Katkis J, Hoff JT: The influence of shock on mortality after head injury. *Crit Care Med* 8:254, 1980.
6. Plum F, Posner JB: *The Diagnosis of Stupor and Coma.* Philadelphia, Davis, 1980.
7. Cushing H: Some experimental and clinical observations concerning states of increased intracranial tension. *Am J Med Sci* 124:375, 1902.

8. Hoff JT, Reis DJ: Localization of regions mediating the Cushing response in CNS of cat. *Arch Neurol* 23:228,1970.
9. Andrews BT, Levy ML, Pitts LH: The implications of systemic hypotension for the neurological examination in patients with severe head injury. *Surg Neurol* 28:419, 1987.
10. Andrews BT, Pitts LH, Lovely MP, Bartkowski HM: Is computed tomographic scanning necessary in patients with tentorial herniation? Results of immediate surgical exploration without computed tomography in 100 patients. *Neurosurgery* 19:408, 1986.
11. Harper AM: Autoregulation of cerebral blood flow: Influence of arterial blood pressure on the flow through the cerebral cortex. *J Neurol Neurosurg Psychiatry* 29:398, 1966.
12. Lewelt W, Jenkins LW, Miller JD: Autoregulation of cerebral blood flow after experimental fluid-percussion injury of the brain. *J Neurosurg* 53:500, 1980.
13. Bruce DA, Langfitt TW, Miller JD: Regional cerebral blood flow, intracranial pressure, and brain metabolism in comatose patients. *J Neurosurg* 38:131, 1973.
14. Simon RP: Breathing and the nervous system. In: Aminoff MJ (ed): *Neurology and General Medicine*, New York, Churchill Livingstone, 1989, pp 1–22.
15. Brown HW, Plum F: The neurologic basis of Cheyne-Stokes respirations. *Am J Med* 30:849, 1961.
16. North JB, Jennett B: Abnormal breathing patterns associated with acute brain damage. *Arch Neurol* 31:338, 1974.
17. Webb P: Periodic breathing during sleep. *J Appl Physiol* 37:899, 1974.
18. Dowell AR, Buckley CE, Cohen R, Sicker HO, et al: Cheyne-Stokes respirations. *Arch Intern Med* 127:712, 1971.
19. Lumsden T: Observation of the respiratory centers in the cat. *J Physiol* 57:153, 1923.
20. Sears TA: The respiratory motoneuron and apneusis. *Fed Proc* 36:2412, 1977.
21. Plum F, Alvord EC: Apneustic breathing in man. *Arch Neurol* 10:101, 1964.
22. Teasdale G, Jennett B: Assessment of coma and impaired consciousness: A practical scale. *Lancet* 2:81, 1974.
23. Marshall LF, Barba D, Toole BM, et al: The oval pupil: Clinical significance and relationship to intracranial hypertension. *J Neurosurg* 58:566, 1983.
24. Selhorst JB, Hoyt WF, Feinsod M: Midbrain corectopia. *Arch Neurol* 33:193, 1976
25. Andrews BT: Management of delayed post-traumatic intracerebral hemorrhage. *Contemp Neurosurg* 10:1, 1988.
26. Meyer A: Herniation of the brain. *Arch Neurol Psychiatry* 4:387, 1920.
27. Obana WG, Pitts LH: Extracerebral lesions. *Neurosurg Clin North Am* 2:351, 1991.
28. Pitts LH: Neurological evaluation of the head injury patient. *Clin Neurosurg* 29:203, 1981
29. Pitts LH, Martin N: Head injuries. *Surg Clin North Am* 62:47, 1982.
30. Ropper AH, Rockoff MA: Treatment of intracranial hypertension. In: Ropper AH, Kennedy SF (eds): *Neurological and Neurosurgical Intensive Care*. Rockville, MD, Aspen, 1988, pp 23–41.
31. Kernohan JW, Woltman HE: Incisura of the crus due to contralateral brain tumor. *Arch Neurol Psychiatry* 21:274, 1929.
32. Bricolo A, Turazzi S, Alexandre A, et al: Decerebrate rigidity in acute head injury. *J Neurosurg* 47:680, 1977.
33. Fink ME: Respiratory care: Diagnosis and management. In: Rowland LP (ed): *Merritt's Textbook of Neurology*. Philadelphia, Lea & Febiger, 1989, pp 871–876.
34. Cross CE, Rieben PA, Barron CI, Salisbury PF: Effects of arterial hypoxia on the heart and circulation: An integrative study. *Am J Physiol* 205:963, 1963.
35. Gray FD, Horner GJ: Survival following extreme hypoxemia. *JAMA* 211:1815, 1970.
36. Refsum HE: Relationship between state of consciousness and arterial hypoxemia and hypercapnia in patients with pulmonary insufficiency breathing air. *Clin Sci* 25:361, 1963.
37. Binnion PF, McFarland RJ: Relationship of cardiac massage and pupil size in cardiac arrest in dogs. *Cardiovasc Res* 3:915, 1967.
38. Katsurada K, Yamada R, Sugimoto T: Respiratory insufficiency in patients with severe head injury. *Surgery* 73:191, 1973.
39. Obrist WD, Langfitt TW, Jaggi JL, et al: Cerebral blood flow and metabolism in comatose patients with acute head injury. *J Neurosurg* 61:241, 1984.
40. Riska EB, Myllynen P: Fat embolism in patients with multiple injuries. *J Trauma* 22:891, 1982.
41. Sunha RP, Ducker TB, Perot PL: Arterial oxygenation: Findings and its significance in central nervous system trauma patients. *JAMA* 224:1258, 1973.
42. Neff TA, Petty TL: Tolerance and survival in severe chronic hypercapnia. *Arch Intern Med* 129:591, 1972.
43. Becker DP, Miller JD, Ward JD, et al: The outcome from severe head injury with early diagnosis and intensive management. *J Neurosurg* 47:491, 1977.
44. Chestnut RM, Marshall LF: Treatment of abnormal intracranial pressure. *Neurosurg Clin North Am* 2:267, 1991.
45. Kantner MJ, Narayan RK: Intracranial pressure monitoring. *Neurosurg Clin North Am* 2:257, 1991.
46. Bullock R, Hannemann CO, Murray L, Teasdale GM: Recurrent hematomas following craniotomy for traumatic intracranial mass. *J Neurosurg* 72:9, 1990.

CHAPTER 3
Intensive Care Unit Monitoring

Philip Villanueva

INTRODUCTION

The term *monitoring* is one which has already been used extensively in this text and will continue to be employed in this chapter which, after all, is *about* monitoring. In this chapter, a monitor is taken to be "a person or thing which warns or instructs, or a device for observing a biological function."[1] Key here is the concept that a monitor may be either a machine or a person. In the intensive care unit (ICU) setting, this is an important concept and will be treated later in this chapter.

Key, too, is an understanding of the nature of the information or data obtained by the monitor. The most familiar is direct, quantitative data. The second is qualitative data. It may be difficult at times to differentiate between the two, but a simple example germane to the neurologic ICU may be seen in the pupillary examination. The pupillary size, assuming it is measured correctly, is an example of direct quantitative data. The reactivity, described as brisk, sluggish, or none, represents a qualitative assessment. In most cases, data obtained from a monitoring device are considered quantitative. However, closer inspection may reveal the data to be more qualitative in nature.

Data may also be differentiated as primary or derived. Primary data are uninterpreted, unchanged, and unmanipulated. Derived data, on the other hand, are the result of some form of data handling or equation; basically, it is second-order information. An example of primary data are intracranial pressure (ICP) readings, while the pressure-volume index represents derived data.

Derived data carry the *risk* of introducing inaccuracies during the derivative process. However, primary data may be too raw or limited in immediate scope to be of significant aid to the clinician. It is the clinician's responsibility, therefore, to understand as clearly as possible the nature of data being gathered and to realize the limitations of such information. In discussions about ICU monitoring, the question of reliance upon the clinical examination versus monitoring data arises. In the neurosurgical setting this is sometimes reduced to a moot point, given the numerous confounding factors introduced into clinical assessment either by the underlying pathology or by various forms of therapy. Hence, this chapter will assume that there is a definite role for monitoring devices and the data obtained from them, although clearly in combination with the results of the neurologic examination, as outlined in Chap. 2.

ICU MONITORING: A RATIONALE

The ICU, whether dedicated exclusively to neurologic patients (neuromedical as well as neurosurgical) or a general medical-surgical ICU which treats a variety of patients, is usually the arena in which much of the struggle is waged to preserve and, hopefully, regain central nervous system (CNS) function. *Monitoring*, or the real-time measurement of critical physiologic parameters, is usually performed in the ICU setting exclusively (although some forms of monitoring may be performed elsewhere, e.g., telemetry units). The restriction of this form of monitoring to the ICU is based upon several principles.

First, the monitoring is usually invasive, i.e., the data desired can only be obtained via physical entry into the patient's body. Invasive monitoring is, therefore, not without certain risks, e.g., bleeding, infection, organ damage. Hence, the monitoring must be carried out in a setting where potential complications may be identified as well as treated; where appropriate surveillance against infection, monitoring device malfunction, and inappropriate patient activity may be maintained; and, most importantly, where the data obtained may be analyzed and acted upon in a timely manner by trained, experienced personnel.

Second, the actual monitoring devices used represent a considerable financial investment by the institution involved. Hence, they must be concentrated in a geographically restricted area so as to optimize their appropriate use.

Third, and perhaps most important, even the most sophisticated monitoring devices are dependent upon skilled, experienced personnel for their operation and for the formulation of decisions based upon the data obtained. The ICU setting is usually the optimal location in an institution where such individuals may be concentrated in appropriate numbers to fulfill these tasks.

When dealing with neurologic intensive care, one is faced with a task almost *double* that which others face who are not dealing with a compromised nervous system. In the latter case, the CNS is usually a stable factor whose homeostatic mechanisms are reasonably intact. However, when the CNS is impaired the care givers must not only be concerned with treating the CNS problem but also with the loss of normal homeostatic mechanisms and their effects upon other systems such as cardiorespiratory function and thermoregulation. Thus, it must be remembered that CNS insults may themselves have systemic sequelae too.

Given the theme of this text, this chapter will discuss monitoring in those patients who already have a CNS insult. Attention will be given to monitoring of CNS function and then to systemic monitoring and management, recognizing that there exist a number of *crossover* areas where the two are closely interrelated.

CNS MONITORING

The primary CNS goal of ICU monitoring is the achievement of an optimal CNS environment which will both preserve existing neurologic function and provide the best circumstances to regain function which has been impaired. Realistically, the present state of the art does not allow for actual recovery of function whose anatomical substrates have been lost. However, there is a significant intermediate zone wherein function is suspended without loss of the anatomical substrate and recovery may realistically occur.[2] CNS monitoring and management is, to a great extent, directed toward this area. Simply seen, this is achieved by maintaining an adequate cerebral perfusion pressure (CPP), where CPP = mean arterial pressure (MAP) − ICP, generally considered to be at least 60 mmHg. Maintenance of such a CPP is felt to minimize the risk of ischemic episodes.

In the past, the end point of CNS monitoring was felt to be the control of ICP within safe levels, i.e., those levels which provided the greatest assurance of an adequate CPP.[3] Subsequently, emphasis shifted to following CPP itself.[4] This topic has been covered elsewhere in this text as part of the general topic of ICP monitoring and management and as such will not be discussed further in this section.

An outgrowth of the concern for the effects of cerebral ischemia has led to the development of CNS monitoring techniques to directly examine parameters of CNS circulation, metabolism, and electrical activity. These topics will be discussed further.

CNS Circulation Monitoring

Evaluation of *CNS circulation* is usually accomplished by measuring *cerebral blood flow* (*CBF*). While these two entities are not identical, the use of CBF monitoring techniques provides valuable information as to the overall circulatory status of the brain. Several techniques may be used, which provide circulatory information to varying extents.

Transcranial Doppler The velocity of arterial blood flow in the vessels comprising the circle of Willis may be measured transcranially using ultrasound. This technique employs the principles of Doppler ultrasonography.[5] Similarly, and for comparison, flow in the extracranial carotids may be measured. This technique provides information regarding the *velocity* of flow in the major cerebral arteries in centimeters per second. It does not provide data regarding quantitative flow, i.e., milliliters per 100 g of tissue per second, nor does transcranial Doppler (TCD) provide data for the more peripheral arteries of the brain. However, knowledge of the blood flow velocities in the major basal arteries can provide valuable information as to the integrity of the intracranial circulation. Normally, the paired arteries studied are, i.e., the middle cerebrals (MCA), anterior cerebrals (ACA), and the posterior communicators (PCoA). The posterior circulation may likewise be examined, i.e., the vertebrals (VA), basilar (BA), and posterior cerebrals (PCoA), but technical considerations in the ICU may limit this aspect of the study. Cerebral vasospasm, characterized by flows > 200 cm/s, may be noted following spontaneous and traumatic subarachnoid hemorrhage. TCD may provide an indication of vasospasm before it becomes clinically apparent.[6,7] Likewise, vasospasm may be followed throughout its time course, using TCD as an indicator of the relative success or failure of therapies initiated to counter this entity.[8] Hyperemic states, as frequently found after trauma, may be identified and followed with TCD.[7] Conversely, the low or no-flow states indicative of brain death may be identified, thus assisting the clinician in the critical determination of this state.[9]

Transcranial Doppler is a valuable ICU monitoring tool which is noninvasive, portable, and reproducible. There is no necessity for a time delay between studies. It does require access to the temporal areas for anterior circulation studies and to the region of the foramen magnum to examine the posterior circulation. The latter approach may be somewhat more difficult in the ICU setting. The presence of a cranial defect, as would be expected, will tend to make vessel localization and study somewhat easier. The portability of the system allows its employment outside of the ICU (and, as such, may help to defray its cost via use in other areas of the hospital). It does, as with most monitoring devices, require that the studies be performed by a technician familiar with its use and who can perform the studies under the varying circumstances which occur in the ICU. Modified probes are now available which may be kept in place for prolonged periods using a headband or other device, so as to permit extended recording over time.

Thermal Dilution CBF Monitoring This technique is designed to permit monitoring of focal CBF.[10] It is based upon the thermal dilution principle and, therefore, can only provide data from a limited area of the brain, such as a single gyrus. It requires careful coplanar placement of the probe on the subdural space and continuous contact with the brain surface. The probe is usually inserted intraoperatively, with data recorded during the surgical procedure. The monitor is then left in place during the postoperative phase.

Because of its geographically limited sampling area, the data (recorded in milliliters per 100 mg of tissue per (minute) may vary from the standard 50 to 55 mL/100 g per min. However, valuable data may be derived from *relative* flow changes, indicating ischemic or hyperemic changes. Usually, the surgeon will place the monitor in a region where flow changes are to be expected. In addition to the intraoperative approach, the probe may be placed via a single-burr-hole technique in nonsurgical cases, such as closed-head trauma. This may be done in the operating room or at the bedside, depending upon the policy of the institution. The probe has also been modified at times to incorporate a subdural ICP monitor. Thermal dilution CBF monitoring is an accurate and reproducible means of following regional CBF. Data collection may be computerized and analyzed as to significant trends. More than one area may be studied, but this requires a second probe and either a second analyzer or one with multiple channels. Expertise is necessary for accurate initial placement and any subsequent adjustment of the probe's position.

Global CBF Measurement While the thermal dilution technique of CBF measurement may provide valuable clinical information, it may not portray an accurate representation of global CBF. Therefore, techniques are required which reflect blood flow in the whole brain.

These methods basically involve the washout or clearance of inert substances from the brain's circulation. The rapidity of the washout correlates with CBF.[11] Two methods currently in use involve nitrous oxide (N_2O) or xenon-133.

The nitrous oxide technique requires the inhalation of a known quantity of N_2O by the patients and subsequent samplings of arterial and jugular venous blood. The rate by which the N_2O is cleared (and so appears in the jugular venous blood), correlates with CBF, which is then computed by means of the washout formula.[12]

The xenon-133 technique involves the introduction of this gas usually via inhalation.[13] Rather than sampling blood at fixed intervals as in the prior method, scintillation counters are placed over the patient's head (usually eight per hemisphere) and the isotope concentration is measured over 15 min. A computer then analyzes the washout curve to provide an estimation of CBF. The results in both cases are presented in milliliters per 100 g per minute. However, CBF at specific $P_{A_{CO_2}}$s may be determined to access the degree of cerebral vasoreactivity.

Both the N_2O and xenon-133 techniques provide accurate measurement of global CBF. Because of the use of multiple sensors, the latter may also provide some general regional information too. The N_2O technique requires multiple blood samplings and analysis via specialized instruments over a fixed time period. The xenon-133 technique, in turn, requires a dedicated radioisotope system for its usage. Both require trained personnel for accurate performance. In either case, there is a necessary rest period between studies to allow for complete clearance of the test gases. This latter fact, therefore, limits the number of studies that may be performed in a day. In the case of xenon-133 there is exposure to a radioactive tracer, but this exposure is felt to be minimal.[13] The N_2O method requires no specific hardware to be brought to the bedside, while the xenon-133 system does require complex hardware which may be somewhat unwieldy and cumbersome in certain ICU settings.

Other Techniques of CBF Evaluation Several other methods of CBF estimation are available to the clinician and are presented for the sake of completeness. However, they do not lend themselves to performance on a portable basis and, in general, require patient transport out of the ICU.

Positron emission tomography (PET) scan,[14] single photon emission computed tomography (SPECT) scan,[15] and dynamic CT scanning[16] provide imaging studies which reflect CBF as well as the metabolic status of the brain. They require the injection of tagged tracers that are taken up by the brain which then undergoes an imaging study. The degree of metabolic activity correlates with the degree of enhancement. They are of significant value in demonstrating regional metabolic dysfunction as well as diffuse changes. However, their value as an ICU diagnostic adjunct has not been fully determined as yet. The need for transport out of the ICU setting is a distinct drawback in the case of the critically ill patient. Likewise, the turnover time needed between studies, due to the need for injectate clearance, prevents frequent repetition.

Closely linked to CBF is, of course, cerebral metabolism. Chemical end products of metabolism may be measured from cerebrospinal fluid (CSF) or from jugular venous blood.[17,18] However, these studies require specialized analytic techniques which may be difficult or impossible to achieve in many circumstances. Rather, it may be of more practical value to determine another parameter by which one may infer the status of the CNS circulation and metabolism. This search initially led to the determination of the cerebral metabolic rate of O_2 utilization (CMR_{O_2}).[19]

However, derivation of this value may be rather unwieldy. Hence, another value was chosen, the mixed-venous oxygen saturation in the jugular bulb ($S\bar{v}J_{O_2}$). This term is a valid indicator of CBF and CMR_{O_2}, as $CMR_{O_2} = CBF \times [(A\text{-}V)_{O_2}/100]$, where $(A\text{-}V)_{O_2}$ is the arterial-venous O_2 difference as applied to the cerebral circulation. $S\bar{v}J_{O_2}$ alone will give *at least* an *indication* of CNS circulatory effectiveness and should range from 60 to 70 percent, although the actual maximal and minimal values have not been agreed upon by researchers in this area. If a CBF monitoring method is also employed, then CMR_{O_2} may be derived and the adequacy of CBF determined at that time.[20] This technique is rather analogous to the determination of cardiac output, O_2 uptake, and O_2 utilization on a systemic basis. Just as a fiber-optic, oximetric catheter is used systemically, a single-lumen, 4 French oximetric catheter is placed into the jugular bulb and the $S\bar{v}J_{O_2}$ is recorded in a continuous fashion. Values outside of the 60 to 70 percent range will alert the clinician for possible alterations in O_2 delivery and utilization by the brain. The major drawback of the technique is its invasiveness. Also, experience in the placement and maintenance in proper position of the catheter is necessary. The catheter itself is a pediatric oximetric catheter, originally used for umbilical vein studies. As with any oximetric system, it requires the appropriate monitor.

$S\bar{v}J_{O_2}$ monitoring's invasiveness has prompted the search for a noninvasive method of cerebral venous saturation monitoring. At this time, no technique exists to measure intracranial mixed venous saturation noninvasively. However, using techniques developed for pulse oximetry, the technique of transcranial cerebral oximetry recently has become available.[21] This is accomplished by a scalp sensor and near infrared light technology. The method does not exclusively measure venous O_2 saturation, but also arterial and capillary O_2 saturation within its field of capture. Nevertheless, because the brain's vasculature is primarily venous, the readings should reflect mainly venous saturation. The system is portable, noninvasive, and primarily designed for ICU use. Although its value over the long run has not been fully proven, it holds significant promise as a bedside indicator of CNS blood flow and metabolic function.

Electrophysiologic Monitoring

In addition to examining the circulatory and metabolic parameters of CNS function in the ICU, the electrophysiologic status of the brain may also provide an effective indicator of the integrity of cerebral function. Originally, electroencephalographic (EEG) monitoring and its primary derivatives were the only means of determining electrical function.[22] However, this has given way to evoked potential (EP) monitoring. These techniques provide definite information as to the integrity of neural pathways and may identify points of interruption or dysfunction due to CNS insults.[23]

At this time, the three most commonly employed methods of EP monitoring examine the visual, auditory, and somatosensory pathways. The latter two tend to be the most frequently used in the ICU setting. In addition to their value as diagnostic aids, EPs may also be of value in following changes in patients' clinical status and may be of assistance in predicting outcome.[24]

Evoked potentials are not yet universally accepted as the optimal means of determining CNS function, but they are of significant help in assessing functional status. With few exceptions (certain anesthetic agents for one), EPs are unaffected by systemic metabolic changes. They can also be done on a portable basis and are easily repeated. EPs, as do most of the monitoring techniques described, require an experienced operator for their setup, performance, and interpretation.

Summary

Neurologic monitoring is directed to assuring that as normal an intracranial milieu as possible be maintained. There has been an evolution in monitoring philosophy from following only those parameters which were associated with correcting a deranged CNS status (i.e., ICP and CPP) to also following parameters which are concerned with maintaining as normal a status as possible (CBF, EP).

It is likely that in the near future there will be a general trend away from the CNS-invasive techniques, like ICP monitoring, toward the noninvasive, such as cerebral oximetry, or, at least, toward those which are systemically invasive only, such as jugular O_2 saturation monitoring. The clinician will have to decide which methods and devices best fit the needs of the population to be studied. Likewise, the methods should be adaptable to the ICU setting, as transport away from the ICU may increase the overall risk of the patient. Finally, in this era of managed care and regulation, the cost-benefit ratio of such monitoring systems must also be considered.

SYSTEMIC MONITORING IN THE NEUROSURGICAL ICU

The key to systemic management is the recognition and prevention of those systemic complications which may lead to secondary CNS injury.[25,26] The major threats encountered in the ICU setting are hypotension [systolic blood pressure (BP) > 90 mmHg], hypoxia (PA_{O_2} > 70 mmHg), hypercarbia (PA_{CO_2} > 45 mmHg), hyperthermia (core temperature > 100°F), and electrolyte disturbance, including hyperglycemia (blood sugar > 150 mg/dL). Therefore, most systemic monitoring techniques are designed to alert the clinician to these potentially harmful states so as to allow timely intervention. This section will examine systemic monitoring in the context of the above-noted problems, i.e., cardiovascular, respiratory, and metabolic.

Cardiovascular Monitoring

Central nervous system insults are frequently associated with cardiovascular instability. This may range from dysrhythmias due to subarachnoid hemorrhage (SAH) to neurogenic shock due to cervical spinal cord trauma.

Cardiovascular monitoring must concern itself with both the electrical and volumetric aspects of the system. The electrical aspect is usually fulfilled by electrocardiogram (ECG) monitoring. A full 12-lead ECG should be obtained as a baseline either prior to or upon admission to the ICU. Constant ECG monitoring should be carried out, usually using lead II. When there is an unexplained abnormality of the ECG and a purely benign CNS cause cannot be assigned to it, echocardiography may help to determine if there is an actual myocardial correlate in the form of a dyskinetic or hypokinetic segment. This problem frequently arises in the case of SAH, where concomitant cardiac enzyme studies may be equivocal or not available in time for subsequent decision making.[27,28] Similarly, in the case of multiple trauma, an associated chest injury may not be ruled out initially. In these cases, portable echocardiography may be of significant value in assessing the cardiac status and guide subsequent decision making.[29]

Volumetric monitoring requires invasive techniques. They may be as simple as the insertion of an indwelling urinary catheter to monitor urinary output as an indicator of volumetric status whereby the output is kept between 0.5 and 1.5 mL/kg per h. Or it may entail a more detailed intravascular monitoring technique. The most common form of volumetric monitoring is central venous pressure (CVP) monitoring. This is done via cannulation of either the superior or inferior vena cava (usually the former) with a multiple (2, 3, or 4) lumen catheter. Access is achieved via the subclavicular or supraclavicular, internal jugular or femoral vein approaches using sterile technique and obtaining a postinsertion chest x-ray to assess tip position and to check for complications, specifically pneumothorax.

The relative risks and advantages of the approaches are listed in Table 3-1. One lumen (usually the distal) is used for monitoring and fluid administration, one for parenteral alimentation (PN) if indicated, and the remaining port(s) for fluids and medications. The distal (CVP) port may also be used for venous blood sampling. These catheters are inserted and maintained under sterile conditions. The sites are routinely changed every 7 to 10 days but may be changed earlier if the line becomes contaminated or infected.

In general, the CVP should range between 0 and 8 mmHg. As noted in Chap. 1, in the cardiovascu-

Table 3-1 Central Venous Access Site Risks and Advantages

	Supra- or subclavian	Internal jugular	Femoral
Insertion risk	IIII	I	I
Patient mobility	III	II	I
Venous thrombosis risk	II	I	III
Infection risk	II	II	III
Accuracy of tip placement	II	IIII	III

larly healthy patient, CVP should represent both right and left heart function. However, in those patients with cardiac and pulmonary compromise, the CVP may not accurately reflect left heart function or volume status.[30]

In such cases, or where more detailed information regarding cardiac and volumetric status is needed, a pulmonary artery catheter (PAC) is used. This is inserted sterilely via one of the aforementioned routes via an 8.5 French sheath introducer with a subsequent chest x-ray to assess placement. The PAC is also a multilumen device, usually No. 7 French, with distal (PA), CVP, and proximal ports. It also contains a separate lumen which connects to a latex balloon at the tip. Another lumen contains a thermistor line which emerges to the catheter surface at a point 5 cm proximal to the tip. A final lumen contains a fiber-optic, infrared cable which runs to the tip of the catheter. The hollow lumina are used for measuring pressures in the pulmonary artery (distal-port) and right atrium (CVP port). The balloon, when inflated, allows measurement via the PA port of pressures in the pulmonary artery distal to the balloon. This reflects the pressures in the left atrium and, therefore, left heart function. The thermistor line is used to compute cardiac output (CO) via the thermal dilution technique, and the fiber-optic/oximetric line permits real-time measurement of mixed-venous oxygen saturation ($S\bar{v}_{O_2}$) using reflex spectrophotometry.[31,32]

Mean pulmonary artery pressure (MPAP) should range from 9 to 16 mmHg, while the pulmonary artery wedge or occlusion pressure (PAP), which reflects left atrial pressures, should be between 8 and 12 mmHg.[33] If the balloon becomes nonfunctional, and PAO pressures cannot be obtained, the pulmonary artery end-diastolic pressure (PAEDP) may be substituted for PAO pressure. The PAEDP should range from 3 to 12 mmHg. However, the $S\bar{v}_{O_2}$ provides the clinician with the best instantaneous indication of cardiac function, just as $S\bar{v}J_{O_2}$ reflects O_2 utilization as a function of the brain's circulatory integrity.

$S\bar{v}_{O_2}$ reflects the heart's ability to provide adequate flow to the tissues. Indirectly, this reflects cardiac output. Normally, $S\bar{v}_{O_2}$ ranges from 68 to 77 percent. However, a change in either direction by greater than 10 percent should alert the clinician to a potential alteration in O_2 delivery to the tissues. If the $S\bar{v}_{O_2}$ is elevated, possible causes may be sepsis, neuromuscular blockade, hypothermia, sedation, or coma. $S\bar{v}_{O_2}$ decreases frequently indicate a cardiac output which is not meeting the metabolic demands of the tissue (see Table 3-2). Several technical errors, however, may influence the $S\bar{v}_{O_2}$ reading, and the clinician must rule these out prior to initiating intervention.[34]

Table 3-2

Common causes of elevated $S\bar{v}_{O_2}$
Cirrhosis
Coma (including pharmacologic)
Elevated cardiac output
Hypothermia
Hyperoxygenation
Muscle paralysis
Sedation
Sepsis
Systemic shunting
Common causes of decreased $S\bar{v}_{O_2}$
Anemia
Depressed cardiac output
Hypoxia

Table 3-3 Cardiopulmonary Parameters Derived via the Pulmonary Artery Catheter

Oxygen delivery: Arterial O_2 saturation (Sa_{O_2}) $\times$ C.O. $\times$ hemoglobin (Hgb) $\times$ 1.34 $\times$ 10
Oxygen consumption: ($Sa_{O_2} - S\bar{v}_{O_2}$) $\times$ C.O. $\times$ Hgb $\times$ 1.34 $\times$ 10
Mean arterial pressure (MAP): $\frac{\text{Systolic BP} + 2(\text{diastolic BP})}{3}$
Systemic vascular resistance (SVR): $\frac{\text{MAP} - \text{CVP}}{\text{C.O.}} \times 80$
Pulmonary vascular resistance (PVR): $\frac{\text{MPAP} - PA_{O_2}}{\text{C.O.}} \times 80$
Stroke volume index (SVI): $\frac{\text{C.O.}}{\text{Body surface area} \times \text{heart rate}} \times 1000$
Right ventricular stroke work index (RVSWI): SVI $\times$ (MPAP $-$ CVP) $\times$ 0.136
Left ventricular stroke work index (LVSWI): SVI $\times$ (MAP $-$ PA_{O_2}) $\times$ 0.136

Note: C.O. = cardiac output.

The PAC also provides the clinician with a number of derived secondary parameters which can aid in assessing the cardiovascular status more thoroughly. These are listed in Table 3-3.

Although these values may be critical to the patient's management, it is relatively impractical to calculate them by hand or on a continual basis. Therefore, the PAC is attached to a bedside computer which does provide $S\bar{v}_{O_2}$ readings continuously and can compute the derived parameters whenever a cardiac output measurement is performed and other measured data are entered.

This is usually done upon insertion of the PAC, and then they may be done more or less frequently depending upon patient stability. As a rule, the PAC may be kept in place for only 3 to 7 days before scheduled changing. This is because of the number of interventions performed via the catheter (i.e., cardiac output determinations) and the occasional need to reposition the catheter tip. As a rule, the fiber-optic sensor is recalibrated in vivo at least daily by obtaining a mixed venous blood gas and determining the oxygen saturation. The system should also be recalibrated in vivo if it is necessary to disconnect the fiber-optic cable from the monitor.

As a rule, when venous monitoring lines are changed on a routine basis, the same access site is used for the first change. Any subsequent change will require a new insertion site. This first change may be performed using a teflon-coated guide wire and exchanging the catheters over the wire. If the line is changed in the course of a fever or sepsis workup, the new line may be maintained for a 7- to 10-day span unless cultures of the original line are positive. In such a case, the line is removed after a new access has been made.[35]

The discussion of cardiovascular monitoring has thus far emphasized volumetrics. It must not be forgotten, however, that careful attention must also be paid to the actual BP. The interrelationship of BP and CNS pathology will be examined elsewhere in this text. Blood pressure measurement permits the clinician to follow the contractile state of the myocardium, as well as the status (to some extent) of the peripheral vascular bed. While the volumetric monitoring techniques described above may give an accurate picture of the cardiovascular system, simple BP and pulse determination provides a real-time indication of the system's status. Usually the BP is monitored via an indwelling 20 or 22 gauge arterial catheter placed in the redial, axillary, femoral, dorsalis pedis, or posterior tibial arteries. The catheter should be placed and maintained using the same sterile technique as a central venous line. Care must be taken prior to insertion to access for adequate collateral circulation especially when cannulating end-arteries. If there exists any doubt, another site should be chosen.

Neurovascular checks should be performed hourly on the extremity where an arterial catheter is placed, keeping in mind the twin complications of vascular thrombosis and embolization. It has been our practice to maintain these lines in place for up to 7 days before changing sites. If a sepsis workup is under way, the site is simply changed without a catheter exchange. The arterial catheter, in addition to BP monitoring data, also provides access for arterial blood gas (ABG) measurement and other blood samplings. It must be remembered that although arterial cannulation may provide accurate, constant BP measurement, there may be several technical pitfalls associated with the technique. Artifacts related to arteriosclerotic changes, pressure tubing elasticity, and the length of the pressure tubing may lead to erroneous values. The clinician must keep these potentials in mind when making judgments based upon data derived from these systems.

In those circumstances where placement of an indwelling arterial catheter is not possible or is contraindicated, an automated sphygmomanometric cuff system may be used. This will obtain cuff pressures at predetermined intervals as short as 1 min apart. It must be noted, however, that the noninvasive technique (NIBP) is not the optimal means of BP assessment when one is infusing either pressors or vasolytic drugs. The rapid alterations in pressure which may be caused by these medications occur too quickly for even the fastest NIBP system to ascertain. Hence, an indwelling arterial system for continuous BP monitoring is indicated in these situations.

In light of the significance of the role of hypotension and ischemia in the compromised nervous system, cardiovascular monitoring is a critical component of the overall ICU monitoring picture. While pulmonary artery catheterization is not indicated in all patients, evaluation of cardiovascular function must go beyond the traditional pulse and portable cuff measurements, with the degree of invasiveness being dictated by the degree of risk at which the patient stands.

Respiratory Monitoring

Avoidance of the twin threats of hypoxia and hypercarbia provide much of the impetus for respiratory monitoring in the neurologic ICU. The most accurate means of determining respiratory status is via a combination of the clinical examination and ABG analysis. The examination, however, may be altered by therapeutic interventions (e.g., controlled ventilation, sedation), and frequent arterial sampling is both costly and potentially detrimental to the patient. Therefore, techniques have been developed to provide a continuous, noninvasive means of assessing respiratory function.

The first technique is the pulse oximeter. This measures red blood cell (hemoglobin) oxygen saturation in the peripheral capillary bed.[36] This is usually the fingertip or the toe. However, if there is any significant degree of peripheral vasoconstriction, a more central site, e.g., ear lobe or nose, may be chosen. The monitor exhibits two numbers: heart rate and arterial oxygen saturation (Sa_{O_2}). The latter is preferentially kept > 95 percent under most circumstances. However, in situations where there exists significant respiratory compromise, Sa_{O_2}s down to 90 percent may be accepted.

While providing an instantaneous indication of respiratory function, the system does not indicate the actual $P_{A_{O_2}}$. If therapy is being titrated based upon the $P_{A_{O_2}}$, then ABG sampling must be carried out. It must also be remembered that certain dyes such as methylene blue and indigo carmine can block the reading by the pulse oximeter. This must be kept in mind when inexplicable data are obtained.

Currently, there are several intra-arterial and transcutaneous systems in the developmental phase which can provide actual $P_{A_{O_2}}$ data. These promise to be of significant value when fully developed.[37]

Noninvasive carbon dioxide monitoring may also be carried out in the ICU setting. This is accomplished by the use of the end-tidal CO_2 monitor, originally developed for anesthetic management.[38] This is usually placed in-line with the expiratory limb of the respiratory circuit. Naturally, if there is no airway circuit in place, this system cannot be used. In addition, there may be a variance of 4 to 5 mmHg between the $P_{A_{CO_2}}$ measured via the end-tidal method and that obtained from the blood gas with the ABG method registering the higher value. The technique is also affected by the degree of moisture in the tubing. However, the technique does allow at least for tracking of trends in $P_{A_{CO_2}}$ without invasive sampling.

Using a technique similar to that being developed for intra-arterial P_{O_2} measurement, systems for P_{CO_2} determination are likewise being evaluated clinically. It is likely that real-time $P_{A_{O_2}}$ and $P_{A_{CO_2}}$ measurement will be achievable via an indwelling probe placed within an arterial catheter. Although this method will be invasive, the increase in data obtained as well as the accuracy of such data should outweigh the negative aspects of such an invasive technique.[37]

Another aspect of respiratory function monitoring is the evaluation of breathing mechanics. Again, in the case of controlled ventilation, this may be a moot point. However, in the case of a patient being weaned from ventilatory support, following such parameters as spontaneous tidal volume, peak flow rates, and negative inspiratory force can be of value in the weaning process. These, along with other parameters, can provide an indication of the respiratory work performed by the patient and may be used to adjust the rate of the wean. Certain ventilator systems, such as the Puritan-Bennett 7200, can mount a display panel which graphically portrays the values measured. These systems can also be interfaced with the bedside monitor and the data included with the rest of the patient parameters.

Temperature Monitoring

Uncontrolled hyperthermia can be a devastating complication of a compromised CNS. Elevations of temperature concomitantly increase CMR_{O_2}. If there is a preexisting compromise of CBF, this further uncoupling of CNS metabolism may seriously jeopardize recovery. Therefore, hypothermia, whether moderate (94 to 98°F) or profound (> 94°F), may help to reduce CNS metabolism and serve as a protectant.[39] The temperature parameter which is followed is the core body temperature, usually measured via an esophageal or rectal temperature probe or via an indwelling bladder catheter incorporating a temperature sensor. Other probes may be secured on the ear lobe, fingertip, or even the nose, but the validity of these surface monitors may be affected by local changes in blood flow. Recent studies which measured intracranial temperature indicate a differential between intracranial readings and their systemic-core counterparts, with the intracranial readings being higher.[40]

Regardless of the system chosen, a continuous, accurate monitoring of temperature is necessary to identify and prevent the progression of spikes of temperature.

Metabolic Monitoring

This term includes the monitoring of electrolytes, blood sugar, urinary waste products, and other parameters which both reflect and influence systemic homeostasis.

Following any significant insult to the CNS, there is a marked shift of metabolism to the catabolic phase. This has been noted clearly in the case of head injury.[41] As the brain is a fastidious consumer of glucose, once the supply of this compound, as well as of glycogen, have been exhausted, the body shifts to protein and, to a lesser extent, lipid breakdown in order to satisfy its glucose need. The full implications of this altered metabolism have yet to be determined. However, studies have shown that such protein-calorie depletion may affect, among others, the immune system. The topic of nutritional and metabolic support has been treated elsewhere in this text. This section will discuss those metabolic parameters which are followed as part of the general ICU monitoring scheme.

Upon admission to the ICU, baseline blood chemistries should be obtained. If the patient has been admitted through the emergency room or is an elective postoperative admission, some or all of these will have been sent. In general, these tests include blood chemistry (profile 6 & 8 or SMS 12/20), live enzymes, serum creatinine, cardiac enzymes (if applicable), serum amylase, cholesterol, triglycerides, magnesium, and transferrin. These last five are especially applicable to trauma patients who may require prolonged parenteral nutrition (TPN).

Additionally, complete blood count, platelets, and clotting studies should be obtained. A 24-h urine collection for urine urea nitrogen should be started if the patient is a major trauma victim or if TPN is expected to last over 5 days. Daily electrolytes should be monitored. These may be sent on a more frequent basis if there is a concomitant problem such as diabetes insipidus or renal insufficiency. Blood sugars should be monitored every 4 h and controlled to a level < 150 mg/dL via a sliding insulin scale while the TPN formula and rate are adjusted to the patient's needs. This minimizes the potentially harmful effect of hyperglycemia on the impaired brain. If the patient is receiving a diuretic or has diabetes insipidus, it may be necessary to monitor serum potassium levels. Intravenous sensors which can determine serum electrolyte concentrations and obviate the need for repeated blood sampling are currently undergoing clinical trials.

Serum magnesium and transferrin levels, as well as 24-h urine urea nitrogen levels, should be followed weekly while the patient remains in the highly catabolic state. These parameters eliminate the costly and cumbersome basal metabolic rate determinations previously used to assess metabolic activity.

DATA MANAGEMENT IN THE ICU

The data collected via all the foregoing techniques and systems is, of course, highly critical to the management of the patient while in the ICU. However, it has become increasingly more difficult to manage the tremendous amount of data generated per patient on a daily, even hourly basis. Most bedside monitoring systems provide 8-, 12-, or 24-h recall capability for some parameters. This may be of value when tracking arrhythmias, ICP spikes, and the like. However, it is not practical to be able to recall *all* the parameters over a 24-h period. Usually, an add-on data management system is used if one wishes to be able to capture and recall extensive numbers of data points.[42] This is the option frequently selected by ICUs wherein a significant amount of clinical research is carried out.

There is a growing trend to acquire patient data management systems (PDMS) for the ICU. These are basically computerized data recording systems which also provide interactive capabilities at the bedside. It may, at a minimum, allow more extensive data retrieval over designated time frames and, in its fully developed format, permit the development of a paperless ICU. That is, it may create a system whereby all flow-sheet data, interventions, documentation, laboratory reports, and other data are fed directly into the PDMS and are made retrievable at the bedside or central computer station.[43]

Additionally, nursing care plans and medication records may be brought up at the bedside. Printed reports and data sheets may be generated at any time. These systems not only provide for more efficient usage of care givers' time and effort but may also be valuable adjuncts for clinical research.

ICU MONITORING: THE HUMAN FACTOR

This chapter has discussed, in varying depth, most of the types of monitoring systems encountered in the neurologic ICU or in an ICU which treats the neurosurgical patient. However, one critical factor remains to be discussed. Regardless of the degree of sophistication and technical development of any monitoring system, there must exist a human component which can interpret and act upon the data gathered.

This role can only be fulfilled by a highly trained and dedicated nursing staff. While the physician certainly formulates and directs the care of the patient, it is the nurse who provides the first line of intervention based upon the data obtained from the monitoring system. It is up to the nurse to receive the data and provide the first level of interpretation. Likewise, it is the nurse's responsibility to troubleshoot the system when there is an apparent malfunction which threatens the validity of the data.

These are significant responsibilities and require that the nurse be well-trained in all aspects of the systems in use. This high level of competence may be ensured by an ongoing program of nursing education, in-services, and bedside teaching. Without such, there will be little or no enhancement of care afforded by the most sophisticated technical advances.[44]

SUMMARY

The ICU phase of neurosurgical care is an extremely critical one. It is in the ICU that the interrelationship of neurologic and systemic pathophysiology may be manifest most clearly. It is the first extended period when all systems may be seen to play a role in the brain's recovery or failure to recover. It is that period when fine-tuning of the body's homeostatic mechanisms may be done most efficiently.

Therefore, in order to make such discrete adjustments in patient management, as detailed a knowledge as possible of that patient's neurologic and systemic status is mandatory. Aggressive and comprehensive monitoring provides this critical aid for diagnosis. It also provides the clinician with a feedback method, i.e., a means of assessing the success or failure of therapy. But even the most sophisticated monitoring array does not permit the patient to be placed on automatic pilot. An intelligent, experienced human factor must be present, too, in order to interpret and act upon the data collected.

The future development of monitoring capabilities in the ICU will likely demonstrate even further the role of systemic stability in the treatment of CNS insults. It will certainly add even greater credence to that statement which summarizes neurosurgical critical care: "The body is a life support system for the brain."[45]

REFERENCES

1. *Webster's New Collegiate Dictionary.* Springfield, Mass., G & C Merriam, 1977.
2. Eisenberg HM, Cayard C, Papanicolaou AC, et al.: The effects of three potentially preventable complications on outcome after severe closed head injury. In: Ishii S, Nagai H, Brock M (eds): *Intracranial Pressure ICPV.* Berlin, Springer-Verlag, 1983, pp 549–553.
3. Narayan RK, Kishore PRS, Becker DP, et al.: Intracranial pressure—to monitor or not to monitor: A review of our experience with severe head injury. *J Neurosurg* 56:650–659, 1982.
4. Rosner MJ, Coley IB: Cerebral perfusion pressure, intracranial pressure, and head elevation. *J Neurosurg* 65:636, 1986.
5. Arnolds BJ, Von Reutern G-M: Transcranial Doppler sonography: Examination technique and normal reference values. *Ultrasound Med Biol* 12:115, 1986.
6. Harders AG, Gilsbach JM: Time course of blood velocity changes related to vasospasm in the circle of Willis measured by transcranial Doppler ultrasound. *J Neurosurg* 66:718, 1987.
7. Weber M, Grolimund P, Seiler RW: Evaluation of posttraumatic cerebral blood flow velocities by transcranial Doppler ultrasonography. *J Neurosurg* 27:106, 1990.
8. Sekhar LN, Wechsler LR, Yonas H, et al.: Value of transcranial Doppler examination in the diagnosis of cerebral vasospasm after subarachnoid hemorrhage. *Neurosurgery* 22:813, 1988.
9. Hassler W, Steinmetz H, Gawlowski J: Transcranial Doppler ultrasonography in raised intracranial pressure and in intracranial circulatory arrest. *J Neurosurg* 68:745, 1988.
10. Carter LP: Surface monitoring of cerebral cortical blood flow. *Cerebrovasc Brain Metab Rev* 3:246, 1991.
11. Bell BA: A history of the study of the cerebral circulation and the measurement of cerebral blood flow. *Neurosurgery* 14:238, 1984.
12. Kety SS, Schmidt CF: The nitrous oxide method for the quantitative determination of cerebral blood flow in man: Theory, procedure, and normal values. *J Clin Invest* 27:476, 1948.
13. Obrist WD, Thompson HK, Wang HS, et al.: Regional cerebral blood flow estimated by 133 Xenon inhalation. *Stroke* 6:245, 1975.
14. Langfitt TW, Obrist WD, Alavi A, et al.: Computerized tomography, magnetic resonance imaging and positron emission tomography in the study of brain trauma: Preliminary observations. *J Neurosurg* 64:760, 1986.
15. Hill TC, Holman BL: SPECT brain imaging: Finding a niche in neurologic diagnosis. *Diagnostic Imaging* 7:64, 1985.
16. Yoshino E, Yamaki T, Higuchi T, et al.: Acute brain edema in fatal head injury: Analysis by dynamic CT scanning. *J Neurosurg* 63:830, 1985.
17. DeSalles AF, Kontos HA, Becker DP, et al.: Prognostic significance of ventricular CSF lactic acidosis in severe head injury. *J Neurosurg* 65:615, 1986.
18. Noseworthy TW, Anderson BJ, Noseworthy AF, et al.: Cerebrospinal fluid myelin basic proteins as a prognostic worker in patients with head injury. *Crit Care Med* 13:743, 1985.
19. Siesjo BK: Cerebral circulation and metabolism. *J Neurosurg* 60:883, 1984.
20. Robertson CS, Narayan RK, Gokaslan ZL, et al.: Cerebral arteriovenous oxygen difference as an estimate of cerebral blood flow in comatose patients. *J Neurosurg* 70:222, 1989.
21. McCormick PW, Stewart M, Goetting MG, et al.: Noninvasive cerebral optical spectroscopy for monitoring cerebral oxygen delivery and hemodynamics. *Crit Care Med* 19:89, 1991.
22. Dow RS, Ulett G, Raaf J: Electroencephalographic studies immediately following head injury. *Am J Psychiatry* 101:174, 1944.
23. Greenberg RP, Ducker TB: Evoked potentials in the clinical neurosciences. *J Neurosurg* 56:1, 1982.
24. Greenberg RP, Newlon PG, Hyatt MS, et al.: Prognostic implications of early multimodality evoked potentials in severely head-injured patients: A prospective study. *J Neurosurg* 55:227, 1981.

25. Marshall LF, Toole BM, Bowers SA: The national traumatic coma data bank. Part 2. Patients who talk and deteriorate: Implications for treatment. *J Neurosurg* 59:285, 1983.
26. Reilly PL, Graham DI, Adams H, et al.: Patients with head injury who talk and die. *Lancet* 2:375, 1975.
27. Larremore T, Markovchick, V: Cardiac sequelae of acute head injury. *Br Heart J* 49:101, 1983.
28. Weintraub BM, McHenry LC: Cardiac abnormalities in subarachnoid hemorrhage: A resumé. *Stroke* 5:384, 1974.
29. Advanced Trauma Life Support (ATLS) Course for Physicians: Instructors' Manual. American College of Surgeons. Chicago, Ill., 1988.
30. DeLaurentis DA, Hayes M, Matsumoto T, et al.: Does central venous pressure accurately reflect hemodynamic and fluid volume patterns in the critical surgical patient? *Am J Surg* 126:415, 1973.
31. McMichan JC, Baele PL, Wignes MW: Insertion of pulmonary artery catheters: A comparison of fiberoptic and nonfiberoptic catheters. *Crit Care Med* 12:517, 1984.
32. Swan HJC, Ganz W, Forrester J, et al.: Catheterization of the heart in man with a flow-directed balloon-tipped catheter. *N Engl J Med* 283:447, 1970.
33. Sprung CL, Rackow EC, Civetta JM: Direct measurements and derived calculations using the pulmonary artery catheter. In: Sprung CL (ed): *The Pulmonary Artery Catheter.* Baltimore, University Park Press, 1983.
34. Nelson LD: Applications of venous saturation monitoring. In: Civetta JM, Taylor RW, Kirby RR (eds): *Critical Care.* Philadelphia, Lippincott, 1988.
35. Hudson-Civetta JA, Civetta JM: Clean and aseptic technique at the bedside. In: Civetta JM, Taylor RW, Kirby RR (eds): *Critical Care.* Philadelphia, Lippincott, 1988.
36. Yelderman M, New W: Evaluation of pulse oximetry. *Anesthesiology* 59:349, 1983.
37. Stasic A: Continuous evaluation of oxygenation and ventilation. In: Civetta JM, Taylor RW, Kirby RR (eds): *Critical Care.* Philadelphia, Lippincott, 1988.
38. Linko K, Paloheimo M: Capnography facilitates blind nasotracheal intubation. *Acta Anaesthesiol Belg* 34:117, 1983.
39. Rosomoff HL: Protective effects of hypothermia against pathological processes of the nervous system. *Ann NY Acad Sci* 80:475: 1959.
40. Sternau LM: Personal communication.
41. Clifton GL, Robertson CS, Grossman RG, et al.: The metabolic response to severe head injury. *J Neurosurg* 60:687, 1984.
42. Johnson P: Personal communication.
43. Augenstein JS, Peterson EA: Computerized intensive care: Transforming concepts to needs. In: Civetta JM, Taylor RW, Kirby RR (eds): *Critical Care.* Philadelphia, Lippincott, 1988.
44. Hudson-Civetta JA, Civetta JM, Weppler D, et al.: Improved nursing efficiency and productivity. *Crit Care Med* 15:351, 1987.
45. Ruben BH: Personal communication.

CHAPTER 4
Pathophysiology and Management of Increased Intracranial Pressure

Michael J. Rosner

This chapter will examine the basic physiologic and pathophysiologic concepts required to understand intracranial pressure (ICP) phenomena. Much of the discussion will be couched in terms of cerebral perfusion pressure (CPP), its relationship to autoregulatory phenomena, and the resultant ICP effects. The therapeutic impact of the manipulation of this interaction will be discussed in detail along with clinical results. Many traditional observations relating ICP and systemic events will be reinterpreted in a broader context which will include CPP effects: This will alter many of the conclusions one reaches about ICP management.

MONRO-KELLIE DOCTRINE

The rigid nature of the brain's container, i.e., the craniospinal axis, introduces the topic of ICP and its pathophysiologic response. Because of its rigidity this volume is fixed. Under conditions of high ICP the spinal dura and nerve root sleeves may expand slightly and represent a true volume change for the intracranial space. The craniotomy with a loose bone flap or one in which the dura has been enlarged or has simply been left open without the bony covering is another situation in which the fixed nature of the intracranial volume may be altered. The neonate and, in particular, the premature infant represent important partial exceptions. However, for the majority of clinical situations the rigid container – fixed volume concept of the craniospinal axis dominates. This has come to be known as the Monro-Kellie Doctrine.[1]

A useful concept is subdivision of the intracranial volume into subcomponents. The first and largest component is the parenchyma of the brain. It represents approximately 1100 to 1200 g and should be considered a constant under most conditions. The vascular component represents blood distributed between arteries, arterioles, capillaries, venules, and the larger venous system. This total volume is approximately 150 mL but varies widely. This variability and, as will be discussed, the ability of the physician to physiologically manipulate cerebral blood volume are critical to the understanding and management of ICP disorders. The cerebral spinal fluid (CSF) compartment also represents approximately 150 mL of volume and has tremendous therapeutic potential since a portion is usually available for removal. When combined, the total volume of the central nervous system is approximately 1500 mL of which the majority (parenchyma) is fixed and 20 percent (CSF and blood) are variable. It is the variability in these latter two compartments that explains most of the phenomena of ICP variation.

We have often been in the habit of thinking that pathologic ICP develops as the result of *volume added* to the intracranial compartment (Fig. 4-1). Clearly, this is not the case. The fixed nature of the craniospinal axis volume mandates that if an additional mass lesion such as hematoma, neoplasm, or parenchymal edema should occur, then a portion of the other components must be displaced. The ultimate volume must remain constant:

$$V_K = V_{\text{blood}} + V_{\text{CSF}} + V_{\text{parenchyma}}$$

where V_K = total craniospinal volume. Since pressure = force/area, pathologic ICP is an estimate of the *force* required to *displace* blood and CSF from the intracranial space in order to accommodate the new volume. Since the area over which

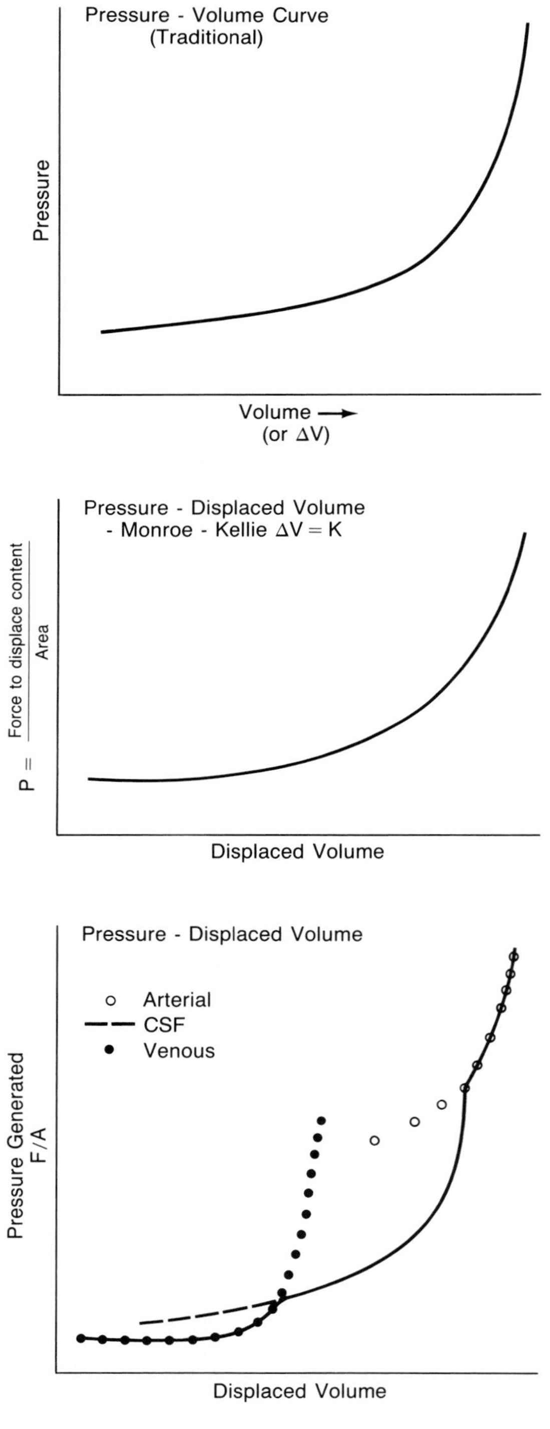

Figure 4-1 The first panel is a traditional view of the response of intracranial pressure to increasing volume within the intracranial compartment. While the general relationship of relatively slowly changing pressure as volume changes is correct, there are errors implicit in the labels. The middle panel suggests that pressure is better defined as the force/area, which can then be replaced by the concept of "force necessary to displace contents." Because volume remains constant, the horizontal axis becomes "displaced volume." The vertical axis then becomes the force required to displace this volume as intracranial pathology evolves. The bottom panel suggests that this simple logarithmic "pressure–volume curve" is actually a composite of curves made up of a curve for "displaced" venous volume superimposed on a curve for displaced CSF volume, which is superimposed on the forces necessary to displace arterial volume. Because these volumes are increasingly turgid, the pressure generated increases rapidly.

this force has been applied is difficult to estimate, we are left with the directly and easily measured pressure.

PHYSIOLOGY AND PATHOPHYSIOLOGY OF VOLUME COMPONENTS

Parenchyma

The glial-neural elements of the cerebral parenchyma have a relatively fixed mass. The parenchyma has also been viewed by some authors as a sponge that can be compressed and therefore act as a buffer for additional volume components in the intracranial space. This is a reasonable model, but the compressible elements of the parenchyma are better thought of as displaceable. They are primarily represented by the vasculature and the CSF components, which will be discussed separately.

The cerebral parenchyma contains no lymphatic circulation. Under normal circumstances this is mitigated by the relative impermeability of the capillary endothelium and related structures constituting the *blood-brain barrier.* Leakage of water from the intravascular into the extravascular extracellular space is minimal and decreases the need for lymphatic drainage. Cerebral capillary pore size has been estimated at 1 μm^2; this is only 1 percent of systemic capillary pore size.[2]

This is not to say that the extracellular space and matrix are unimportant in the function of cerebral parenchyma. The extracellular matrix of the parenchyma acts as a sink for various molecules diffusing or being pumped out of glial-neural cell bodies. These compounds flow with extracellular water into the ventricular system. Lactate reaches the ventricular CSF in this manner. Under normal circumstances, this system functions as lymphatic drainage for the brain.

Pathophysiology of the Parenchyma Many pathologic conditions affect the cerebral parenchyma, though rarely in the absence of effect upon the vasculature or CSF components. However, it is useful to separate effects on the different components and later discuss their interaction.

Cerebral *edema* is the prototypical process capable of increasing the parenchymal component of the intracranial volume. Cerebral edema is an increase in the water content of the brain. Cerebral edema itself has been separated into two types of brain water accumulation based on histologic location:[3] cytotoxic and vasogenic.

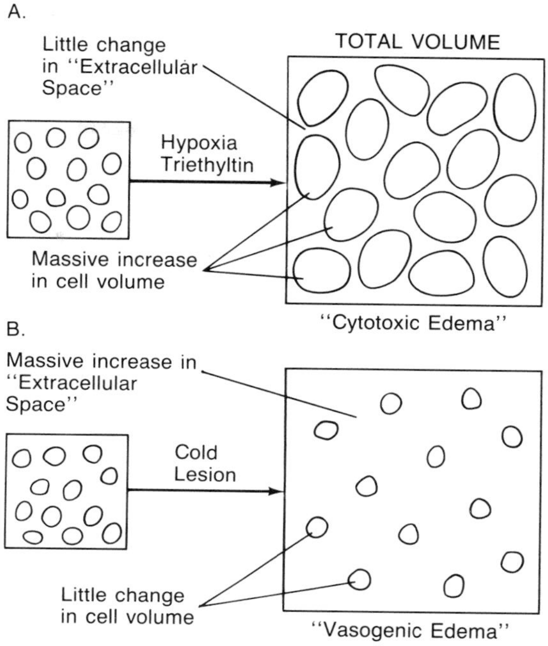

Figure 4-2 The concepts of "cytotoxic" edema and "vasogenic" edema are illustrated here. These are simplistic concepts but serve to illustrate that certain pathophysiologic events differentially affect parenchymal volume in different ways. Clearly both cellular and interstitial "swelling" may occur. Cerebral ischemia may ultimately lead to both processes, and hyponatremia is another process which leads to an increase in the volume of both spaces.

Cytotoxic edema (Fig. 4-2) has been used to refer to the accumulation of primarily intracellular water. Hypoxic injury and many experimental toxins damage the cell's ability to pump water out of the intracellular space. While the process may or may not be reversible, edema accumulation is primarily intracellular.

It is differentiated from vascogenic edema which represents an ultrafiltrate of plasma leaking at a greater than normal rate into the cerebral parenchyma. This is generally due to insults that affect primarily the vasculature at the capillary endothelial level and the integrity of the blood-brain barrier. Cold lesion edema models are the prototypical method for creating vasogenic edema. Neoplastic and infectious processes such as a brain abscess tend to be associated with abnormally "leaky" vasculature and will produce a vasogenic type of edema. Starling's law relating the movement of fluid across the capillary membrane is useful in visualizing how alteration in the blood-brain barrier may enhance fluid movement into the parenchyma (Fig. 4-3).

To the extent that cytotoxic processes are going to be primarily intracellular and presumably respond to those therapeutic events aimed at cellular mechanisms for maintaining intracellular salt and water balance, they can be viewed as metabolic processes requiring therapies aimed at cellular metabolism. They can be slow to respond and difficult to treat. The vasogenic forms of edema can be viewed as more mechanical in their formation, and therapies aimed at vasogenic edema will tend to be more mechanically based and directed at the blood-brain barrier.

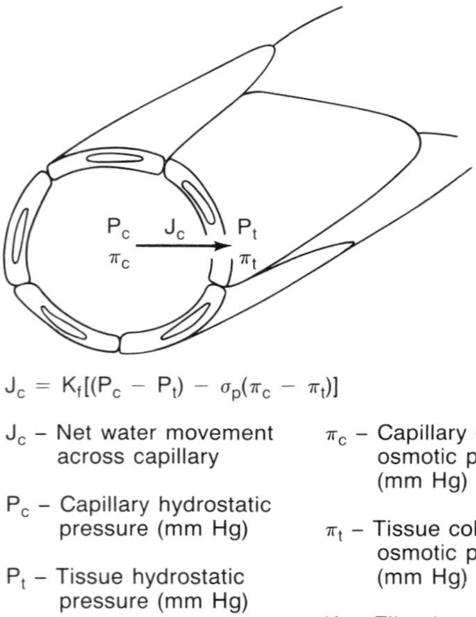

$$J_c = K_f[(P_c - P_t) - \sigma_p(\pi_c - \pi_t)]$$

J_c – Net water movement across capillary

P_c – Capillary hydrostatic pressure (mm Hg)

P_t – Tissue hydrostatic pressure (mm Hg)

π_c – Capillary colloid-osmotic pressure (mm Hg)

π_t – Tissue colloid-osmotic pressure (mm Hg)

K_f – Filtration coefficient

σ_p – Reflexion coefficient

Figure 4-3 Starling's equation demonstrates how high capillary pressure can potentiate transcapillary flow. However, it also demonstrates how very high tissue hydrostatic pressure (P_t) could counteract high capillary hydrostatic pressure (P_c) and lead to little net flow. Breakdown of the blood brain barrier has the effect of increasing filtration coefficient (K_f) and decreasing reflexion coefficient (σ_p).

To the extent that the two coexist and interact, the distinction becomes artifactual. For instance, vasogenic edema may lead to a general increase in ICP, or local decreases in tissue perfusion such that tissue hypoxia occurs and cytotoxic edema results. Cytotoxic events may not limit their toxicity to neuroglial metabolism but may also affect vascular membranes and lead to increasing tissue water; toxic by-products of abnormal parenchymal metabolism may damage endothelial membranes and lead to an increase in their permeability and therefore vasogenic edema.

Storage disease with the accumulation of intracellular products of abnormal metabolism clearly increases parenchymal intracellular volume. Neoplastic processes also augment parenchymal volume but in addition contain abnormally permeable vasculature resulting in vasogenic edema. As parenchymal mass increases, either as the result of abnormal storage, neoplasia, or edema, some other component must be forced out and ICP will usually increase.

There are circumstances in which cerebral parenchyma actually decreases. The most frequent is the normal aging process, though it is unclear what happens with the associated vasculature. Here the Monro-Kellie doctrine continues to hold, however, and the decreased parenchymal mass is offset by an increase in CSF volume. Age can be viewed as a generalized atrophic process, but localized processes do occur. Atrophy of underlying cerebral tissue seen with slow-growing neoplasms such as meningiomas is typical. But encephalomalcia following cerebral contusion or ischemic infarct also reduces the mass of the brain, and, in general, this will also be offset by an increase in CSF volume.

Sodium is not only the primary ion involved in maintaining vascular volume, it is also the primary ion in maintaining the extravascular, extracellular volume as well. So while we discuss the accumulation of water in the extracellular space as a result of vasogenic edema, it is important to note that this water contains sodium, and the sodium itself may be manipulated as a treatment of vasogenic edema.

Pseudotumor cerebri is a disease process easily viewed as vasogenic cerebral edema of uncertain etiology. While pseudotumor cerebri probably represents the manifestation of several different disease processes, it is clear that there is a subset of patients whose increased brain water is secondary to increased total body salt and water. While in some patients this is simply a function of massively increased salt intake, in others it is probably more complex. The importance of this form of pathologic water accumulation is in the insight that it gives us for treatment of more common forms of intracranial hypertension. Most patients with pseudotumor cerebri can be effectively treated by sodium restriction alone. It is not necessary to dehydrate them nor to make them hyponatremic.[4,5]

Cerebrospinal Fluid

Under normal circumstances CSF volume in the adult is 150 mL. It is produced at a relatively constant rate by the choroid plexus as an ultrafiltrate of plasma. This fluid is secreted directly into the ventricles. Under normal circumstances the choroid plexus is the source for about 70 percent of CSF production; movement of water through the extracellular matrix and into the ventricular system may account for 30 percent. Total CSF production is a relatively constant 20 mL/h or nearly 500 mL/day.

Ventricular volume is approximately 40 to 50 mL with the remainder of the CSF volume being in the spinal and cerebral subarachnoid spaces. The most important aspects of CSF circulation are production in the ventricular system, flow into the posterior fossa subarachnoid space, sluggish flow through the spinal subarachnoid space and then through the cerebral subarachnoid space to be absorbed into the systemic venous circulation via the arachnoid granulations.[6]

These arachnoid granulations are located in association with venous lacunae and the sagittal sinus. The function of the arachnoid granulations is complex in that they have a semiactive mechanism for movement of normal amounts of CSF under normal pressure gradients; vesicles form that move from the CSF side of the membrane to the venous side thus keeping the two compartments separate (Fig. 4-4). Under stable conditions CSF is absorbed at the same rate it is produced, and the arachnoid granulations can thus handle 20 mL/h of CSF. Under conditions of higher pressure, CSF will be absorbed more rapidly and the arachnoid granulation mechanism forms a series of transcellular tubules that allow direct flow into the venous compartment. It is unclear whether there is absorption of CSF into or from the parenchyma under normal circumstances.

Pathophysiology of Cerebrospinal Fluid Hydrocephalus is loosely defined as "large ventricles." However, while the classical terminology remains, our understanding of both the normal and abnormal physiology of CSF has increased tremendously. As a result, we will evolve the concept of hydrocephalus to include other conditions that may not always include ventriculomegaly.

Hydrocephalus has traditionally been divided into communicating and noncommunicating hydrocephalus. Communicating hydrocephalus was inferred when dye placed in the ventricular system was recovered by lumbar puncture. This implied communication between the ventricular and the spinal subarachnoid spaces. When ventriculomegaly was present, the concept of communicating hydrocephalus was advanced. Noncommunicating hydrocephalus implied that ventricular dye was not recovered after lumbar puncture. A physical block to ventricular outflow was implied.

A third term that is occasionally used is *external* hydrocephalus. This implies that CSF is accumulating in spaces other than the ventricles, yet the accumulation still results in increased ICP on the basis of hydrocephalus. This process can be seen after transventricular surgery where CSF is allowed to move directly to and collects in the subarachnoid or subdural space. Ventricular size is normal or reduced but may still result in elevated ICP and in CSF collecting elsewhere with both local and general consequences.

Physiologic Concepts There are several physiologic concepts that are necessary for the understanding of the development of ventriculomegaly

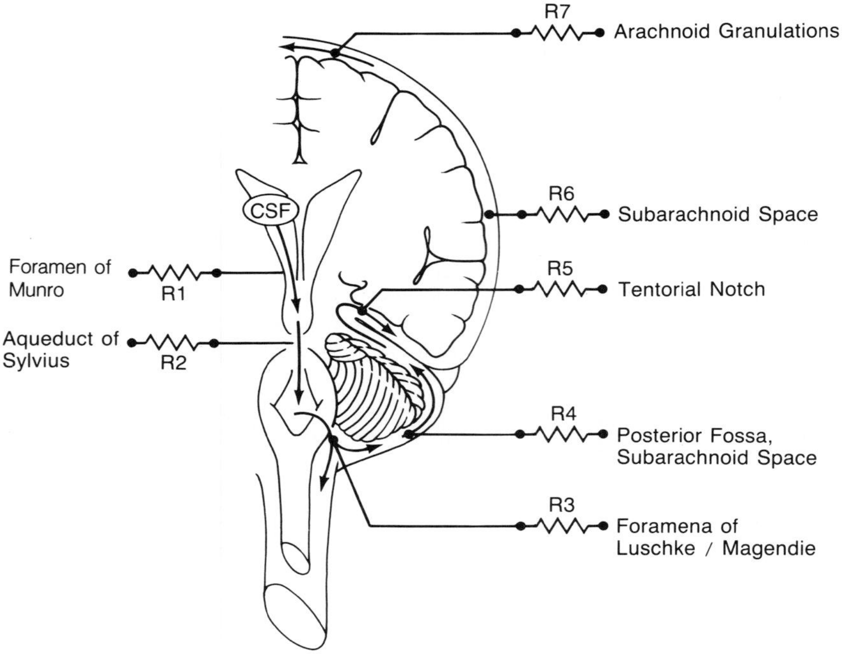

CSF "Outflow Resistance" $= R_1 + R_2 + R_3 + R_4 + R_5 + R_6 + R_7$
$= \Sigma R_x$

Figure 4-4 The resistance to the outflow of CSF is the sum total of the resistance offered at the foramena of Munro, the aqueduct, the foramen of Luschke and Magendie, the subarachnoid spaces of the infra- and supratentorial regions, the tentorial notch, and the arachnoid granulations of the venous sinuses. It is easy to understand that multiple small increases in resistance at several areas may yield hydrocephalus. Meningitis and subarachnoid hemorrhage may act in such a manner, while a colloid cyst at the foramen of Munro may cause a very large increase in resistance at a single point (foramen of Munro). Depending on the location and the degree of resistance increase, we may observe hydrocephalus which is communicating, noncommunicating, or a combination of both.

and abnormalities of CSF absorption. Perhaps the most important is that of *resistance* to absorption of CSF. As mentioned, most of CSF absorption occurs at the arachnoid granulations and venous lacunae; the normal pressure gradient here will be the CSF pressure minus the sagittal sinus pressure. This gradient is 5 to 10 mmHg or less under most normal circumstances and body positions, with CSF absorption of 20 mL/h. Therefore, we can estimate a resistance to CSF or absorption by Ohm's law of about 0.5 mmHg/mL per hour. If this resistance should increase by a factor of 3, and CSF production remains a constant 20 mL/h, then the ICP would increase to 30 mmHg if all else remained constant.

That intracranial hypertension can result from as simple a process as increasing the resistance to absorption of CSF is very important. Meningitis, encephalitis, red cells, and protein from subarachnoid hemorrhage can all directly affect the arachnoid granulations, increasing the resistance to the absorption of CSF.

When combined with cerebral edema, the ventricular system will be compressed (Fig. 4-5). The tendency for ventricular collapse will be countered by increased CSF pressure tending to dilate the

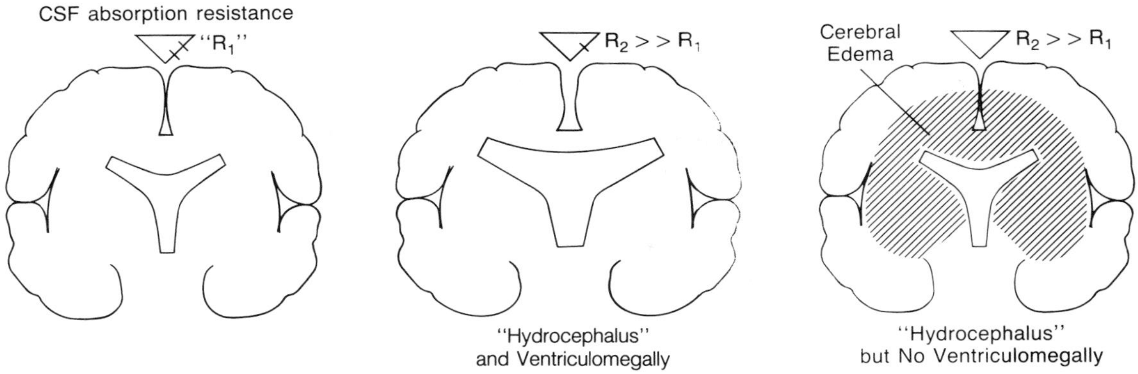

Figure 4-5 This figure reduces the multiple points of CSF outflow resistance demonstrated in Fig. 4-4 to the single value R_1. When R_1 is replaced by a larger value of CSF outflow resistance (R_2), resistance to CSF absorption increases, which generally will result in ventriculomegaly. However, if parenchymal tissue pressure is higher than normal, then the forces generating ventriculomegaly will be counterbalanced, and even though outflow resistance is high at R_2, tissue pressure may force ventricular size toward a more normal value. This is a common event in the early stages of traumatic brain edema, but also occurs in subarachnoid hemorrhage, pseudotumor cerebri, and inflammatory processes such as encephalitis and meningitis. Therefore, relying on CT scan determination of ventricular size to "rule in or rule out" hydrocephalus is fraught with danger if one does not remember that ventriculomegaly may occur late in the process as the high tissue pressure of cerebral edema resolves.

ventricles. The net result may be no change in ventricular size. If the edema resolves before CSF absorption returns to normal, ventriculomegaly will occur. This is a common series of events in the severely brain injured patient.

A second form of resistance increase can occur at any of the channels for CSF circulation, including the foramen of Monro, the aqueduct of Sylvius, the foramina of Magendie and Luschka, the tentorial incisura, and the subarachnoid spaces over the cerebral hemispheres (Fig. 4-4). If we apply Ohm's law to these channels, then we see how a narrowed aqueduct of Sylvius increases resistance to flow and the pressure generated in order to maintain flow will be higher. The same principle applies to the subarachnoid space in general. If the arachnoid is densely scarred by infection or other processes, then the resistance to flow of CSF through the subarachnoid space will also increase. Higher CSF pressure will be necessary to allow the 20 mL/h of flow required.

Implicit in the above is the possibility that many pathophysiologic events damage not only arachnoid granulations, but lead to scarring in the subarachoid space as well as narrowing of the intraparenchymal CSF channels flow such as the Foramen of Monro and Aqueduct. Herein lies one of the many reasons that simple diversion of CSF from the ventricular system to the subarachnoid space by Torkildsen's shunt worked in only limited fashion. Choroid plexectomy may reduce the total production of CSF but may not eliminate abnormal resistance to absorption. Even at low flow rates, high intracranial pressures can be generated.

Transependymal Flow With the advent of computed tomography (CT) and magnetic resonance imaging (MRI), increases in periventricular lucency or evidence of water around dilated ventricles, particularly the frontal horns, had been interpreted as transependymal *absorption.* The concept is appealing and seems to be based on the idea that pressure in the ventricle is higher than pressure in the tissue and therefore fluid will be forced into the tissue where it can be absorbed from the spongelike cerebral matrix. However, this is unlikely to be the case.

As pressure within the ventricular system rises

due to an increase in downstream resistance, one can view the pressure gradient from the extracellular matrix to the ventricle as having been decreased and therefore *slowing* the movement of extracellular water into the ventricular system. This would result in periventricular lucency on CT scan. It makes more physiologic sense to view periventricular, white matter lucency as representing *hindered* movement of water into the ventricle rather than a reversal of flow.

Two other concepts are also very useful in understanding the relationship of ventricular size, CSF pressure, and hydrocephalus. They are the law of LaPlace and CSF pulse pressure.

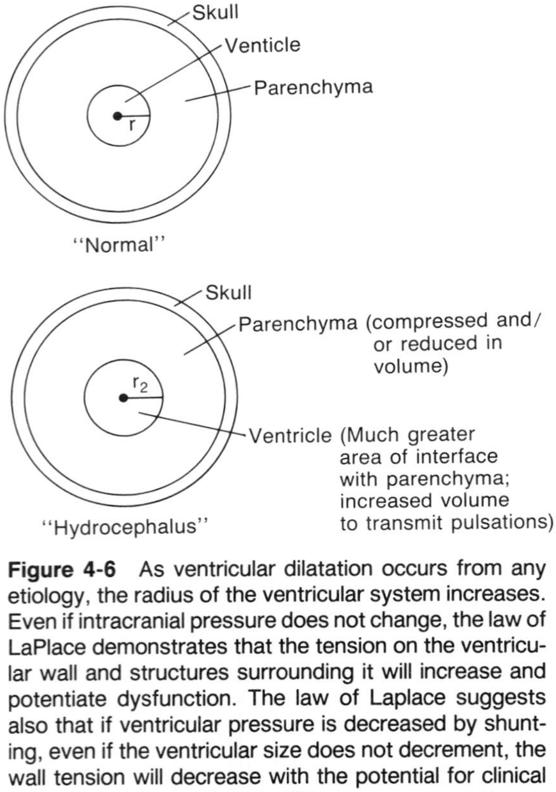

Figure 4-6 As ventricular dilatation occurs from any etiology, the radius of the ventricular system increases. Even if intracranial pressure does not change, the law of LaPlace demonstrates that the tension on the ventricular wall and structures surrounding it will increase and potentiate dysfunction. The law of Laplace suggests also that if ventricular pressure is decreased by shunting, even if the ventricular size does not decrement, the wall tension will decrease with the potential for clinical improvement even though CT scans may remain unchanged. A larger ventricular system will consist of incompressible fluid that will more effectively transmit CSF pulsations and lead to increased CSF pulse pressure. This will be true even if absolute intracranial pressure does not increase.

Law of LaPlace The law of LaPlace relates the wall tension T in a structure to the diameter D and pressure P within the structure:

$$T = 2PD$$

The relationship is very useful in hydrocephalus. The wall of the ventricular system is bounded by white matter tracts that can be placed under tension by abnormalities of *either* ventricular size *or* pressure (Fig. 4-6). The white matter tracts from the mesial frontal lobe and, in particular, the leg and bladder areas wrap superiorly around the ventricle, sweeping laterally and then down into the internal capsule, and can be placed under great tension by an increase in pressure *or* size (radius) of the ventricular system. An immediate clinical correlate exists with urinary incontinence and gait ataxia.[7]

It is apparent from the law of LaPlace that an increase in diameter of the ventricle *without* an increase in the pressure within the ventricle is capable of increasing the *tension* on the ependymal structures of the wall as well as the tracts related to the ventricle. As these tracts are placed under greater tension either through an increase in ICP or ventricular dilation, they become more dysfunctional and clinical symptoms result.

It is, in addition, the *transmural pressure gradient* that is important and not the absolute ICP. Therefore, one can have a process such as pseudotumor cerebri where intraventricular pressure is quite high but balanced by the relatively high tissue pressure of parenchymal edema. This will tend to compress the ventricular system, and ventricular size will often be small in these individual patients. The result is that the actual transventricular pressure gradient is not high even though the absolute ICP is.

It also implies that if CSF pressure were reduced by a shunting procedure, wall *tension* will be reduced even if there is no reduction in ventricular size. As tension on the periventricular structures is reduced, neurologic function may improve even with little or no change in ventricular size. This may seem puzzling; however, it has a sound physical and physiologic basis.

CSF Pulse Pressure There is substantial evidence that the dilation of the ventricular system under many conditions associated with ventriculomegaly and hydrocephalus is strongly influenced by the CSF pulse pressure (systolic ICP − diastolic ICP).[8] The pulse pressure will be generated by cardiac systole and diastole as it is transmitted to the ventricular volume via the vasculature of the choroid plexus and cerebral parenchyma. Normally the CSF pulse pressure is 2 to 3 mmHg. Under conditions of brain edema and increased resistance to CSF flow and absorption, this pulse pressure may rise 10- to 20-fold.

While accompanied by an increase in the mean CSF pressure the increase in pulse pressure is disproportionate because of an increase in brain stiffness. As CSF volume increases as a result of ventriculomegaly the effect on the ventricular wall is further magnified by the large surface area against which the pulse pressure acts. The pulse pressure is further magnified by the increase in noncompressible CSF and the reciprocal reduction in volume of the compressible vasculature and parenchyma.

Ventricular size is therefore a balance between parenchymal forces tending to compress and collapse the ventricles versus intraventricular forces (CSF pressure and pulse pressure) which tend to enlarge the ventricular system. This balance may shift in various directions depending upon the evolution of the disease process.[9]

Intracranial Hypotension Intracranial hypotension is an ill-defined syndrome usually consisting of disturbance in level of consciousness, cranial nerve palsies (most often cranial nerve VI), vertigo, dizziness, confusion, etc. It has three primary etiologies:

1. CSF leak usually of traumatic but occasionally of postsurgical origin. It is often difficult to separate the positional vertigo of an individual with a basal fracture and an active CSF leak from traumatic labyrinthine dysfunction. It becomes clearer that intracranial hypotension is the cause of these symptoms when they are present primarily during periods of active CSF leakage.

2. Large decompressive craniectomies can also result in similar signs and symptoms; patients who are alert and conversant when supine may become lethargic, with increased focal deficits when upright. The craniectomy "sinks" when the patient moves upright; presumably, the mechanism is brain shift caused by negative pressure gradients in the upright position.

3. The use of a CSF shunt that drains either too rapidly or to an excessively low pressure can result in positional headaches, occasional disturbances of consciousness, sixth and seventh cranial nerve palsies. The mechanism for these symptoms is often unclear though most are reversible when CSF drainage is reduced.

The concept of negative ICP gradients is fascinating. They may occur in the absence of CSF diversion. Gravity both via the venous system and directly via the parenchyma exerts forces that tend to pull the cortex away from the inner table of the skull and the dura. This is counteracted by negative pressures due to the rigidity of the skull, and these pressures allow little if any movement under normal circumstances. The process seems exaggerated in individuals with decreased brain mass as the result of age or other atrophic processes. These negative forces are probably important in the generation of chronic subdural hematomas that are the result of repeated hemorrhages. Negative pressure gradients are likely to potentiate both the severity and frequency of these hemorrhages as well as the movement of fluid into the subdural space. Accumulation of CSF in the subarachnoid and subdural spaces to fill the void occupied by a prior hemorrhage is a practical consequence of negative pressures within the subdural spaces.

The Vascular Compartment

While total cerebral blood volume under resting circumstances may be as much as 150 mL, only 25 to 50 mL of this volume will be found in the arterial system. Functionally, the arterial system can be divided into large, medium, and small arteries. The large arteries will include the internal carotid artery, the vessels of the circle of Willis, and the majority of the vessels easily visible down to approximately 250 to 350 μm in diameter. These large vessels are primarily conducting channels with relatively little absolute constriction potential. However, if blocked, thrombosed, or when affected by arterial spasm, the pressure transmitted to the medium arteries and arterioles may be greatly reduced. During autoregulatory responses the larger arteries dilate early, but this dilation is usually no more than 15 to 40 percent. Mean pressures measured distally in normal large cortical arteries are 80 to 90 percent of systemic pressure. However, arterial pulse pressure is greatly reduced.[10,11]

Medium arteries ranging in diameter from 50 to 350 μm are much more reactive and capable during autoregulation of changing their diameter by nearly 100 percent. Pressure delivered distally in these vessels is approximately 60 to 70 percent of systemic pressures measured at the internal carotid artery (Fig. 4-7).

The most important vessels in terms of both autoregulation and its interaction with ICP are the cerebral arterioles. These vessels are approximately 50 μm in diameter and are capable of diameter changes of 200 to 300 percent. It is this very large diameter change that is responsible for the arteriolar component of cerebral vascular resistance, which may be as much as 85 percent of the total resistance to flow offered by the cerebral circulation. From an ICP standpoint, this is also the most important component of the cerebral vasculature. The ability of the arteriolar system to increase diameter by 200 to 300 percent subserves a potential increase in blood volume of 400 to 900 percent (Fig. 4-8). Blood volume will increase as the square of the diameter, and the very large diameter changes possible in this group of vessels allow very rapid and important increases in the vascular volume subserved by them.

Cerebral Perfusion Pressure Often not appreciated but absolutely crucial to understanding blood flow and its interaction with ICP phenomena is the pressure gradient across the vasculature tree: the cerebral perfusion pressure. CPP is the stimulus to cerebral autoregulation, *not* the absolute systemic arterial pressure.

When systemic arterial pressure is normal and the ICP is normal, the difference between CPP and systemic arterial pressure is minimal and probably unimportant under most circumstances. These conditions fail to hold in the damaged brain and/or in the face of intracranial hypertension.

Another implication is that the arterial system must be *patent* and that the CPP both regionally

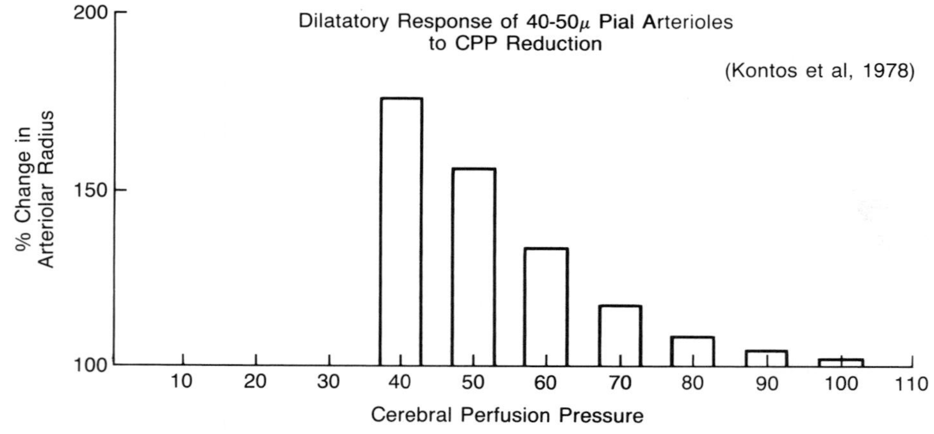

Figure 4-7 To be noted is the relatively small change in average pial arterial diameter as cerebral perfusion pressure decrements toward 90 to 100 mmHg. As this decrement increases, there is a rapid increase in average vascular diameter, which is maximal in the range of 40 to 50 mmHg. It is important to recognize that the horizontal axis is the pressure gradient across the vasculature and not the absolute arterial pressure. Under normal circumstances, CPP and mean arterial pressure are virtually identical; however, under pathologic circumstances, both regionally and generally, the CPP becomes the relevant variable. While it is difficult to estimate a regional cerebral perfusion pressure, it is still important to recognize that the vasodilatory response occurs regionally to the local circumstance. (This is derived from observations of the pial arterial circulation by Kontos et al.[11])

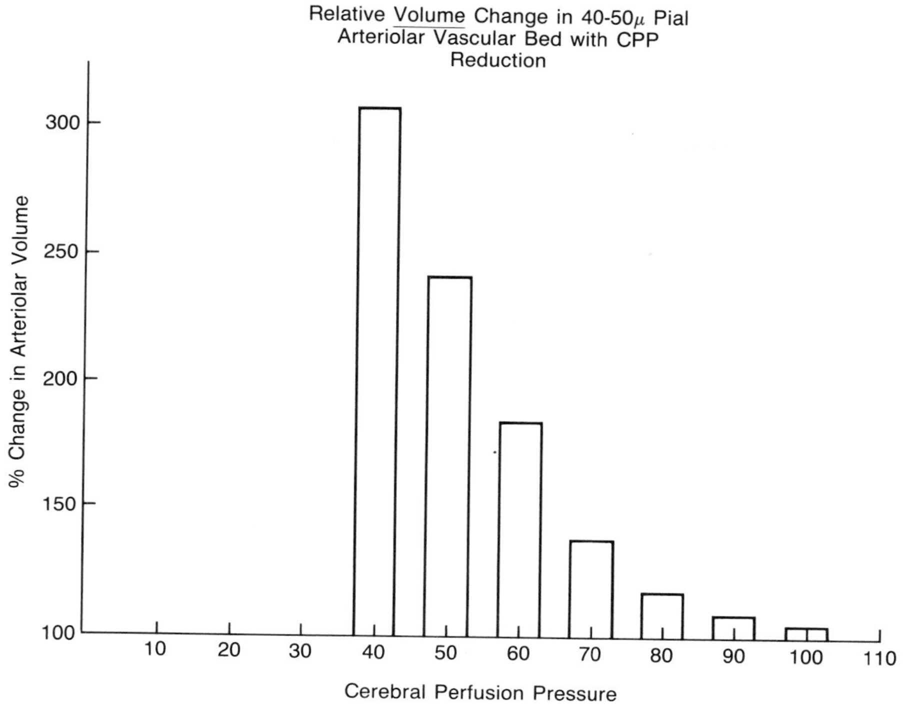

Figure 4-8 This figure relates to relative volume change in the same vascular bed as described in Fig. 4-7. Note that the volume increase is quite rapid and massive as perfusion pressures drop into the range of 80 and 70. Again, note that this represents normal vascular response and that pathophysiologic conditions shift this curve to the right, with vasodilatation occurring at higher pressure gradients rather than lower.

and generally must be within the autoregulatory limits of the vascular bed before judgments as to the integrity of the autoregulatory response can be made. For instance, if the middle cerebral artery is occluded by embolus, surgical clip, etc., then before one concludes that the vasculature distal to the occlusion no longer autoregulates, one must know that the intraluminal pressure is in fact within a range where the vasculature could be *expected* to respond.

Another important but often unrecognized concept is that of the *critical closing pressure.*[12] This refers to the tendency of the vasculature to collapse as intraluminal or transluminal pressure gradients decrease. Functionally it means that cerebral blood flow (CBF) will cease at a pressure somewhat above zero, often as high as a 5- to 10-mmHg pressure gradient in normal individuals. The importance of this concept is that CBF will cease at perfusion pressures above zero. Injury of the brain and vasculature will increase this critical closing pressure, and CBF will decrement sooner and at a higher CPP than normal.

Hysteresis is the concept that *work* is required to overcome the elasticity of the vasculature in order for it to dilate and allow flow. Once the perfusion pressure gradient has increased sufficiently and the vasculature is operating within the autoregulatory range, the pressure can be reduced and blood flow will be maintained at lower pressures than those at which it was established. The requirement that *work* be expended to expand the cerebral vasculature (hysteresis) becomes very important but often unrecognized under conditions of high ICP where the vasculature may, for awhile, be exposed to very low perfusion pressures.[13]

While CBF is dealt with in other chapters, there are a number of points worth reiterating in terms of ICP. Normally, cerebral metabolic rate for oxygen ($CMRO_2$) is very closely matched by oxygen delivered by CBF. Thus, if a patient should go from an aroused, awake state to deep sleep or coma, cerebral metabolic rate is reduced to approximately 50 percent of the baseline state.[14] Cerebral oxygen requirements are only 50 percent of the awake oxygen requirement and therefore are met by 50 percent of the awake blood flow. This is indeed one of the means by which the brain responds to and protects itself from injury.[15]

While the abnormal brain may no longer be able to match blood flow to metabolic rate, this is true only in extreme circumstances. The vast majority of cerebral injuries leave both the autoregulatory response and the matching of blood flow and oxygen delivery to metabolic need *relatively* intact.[16-20] These relationships are often blurred and may regionally be more abnormal, but they still are maintained.[21,22] The relevance of these relationships to ICP phenomena is profound.

Poiseuille's law relates flow *directly* to the pressure gradient across the vessel, the fourth power of the radius, and *indirectly* to blood viscosity and length of the vessels involved. The pressure gradient becomes CPP when we speak of the cerebral vasculature. Poiseuille's law is stated as follows:

$$F = \frac{8dPr^4}{\pi nl}$$

where F = flow
dP = pressure gradient (CPP)
r = vessel diameter
n = viscosity
l = vessel length

When $CMRO_2$ is relatively well matched to blood flow, we can gain insight into expected ICP effects by examining the reciprocal relationships betwen the pressure gradient (CPP) and vessel radius. If blood flow requirements are reduced by half *and* the pressure gradient (CPP) is held constant, then vasoconstriction or a reduction in vascular radius must occur. A reduction in cerebral blood volume will follow and result in a reduction in ICP. Similarly, if $CMRO_2$ or CBF requirements are *increased* and CPP is held constant, then the opposite change must occur in the vasculature resulting in vasodilatation. Cerebral blood volume will increase and ICP will tend to follow.

Other Influences The most potent cerebral vasodilator is reduced oxygen delivery. Oxygen delivery is a function of blood flow and the oxygen content of arterial blood. Therefore, it is a function of hemoglobin, blood flow, and the saturation of the hemoglobin. A Pa_{O_2} as low as 70 mmHg is normally not associated with reduced oxygen delivery because the hemoglobin oxygen dissociation curve is relatively flat in this range. If $CMRO_2$ requirements are to be met, then further decreases in Pa_{O_2} saturation or a reduced amount of hemoglobin will require either an increased CPP or increased vasodilation. The latter will elevate ICP.

Hypercapnia is a well-known cerebral vasodilator and will result in an increase in cerebral blood volume and potentially an increase in ICP. Hypocapnia induced by controlled hyperventilation has traditionally been used as a cerebral vasoconstrictor for the purposes of lowering cerebral blood volume and therapeutically reducing ICP. Several observations need to be considered before the therapeutic use of hypocapnia as a modality is discussed.

There is strong evidence that the cerebral vasculature adapts to chronically low Pa_{CO_2},[23] resulting in progressive vasodilation or return toward normal diameter. This adaptation may require several hours or even a day or so before the baseline vessel diameter is reached. Given a constant CPP, the vessel will have returned to a state where cerebral blood volume is once again at baseline and ICP is stable. At this point, if the Pa_{CO_2} is returned to normal, the vessel will then react as if it were seeing hypercapnia and will vasodilate further (Fig. 4-9). Cerebral blood volume will increase. This phenomenon will also resolve over the next several hours; however, the patient may deteriorate before it does. This phenomenon has been interpreted to mean that continued hypocapnia was still having a useful effect, a conclusion that should be reached with great caution.

Cerebral Blood Volume Within the context of ICP it is crucial to recognize that CBF and cerebral

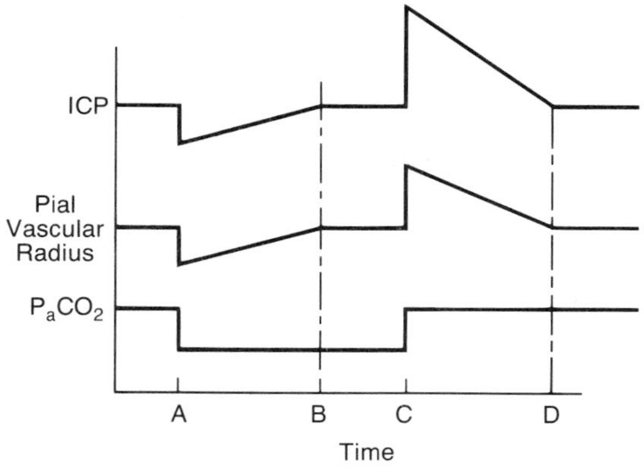

Figure 4-9 When $PaCO_2$ is lowered, vasoconstriction results but gradually returns to baseline within hours (A to B). If all else were constant, ICP would and does return toward its baseline (A to B/C). When $PaCO_2$ is increased, the vasculature dilates as if it were seeing hypercapnia and ICP increases, even though $PaCO_2$ is only raised toward the baseline (C). The ICP increase has the potential to lead to a fatal outcome in "marginal" situations.

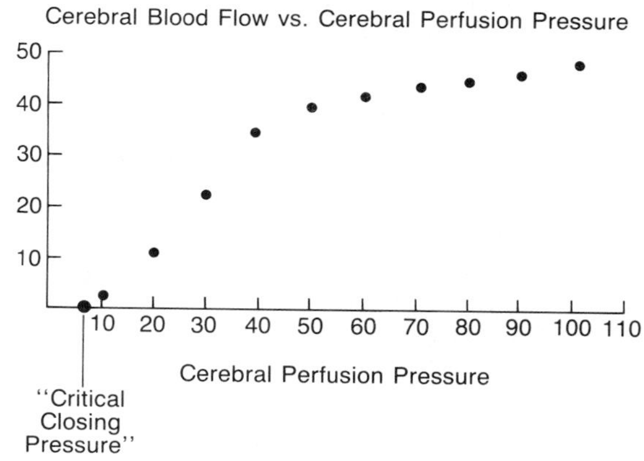

Figure 4-10 Cerebral blood flow is relatively consistent across a wide range of pressure gradients. Under normal circumstances, systemic arterial blood pressure (SABP) and cerebral perfusion pressure (CPP) are effectively the same. However, when intracranial hypertension is present, it is more accurate to use CPP on the horizontal axis. This simplified curve contains at least two important points: (1) As CPP decrements, there is a *slight* decrement in CBF which will normally be about 15 to 20 percent of "normal flow" by the time the lower limit of autoregulation is reached. (2) Cerebral blood flow becomes "O" at a cerebral perfusion pressure above zero. This is the "critical closing pressure" of the vasculature. Both phenomenon are altered in the face of injury. The slope of CBF versus CPP will increase as will the critical closing pressure. Therefore, greater than "normal" CPP will be required to achieve "normal" CBF after cerebral damage.

blood volume are *completely* independent of each other. High CBF does not necessarily mean high cerebral blood volume. Failure to recognize this independence has led to misinterpretation of experimental data and futile therapeutic paths.

Figures 4-10 to 4-13 demonstrate the relationship between pial arterial diameter, CBF, cerebral blood volume, and ICP as a function of CPP. As CPP is reduced, the autoregulatory response demands that the arteriolar system dilate, reduce its resistance, in order to maintain blood flow and oxygen delivery. The rate of vasodilation is not linear. Only 10 to 20 percent of ultimate vasodilatation has occurred by the time CPP has been reduced to 85 mmHg. As CPP decreases through the range of 70 to 80 mmHg, vasodilation occurs logarithmically and reaches a maximum at about 55 to 60 mmHg CPP. The vascular smooth muscle is concentrically arranged and can only *constrict* or *relax* to adjust vessel radius. As CPP decreases, the smooth muscle relaxes, which causes the vessel to dilate.

As smooth muscle relaxation achieves its maximum (one definition of the lower limit of autoregulation), further reductions in the transluminal gradient will result in vascular collapse. Intracranial pressure will decline; however, CBF and oxygen delivery will also be impaired. Recognizing that ICP may appear to improve but that the overall circumstance may worsen is crucial to ICP-CPP management; a *critical minimum* CPP of 55 to 60 mmHg should always be maintained to avoid a reduction in CBF and oxygen delivery.

Abnormality of Cerebral Autoregulation The way in which the autoregulatory response is altered by injury and disease is also vital to understanding and avoiding misinterpretation of CBF, ICP, and CPP information.

In the face of intracranial pathology of virtually any etiology, to varying degrees a similar alteration

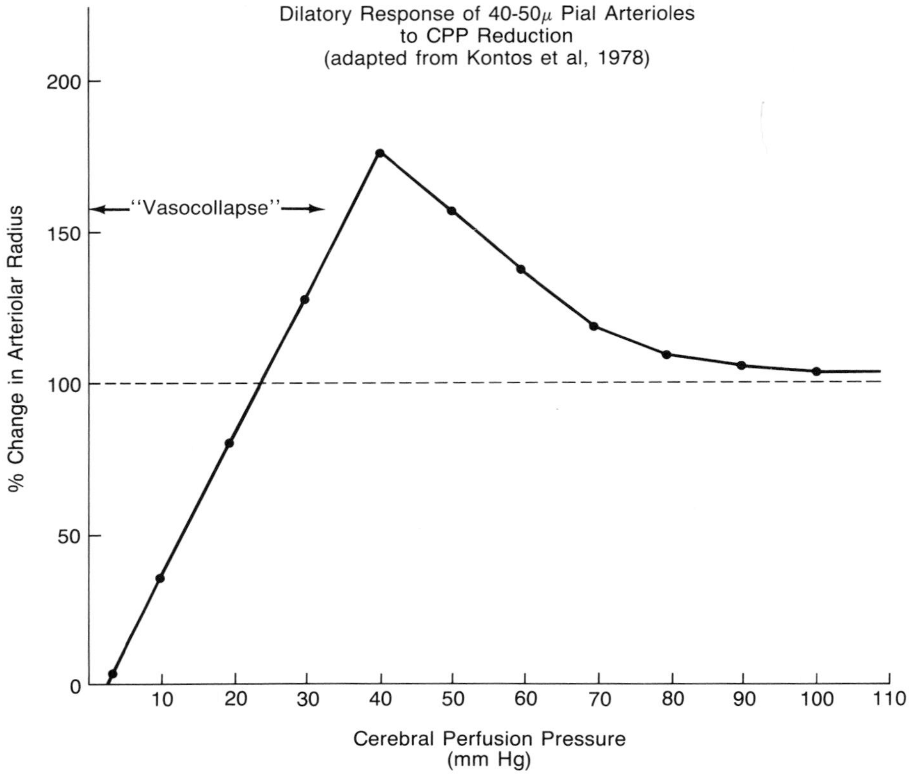

Figure 4-11 Cerebral autoregulation of blood flow is affected by change in cerebrovascular resistance. Over short periods of time and constant metabolic rate, these resistance changes are brought about by change in vascular radius. As CPP decrements toward the lower limit of autoregulation, the vessels dilate. However, the rate at which they dilate is logarithmic and is very important for concomitant ICP effects. With decrementing CPP, the vascular smooth muscle reduces its tone (vasorelaxation) which allows the *transmural pressure gradient* to *dilate* the vessel. Once the vascular muscle is completely relaxed, further decrements in the transmural pressure gradient will *allow* the vessel to passively *collapse* ("vaso collapse"). Again, collapse will be complete slightly above a zero pressure gradient due to the elastance of the vasculature. If CPP (or the transmural pressure gradient) is increased from near zero, the vessel will expand, flow will increase passively until a sufficient pressure gradient is reached, which will allow the smooth muscle to develop tone and hold CBF relatively constant by increasing resistance to flow.

in the relationship of the CPP-CBF curve occurs.[21,24–26] The slope of the CPP-CBF curve increases, and the pressure gradient driving flow through the cerebral circulation is decreased. This abnormality tends to be greatest after traumatic brain injury and subarachnoid hemorrhage and gradually returns to normal over time. The absolute height of the curve may well be depressed. In other words, given any CPP there will tend to be a decrease in flow. It is not always clear whether these measurements represent a decrease in metabolism or continued matching of flow to decreased metabolism.

Perhaps most importantly, the lower limit of autoregulation is elevated to 70 to 90 mmHg or more.[22,27,28] The implications of this increase are

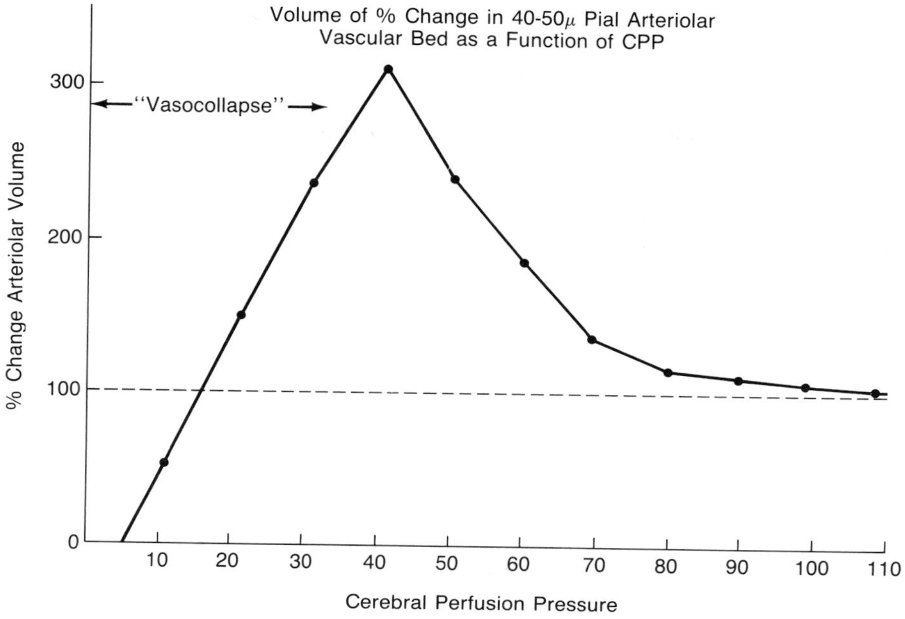

Figure 4-12 Since the cerebral vasculature accomplishes autoregulatory phenomena by vasodilation and vasoconstriction, i.e., by a change in vascular radius, there must be a concomitant *volume* change in the vascular bed. This figure depicts the volume change expected in the 40 to 50 μm arteriolar bed as the lower limit of autoregulation is approached. Note that the logarithmic radius change is further amplified on this "volume change" graph. The volume occupied by a vessel will *double* as CPP drops from "normal" to the lower limit of autoregulation. However, once smooth muscle tone is completely gone (flaccid), the vessel collapses with further reductions in CPP (transmural pressure). In this pressure range, the potential volume change is 300 percent. Therefore, the ICP effects of lowering CPP below the lower autoregulatory limit are profound and quantitively greater (50 percent) than the change from the lower limit to midrange of autoregulation. This curve *under*estimates the volume changes because it is based *only* upon radius change and does not account for the expected, simultaneous change in *length* of the vessel. It also assumes a *linear* rate of vasocollapse which probably is not completely true.

profound. A CPP of 80 mmHg would normally be well within the autoregulatory limits of a normal brain. However, under pathologic circumstances this same 80-mmHg perfusion pressure may well be *below* the now elevated limits and blood flow would be decreased and inadequate: ischemia would result.

When CPP varies below the lower limit of autoregulation, the vasculature dilates or constricts passively and directly with CPP. ICP will thus vary directly with CPP (Figs. 4–11 to 4–13). Since the process is passive, the terms dilation and constriction should be avoided since they imply active vascular response.

Four closely related vascular phenomena needed to understand ICP phenomena are:

1. An increase in critical closing pressure of the vasculature
2. An increase in hysteresis or work to overcome vessel elasticity to allow flow
3. An increase in the autoregulatory lower limit
4. Prolongation of the autoregulatory latency

The increase in critical closing pressure combined with hysteresis means that as CPP is decreased, not only does blood flow drop off very rapidly but elevating CPP from a significant decrease will have to

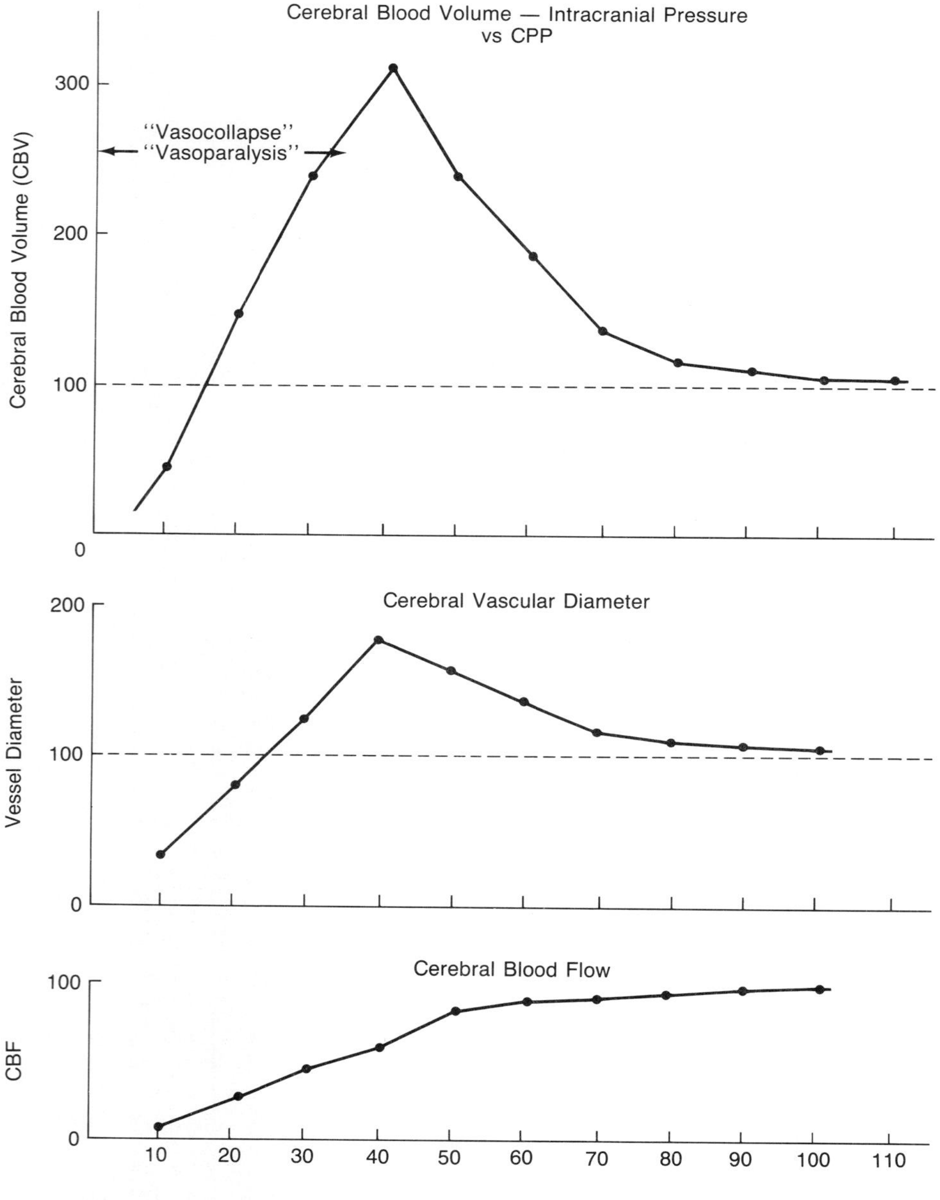

Figure 4-13 This figure integrates the simultaneous factors involved in an autoregulatory response: CPP, CBF, vascular diameter, CBV, and ICP under conditions of constant CMR-O_2 and blood viscosity. The top panel represents CBV changes in the 40 to 50 μm vascular bed. If all other factors are constant, these CBV changes will directly relate to ICP change. The graph allows us to visualize the massive CBV changes which occur with little change in CBF. Once the lower limit of autoregulation is passed, further CPP decrements *decrease* CBV via vasocollapse. Below the lower limits of autoregulation, vessel radius, CBV, and ICP vary *directly* with CPP. Within cerebral autoregulatory limits, vessel radius, CBV, and ICP vary *indirectly* with CPP. Iden-

be done very aggressively. CPP will have to be elevated to supranormal levels in order to reexpand the vasculature and reestablish flow. It is very much analogous to the higher pressure requirements for ventilation and reexpansion of the atelectatic lung.

Normally the cerebral vasculature has a single layer of elastica and relatively sparse musculature. It is easily expanded, requiring relatively little work. But in the face of pathophysiologic events, such as trauma, the diffuse vascular damage generated by free radical release causes the vessels to become less compliant: more work is required.

The elevation of the lower autoregulatory limit in the face of pathology will increase the range over which passive phenomena occur. A normal autoregulatory response may not be seen until CPP is raised *above* the new lower limit; this may not occur until CPP reaches 90 to 100 mmHg or more in severe injury.

Normally, the vasculature actively dilates or constricts to pressure change within 3 to 5 s of the change. This normal latent period may be *prolonged* after injury. The response to changes in CPP may not be observed for 10 to 20 s or longer. During this latent period, the vascular, and therefore ICP, effect will be passive.

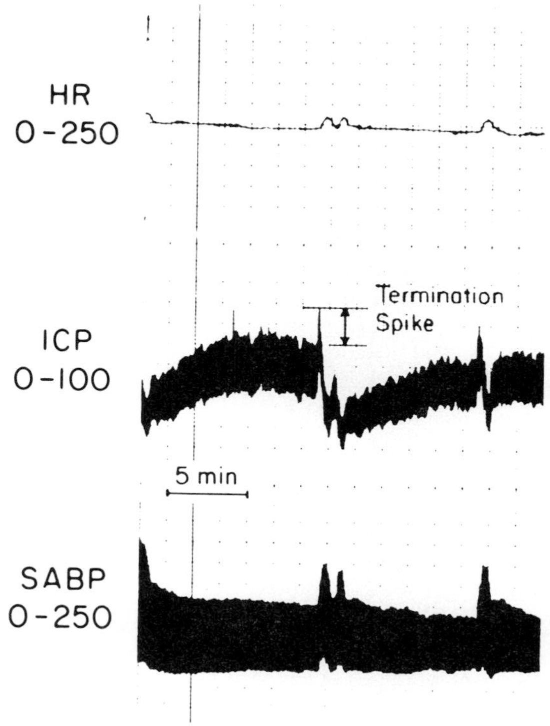

Figure 4-14 This is a trace demonstrating pulsatile recordings of heart rate, ICP, and SABP. Note the intense termination spike generated by the short duration Cushing responses seen in the bottom SABP trace. As SABP declines from higher levels (first half of the frame), the ICP rises. Note how difficult the relationship between SABP, ICP, and cerebral perfusion pressure is to visualize in the absence of a continuous CPP output.

Cerebral Spinal Fluid Pressure Waves CSF pressure waves are extremely useful in understanding many of the pathophysiologic events that occur in the face of intracranial hypertension. CSF pressure waves are relatively sudden increases in ICP reaching levels well above those of baseline pressure before returning toward baseline. These events seem to fall into two broad categories.

The first are *cyclic waves* that have a recurrent pattern with a relatively stereotyped form. There are the *plateau* (A) (Fig. 4-14) and B waves (Fig. 4-15) described by Lundberg (Fig. 4-16). There are also noncyclic CSF pressure waves that are less easily described. These are often single, unique events of varying morphology.

Both cyclic and noncyclic types of waves can be understood at least in part by referring to the vasodilatory cascade model (Fig. 4-17). This model

Figure 4-13 (continued)
tification of this indirect relationship is one method of knowing that the patient is *within* his autoregulatory limits. Note also: (1) Variation of SABP/CPP below the lower limit of autoregulation will lead to ICP changes identical to those earlier described as "vasoparalysis". (2) The lower limit of autoregulation *increases* with injury. This means that "passive" ICP phenomena will occur over a wider range of CPP and indirect responses may not occur until a CPP of 80 to 90 or higher is reached. (3) CBF always varies directly with CPP even though the slope of the curve changes.

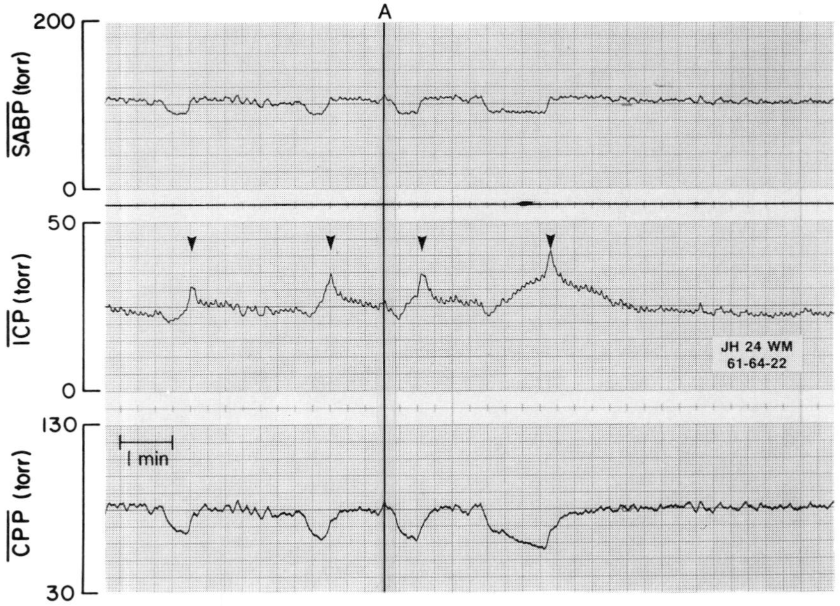

Figure 4-15 This is a series of four "B" waves of slightly varying duration and amplitude. The arrowheads all demonstrate the termination spike which represents a major component of the "B" wave amplitude. In this case, probably 40 percent of the total amplitude is composed of the termination spike. Again, the termination spike is a *passive increase in ICP* occurring with *zero latency* between the SABP and CPP changes, and reversing its direction decrementing the ICP after approximately 10 s (which represents the autoregulatory latency to vasoconstriction). The heavy line (A) marks the time relationship between the decrement in SABP, CPP, and ICP. Note that this initial decrement was associated with a passive decline in ICP. As CPP declined, the decrement in CPP to vasodilatation which reversed the ICP declined and initiated the B wave. Both the termination spike and the decrement in ICP prior to the actual vasodilatory increase are purely passive with a direct relationship between SABP and ICP change.

demonstrates how a reduction in CPP can act as a vasodilatory stimulus leading to an increase in cerebral blood volume and ICP. The ICP increase leads to a further reduction in CPP and therefore a further vasodilatory stimulus. This process, *once initiated*, becomes self-sustained (Figs. 4-18 to 4-20). The cycle continues until vasodilatation is maximal (lower limit to autoregulation) and then ceases. The cycle may be interrupted by counterbalancing events that increase CPP such as an increase in blood pressure, CSF drainage, perhaps hyperventilation, and others.

The events of this cycle demand that the CPP originate far enough *above* the lower limits of autoregulation of a given patient. Otherwise, only passive responses will be observed since autoregulatory phenomena will not occur outside of the autoregulatory range.

Figure 4-23 is a slightly more complex version of the same model and shows how stimuli that affect systemic arterial pressure, the cerebral vasculature primarily, and the ICP component can initiate this cascade. The vasodilatory cascade can be initiated at the systemic arterial pressure side of the model, at the level of the cerebral vasculature, or at the level of the CSF. If the stimuli initiating the cascade are cyclic and relatively stereotyped, then the result will be cyclic, stereotyped CSF pressure waves. When cyclic waves are observed, the vast majority are related to cyclic variation in the systemic arterial blood pressure.

Figures 4-16 and 4-22 demonstrate simultaneous recordings of systemic arterial blood pressure, ICP, and a continuous display of CPP. Early in the recording there is relative stability in systemic arterial pressure coupled with stable CPP of approximately 80 mmHg and a stable ICP. Systemic arterial pressure then begins to decline, CPP declines, and ICP increases. In this case, the systemic arterial pressure stabilized only slightly below the baseline level. This demonstrates the self-sustaining nature of the vasodilatory cascade model. Increases in ICP led to further reductions in CPP because systemic arterial pressure did not increment. Increases in ICP (via vasodilation) occurred and CPP continued its decline. Theoretically, maximal stable ICP will occur at maximal vasodilation.

The increase in ICP was aborted in this case by a sudden increase in systemic arterial pressure that reversed the CPP decrement. An initial rise in the ICP that we have previously termed *termination spike* occurred due to the latency of autoregulatory response. Within 10 s, the ICP increase ceased and ICP fell. Even though systemic arterial pressure stabilized, the falling ICP increased CPP; the

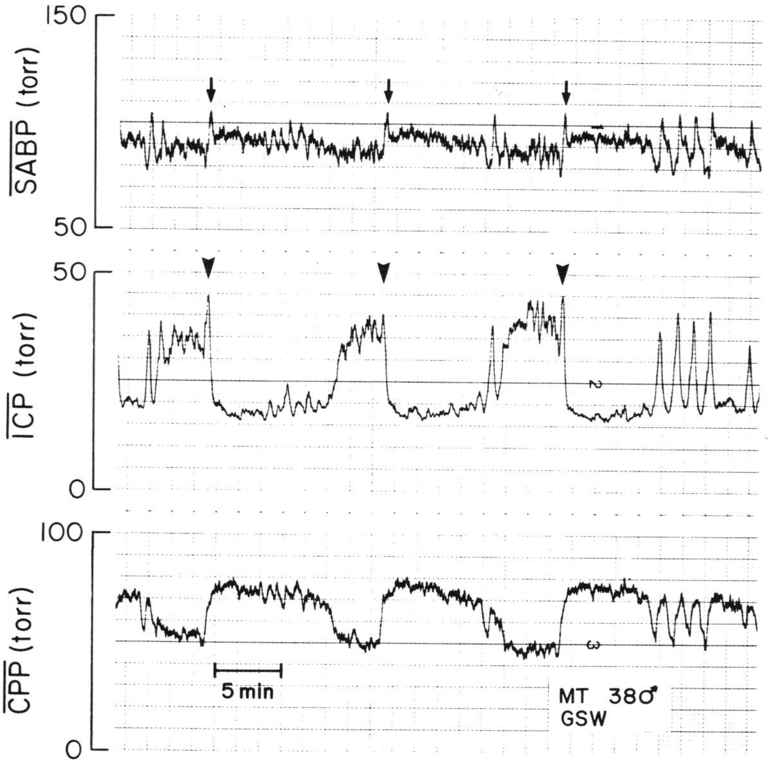

Figure 4-16 This trace demonstrates three plateau waves each terminated by a Cushing response (marked by the small vertical arrow on the SABP trace). Exactly in phase with this Cushing response is the termination spike on the plateau wave (arrowheads). Note how easy it would be to miss these relationships if the recordings were pulsatile in nature and done at a slower speed. Note the five B waves at the end of the trace, each causally related to SABP change which was rapidly cycling. Note also the very narrow range over which the Cushing response occurred: between 45 and 50 mmHg in nearly every case. This is useful information in that this response is due to brainstem ischemia.

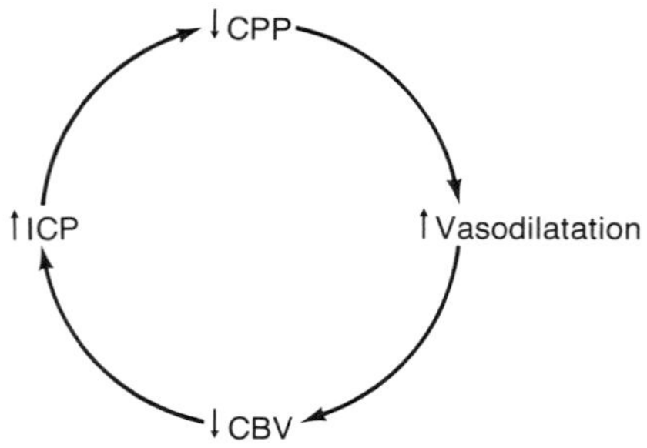

Figure 4-17 Vasodilatory cascade model helps visualize the manner in which a decrement in CPP (SABP-ICP) can initiate a CSF pressure wave. The CPP decrement stimulates vasodilatation, which increases cerebral blood volume (CBV), which forces an increase in ICP. If SABP remains constant, CPP will decline again, further stimulating vasodilation and increasing ICP. The cycle will continue until vasodilation is maximal (about the lower limit of autoregulation) or until SABP forces an increase in CPP. The patient must be well above their lower limit of autoregulation for this mechanism to operate.

higher CPP acted as a vasoconstrictor stimulus, further reduced ICP, and the process continued to cycle.

A minimal ICP will occur when vasoconstriction is maximal. This will usually be associated with a CPP of 100 mmHg or slightly higher. This process, the reciprocal of the vasodilatory cascade, has been termed the *vasoconstriction cascade.*

Termination Spike and Autoregulatory Latency There is a latent period between CPP changes and the autoregulatory response of the cerebral vasculature (Figs. 4-18 to 4-22). The time lag between a pressure change and the metabolically mediated vascular diameter change is 3 to 10 seconds under relatively normal circumstances and significantly prolonged under pathologic circumstances. Thus, during this latent period, the vascular diameter will vary directly or passively with cerebral perfusion pressure. Cerebral blood volume will vary directly with CPP during this latent period and intracranial pressure will appear to vary passively with blood pressure changes. As the metabolic mediators of the vasculature response bring about active vasoconstriction or vasorelaxation, the response of the intracranial pressure will vary *indirectly* with cerebral perfusion pressure. It is quite easy to estimate this time lag from appropriate recordings and is usually 5 to 15 seconds.

Because of autoregulatory latency, the termination spike occurs with *zero* time lag and *directly* with the systemic arterial pressure: the termination spike is a passive phenomenon. Within 10 s it has ended and ICP rapidly falls, as autoregulatory vasoconstriction occurs. The same process may occur at the beginning of the wave with a decrease in ICP due to the rapid reduction in CPP brought about by the systemic arterial pressure drop. The passive nature of this response is manifest by the zero time lag between the reduction in systemic arterial pressure and ICP. Notice that even though the ICP is reduced, cerebral perfusion pressure decreases to an even greater degree.

One can easily see how a physician or nurse standing at the bedside watching an ICP increase as a patient is stimulated might easily conclude that this stimulus was not in the patient's best interest since the ICP increased. It can be difficult to stand and continue to apply that same stimulus for the next 10 to 15 s or longer and await the termination of the ICP wave.

If reductions in systemic pressure are associated with a rapid reduction in ICP, then it is easy to conclude that control of systemic hypertension may be a good thing in terms of ICP management. Subsequent ICP elevation due to inadequate CPP is less likely to be linked to the reduction in systemic pressure because of the time delay between the interaction of systemic arterial blood pressure, CPP, and ICP. If the individual patient falls below his or her autoregulatory limits, then the natural response of the vasculature will be *passive* and further reductions in systemic pressure will result in passive ICP changes: ICP will decline. This reduction will not be associated with spontaneous reversal as it is when a patient is within his or her autoregulatory range. These changes will be sustained and are potentially harmful.

Observations of termination spike phenomena associated with different medical and nursing maneuvers have led to many of the traditional methods of ICP control. Attending to the true autoregulatory response to changes in CPP will invariably lead to diametrically opposed conclusions.

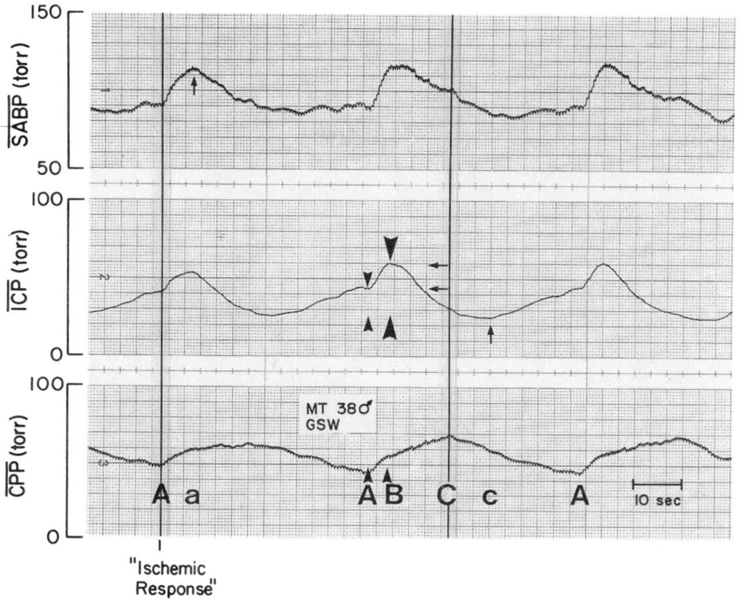

Figure 4-18 Rapid recording (1.5 mm/s) of B waves. The "ischemic response" (A) occurs at a CPP of 50 mmHg. Because the response is rapid (25 mmHg over 5 to 7 s), the ICP increases passively as a "termination spike." Note that the SABP and ICP increase exactly in-phase (heavy line at A on left); there is no latency between "passive" ICP increases/decreases and the SABP change that drives them. However, by "a" the cerebrovasculature has "sensed" the increase in CPP and autoregulatory vasoconstriction occurs to the point that the ICP begins to decline for the next 15 to 20 s. CPP is restored, and though the SABP also declines, the net result is CPP maintenance. This allows the vasculature to continue to constrict and further reduce ICP. The process reverses when the SABP fall finally leads to a net reduction in CPP (point C). The decline in ICP slows and reverses. Even though SABP stabilizes, the CPP reduction stimulates vasodilation and an ICP increment. The ICP increment lowers CPP, further stimulating vasodilation and ICP increase. The process terminates when CPP reaches a point (45 to 50 mmHg) when an "ischemic response" occurs. Note that this potentiates the ICP rise by adding the passive termination spike amplitude (between horizontal arrows) to the *active* autoregulatory vasodilation component (amplitude between small arrowheads). The total "wave" amplitude (large arrowheads) is a combination of active and passive vasodilation but with completely opposite CPP behavior. Note the passive decrement in ICP (C to c) preceding the active vasodilation phase.

The type of recording necessary to visualize the relationships between systemic arterial blood pressure, ICP, and CPP is simple yet historically uncommon. These changes are only apparent when systemic arterial blood pressure and ICP are recorded as means, and the CPP is displayed as the continuous difference. The recording rate must be rapid enough to discriminate events that may be separated by 5 s or less. Recordings done at slow rates and using pulsatile pressures are often impossible to analyze (Fig. 4-14). Variations in systemic arterial pressure that causally lead to the generation of cyclic CSF pressure waves are often lost in slow recording and appear to be noise. Figures 4-24 and 4-25 are examples of such recordings. Failure to continuously display CPP makes the relationship between the CPP and ICP changes extremely difficult to visualize. Often the decrement in systemic arterial pressure that is capable of initiating the CSF pressure wave is lost because of in-

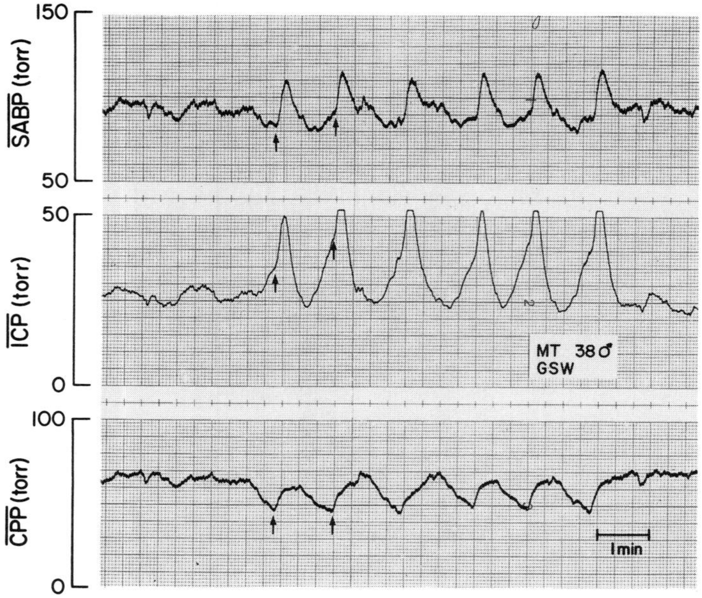

Figure 4-19 Somewhat slower recording (15 mm/min) of B waves demonstrating their rhythmic nature, but driven by the SABP. The vertical arrows (first two waves only) mark the point where the "ischemic" or Cushing response occurs. Note: (1) The very narrow CPP threshold, 46 to 48 mmHg, over which this patient's "Cushing" response occurs. This value is highly stereotyped for given patients and may vary from 45 to 100 mmHg or more in any individual. (2) Note the "shoulder" on the ICP B wave where active vasodilation converts to the passive but intense termination spike characterizing the B wave. Recognition of this shoulder as the beginning of the termination spike allows one to look for the Cushing response driving it. Again, the latency between the ischemic/Cushing response and "termination spike" is zero. The CPP always increases during this phase regardless of the degree of termination spike ICP increase. Note also the absence of B waves in the few min prior to the first arrow. This was because the SABP never decremented enough or long enough to initiate the vasodilatory cascade.

sensitive scales; a decrement of only 10 to 15 mmHg in the systemic arterial pressure may be unrecognized or dismissed as insignificant.

Figure 4-15 demonstrates that the decrement in systemic pressure from 100 to 85 mmHg occurred quickly and then became stable. Neither of these values are hypotensive, and it is easy to overlook the importance of the change. The continuous recording of these variables using mean pressures recorded with a rapid paper speed make the relationships and interrelationships obvious.

Cyclic CSF Pressure Waves

Lundberg described three types of cyclic CSF pressure waves. The most famous is the A wave or what has been known as the *plateau wave* (Figs. 4-14 and 4-16). This is an increase in ICP that comes about relatively suddenly and rises to very high levels (50 to 100 mmHg) that are sustained for periods of several minutes to an hour or so and then may abort equally suddenly. These may well be repetitive with a very stereotyped shape in any given patient. They are easily explained by the vasodilatory cascade model. Careful recordings demonstrate a reduction in systemic arterial pressure occurring before the initiation of the CSF pressure increase. CPP will drop, and ICP will increase and remain so until CPP is restored. Variations in the systemic arterial pressure occurring at a rate that cycles faster than the autoregulatory response time, or variations that are inadequate to restore

CPP will produce superimposed ICP variation. However, it will only be when CPP is restored to a level where autoregulation becomes active that the wave will terminate.

Termination of the plateau wave is probably best viewed as a sympathoadrenal event, or Cushing's-type response, that will often be associated with hypertension, tachycardia, tachypnea, hyperventilation, and shivering. The clinical observations that spontaneously breathing patients tend to become diaphoretic, tachypneic, agitated, and tend to hyperventilate, complain of headache if they are awake enough, and may demonstrate shivering are consistent with the autonomic events associated with plateau waves.

There may well be a complementary interaction between hyperventilation and hypertension and the termination of plateau waves in spontaneously ventilating patients, but the same sequence of events occurs in pharmacologically paralyzed and ventilated patients where Pa_{CO_2} is held constant (Fig. 4-27). Changes in Pa_{CO_2} are not necessary for the occurrence nor the abolition of CSF A-waves, though synergism may occur.

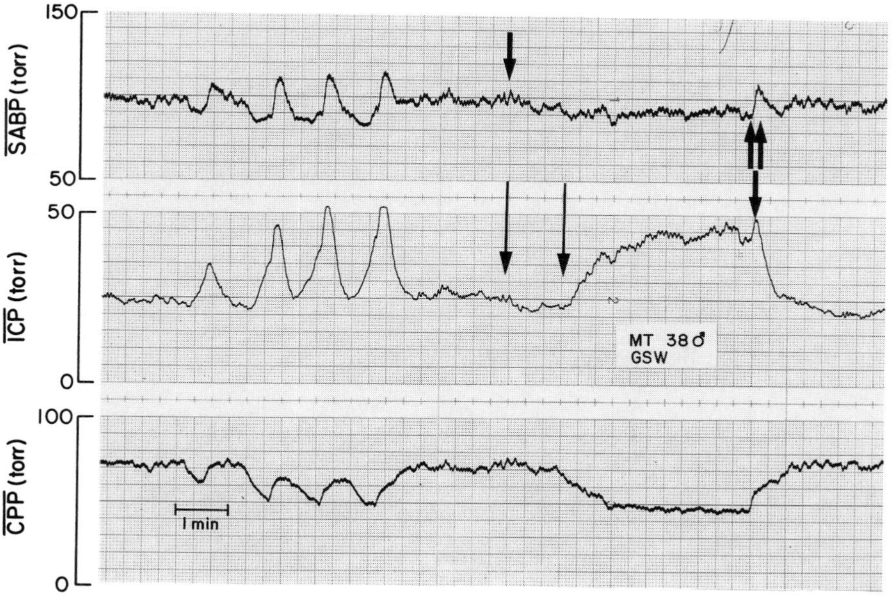

Figure 4-20 A "plateau" or A wave lasting about 4 min demonstrates the decline in SABP preceding the ICP rise. The decline in SABP (heavy arrow) was gradual and amounted to 10 mmHg over 2 min. The ICP initially responded with a slight passive decline (narrow arrows) until the CPP declined enough to stimulate the autoregulatory, vasodilatory cascade at a threshold of about 65 torr. Note that the SABP decline continued and CPP declined 15 s *before* the ICP rise of the plateau wave. The SABP then stabilized at about 90 mmHg, but the ICP continued to rise because the vasodilatory cascade had been initiated. This rise continued for two min until the plateau ICP was reached at a stable CPP of 48 to 50 torr. Note the Cushing response at 45 torr (double heavy arrows) which raised CPP, caused a 10 s termination spike (ICP trace, heavy arrow) in-phase with the Cushing response, and was followed by abolition of the plateau wave. Note that the four B waves preceding the A wave are qualitatively identical to the plateau wave. The B wave differs only in the time course of the SABP change that drives them: B waves are associated with rapid, intense SABP change compared to the more slowly evolving A wave.

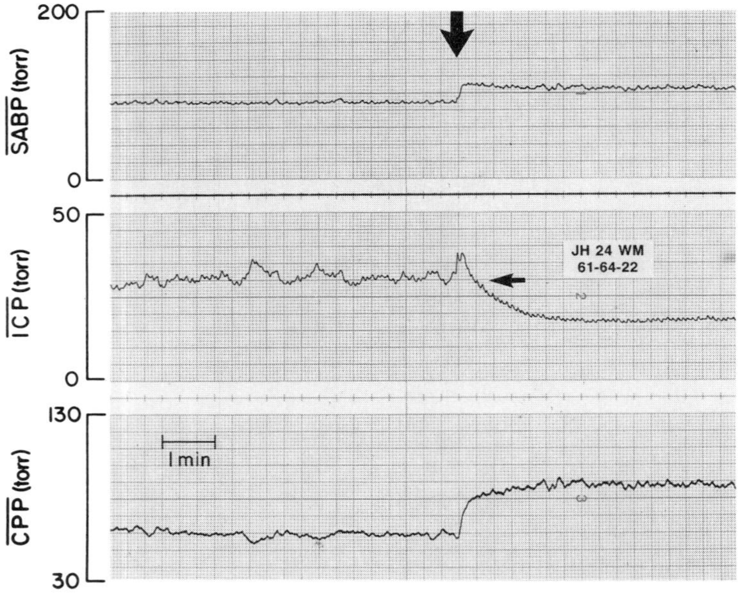

Figure 4-21 This trace demonstrates a spontaneous increase in systemic arterial blood pressure from approximately 90 to 110 torr. CPP increased from 60 to approximately 90 mmHg over the next two min. Note the sharp increase in intracranial pressure at the point where SABP increases (heavy vertical arrow). This termination spike increased ICP from approximately 30 to 37 mmHg over about 10 s before the ICP began to decline. The "vasoconstriction cascade" model nicely explains the subsequent ICP decline. As perfusion pressure is restored, the cerebral vasculature begins to constrict, cerebral blood volume declines, and intracranial pressure declines. Even though the SABP did not change further, the reduction in ICP led to further increases in CPP, which continued to act as a vasoconstrictor stimulus. This cycle continued until vasoconstriction was maximal, which occurred at a CPP of approximately 90 mmHg. ICP stabilized at approximately 18 mmHg. Note that if an observer was merely standing at the bedside and a stimulus was applied to the patient, the observer would have seen the ICP rise. It is natural to assume that the stimulus raising the blood pressure had led to an increase in ICP and that this was therefore the wrong thing to do. Correlating the increase in blood pressure, the improvement in perfusion pressure, and the *subsequent* reduction in intracranial pressure is extremely difficult to do without continuous multimodality recordings.

The relationship between brain electrical activity and plateau waves is more complex. However, CSF pressure waves may and do occur with no change in brain electrical activity. Brain electrical activity and metabolic change is not required for these cyclic variations in CSF pressure to occur but, again, may be synergistic.

B-Waves B-waves were also described by Lundberg as cyclic waves occurring at a rate of 0.5 to 1 per min. They would often reach peaks of 50 to 75 mmHg. They also can be described and understood best using the vasodilatory cascade model (Fig. 4-17). Figures 4-18 to 4-20, 4-26, demonstrate B-wave recorded in association with continuous recording of the systemic arterial pressure. The increase in ICP associated with a decrease in mean arterial pressure leading to a reduction in CPP is clear. Equally clear is the autoregulatory latent period during which time the ICP and CPP vary directly. This is in the neighborhood of 5 to 10 s, and the indirect portion of the ICP increase as a result of vasodilation is obvious. What is prominent about the B-wave is the very large component of its total amplitude that is the result of its termination spike. When B-waves are identified, the termination spike may represent 50 percent or even more of the actual total amplitude. This is a result of the very intense, rapid systemic arterial pressure changes that drive these waves.

The decrease in systemic arterial pressure tends to occur more rapidly and to a greater degree than those observed during plateau waves. Similarly, as the systemic arterial pressure returns to baseline levels, the rate of restoration and the degree of change also tend to be more vigorous. Although the termination spike is more prominent with B-waves than A-waves, qualitatively, the two are virtually identical.

The CPP range at which the CPP is restored is remarkably narrow in B-waves. The threshhold range for this restoration is highly specific to individual patients. The increase in blood pressure that is associated with termination of both B-waves and plateau waves can be viewed as an ischemic response or a Cushing's response. This is purely sympathoadrenal in nature, associated with an increase in circulating catecholamines and vasoconstrictor tone. It is most likely generated in the rostral medulla and occurs in response to a de-

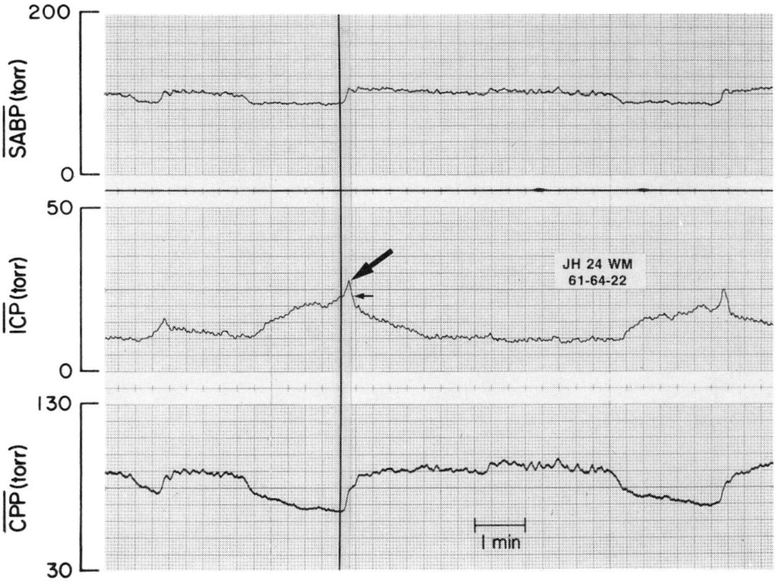

Figure 4-22 This figure demonstrates three ICP waves. The first wave was extremely short flived and of low amplitude. Most of its amplitude consisted of a "termination spike." The second wave lasted for approximately two min. Note that all three waves were terminated by spontaneous SABP increases. On the second wave this is marked by the heavy black line. Note the termination spike peaking at the large arrowhead with the amplitude being marked by the difference between the arrows. Even though the termination spike increased the ICP by 5 to 6 mmHg, no decrement in CPP occurred. Note that the difference between the first and the next two waves on this trace is the *duration* and not the degree of SABP decrement. The degree of change needed to stimulate the vasodilatory cascade is on the order of 10 mmHg in this and many other patients. This is often considered a trivial degree of blood pressure change and often ignored by the clinical staff. However, when the change is consistent and long lasting enough, the vasodilatory cascade is activated and a pressure wave generated.

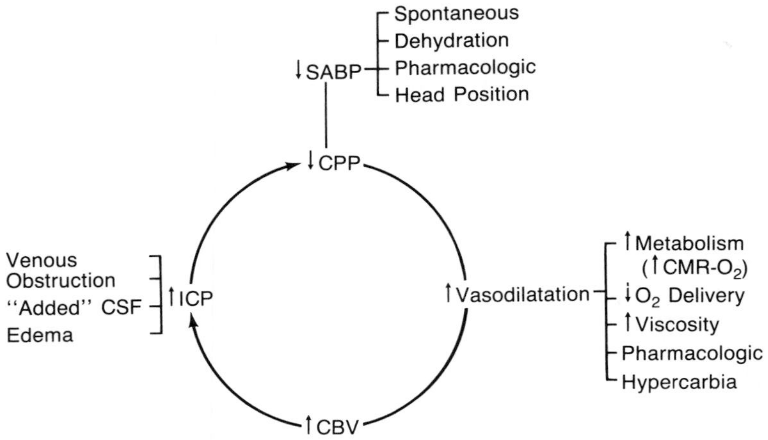

Figure 4-23 "Complex Vasodilatory Cascade" model helps explain many contradictory events and demonstrates how the cycle can be stimulated at any of the main components. For example, raising the head of the bed may decrease SABP and initiate a pressure wave, but if this were countered by decreased venous congestion, then the CPP and ICP may actually decline. Barbiturate therapy may decrease CMR-O_2 and potentially abort a CSF pressure wave, yet if SABP declines as a result of the barbiturate, a net decrement in CPP could result and potentiate intracranial hypertension. An offshoot of this model suggests the minimum requirement for demonstrating primary pharmacologic effects on the cerebral vasculature: constant CMR-O_2 and constant SABP, as well as constant $PaCO_2$.

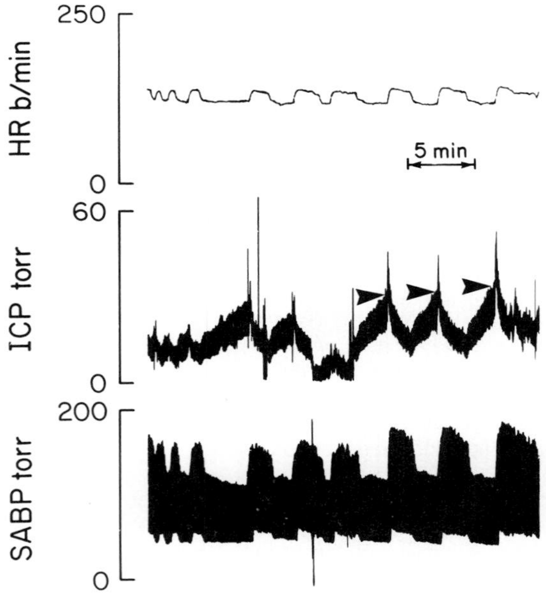

Figure 4-24 This is another pulsatile recording demonstrating the termination spike in the B waves. Note the increase in heart rate with each increase in blood pressure. This is a sympathoadrenal response generated by the rostral medulla in an effort to maintain medullary blood flow. It is associated with increased levels of epinephrine and norepinephrine, as well as increased vasoconstrictor sympathetic nerve activity.

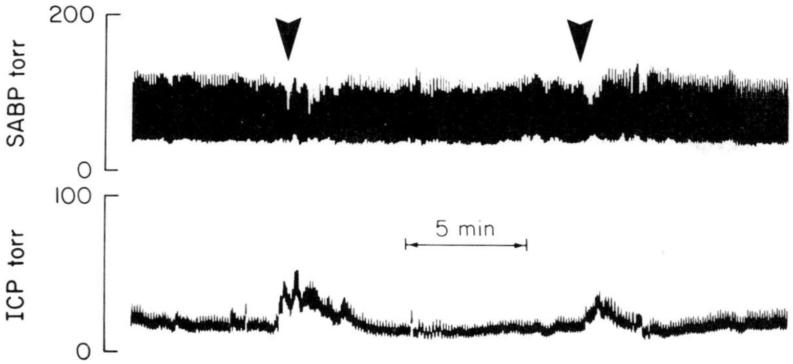

Figure 4-25 This figure demonstrates the difficulty with very slow pulsatile recordings of ICP and SABP in detecting the relationship between SABP and ICP change. The large arrowheads mark decrements in SABP which are "real." These are associated with the generation of ICP waves. However, it is easy to dismiss these SABP changes as "noise." Faster recording rates as well as the use of mean pressures in the recording make these relationships much clearer. Recording rates which allow the discrimination of events within one to 2 s are extremely important. Mean SABP scales should be such that changes of ≤ 10 mmHg in SABP are readily apparent. The simultaneous presentation of CPP traces is also extremely useful in identifying the temporal relationships and the direction in which they are occurring.

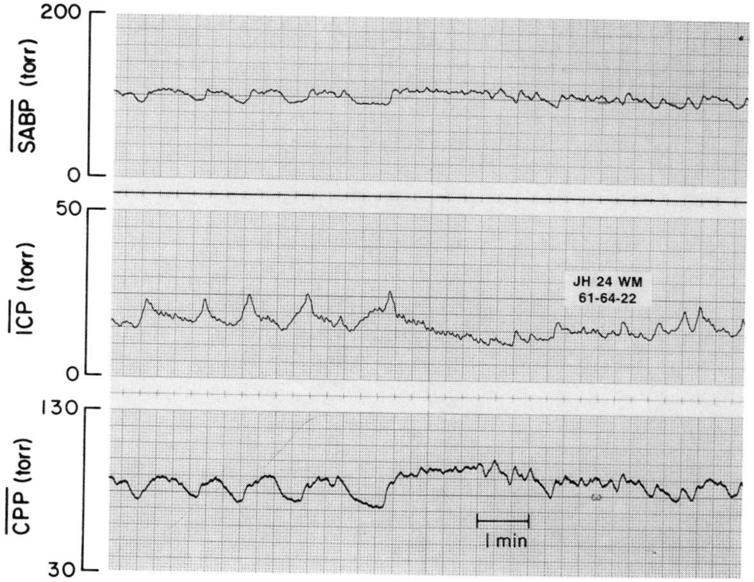

Figure 4-26 Another series of ICP waves (B waves), each generated by spontaneous decrements in SABP. Note (the middle of the trace) where SABP remained constant for 2 to 2.5 min, the ICP decremented, and wave behavior disappeared. As the SABP became more unstable, ICP waves of both a passive and active sort began to reappear.

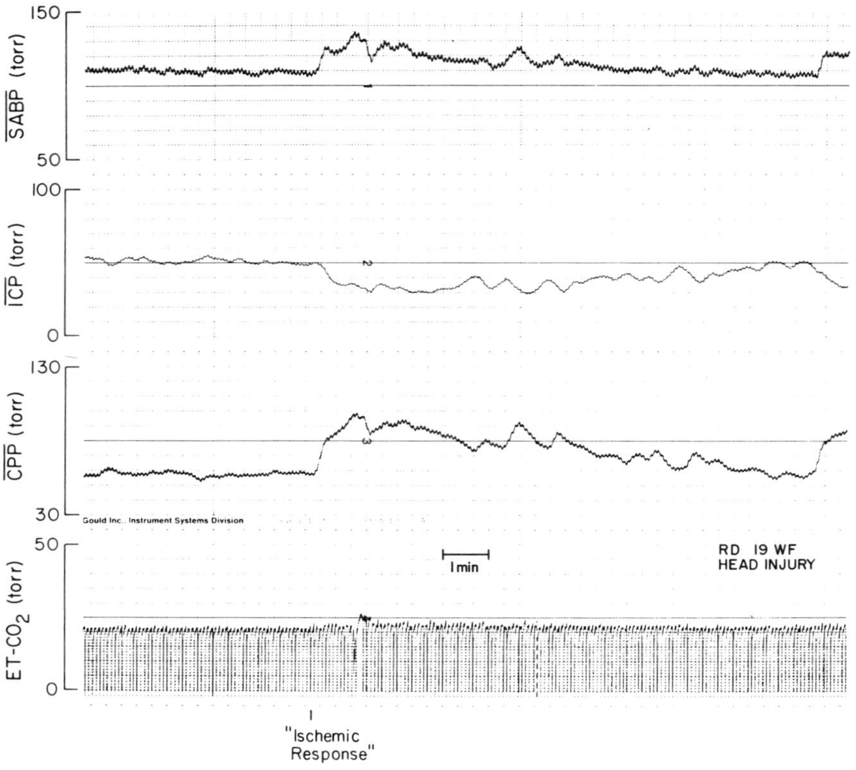

Figure 4-27 A Cushing response occurred in this head-injured patient at a CPP of 60 torr. Blood pressure elevated from approximately 110 mmHg to 125 to 135 torr. Intracranial pressure came down to approximately 30 to 35 torr. As the hypertension decayed toward baseline levels, CPP also decayed and ICP returned to 50 mmHg. Note that at the time of the ischemic response, end-tidal CO_2 actually increased. The increase was due to increased CO_2 *production* as the result of a surge in circulating catacholamines. Note that even in the face of this slight CO_2 increase, the intracranial pressure still decremented.

crease in pontomedullary blood flow.[29] When this decrease is sufficient, the region will be stimulated to raise systemic arterial blood pressure. This will restore blood flow to the region and simultaneously reverse the ICP wave phenomenon. As blood flow is restored, the stimulus to systemic hypertension is eliminated and vasomotor tone decreases. The decrease in vasomotor tone and circulating catecholamines will result in a decrease in systemic arterial pressure that will reduce CPP and initiate an ICP wave, and the entire cycle will repeat.

C-Waves C-waves, also described by Lundberg, are clearly related to systemic Traube-Herring-Meyer waves. These cycle at the rate of approximately 4 to 5 per min. The corresponding ICP changes are often direct and passive. The cycle time often precludes the development of the indirect vasoconstrictor and vasodilatory components of the wave, and given rapid enough systemic variation, the ICP and systemic waves are completely in sync. There may be minimal variation in CPP with these waves. If the Traube-Herring-Meyer waves are slow enough, then the cerebral vasculature will respond and the same qualitative events as those occurring in the B-waves will be seen. Because of the relatively rapid cycle time of the blood pressure change, and the relatively low amplitude of the change, the clinical import of these waves is usually minimal.

NONCYCLIC INTRACRANIAL PRESSURE EVENTS

Noncyclic events are not infrequent in both laboratory and clinical observations of ICP phenomena. The vasodilatory cascade is capable of being activated by any number of these events (Fig. 4-23), and the resulting ICP wave can be the result of both primary stimuli and the interaction of secondary CPP changes.

Perhaps the most potent and clinically relevant cerebral vasodilator is decreased oxygen delivery. The occurrence of a mucous plug in a major bronchus can cause rapid hypoxemia, decreased oxygen delivery, and cerebral vasodilation. This cerebral vasodilation can then activate the cerebral vasodilatory cascade and potentiate high ICP and low CPP. The ICP rise may actually be mitigated in its effects by simultaneous systemic hypertension, but if the systemic hypertension does not occur or is actively blocked, then major reductions in CPP may occur and injury potentiated.

In contrast, endotracheal suctioning often produces intense cough and systemic hypertension, which will appear to increase the ICP (passive ICP response, zero latency). These are usually brief, passive events associated with an increase in CPP and are usually of little consequence. However, if one is only attending to the ICP, then therapeutic decisions such as blocking the hypertensive response may evolve. The result may be an ICP that remains stable but a CPP that decreases.

Other events that may lead to the generation of relatively isolated ICP increases are those associated with a change or alteration in $CMRO_2$. The simplest of these is brain arousal. If a patient is stimulated or awakened, $CMRO_2$ will increase. Normally this is accompanied by an increase in systemic arterial pressure, and little change in ICP occurs. If the systemic arterial pressure change does not occur, then the increased needs for oxygen delivery will be met via vasodilation that will increase ICP.

Seizures, either clinical or purely electrical, are capable of a regional or generalized increase in $CMRO_2$ and blood flow.[30] Net cerebral vasodilation virtually always occurs and will raise ICP. It is important that this increase in ICP be counterbalanced with an increase in systemic pressure to maintain CPP as best as possible to avoid ischemic change.

Carotid dissection, cerebral emboli, and other occlusive events that may occur as a concomitant of either trauma or natural disease may again reduce CPP within a given region or globally. Even though systemic arterial pressure might appear to be adequate, the regional CPP may well be low, leading to vasodilation and, potentially, elevated ICP.

Antihypertensive agents, either given for control of what often appears as excessive levels of systemic hypertension, or drugs that are given for diuresis may have secondary effects on blood pressure. Hemoconcentration with volume depletion or the vasculature effects of furosemide may stimulate ICP waves.

Reductions in CPP either locally or generally will also occur if venous sinus thrombosis or cerebral venous thrombosis occurs either as a result of trauma, infection, hypercoagulable states, or other events. Here again, systemic hypertension is often prominent but may still be inadequate to perfuse the brain in the face of an occluded or partially occluded venous system. When this occlusion is total, the results are invariably fatal; but when it is partial or progressive, then ICP events may occur as a single isolated event with gradual resolution. It is important to recognize that impairment of venous drainage, not generally via the patient in the flat position but more by tracheostomy tapes that are too tight, or excessive torsion of the neck are important clinically and should be sought when ICP increases.

The literature with regard to anesthetic effects on ICP is thus extraordinarily difficult to interpret. Most anesthetics lead to a decrease in systemic arterial pressure, as well as to a reduction in $CMRO_2$. When these events occur together, there may be little change in ICP. If the decrease in arterial pressure is great enough, however, an increase in ICP may result. It is dangerous, however, to assume that the increase in ICP has a direct effect on the cerebral vasculature when the arterial pressure is also changing. While primary cerebral vascular effects may occur, it is difficult to separate them from systemic events. A requirement for identifying an ICP or cerebral vasodilator effect of any drug would be that systemic arterial pressure *and* $CMRO_2$ must be constant. These are not easy conditions to establish. Much confusion about ICP effects of various drugs can be traced to the failure to recognize this necessity. In addition, the degree of arterial pressure change necessary to activate the cerebral vasodilatory cascade and generate ICP waves is often on the order of 10 to 15 mmHg or less; so small a change is frequently not obvious from pulsatile recordings carried out with blood pressure measured on scales of 0 to 200 mmHg. If the change is noted, it is often dismissed as being of no consequence because the degree of change is so small.

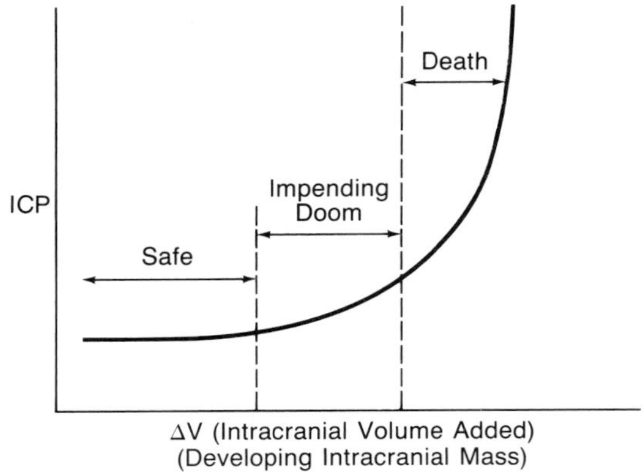

Figure 4-28 "Classical" approach to volume injected into intracranial compartment demonstrates the relative stability of the ICP over the early stages of "dV." The clinical need has been to clearly identify and retrieve the patient from the "impending doom" zone prior to major deterioration. The VPI, PVI, and other derivative measures have been derived for this purpose to counter the relative insensitivity of the ICP alone (a poor predictor).

DERIVATIVE MEASURES

As an intracranial mass is expanding, relatively little change in ICP occurs until some point is reached at which the ICP increases rapidly (Fig. 4-1). This observation has its parallel in the clinical situation where patients have been noted to be relatively stable for long periods of time and, without warning, suddenly deteriorate. It often seemed that their intracranial reserve had been exhausted and thereafter only minimal additional changes led to major clinical deterioration (Fig. 4-28). Intracranial pressure per se predicted only poorly such deterioration. In order to better predict which patients were at risk for such deterioration, derivative measures of ICP were advanced.

Volume-Pressure Response

The simplest of these measures was the volume-pressure response (VPR) suggested by Miller and associates.[31] This involved the injection of 1 mL of saline into the ventricle over a period of 1 s. ICP was measured at baseline and after the injection of 1 mL. If the ICP rose less than 4 mmHg, then the suggestion was that the patient was far to the left on the volume-pressure curve and therefore was in little imminent danger of deterioration and still possessed adequate intracranial reserve. If the rise in ICP were greater than 4 mmHg, then one concluded that the patient was further to the right on the curve and was in danger because most of his or her intracranial reserve had been used up.

While attractive, this measure correlated poorly with the timing of clinical deterioration. It also tended to be reassuringly low during periods of very high ICP, e.g., during plateau or Lundberg A-waves, and it did not take into account baseline ICP. The VPR did not differentiate between the results that might occur at an ICP of 35 versus 90 mmHg.

Pressure-Volume Index

The more widely used measure is the pressure-volume index (PVI) defined by Marmarou.[32] This measure does take into account baseline ICP and because of the logarithmic term provides a measure that estimates the *volume* that would have to be injected to increase ICP by a factor of 10.

Regardless of the ultimate clinical utility, the development of the VPR and the more commonly used PVI have systematized the concept that there is a relationship between change in intracranial volume and change in ICP.

This has led to the concept of brain compliance. *Compliance* is a quantitative estimate of the amount of pressure needed to induce a given volume change within a system. This works quite well for balloons, lungs, and other expansile structures.

Volume Tolerance and Brain Stiffness

The Monro-Kellie doctrine holds that the craniospinal axis has a fixed volume. There is *no* defineable *additional* volume added to the intracranial cavity. If 1 mL of saline were rapidly injected into the ventricular system, 1 mL of some other component must be displaced. With rapid injection, this is almost exclusively cerebral venous blood. The venous blood volume will return to normal as the additional fluid is absorbed as CSF.

Therefore, the graph in Figs. 4-1 and 4-28 is in itself a basic misconception. There is no increasing volume because the volume is constant. There is no question that patients clinically act as if this curve has a real basis. Indeed it does, but it is not in the concept of compliance nor its inverse: *elastance*. What is actually being measured as a given volume element is added to the intracranial compartment is the pressure or force per unit area required to *displace* vascular volume and/or to more rapidly absorb CSF.

While the point may seem trivial, the use of the term *compliance* implies specific mathematical definitions and predictions based on those mathematic manipulations. A concept such as *brain stiffness* or *volume tolerance* as used by Schrader et al is preferable because these terms do not imply a specific mathematic treatment for their derivation and manipulation.[33]

Arguments have been made that as a volume is injected into the ventricle, the craniospinal dura may expand slightly to allow for this additional volume. However, the actual volume change accommodated by the craniospinal axis is unknown, and it becomes unmeaningful to assume that the entire injected volume was accommodated by a true expansion of the craniospinal dura across a wide range of CSF pressures.

The newborn infant and in particular the premature infant are minor exceptions. In these cases the flexible skull does accommodate additional volume. Here again the concept is quite interesting in terms of the actual measured variable. We speak of brain compliance just as we might of pulmonary compliance. However, at least 50 percent of measured pulmonary compliance represents the actual compliance of the chest wall. The concept that the container contributes part of the compliance or elastance of the system is very important. In the newborn, the skull is quite flexible. The actual measure does not necessarily relate to brain compliance but represents brain + skull + scalp compliance. In fact, the brain, once removed from the rigid calvaria, is an extremely compliant structure.

These conditions are more relevant to clinical practice than one might suspect. Expansion of the brain into cranial defects, herniation, or relaxation at the time of surgery, and its response to retraction all suggest a very compliant structure. The difficulty lies in its measurement. If we accept that these traditional measures of brain compliance measure neither brain nor compliance, there is still useful information to be gained by the injection of a known volume with measurement of the subsequent ICP response.

Work by Marmarou and associates has suggested that 80 to 90 percent of the PVI represents vascular factors.[34] Much of this response is venous, but capillary and arterial components of the response cannot be neglected. Presumably the remaining 10 to 20 percent of the PVI response represents CSF absorption and displacement of parenchyma. However, PVI has failed in clinical use for predicting deterioration and outcome partly because of the assumption that it was constant across wide ranges of intracranial conditions. This is not the case. Just as Miller and colleagues noted that the VPR may well be very low (safe and comforting) during periods of very high ICP, others have noted that both the PVI and pulse pressure analysis (of Avezatt) yield similar results; i.e., they looked good when the patient looked bad.[35]

The reason for this is that they are nonlinear with respect to CPP.[36] Figure 4-29 relates successively determined PVI values as CPP was decremented.[28] In fact, PVI decreases as CPP is lowered to a region close to the lower limits of autoregula-

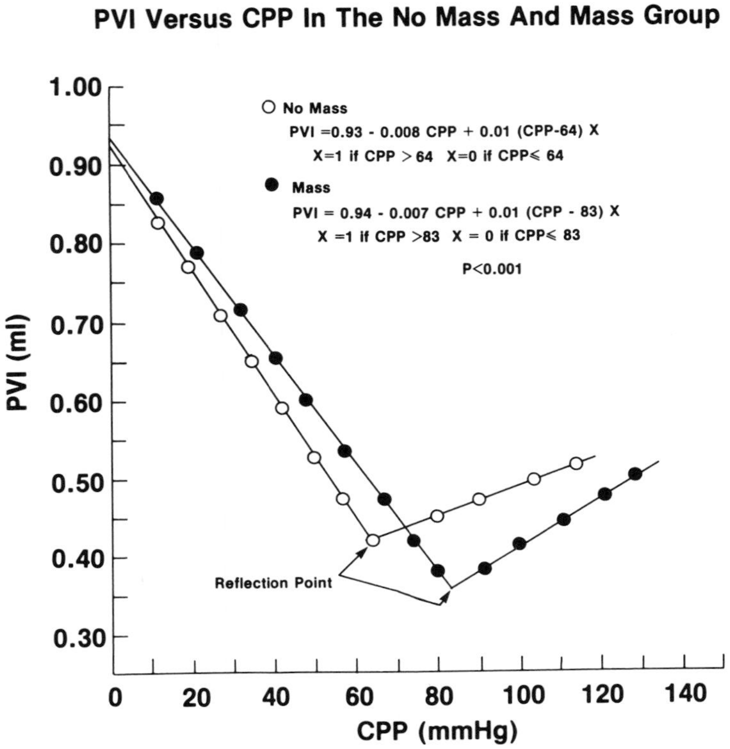

Figure 4-29 This plot is from a study of intracranial hypertension induced by cisternal infusion (no mass) versus an epidural balloon (mass).[28] Though not shown, CBF was monitored by H_2 clearance at each CPP. The relationship between PVI and CPP is complex. Below the lower limit of autoregulation, the CPP-PVI slope is negative; above this limit, the slope is positive. The point at which the slope changes from negative to positive is the "reflection point." As pathologic processes progress, the reflection point shifts to the right toward a higher CPP. Not shown is the reflection point for a normal brain which is further to the left at about 50 mmHg CPP and occurs at a higher (better) PVI than the "pathologic" conditions.[27,41] [Reproduced with permission from El Adawy Y, Rosner MJ: Cerebral perfusion pressure, autoregulation, and the PVI reflection point: Pathological ICP. In: Hoff JT, Betz AL (eds): *Intracranial Pressure VII*, Springer-Verlag, pp 829–833.]

tion; the brain becomes *less* volume-tolerant or stiffer as CPP is reduced. Concomitant blood flow measures demonstrate that when the lower limit of autoregulation is passed and blood flow begins to rapidly decline, the PVI actually improves. In other words, the brain becomes more volume-tolerant or less stiff. Most likely the decreased turgor of the vasculature under conditions of low perfusion pressure allowed not only venous blood but now *arterial* blood to be displaced in order to accept the additional volume.[27,28] Barbiturate anesthesia tends to flatten this curve, making the dependence of PVI on CPP less obvious.[36]

For predictors such as PVI or VPR to be useful, one must clearly understand the CPP at the time the value was derived. In addition, it may be possible to do multiple measures at different CPP levels to improve the validity of PVI. This has yet to be accomplished but makes rational use of these measures.

MANAGEMENT OF INCREASED ICP

Management of intracranial hypertension is little different than many other management schemes in general medicine and surgery: It is to eliminate the cause of dysfunction and to support the brain and patient while reparative processes take place. Ischemia more than any other insult potentiates intracranial hypertension, cerebral edema, and irreversible tissue damage (Fig. 4-30). Even in settings where cerebral hyperemia is purported to be an important manifestation of cerebral injury, it is ischemia from which the patient dies.[37–42]

This discussion will be focused on CPP management as an end point in itself. This is in contrast to management of the ICP, per se, as the specific end point. Already outlined in some detail are basic physiologic principles that will be applied as a basis for CPP management.

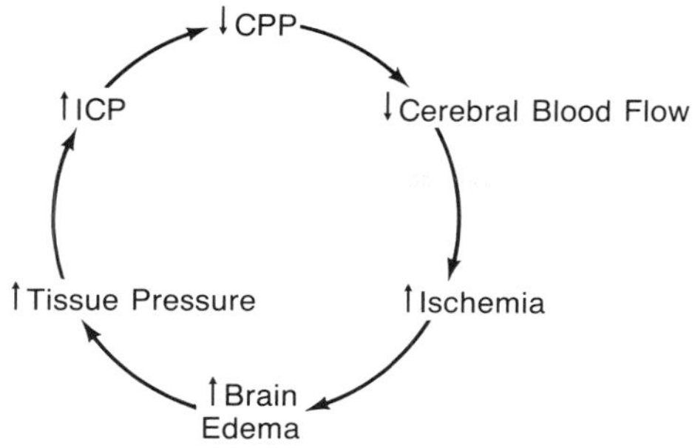

Figure 4-30 A derivative of the vasodilatory cascade model demonstrates the interaction of several factors which both locally and generally potentiate brain edema. By allowing areas of ischemia to develop, this cycle leads to enlargement of edematous areas. Another way to visualize the problem is to ask, "How can we expect brain edema to resolve if there is continuing ischemia?"

Brain Shift

Mass effect, especially from hematoma, alters cerebral vascular reactivity in a major way, shifts the lower limits of autoregulation to very high levels, and contributes more to avoidable mortality and morbidity than most other specific events.[28,40-42] There is little debate about the wisdom of removing large epidural and subdural hematomas. There is more debate about the debridement of focal contusions and small traumatic intracerebral hemorrhages.

When frontotemporal contusions are large and associated with mass effect, many neurologic surgeons debride them. There has been hesitancy in the neurosurgical community with regard to the debridement of dominant hemisphere temporal and frontal contusions due to concern of potentiating damage to eloquent brain areas. However, resection of necrotic tissue with preservation of healthy adjacent tissue should not potentiate damage if done with basic finesse. At the same time, removal of this hemorrhagic, necrotic nidus will tend to speed resolution of edema, will do much to control intracranial hypertension, and will ultimately *preserve* eloquent brain regions. If a contusion acts as a mass lesion, reduction will allow the lower limit of autoregulation in the adjacent areas to begin to shift into a more normal region. Even if the ICP were not to decrease or CPP were not to increase, blood flow both globally and especially to the area surrounding the contusion site will improve toward more normal levels. In other words, the cerebral vasculature becomes more effective.

Many contusions appear relatively small or are of an intermediate size and have a related brain shift of only a few millimeters, and it is not easy to know whether these should be debrided. This is particularly true of balancing bifrontal contusions where brain shift is often manifest primarily by coaptation of the front horns. In these cases, when CPP is 70 to 80 mmHg and ICP is consistently 30 mmHg or greater, then consideration should be given to surgical debridement. The CPP must be low to stimulate *vasodilation* and elevate ICP per se. If ICP is to be a criteria for surgery, one must be certain that intracranial hypertension is primarily the result of the mass lesion rather than low CPP.

Reversal and Prevention of Ischemia A basic principle is that cerebral edema will never resolve in the presence of continued ischemia, and the ischemic brain will not be capable of adequate healing or recovery. A major problem with many previous studies of CBF was that an external xenon counting technique was used that scanned a relatively large volume of tissue at one time.[43] A nidus of ischemia may well exist within the region examined surrounded by a much larger volume affected by reactive hyperemia. Because the volume of hyperemia would be much larger than the ischemic nidus, the net result would be abnormally high CBF (Fig. 4-31).

The potential for falsely concluding that the pathophysiologic change is due to excess blood flow or luxury perfusion seems obvious. If steps are taken to reduce the blood flow, such as the use of blocking agents to treat hypertension, or hyperventilation to induce vasoconstriction, then indeed the hyperemia may be reduced, but the area of ischemia would be left untreated and would likely enlarge, potentially becoming generalized.[37-42,44-46] Ultimately, CBF would decline globally with a morbid outcome.

If these hyperemic areas are alternatively viewed as a worthwhile reaction to ischemia rather than part of the injurious process, then one may con-

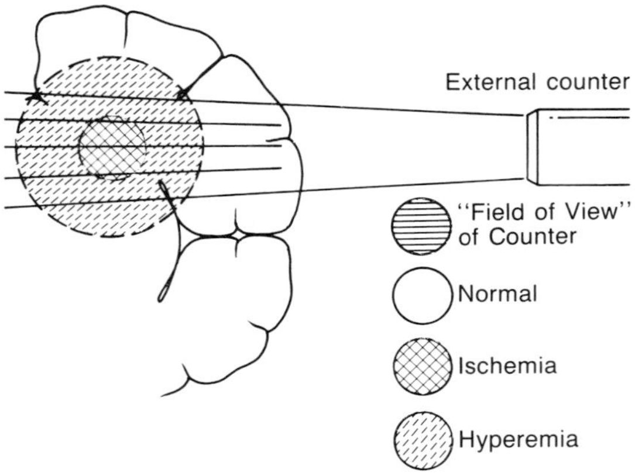

Figure 4-31 External, nontomographic technique of CBV measurement average the radiation from the isotope, usually Xenon, passing through the "field of view" of the counter. The ischemic zone will be surrounded by a much more voluminous zone of reactive hyperemia. When averaged, the result will be hyperemia. One might then, erroneously, conclude that the dangerous pathology is hyperemia rather than ischemia.

clude that many traditional therapies are potentially dangerous.

Cerebral Blood Flow and Poiseuille's Law In the manipulation of ischemia Poiseuille's law is probably the most important for establishing a rational basis for the selection of therapies and for understanding what to expect from each. There are three elements in Poiseuille's law that are amenable to manipulation. They are the pressure gradient across the vascular bed (CPP), vessel radius (r), and viscosity (n).

Pressure Gradient (CPP) When other factors are held constant, CBF will *always* be directly proportional to CPP (Fig. 4-10). In any short-term observation where CPP has decreased or increased, CBF will have followed to some degree. Therefore, maintenance and induction of elevations in systemic blood pressure or in the reduction of ICP will result in improvement in cerebral blood flow if CPP increases. This increase is likely to most affect areas least damaged, and unless blood flow is being monitored tomographically it will be difficult to judge whether the increase is adequate for injured areas.[47,48] Methods of determining the adequacy of the induced hypertension will be discussed below. In general, it is easier to elevate blood pressure than it is to reduce ICP in a constant and prolonged fashion.

Vessel Radius Vasodilation of even slight degree will increase blood flow *if CPP does not decline.* In general, this has not been clinically attempted since even modest increases in vascular diameter are likely to potentiate increased ICP and further reductions in CPP. This may in fact activate the vasodilatory cascade and stimulate the generation of Lundberg A or plateau waves (Figs. 4-20 and 4-32). Vascular radius is probably the least amenable to direct manipulation, and the essence of the manipulation of vessel diameter is that it be done in a manner in which CBF is not reduced.

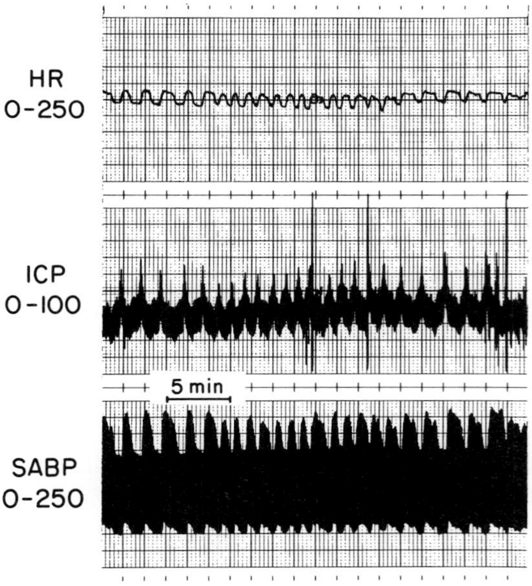

Figure 4-32 This trace demonstrates a classic recording of "B waves." While this trace makes the relationship of the B wave, and in particular, the termination spike, relatively straightforward, the reason for showing it is to demonstrate how difficult the ICP/SABP/CPP relations, as they have been described in this chapter, are to define with classical recording. When the time frame is even slower than this recording, the changes in blood pressure and intracranial pressure are virtually impossible to distinguish and these relationships will always be missed.

Viscosity and Rheology The two most important factors in determining viscosity are hematocrit and fibrinogen.[49] As hematocrit is reduced, blood flow will increase. However, oxygen delivery becomes an important factor in limiting the utility of viscosity reduction; once hematocrit drops below 30 percent, oxygen-carrying capacity begins to decrease. Therefore, to maximize oxygen delivery in order to meet metabolic needs of the injured brain, hematocrits in the range of 30 to 35 percent seem best.

The elements of Poiseuille's equation, if we assume a normal vessel reactivity and hold CBF constant, suggest that if we increase the CPP through systemic hypertension, the radius of the vasculature *must* decrease. This will result in a reduction in cerebral blood volume and a lower ICP.

Intravenous infusion of mannitol causes influx of extravascular water and will *hemodilute* the red cell mass reducing viscosity. When other factors are held constant, Poiseuille's law demands a reciprocal change in vascular radius. This will lead to a reduction in cerebral blood volume and a reduction in ICP. Some studies have suggested that mannitol acts by inducing vasoconstriction, but a more correct explanation is that mannitol *allows* the same CBF and oxygen delivery to be maintained via *smaller* vessels.[50–52] More will be discussed about the effects of mannitol later in this chapter.

Hemodilution due to mannitol or other mechanisms can be expected to be effective only when hematocrit is relatively high. When hematocrit is in the range of 30 to 35 percent, and further hemodilution occurs, oxygen delivery will decrease and stimulate vasodilation. Many ill patients are already mildly anemic with hematocrits of 30 to 35 percent but may still benefit from mannitol administration because mannitol has at least two other effects upon the hemodynamic and rheologic systems. First, mannitol causes red cells to shrink by approximately 15 percent and improves deformation and cell wall flexibility. Therefore, red cell effectiveness at delivering tissue oxygen improves after mannitol administration. Thus oxygen requirements are satisfied at either lower CPP or with greater vasoconstriction. It is easiest to visualize the vasculature as being *allowed* to constrict, with constant flow and CPP.[53,54] However, this is unrealistic. Intravascular volume increases massively after mannitol, cardiac output will increase, and blood pressure will increase.[55] Not only does mannitol make oxygen delivery to tissue more effective, it also *increases* the pressure gradient across the cerebral vasculature which further potentiates blood flow oxygen delivery and even greater vasoconstriction is allowed.[56] As the vasculature constricts and maintains blood flow and oxygen delivery constant, ICP decreases and CPP increases even further.[57] This allows continued vasoconstriction and, indeed, the events described by the vasoconstriction cascade (Figs. 4-33 and 4-34).

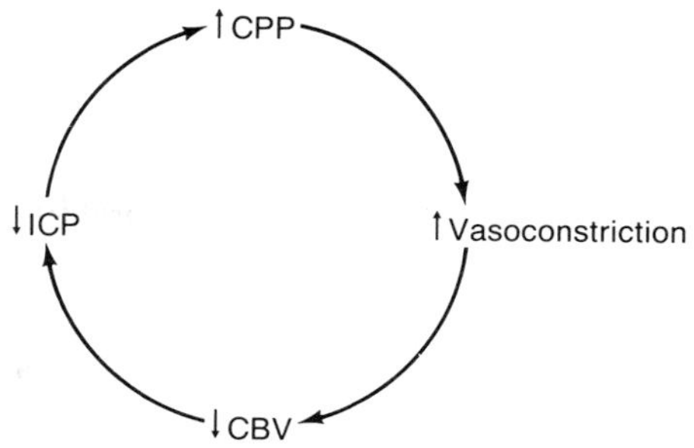

Figure 4-33 Vasoconstriction cascade model helps demonstrate the self-sustaining nature of incrementing the CPP. Given constant PCO_2, CMR-O_2, etc., an increment in the CPP stimulates vasoconstriction, lowers CBV and ICP, and potentiates CPP. The cycle continues until vasoconstriction is near maximal. Again, the patient must be "operating" within, or brought up to, *their* autoregulatory range.

Cerebral Metabolic Rate Much of this discussion has assumed the need for constant CBF. The demand for CBF is the cerebral metabolic rate for oxygen. If the $CMRO_2$ increases, then blood flow must increase. A common example occurs with arousal of a lethargic patient to a state where he or she obeys commands.[58,59] This change in arousal will be associated with an increase in $CMRO_2$ and must be subserved by an increase in oxygen delivery. Poiseuille's law shows that if flow is to increase, there must be a reduction in viscosity, an increase in pressure gradient (CPP), or an increase in vascular diameter. In the majority of clinical situations, the change to an aroused state is

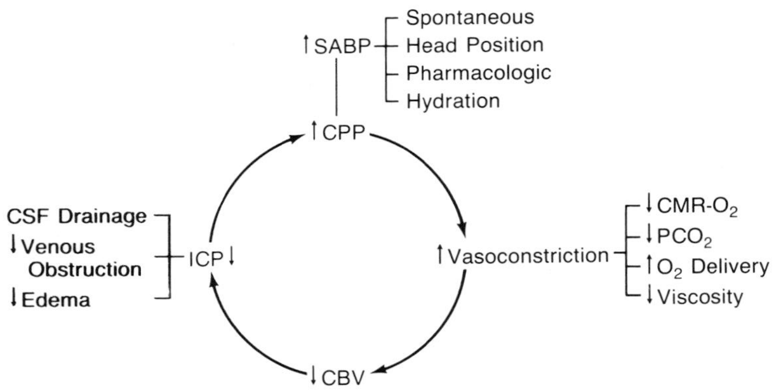

Figure 4-34 Complex vasoconstriction cascade model allows easier conceptualization of the *therapeutic* potential of this model system. CSF drainage can potentiate CPP by primarily lowering ICP. Mannitol potentiates (at least transiently) both O_2 delivery via decreased viscosity *and* SABP through vascular expansion. It becomes apparent that if mannitol is allowed to *dehydrate* the patient, then *vasodilatory* effects would predominate and mannitol "rebound" might occur. The "double-edge sword" nature of many neurosurgical interventions becomes apparent with this model.

accompanied by systemic blood pressure increases.[60] The CPP thus increases and subserves the increase in blood flow. If the increase in pressure is adequate, no change in vascular diameter will be required and ICP will remain constant. However, if the increase in systemic blood pressure does not occur, or is blocked pharmacologically, by the sympathectomy of quadriplegia, or inadequate vascular volume, etc., then the required CBF increase must be associated with vasodilation. (Fig. 4-33). An increase in ICP will follow. When ICP is low, this increase will be minimal and quickly buffered by CSF absorption, but when the volume tolerance of the brain has been consumed, such arousal can lead to a major increase in ICP and potential activation of the vasodilatory cascade. A plateau wave may result. It follows that the ability to *decrease* $CMRO_2$ is potentially useful in therapy.[61,62] The brain can reduce metabolic need by becoming comatose. The extreme of this situation is death of portions of the brain, which indeed reduces its metabolic needs. An example of this are patients who have transient ischemic attacks (TIAs) until they eventually have an infarct and the TIAs cease. Here the amount of brain has been reduced to accommodate the amount of blood flow available: The ultimate in matching of metabolism and flow.

The pharmacologic reduction in $CMRO_2$ is capable of reducing ICP under given circumstances.[61,62] If $CMRO_2$ is to be reduced, then blood flow can be reduced. Given constant viscosity, the reduction in flow can be brought about by a reduction in either CPP (which will leave the vascular radius and ICP unchanged) or the vasculature can constrict. This will reduce ICP and potentiate adequate perfusion pressure. Barbiturates are a class of drug that brings about these changes. These phenomena have been observed and occasionally attributed to a vasoconstrictive action of barbiturates. This is probably incorrect and the effect is better viewed as one analogous to the vasoconstriction allowed by mannitol: adequate oxygen delivery can be maintained with smaller caliber vessels. The action of barbiturates and other metabolic depressants is best viewed as *allowing* the vasculature to regulate itself to a smaller size yet maintain flow adequate for oxygen delivery.

As with most effective drugs there are side effects, and the barbiturates also reduce systemic arterial pressure (Fig. 4-23). Poiseuille's law predicts that if the pressure gradient is reduced, then either no effect on ICP may be realized, or if the reduction is great enough, then intracranial hypertension may be potentiated. This in fact has been described by Nakatani et al as a "parodoxical response to barbiturate therapy."[63] Clearly, reciprocal changes *must* exist between the pressure gradient in the vasculature and vascular radius.

The intraoperative use of barbiturates of various types to mitigate brain swelling is an extraordinarily useful maneuver. Pentothal 500 to 1000 mg given over a few minutes is profoundly effective at controlling brain swelling even under the most severe circumstances. However, to be effective, there must be careful attention to the systemic arterial blood pressure, often requiring support with pressor agents. Only then, with a decrease in $CMRO_2$ and thus the need for CBF, can the cerebral vasculature be allowed to constrict, reducing ICP.

Delineation of Adequate Cerebral Perfusion Pressure

If a decision is made to manage CPP as the primary goal of therapy, one must decide the CPP level at which active therapy is going to be invoked. In other words, what level should the CPP not fall below?

This is a complex question because CPP, as already discussed, is not necessarily uniform throughout the intracranial space. It is not necessarily the same between the supratentorial and the infratentorial spaces; in regions of tissue compression it may be substantially lower than in areas without edema, contusion, or other mass effect and will be lower distal to an arterial occlusion. So the first rule of CPP management becomes one of recognizing the limitations of the measure. CPP is best viewed as an *estimate* rather than an absolute value that is homogenous throughout the intracranial space. Several factors can serve as guidelines.

Guideline 1 The abnormal brain will always require higher CPP than the normal brain.[21,28,41,64] Accepting CPP levels of 50 or 60 mmHg (which represent the lower limits of autoregulation in normal, healthy individuals) will virtually *always underestimate* the ideal CPP level for the sick patient. Increasing severity of injury and the presence of brain shift both increase CPP requirements rather than decrease them. Focal mass lesions will be associated with regionally reduced CPP. To meet the needs of this tissue, greater than normal CPP levels will be required.

Guideline 2 Implicit within the patient's own physiologic response, is most of the information needed to estimate initial CPP limits. Schrader and associates have shown that the *Cushing response* is a response to inadequate blood flow affecting the rostral medulla and caudal pontine region.[29] When this region becomes ischemic, a sympathoadrenal discharge is generated manifest by increased systemic vasoconstrictor tone and circulating catecholamines. Systemic hypertension results, which improves blood flow to needed levels. The rostal medulla thus provides feedback control that serves to keep the arterial blood pressure centered about an adequate CPP. Thus, if CPP is less than adequate, a Cushing response can be observed.

The chronic hypertensive patient will have a much higher set point than the usually normotensive patient. The patient with hypertensive hemorrhage may require mean CPP $\geq$ 110 to 140 mmHg. The characteristic of a chronic hypertensive patient is that these apparently extreme levels of systemic pressure are frequently maintained quite well, as long as the physician does not interfere. Blood pressures of 240/120 (mean = 160) may occur. If the ICP is 30 to 40 mmHg, then the CPP is 120 to 130 mmHg. This is quite an acceptable circumstance when managing CPP; however, it may be troubling to the visiting internist or intensivist.

Physicians may attempt to lower the systemic arterial pressure slightly in order to "take the edge off" the blood pressure. Our observations suggest that this systemic hypertension is quite closely titrated to cerebral need and that this so called edge does not exist: These patients are already on the edge of adequate CPP. (Figs. 4-14 to 4-16, 4-18 to 4-20, 4-24 to 4-27). Another characteristic of this medullary-driven hypertension is that it can be extraordinarily difficult to treat as the result of continued sympathoadrenal discharge. The institution of low doses of sodium nitroprusside, nitroglycerin, and other antihypertensives may be virtually without effect until the blood pressure suddenly declines. The patient neurologically worsens, and often the baseline neurologic state cannot be regained by withholding these drugs or even raising the pressure further.

A similar situation exists in young children

where medical personnel expect much lower systemic arterial pressures. However, when young children are injured, they become quite hypertensive, and again this hypertension is a clear-cut guide to what their brains seem to require at any given moment. In children 1 to 2 years old, this often approaches adult blood pressure levels, and experience has shown that the same guidelines useful for adults also apply to children. There is a tendency for infants less than 6 to 12 months to require CPP closer to 60 mmHg than the adult levels of 70 to 90 mmHg.

Guidelines 3 to 8 are more specific techniques of identifying adequate CPP.

Guideline 3 Cyclic variations in ICP of significant degree, i.e., Lundberg A-waves or plateau waves of B-waves indicate that CPP is *inadequate.* The presence of these waves occasionally can be suspected from examination of the flowsheet and when there are wildly varying ICP levels recorded, or when CPP is relatively low. The presence of CSF pressure waves can be better detected with continuous recorders that allow moment-to-moment examination of ICP and their correlation with systemic arterial pressure and continuous estimates of CPP. The newer bedside monitoring systems with many hours of memory and the ability to resolve 1- to 2-s increments are ideal for this purpose.

Guideline 4 Artificially raising or stabilizing CPP at a constant level above the threshold will eliminate these waves (Figs. 4-14 to 4-16, 4-18 to 4-27, and 4-33 to 4-35, 4-37). A stable and lower ICP strongly suggests that the new threshhold CPP value is more appropriate for the patient.

Guideline 5 Figure 4-13 suggests that if CPP is above the lower limits of autoregulation, then ICP will vary inversely with CPP. Precipitating an increase in systemic arterial pressure is one of the mechanisms that can be used to increase CPP. If ICP should decrease or remain constant with an increase in CPP, then the patient is on the healthy side of the autoregulatory curve. This increase in pressure can be brought about by pharmacologic means such as infusion of a pressor agent such as phenylephrine or epinephrine. (Figs. 4-34 and 4-35). If ICP increases and CPP does not change with the increase in systemic arterial pressure, then the patient is low on the cerebral autoregulatory curve. Most often this will occur with a CPP of less than 50 to 70 mmHg, which will usually be inadequate for the patient with a severe injury.

Guideline 6 Another technique that *can* be very useful if it is understood is to use a pain stimulus to induce transient hypertension. The advantages are that it is a bedside technique, it is part of the normal neurologic examination of comatose patients, does not require the use of drugs or other potentially toxic agents, and it is quick. If painful stimulus is applied, systemic arterial pressure increases, and CPP increases with a concomitant reduction or stability of ICP, then this information can be used to determine where on the autoregulatory curve that patient is functioning.

There are two limitations using this technique. First, with rapid and acute increase in systemic arterial pressure elevating CPP the cerebral vasculature will require 5 to 10 s or more to respond with vasoconstriction. In the interval before vasoconstriction, there may occur what has been termed the *termination spike* of the ICP (Figs. 4-14 to 4-16, 4-18 to 4-22, 4-24, 4-36, 4-37). If only ICP is being monitored, then those unfamiliar with the manipulation of CPP may conclude that the painful stimulus led to an ICP increase and was the wrong thing to do. To judge the ICP response, adequate time, usually 1 to 2 min, must be allowed for the resolution of the termination spike and the response of the ICP. Throughout this period of time, the stimulus must be applied in order to maintain the systemic arterial pressure. If the pressure is only driven up and then rapidly drops back to or even below baseline before the generalized vasoconstriction of the cerebral vasculature has had a chance to come into effect, one can misinterpret this test (Fig. 4-36).

Second, depending upon the neurologic status of the patient, the painful stimulus may be associated with *arousal* and an increase in $CMRO_2$. If $CMRO_2$ and blood flow requirements should increase, then the increase in systemic pressure associated with the arousing stimulus may be only barely adequate to supply this increased flow. Poiseuille's law suggests that the radius of the vessel will then not change and there may be little if any change in ICP. If indeed the degree of $CMRO_2$ in-

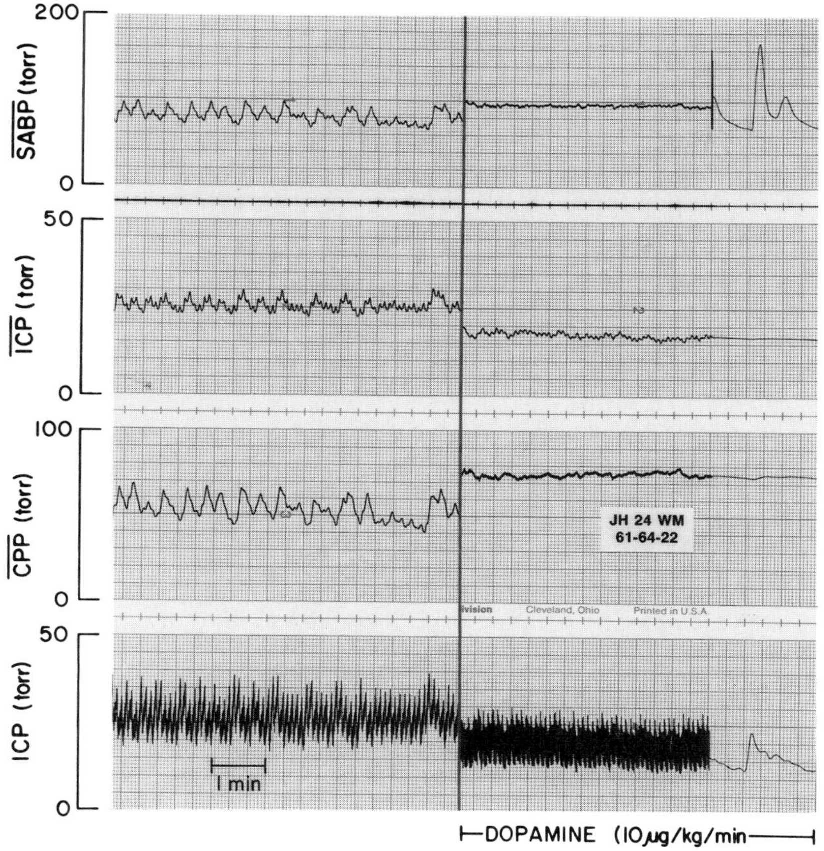

Figure 4-35 The left panel of this photograph is the spontaneous SABP/ICP/CPP trace. The SABP varied between 70 and 100 torr. Intracranial pressure varied about 25 torr. Neither of these values are particularly extreme nor is the mean SABP particularly low. However, when we examine the CPP, we realize that it is varying between 45 and 65 mmHg, which represents the lower limit of autoregulation of a *normal* individual. By starting a dopamine infusion and stabilizing the systemic arterial pressure at a level which was equal to the highest level reached spontaneously, CPP improved to approximately 75 torr and intracranial pressure actually stabilized at approximately 17 torr. This latter effect was due to the vasoconstrictor stimulus induced by elevation in the CPP. This effect of pressors on the SABP/CPP/ICP is nonspecific. Any method of elevation of the blood pressure (phenylephrine, epinephrine, norepinephrine) will produce the same effect. The goal is to use the least toxic agent.

crease is greater than the relative increase in SABP, then ICP may actually increase: in this case stimulating the patient may be detrimental.

Guideline 7 CPP versus PVI. Figure 4-29 suggests that PVI calculated at multiple different cerebral perfusion pressures may provide a quantitative estimate of whether a patient is on the healthy versus low side of the autoregulatory curve. If PVI is plotted at multiple CPP levels and the slope is positive then the suggestion is that the patient is on

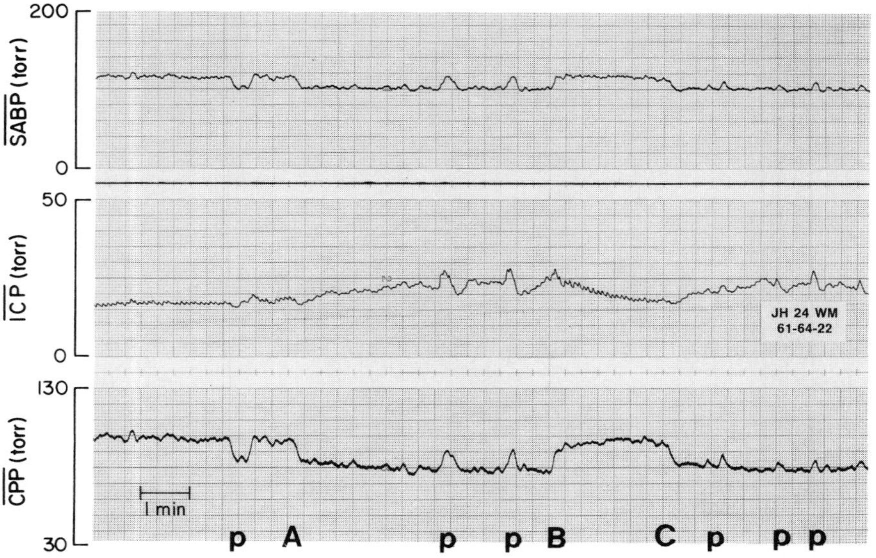

Figure 4-36 This figure demonstrates the importance of the duration of SABP change. At point A the SABP declines from approximately 115 mmHg to 100 mmHg and CPP decrements. The ICP rises slightly and then begins to decline at point B as the SABP returns to baseline levels, and by C the perfusion pressure and ICP have returned approximately to baseline. Note that there are perturbations in SABP which are of very short duration. They are associated with generally passive changes in ICP and CPP. In general, these changes are direct in nature because they cycle too quickly to allow active vasodilatation or vasoconstriction. Note the difference between the two ICP peaks just before point B. These are both marked with p and in essence represent termination spikes which are not associated with a long enough duration SABP response to continue the vasoconstriction cascade as appeared at point B. The decrement in SABP occurring just before point A was also of too short a duration to significantly affect the ICP trace, though it did vary somewhat.

the healthy side of the autoregulatory curve. If the slope is negative, regardless of how good the PVI values appear, then the patient is on the low side of the curve. This remains a highly promising technique for determination of CPP thresholds in individual patients.

Guideline 8 Jugular oxygen saturation. The technique of placing a catheter in the jugular bulb and continuously monitoring SjO_2 is appealing. It provides a continuous moment-to-moment measure that when combined with arterial oxygen saturation measures may allow estimates of the adequacy of cerebral oxygen delivery relative to oxygen consumption. Little information has accumulated using this technique in CPP management, though some results are consistent with the threshold values identified using the other techniques already noted. Most patients with significant brain injury and intracranial pathology require a CPP of 70 to 80 mmHg using this technique as a criterion.

The potential difficulties of SjO_2 monitoring are similar to other techniques that volume average large areas of the brain. Significant focal areas of ischemia may not be represented. If ischemia is severe enough, the tissue will be nonfunctional and contribute neither to oxygen consumption nor desaturation of cerebral venous blood, though these areas may well contribute to further brain edema, local compression, and potentiation of ischemia.

So this global measure may in fact suggest adequacy of CBF and oxygen delivery but *underestimate* the specific needs of subfrontal, temporal, or other areas inadequately perfused.[65]

To some extent this is a potential difficulty with all the techniques mentioned above. These reduce to a single number, CPP, the entire intracranial content. Those that rely solely on the threshold of the Cushing response may also underestimate the CPP required. The results of CPP management will be discussed in greater detail and in comparison with traditional forms of management. However, those techniques that rely solely on the Cushing response are using a technique that is sensitive to caudal pontine and rostral medullary blood flow. While clearly CPP must be adequate to supply the brainstem, the adequacy of that may be insufficient for perfusion of contused and otherwise damaged supratentorial structures.

Systemic Arterial Blood Pressure Management

An important aspect of management of the systemic arterial blood pressure to improve CPP is recognition that systemic hypertension is required for survival in the face of intracranial hypertension. The degree of hypertension closely relates to the required CPP for the individual under observation. This systemic arterial blood pressure is often somewhat unstable. Natural variations will be magnified in the presence of inadequate vascular volume.

Maintenance of adequate *vascular* volume is the mainstay of management of the systemic arterial pressure component of CPP therapy. In some ways this is similar to the approach used for treatment of cerebral vasospasm. As in that disorder, the monitoring of adequate vascular volume becomes paramount. The presence of the highly adrenergic state characteristic of traumatic brain injury and other CNS insults makes the use of the systemic arterial pressure alone a poor measure of adequate vascular volume. Most patients are tachycardic; therefore, the heart rate becomes less useful. However, both of these must be assessed. Wide variations in systemic arterial pressure or heart rate suggest the need for increased intravascular volume. These clinical observations must be combined with clinical assessment of the patient, including tissue turgor or edema, urine output, and specific gravity. Monitoring of systemic vascular volume can be augmented by central venous pressure measurements and pulmonary artery catheter measurements as reviewed in Chap. 1.

The use of serum sodium to estimate the degree of hydration is problematic. Dehydration may be associated with hyponatremia or hypernatremia. A decrease in urine output or changes in blood urea nitrogen and creatinine occurs only *after* inadequate volume and inadequate renal perfusion have become established. The problem of inadequate vascular volume once well established is easily recognized. However, the real essence of brain injury therapy is the anticipation and prevention of such events.

Natural CPP homeostatic mechanisms are relatively effective though not always adequate or consistent enough for stable systemic hypertension. The use of pressors to stabilize systemic arterial pressure at or slightly above what appears to be the needed CPP threshold for a particular patient is extremely useful. Certain drugs are more reliable than others in stabilizing the CPP via the systemic arterial pressure side. Experience with phenylephrine in doses not exceeding 2 to 4 μg/kg per min has shown this drug to be fairly reliable. When CPPs are stabilized using phenylephrine, dopamine at 2 μg/kg per min has been instituted to help protect the kidneys from the vasoconstrictor effects of phenylephrine. This helps reduce the renal and systemic toxicity of this drug. Levophed at 0.04 to 0.1 μg/kg per min is proving more reliable and predictable than phenylephrine (Figs. 4-35 and 4-37); however, the peripheral vascular side effects of Levophed may prove unacceptable.

The use of pressors does complicate the issue of adequate vascular volume. Vasoconstrictor agents such as phenylephrine increase afterload on the left ventricle and tend to increase the pulmonary capillary wedge pressure (PCWP). If the vasoconstrictor were not present, the PCWP would be lower. Because these agents also increase preload on the right ventricle, the central venous pressure is also elevated. These elevations are real but do not represent true vascular volume. Thus, if the PCWP and the CVP appear to be normal in the face of phenylephrine or other vasoconstrictor

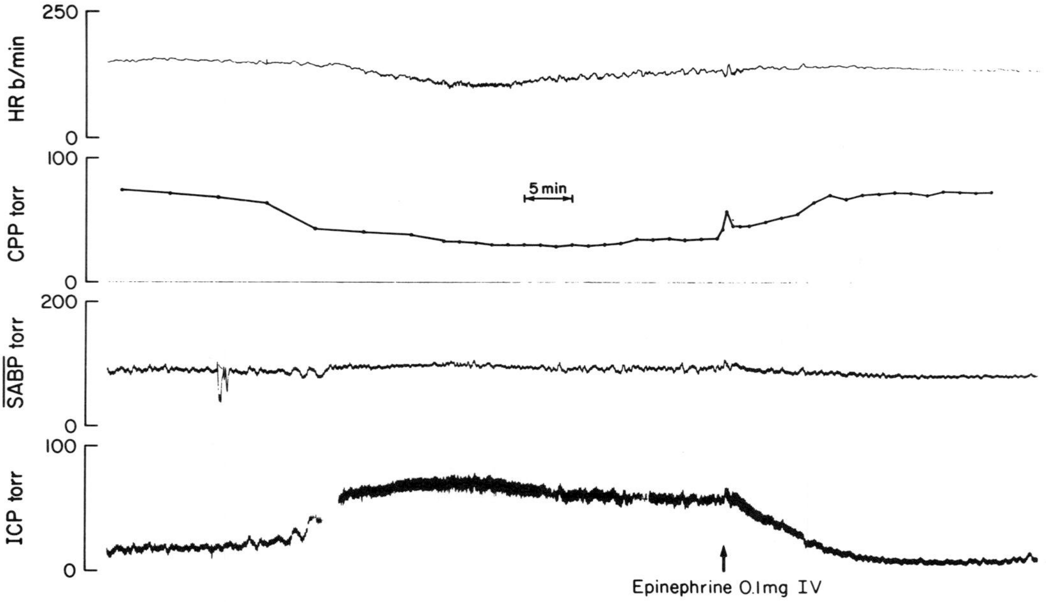

Figure 4-37 This was a plateau wave reaching nearly 70 mmHg in a patient with a CNS neoplasm. The CPP trace is hand-plotted and many of the transient variations are missed. However, the CPP trace gives an approximation of this estimate. Note the plateau wave was terminated by a small dose of intravenous epinephrine which raised the blood pressure 10 to 15 mmHg. CPP improved by 15 to 20 mmHg and then continued to improve as the plateau wave was aborted. While continuous CPP recordings would have been of utility, the phenomenon is well explained. Note that as the plateau wave developed, the blood pressure was becoming more unstable and then stabilized at a baseline level. However, this was not adequate to reverse the continued decline in CPP brought about by earlier SABP changes, and therefore, the plateau wave continued to evolve. The decrement in heart rate during the midst of the plateau wave can be viewed as reflex bradycardia.

therapy, there is probably a need for increased vascular volume.

The best vascular expander is red blood cells although concentrated albumin is also very effective. A signal that a patient may be a candidate for red cell transfusion is unstable blood pressure in the face of normal CVP and PCWP, on pressors with a hematocrit of 30 percent or less. The total red cell mass in these patients is usually 50 percent or less of normal though the hematocrit appears adequate. Measurement of the circulating plasma and red cell volumes can be useful although this test is not universally available.

Adequate fluid intake does not guarantee adequate vascular volume. The neurosurgical fluid problem is vascular expansion without overhydration. It is quite possible for a patient to be 5 or more liters overhydrated but with inadequate vascular volume. This is best treated with transfusions of blood and concentrated colloid, which tend to remain in the intravascular space.

Intracranial Pressure

The treatment of ICP in a CPP context is quite important. However, this is more complex than may first appear because therapies that affect ICP beneficially without simultaneously decreasing the systemic arterial pressure side of therapy must be used (Figs. 4-33 and 4-34). This means eliminating certain therapies that may be traditional in some units and modifying the manner in which other modalities are utilized. This theme is well illustrated when we examine mannitol and its effects.

Mannitol

Mannitol has at least three putative mechanisms of action that are mutually complementary: blood pressure elevation, improvement of rheologic aspects of the circulation, and dehydration of the brain.[51,55,57,66] The mechanism for which there is the least amount of evidence is cerebral dehydration.[63,67] Lastly, the infusion of a large osmotic load of mannitol will quickly raise serum osmolality. This osmolar gradient is necessary if water is to be moved out of the brain or any other organ. However, within 5 min or so of mannitol administration, the serum osmolality will drop to only slightly above normal levels. This is secondary to the movement of extravascular water into the vascular space which effectively dilutes the serum osmolality toward normal.[68,69] In the meantime, the osmotic gradient that is encouraging water to move out of the brain is rapidly disappearing as the result of very rapid movement of systemic water through capillaries into the vasculature. While unconvincing in terms of cerebral water removal, the movement of the vascular water into the circulation dilutes hemoglobin and fibrinogen. This will reduce blood viscosity, which will allow the same blood flow to occur with a smaller caliber cerebral vessel (Poiseuille's law). Thus there is vasoconstriction that will tend to lower ICP. Concomitantly, the red cell shrinks and becomes more deformable and, therefore, is more effective at delivering its oxygen load to tissue. This is probably quite important for marginally perfused and damaged tissue. This will potentiate the ability of the vessel to deliver adequate nutrition at a small vessel diameter.[70] Again, mannitol seems to *allow* rather than cause vasoconstriction (Figs. 4-38 and 4-39).

The tremendous influx of extravascular water into the vascular space has the very real advantage of potentiating or stabilizing systemic arterial pressure. As cardiac output increases so will blood pressure, and this will affect the CPP in a positive manner.[55]

As with all drugs, mannitol has potential difficulties and complications. First, it is an osmotic diuretic. It is extremely effective at inducing negative fluid balance, and most of its mechanism is

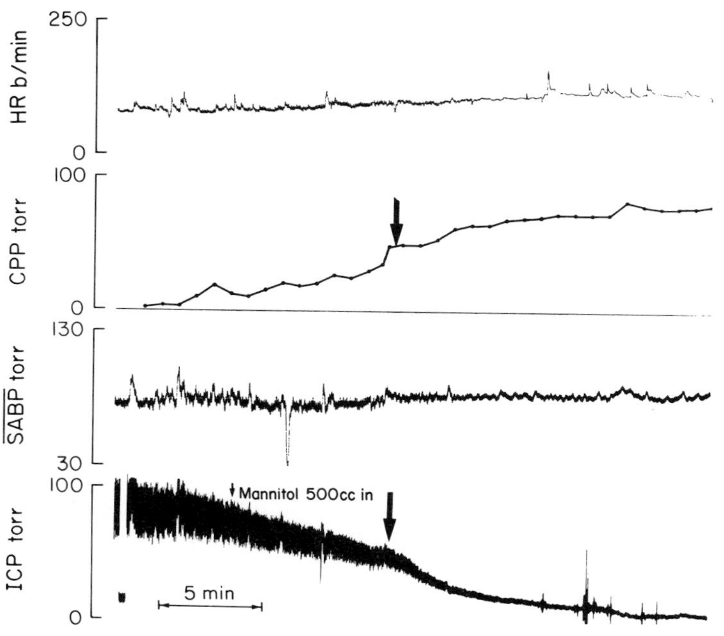

Figure 4-38 This trace demonstrates the ICP reduction following mannitol. At the small vertical arrow, 500 mL of mannitol has finished infusing. The infusion had begun approximately 10 to 15 min before this point. The ICP was decrementing very slowly and SABP remained relatively constant. This is an example of viscosity changes, red cell changes, and perhaps minimal SABP changes which were improving oxygen delivery and allowing vasoconstriction to occur. At the large vertical arrow, the CPP threshold for vasoconstriction was passed and the *slow* decline in ICP rapidly accelerated. Note that this was at a CPP of approximately 60 mmHg, which suggests that this patient is actually moving into the "benign" side of his autoregulatory curve. It was at this point that autoregulatory vasoconstriction became effective. The vasoconstriction cascade began to cycle and further reduced ICP to very low levels.

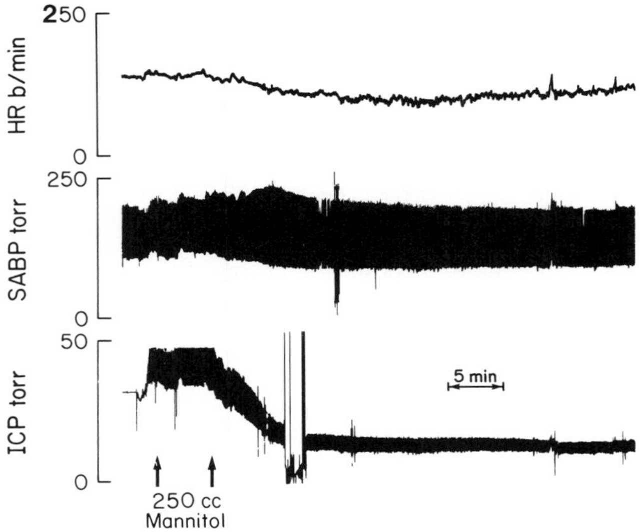

Figure 4-39 Note the effect of 1 g/kg of mannitol infused in this patient with CNS lymphoma. There was an increase in SABP and a decrement in heart rate due to the vascular expansion induced by mannitol. This vascular expansion is a function of transiently high serum osmolality which draws extravascular water into the vascular compartment. This will increase cardiac output, increase systemic arterial blood pressure, help decrement the pulse, and improve cerebral oxygen delivery. Under these conditions, the result will be increased vasoconstriction and a reduction in intracranial pressure. Note the very rapid reduction in ICP after mannitol was infused. This was most compatible with hemodynamic and other "vascular" effects of mannitol. While they are not incompatible with "cerebral dehydration," the latter mechanism is much less likely.

due to its vascular expansion effects. As negative fluid balance evolves, the result will be hemoconcentration and intravascular depletion. Some of the water will move back into the extravascular space, but much will have been lost via renal excretion. Thus, hemodilution or the positive effects on viscosity are lost and even *reversed* as the circulating blood volume decreases. This will reduce the cardiovascular system's ability to maintain adequate perfusion. Poiseuille's equation predicts that vasodilation will be required in order to maintain constant oxygen delivery and blood flow. If the increase in viscosity and decrease in perfusion pressure are great enough, an actual increase in ICP beyond that originally seen (mannitol rebound) will be encountered.[51] This may not be obvious after only a single dose of mannitol in the newly resuscitated and perhaps overhydrated polytrauma patient, but as net dehydration evolves, the clinician will note that mannitol first becomes less effective, later associated with mannitol rebound, and then not effective at all.

If fluid therapy has been inadequate to negate the diuretic effects of mannitol, renal tubular toxicity will be potentiated. Even in the face of relatively normal hydration, mannitol is toxic to the tubular system of the kidney. This toxicity is reversible, but not necessarily quickly or easily, and mannitol toxicity is cumulative, usually requiring several hundred grams over 2 to 3 days before it is manifest. If frequent high-dose mannitol is combined with vasopressors for the stabilization or induction of systemic hypertension, aminoglycoside or other nephrotoxic antibiotics and drugs, and a history of an hypoxic and/or hypotensive episode, the result can be devastating to the kidneys. Acute renal failure is a frequent consequence in this scenario and is further potentiated by inadequate vascular volume.

Therefore, when patients are judged to be euvo-

Table 4-1 Comparison of Traditional Versus CPP Management

Modality	Traditional ICP therapy	CPP Management
Position	Elevate HOB ≥ 30°	HOB = 0°: Patient flat
Fluids	⅔ Maintenance BUN 35 mg/dL	Hydrate normally I = O + losses
Hypertension	Prevent Use sedatives Use antihypertensives Use blockers Avoid stimulation	Facilitate Vascular expansion Vasopressors Active stimulation
Mannitol	Osmolality 310–320 mOsm Replace ⅔ diuresis	Normal osmolality Replace mL/mL if patient euvolemic I = O + losses
Barbiturates	Burst suppression	Avoid cardiac depressants
Hyperventilation	P_{CO_2} 25–28 mmHg	P_{CO_2} 35–40 mmHg "Bag" acutely only

HOB = head of bed; I = intake; O = output.

lemic, the diuresed fluid after mannitol administration must be replaced mL for mL. This is a point where the decision to manage CPP deviates widely from traditional therapy (Table 4-1).

Because most of the identified mechanisms of mannitol relate to hemodynamic and rheologic effects that are based on the rapid change in serum osmolality brought about by rapid infusions, there is little rationale for the establishment of a continuous infusion or frequent intermittent doses designed to maintain serum osmolality in the 310- to 320-mOsm range. The potential for cumulative toxicity is also increased, since a large percentage of this hyperosmolality may come from dehydration.

Diuretics

The use of furosemide in neurologic surgery has been widespread for many years. The best accumulation of data suggests that furosemide combined with mannitol is able to potentiate the duration of the ICP reduction though not necessarily the degree of the reduction.[69]

With regard to CPP management, it must be remembered that furosemide is not only a loop diuretic capable of inducing negative sodium and fluid balance, but it is also an antihypertensive. Furosemide may therefore have a net advantage *or* disadvantage. Furosemide is extremely effective, especially when combined with mannitol, when the patient is overhydrated. It should be pointed out that all states involving overhydration involve an *increase* in the total body sodium. Furosemide and mannitol are synergistic at inducing diuresis *and* natriuresis and result in a proportionate decrease in the component of overhydration affecting the brain.

Because furosemide is an antihypertensive and mannitol is a volume expander, adding the latter may avert deleterious CPP effects as well as potentiate diuresis and natriuresis. These are desirable *only* if the patient is overhydrated. In the absence of overhydration and excess total body sodium, furosemide has only a limited role to play in CPP management, and if diuresis leads to volume depletion, the drug may have a distinct disadvantage.

Ventilator Management

Manipulation of the ventilator interacts with nearly all aspects of ICP and CPP control. Appropriate oxygenation and hemoglobin saturation and establishment of a stable Pa_{CO_2} are critical. But less recognized are the negative effects of overventilation and excessively high positive end-expiratory pressure (PEEP), excessive ventilator rate, and tidal volume, which reduce systemic arterial blood pressure and decrease CPP.

The most obvious neurosurgical manipulation of the ventilator relates to regulation of the Pa_{CO_2}. Because of the rapid equilibration of the vasculature to hypocapnia and return to near-baseline vascular diameters and cerebral blood volume, CPP management has usually been accomplished within the context of normocapnia, with Pa_{CO_2} maintained at about 35 mmHg.[23] Maintenance of higher P_{CO_2} levels also allows reduced mechanical ventilation. Reduction in tidal volume (V_t) and therefore mean and peak inspiratory pressures (PIP) is accomplished. Accepting hemoglobin saturation of 90 percent (Pa_{O_2} 60 to 70 mmHg) also reduces the need for PEEP and high Fi_{O_2}.

Given less of a demand in terms of mechanical ventilation, the hemodynamic effects of mechanical ventilation are minimized. High volume–high rate ventilation has a tendency to reduce preload and reduce systemic arterial blood pressure. This is counterproductive to the maintenance of CPP.

While hyperventilation has no demonstrated benefit in terms of long-term cerebral vasoconstriction and maintenance of ICP control, it does have utility when ICP rises and requires acute intervention. However, the nursing and physician staff must recognize that vigorous "bagging" or aggressive elevation of the rate of mechanical ventilation can result in a decrease in systemic pressure. Even temporary benefits that might be derived from hypocapneic induction of vasoconstriction may be lost if systemic arterial pressure decreases and reduces CPP. At best, this may result in no change in ICP because both effects cancel. At worst, ICP may continue to rise and CPP to decline. When this circumstance is encountered, the alternatives are use of a bolus of mannitol and increasing CPP with fluids, blood, colloid, or pressors.

Positive End-Expiratory Pressure

The use of PEEP in the head-injured patient has been controversial. The rationale for avoiding PEEP was that this pressure would be transmitted to the venous system, then to the sagittal sinus, and thus to the cerebral venous system, which would raise ICP. Actual evidence suggests that PEEP only affects ICP when it interferes with the systemic arterial pressure.[71,72] The mechanism would be by the induction of arteriolar vasodilation due to reduced CPP as opposed to increased venous back pressure. Venous back pressure is probably only important in ICP dynamics when ICP is relatively low. Even high levels of PEEP (15 to 20 cmH_2O) represent only 10 to 15 mmHg, which is trivial within a cerebral venous system that may be draining at a pressure of 30 to 40 mmHg or greater.

However, not all the PEEP is transmitted to the central venous system. Under conditions characterized by poor pulmonary compliance, PEEP is *not* transmitted directly to the central venous system and potentially to the cranial venous systems. On balance, the patient is better off being treated with the PEEP sufficient to maintain lung volume and adequate oxygenation.

Head Position

Perhaps no aspect of CPP management has yielded more controversy than one of its simplest and most effective components, flattening of the head of the bed. The rationale for elevation of the head is reduction of sagittal sinus pressure, potentiation of cerebral venous drainage into the cerebral venous sinuses and thence into the systemic circulation. The decrease in cerebral venous volume should lower the ICP.[18,73–77] Indeed, the ICP in 50 to 70 percent of patients is approximately 7 to 10 mmHg higher with 0° of head elevation than with 30 to 50° of head elevation.[78]

But when the head is elevated above the heart, the hydrostatic pressure in the carotid artery at the level of the head is diminished by an amount roughly equal to the distance between the point of measurement at the level of the head and the reference level at the heart.[79] This hydrostatic difference in systemic arterial blood pressure is often greater than the 7-mmHg reduction in ICP attained by elevating the head of the bed; the net result is a reduction of CPP. When assessing this phenomenon, it is very important that the ICP and systemic arterial blood pressure transducers be at the same level. When using monitors such as the fiberoptic techniques, the zero point is at the tip of the fiber-optic cable and is not influenced by other factors. The same is true of epidural monitors. The arterial transducer (usually fluid coupled to the arterial system) must be raised not to the base of the skull or to the foramen of Monro, but to the zero level of these transducers. Failure to do this can give a false sense of security in terms of CPP values. Misinterpretation of CPP and ICP information as a result of body position changes is frequent. If the head is raised with a concomitant reduction in arterial pressure at the level of the head, and ICP falls *without a change* in CPP, then the ICP reduction is the result of vasocollapse.[80]

It is likely that when ICP is only modestly elevated and cerebral blood volume is available for displacement into the systemic circulation, that the two effects (decreased venous volume and lower CPP) *may* neutralize each other. However, when severe intracranial hypertension exists, this is not likely to be the case. Direct-observation studies show venous system collapse as ICP is increased: little additional venous volume is available for displacement.[14,81–83] It is our practice, with a patient that has severe intracranial hypertension, to nurse them in the flat position, with all the transducers referenced to the same level. Continuous estimates of CPP, ICP, systemic arterial blood pressure, central venous pressure, and pulmonary artery pressure may easily be interrelated. One-third of the patients demonstrate an increase in intracranial hypertension when the head of the bed is elevated.[77,78] This can be viewed as the result of decreased CPP and activation of the vasodilatory cascade, with the generation of ICP waves. These waves can then be aborted by placing the patient supine.

CSF Drainage

Ventricular drainage is extremely useful once the potential complications of ventriculostomy placement have been passed. However, ventricular drainage is limited when ICP begins to reach the range of 30 mmHg and greater. This is secondary to compression or coaptation of the ventricular system around the catheter tip and obstruction or lack of drainage. There is some evidence that CSF production may be decreased at ICPs of 30 mmHg or more, although this is controversial. Regardless of the actual mechanism, CSF drainage is most effective when ICPs can be maintained at less than 25 to 30 mmHg. Drainage of CSF should be employed liberally to maintain CPP at the highest value possible.

Fluid Management

The fluid management techniques necessary for maintenance of a CPP regimen are substantially different from the dehydration techniques used in traditional ICP management. One can view the basic difference as analogous to the treatment of ARDS with the two primary theoretical approaches. One is a low PEEP-dehydration technique aimed at minimizing fluid movement into the lung by minimizing fluid available. The other is a high-PEEP, high-fluid technique designed to support the cardiovascular and pulmonary systems while the process evolves and resolves. CPP management is analogous to the latter; traditional ICP management relates to the former.

The primary goal of CPP fluid management is euvolemia or slight hypervolemia but avoiding systemic overhydration. In other words, the goal is to maintain the vascular space in a well-expanded state without creating excessive extravascular water. When a patient is overhydrated, the brain will equilibrate with the rest of the body and eventually take part in that overhydration. This may potentiate brain edema and intracranial hypertension.

The advantages of a euvolemic, normally hydrated patient are clearly apparent in the cardiovascular system's ability to maintain the hypertension needed to perfuse the damaged brain. Euvolemia will allow more stable blood pressure, require less in the way of pressor support, and minimize systemic arterial blood pressure changes due to ventilator manipulation. By adequately perfusing the kidneys, nephrotoxic effects of mannitol, pressors, and sepsis are minimized.

The disadvantages of attaining euvolemia related to the greater sophistication required on the part of the clinician. Most of the simple indicators such as blood pressure, heart rate, blood urea nitrogen (BUN), creatinine, and urine output do not apply. They either are artificially elevated or only change late in the course of evolving volume depletion as has been discussed previously. Because of the sustained systemic hypertension and, in particular, when it is combined with the use of systemic pressors and dopamine, the urine output will be falsely high often reaching 200 to 250 mL/h. This must be replaced mL for mL with care to avoid overhydration and significantly positive sodium balance. Again the sophistication required is much greater than simply writing an order for 50 mL/h.

The primary advantage of dehydration techniques is that many neurosurgeons know what to expect from the gradual volume depletion and dehydration of patients. This is occasionally titrated to BUN levels of 35 mg/dL. There is *no evidence* that dehydration in any form has actually improved outcome.

The disadvantages of dehydration are manifest in multiple organ systems. Clearly dehydration makes patients more susceptible to unstable and inadequate systemic and cerebral perfusion. If the blood pressure is inadequate to maintain cerebral perfusion, then the brain will suffer. The dehydrated patient is more susceptible to orthostatic changes in blood pressure as the head of the bed is raised. In traditional neurosurgery these two therapies have frequently been combined. The renal toxicity of virtually all drugs commonly used in the neurosurgical patient such as aminoglycoside antibiotics, mannitol, transfusion reactions, other diuretics, and most other nephrotoxins are amplified and potentiated by dehydration. Dehydration also leads to hemoconcentration, to the false sense of security that red cell mass is actually adequate because the hematocrit is high, and to the adverse effects on viscosity of higher hematocrits. When dehydration is well established, the patient will become refractory to mannitol therapy. The *diagnosis* of clinical dehydration can frequently be made in the face of a patient who has over a 24-h period or so stopped responding to mannitol. A substantial degree of mannitol's mechanism of action is dependent upon its ability to draw extravascular water into the vascular space, and if the extravascular water does not exist, mannitol will have only a minimal effect. But toxicity will be amplified.

Sodium

The sodium ion is of primary importance in maintenance of the intravascular and extravascular, extracellular spaces. In essence, where sodium goes, water will follow. The kidneys function more efficiently to excrete a water load than they do a sodium load. This suggests that as positive sodium balance develops there will be an element of water retention. It is clinically useful to view all overhydrated patients as having an increase in total body sodium. Sodium will move into the extravascular space of the brain. This movement is normally quite slow, but in the face of abnormalities of blood-brain barrier function, contusions, and other foci of edema, this movement is quite rapid. Cerebral edema fluid is sodium-rich.[84,85] It is the sodium that will help hold water and draw water into edematous areas as well. While this is inevitable to some extent, the process can be potentiated by significantly positive sodium balance.

In the practical management of the fluid status during CPP management, regular urinary sodium values are obtained. If the patient is judged to be euvolemic with an adequate but not excessive sodium load, then these values are used to select which intravenous fluid will be used for the subsequent fluid replacement. If a patient has received very large amounts of crystalloid as part of resusitation and has large third-space fluid sequestration, then as the patient improves he or she may well become hypernatremic because of the relative ease with which the kidney excretes a free-water load. In this case hypernatremia is a stage in resolution of the overhydration; it represents excessive total body sodium that will eventually be excreted. Fluid management during this stage should consist of free water only.

Pseudotumor cerebri has already been eluded to as a disease precipitated in susceptible individuals by excess total body sodium. In most of these patients, restriction of salt intake has effectively controlled both papilledema, headaches, and lumbar CSF pressures without the need for shunting. While compliance with this therapy is difficult and may limit its applicability in some patients, the insights gained into the potential of sodium alone to lead to intracranial hypertension and/or to potentiate it are extremely useful.[4,5]

This issue has received little attention when the mechanism of action of furosemide and other diuretics has been considered.[84–87] Virtually all diuretics including acetazolamide are capable of inducing natriuresis. This is particularly true when there is an excess of sodium available for excretion. Experience with the combination of mannitol and furosemide in the face of overhydration has shown the combination to be very effective at mobilizing tissue salt and water. Experience in the absence of overhydration with furosemide has shown it to be not helpful but detrimental.

Traditional Management

Traditional management techniques are directed at reduction of ICP only. This is most important in understanding their evolution and application.

Head Position Traditionally, patients have had their heads elevated to approximately 30° for much of the last 2 decades. This serves to lower ICP and in most studies will reduce this value on average by approximately 7 mmHg. This applies to approximately two-thirds of the patients. It should be pointed out that studies that examine the effects of moving from the supine to the upright position or vice versa demonstrate that approximately one-third of patients may actually have intracranial hypertension potentiated by this maneuver. No study has shown improved clinical outcome with head elevation.

Systemic Arterial Pressure Management The concept of vasoparalysis, i.e., the utter inability of the cerebral vasculature to react to pressure changes in a normal or near normal fashion, has lead to the concern that systemic hypertension potentiates vasodilation that will lead to cerebral hyperemia, further progression of cerebral edema, and death. Given this concern, control of systemic hypertension has been considered important and aggressive pharmacologic management has often been carried out. This has included the use of beta-blockers and some of the derivative agents both of shorter and longer duration. Sodium nitroprusside and other intravenous titratable drugs have also been used.

Related to the pharmacologic control of systemic hypertension is a wide variety of patient manipulations that are avoided because of their potential to increase ICP. Bathing, rectal temperatures, endotracheal and nasotracheal suctioning, family visitation, bright lights, neurologic exams, and painful stimulation have all been associated at one time or another with the potentiation of intracranial hypertension.

Fluid and Electrolyte Management Dehydration therapy based upon the concept that if there is less water available in the body, there will be less water available to potentiate cerebral edema, has been standard in many centers for the last 2 decades and longer. The recommendation that this be titrated to a BUN of 35 mg/dL has been made. The replacement of urine volume lost after mannitol administration has been recommended to be limited to two-thirds of the diuresed amount. Closely related to this is the clinical observation that mannitol and furosemide used together result in a greater diuresis than either agent alone and that this is a desirable end point of therapy.

Closely related to the induction of negative fluid balance has been the avoidance of hypoosmolar states. The traditional recommendation has been to maintain serum sodium in the 145- to 150-meq/L range. This is closely related to the maintenance of serum osmolality at 310 to 320 mOsm, often with the frequent use of mannitol. The rationale is that if a slightly hyperosmolar serum condition is maintained, then brain water will be encouraged to move into the systemic circulation; therefore, cerebral edema will not be worsened and may be improved. To this end, free water and hypotonic/hypoosmolar fluids should be avoided.

Hyperventilation Hyperventilation constricts cerebral arterioles, the cerebral blood volume will be reduced, and intracranial hypertension will be mitigated. Chronically low Pa_{CO_2} levels of 25 to 30 mmHg or lower have been advocated.

Hyperventilation is another traditional modality that has its basis more in theoretical potential rather than demonstrated utility. Hyperventilation, defined as the reduction in arterial partial pressure of carbon dioxide, has the potential to reduce arteriolar radius, which will tend to reduce cerebral blood volume and therefore ICP.

After 2 decades with hyperventilation to arterial P_{CO_2} values of 25 to 30 mmHg or less, no evidence has been accumulated to demonstrate improved mortality or morbidity. In fact, there is no evidence to suggest that intracranial hypertension is actually more effectively controlled in hypocapneic patients as opposed to those maintained normocapneic.

Jennett and associates found that hyperventilated patients when compared to those not intubated, faired slightly worse.[88] Clearly there was no major improvement in outcome. Ward and associates suggest that patients treated with hypocapnia did less well than those who were managed at a higher P_{CO_2}.[89] In the series managed using CPP techniques, mortality was 30 to 35 percent yet mean P_{CO_2} was 35 mmHg.[90] While not a comparative study, hyperventilation clearly was not a component of improved outcome. Hyperventilation is still practiced in many units and is medically acceptable on the basis of tradition, but it is also difficult to justify. Potential detrimental consequences include increased cerebral and systemic tissue lacticacidosis.[90,91] Hypocapnia also decouples oxidative phosphorylation and aerobic metabolism. In a study of intracranial hypertension induced via cisternal infusion of artificial CSF, Proctor and colleagues found no significant reduction in intracranial hypertension, but a profound reduction in the cytochrome a-a_3 system to 50 percent of normal values. Originally such observations were attributed to a reduction in CBF because of vasoconstriction, but in their study the reduction in CBF was only 7 percent: detrimental metabolic events occur at the level of the mitochondria induced by hypocapnia.[90,91]

Barbiturate Therapy Administration of sodium pentobarbital to the level of "burst suppression" has the potential to lower ICP. However, after the reports of three different randomized clinical trials demonstrated no improvement in morbidity, mortality, or ICP control, this therapy has generally been avoided as a routine.[92] However, it is still used with varying levels of enthusiasm when all other measures have failed. Eisenberg and associates have repeated a series of patients where intracranial hypertension had progressed to a profound degree, the situation seemed hopeless and patients were then treated with barbiturate coma.[93] Approximately 50 percent of these patients seem to have been salvaged. A rationale on this basis can be generated for the use of barbiturate therapy in the patient group where all else has failed.

Weaning from Intracranial Pressure Therapy

Hydrocephalus As patients with intracranial hypertension, and cerebral edema improve, there is a natural period of transition between one of aggressive support and a more sanguine, tolerant approach to physiological variation. There is always a degree of urgency felt by the clinician in terms of removal of a ventriculostomy or other invasive ICP monitoring device. The concern is of intracranial infection, ventriculitis, meningitis, and brain abscess.

The coexistence of an increase in CSF outflow resistance with an increase in brain water or cerebral edema has already been pointed out. The cerebral edema will often counterbalance the hydrocephalic component and lead to relatively normal appearing ventricular size. This is often associated with relatively high ICP. As cerebral edema resolves, resolution of CSF outflow resistance may lag behind, and ventriculomegaly may occur (Fig. 4-5). This may well occur at CSF pressures that are well below those that had been extant for the more acute period of illness. Hydrocephalus may in fact persist and require shunting, even when ICPs are only 10 to 15 mmHg. This problem is indeed separate from that of CPP management. Ventriculomegaly may well become profound in the face of perfectly adequate CPPs.

The problem can be managed by following quantitative CSF drainage on a day-by-day basis. If the criteria for drainage are kept constant, and the pressure gradient against which the ventriculostomy is opened are held constant, then ventricular size differences monitored by CT become meaningful. If ventricular size remains constant in the face of decreasing volumes of CSF drainage against a CSF pressure gradient of 20 mmHg, then the amount of drainage or the pressure against which the drainage occurs can be reduced in a systematic fashion as long as ventricular size remains constant. However, simply raising the level of the drainage pressure until CSF no longer drains is not particularly rational. The pressure gradient can be increased to a point where CSF drainage will be zero, but the result will be intracranial hypertension, potential CPP insult, and ventriculomegaly.

Weaning from Hypocapnia

The important issue in those patients who are hypocapneic and have been for 24 h or longer is that the cerebral vasculature will readjust to new levels of Pa_{CO_2} (Fig. 4-9). However, if intracranial hypertension is still extant and/or CPP is marginal, P_{CO_2} adjustments must be made very slowly. Decreases in minute ventilation of approximately 10 percent will usually lead to P_{CO_2} increases of 1.5 to 2.5 mmHg. Four to eight hours or sometimes longer at this new minute ventilation and higher Pa_{CO_2} should be allowed for the cerebral vasculature to equilibrate. Occasionally this can only be accomplished with small changes made on a daily basis. There is often a slight increase in ICP that is perfectly acceptable if CPP is maintained. Over the next several hours ICP will fall toward its baseline value with maintenance of CPP.

If minute ventilation is reduced too quickly (Pa_{CO_2} increased rapidly), then the vasculature will respond as if the patient were significantly hypercapneic with generalized vasodilation. This can induce major intracranial hypertension and low CPP states. If these events are not recognized, or the patient's ventilatory management is carried out by a team unconcerned with the patient's ICP and CPP status, then the results can be fatal.

Weaning from Pressors

When pressors such as phenylephrine, epinephrine, or norepinephrine are used, then they too must be weaned. This weaning can often be best accomplished with recognition that any agent that increases systemic vascular resistance or left ventricular end-diastolic load will tend to increase the PCWP as well as the central venous pressure. If this interaction is not considered, the withdrawal of pressors may result in relative hypotension as a result of hypovolemia. Often this problem can be countered by giving a concentrated colloid solution such as 25% albumin or packed red cells. Occasionally, additional fluid can also be used. It is very difficult to wean pressors without adversely affecting CPP in a hypovolemic patient.

The nephrotoxicity of these drugs is also magnified in the face of hypovolemia. The actual dosage used can often be minimized by giving blood or concentrated albumin as a very rapid bolus while the vasoconstrictor is rapidly decreased. The vasoconstrictor reduction can be viewed as allowing systemic vasodilation that increases the potential systemic vascular volume. If this vascular volume is not replaced, relative hypotension can result. Using colloid and blood as a very rapid infusion or bolus can allow maintenance of CPP at much lower pressor doses with relatively little in the way of overhydration.

If a patient has been on low-dose dopamine for renal protection for long periods of time, he or she may be difficult to wean from this drug. Dopamine can be viewed as a precursor to systemic epinephrine and norepinephrine and in particular norepinephrine in vasoconstrictor terminals. If low doses of dopamine are further reduced and the result is mild hypotension that seems inappropriate to the dosage change, consideration should be given to repleting catecholamine stores by nasogastric administration of L-Dopa (250 mg every 6 to 8 h for 24 to 48 h). Consideration should always be given to the possibility of hypovolemia.

RESULTS

The principles of CPP management outlined in this chapter are applicable to all forms of cerebral injury. However, outcome data are available that allow more or less direct comparisons between CPP management and traditional management. These data are summarized in Figs. 4-40 and 4-41 and relate to both mortality and morbidity in patients with traumatic brain injury.

Marshall and associates present the results from four cooperating centers in the care of the severely brain injured (National Traumatic Coma Data Bank). For a Glasgow coma score (GCS) ≤ 7, overall mortality was 40 versus 31 percent for CPP-managed patients.

More importantly, only 37 percent of traditionally managed patients had a favorable outcome ("good" or "moderate" disability) versus 55 percent of the CPP patients. Figure 4-41 breaks these outcome figures down by postresuscitation GCS. At all GCS levels, CPP management yielded a major improvement in morbidity by reducing mortality, persistent vegetative states, and severe disability.

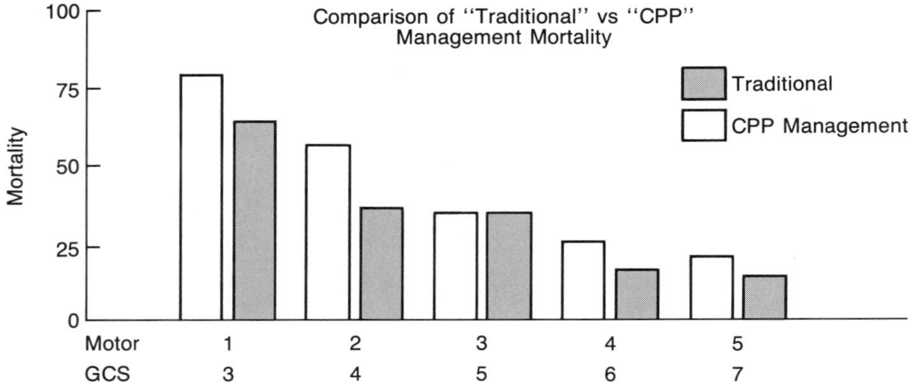

Figure 4-40 Management results are broken down by Glasgow coma and Motor scores. Traditional results are from Marshall et al and are similar to other reports over the last two decades. CPP results are from 120 patients and include deaths for all reasons, occurring anytime up to 1 year. Fifty percent of the patients are polytrauma patients.

The same results apply to patients with surgical mass lesions (epidural, subdural, and intracerebral hematomata) (Fig. 4-42). Mortality with surgery plus traditional management approaches 39 percent with only 23 percent making a satisfactory outcome. Mortality in patients treated with surgery plus CPP management was 75 percent of that in traditionally managed patients (29 versus 39 percent). Satisfactory outcomes were achieved in nearly 60 percent.

Proportionally, the patient with a surgical mass lesion benefits as much and perhaps more than the

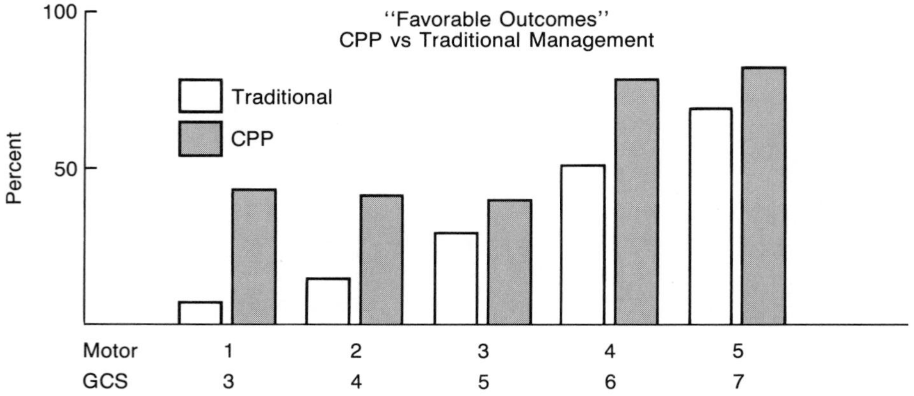

Figure 4-41 Comparison of outcomes from TCDB patients as representatives of traditional therapy as a function of post-resuscitation GCS is shown. CPP techniques have markedly reduced morbidity across the spectrum of severity. As expected, as injury severity declines, the difference between techniques decreases but does not disappear. Favorable outcomes = Good and moderate disability.

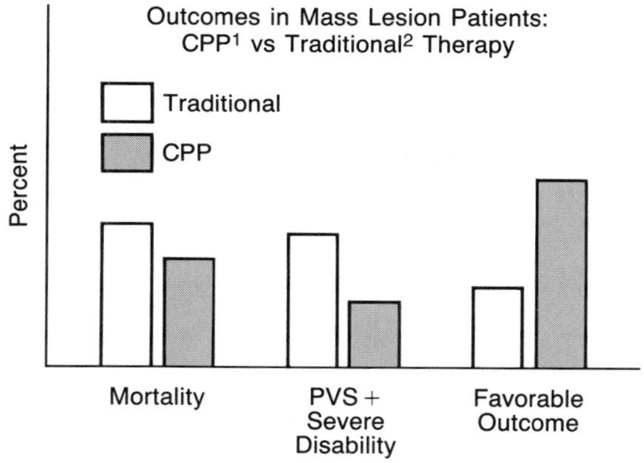

Figure 4-42 Outcome in patients operated upon for surgical mass lesions in CPP versus traditional management schemes. CPP group had average GCS = 5.1, all with GCS ≤ 7. TCDB patient population included 17 percent GCS ≥ 8. Breakdown by GCS in TCDB data was not possible. Therefore, the morbidity in "mass lesion" patients treated using CPP techniques is even better than that suggested above. (1) GCS ≤ 7 postresuscitation (GCS 5.1); (2) Traumatic Coma Data Bank includes GCS 8, and ≥ 9.

patient with the closed head injury. Similar results can be achieved in the treatment of hypertensive hemorrhages, aneurysmal subarachnoid hemorrhage, and neoplastic processes. Clinical results are continuing to improve.

CONCLUSION

The discussion in this chapter has centered about cerebral perfusion pressure. The purpose for this orientation has been at least threefold:

1. The concept of the pressure gradient across the vasculature has been frequently neglected in discussions of the pathophysiology of the cerebral circulation and its interaction with intracranial pressure. It is imperative that the effects of this pressure gradient, CPP, be understood before one can attempt to understand the effects of drugs and other manipulations upon the intracranial space.

2. Approaching the intracranial space's pathophysiology in terms of CPP immediately introduces much basic physiology such as Poiseuille's law that is directly relevant to an understanding of normal and abnormal physiology and its therapeutic manipulation.

3. Lastly, when these principles are pursued, a general theoretical structure begins to emerge that serves as a rational basis for therapy. Early results in the use of this theoretical approach based upon CPP have been encouraging.

REFERENCES

1. Miller JD: Normal and increased intracranial pressure. In: Miller JD (ed): *Northfield's Surgery of the Central Nervous System,* 2d ed. Edinburg, Blackwell, 1987, chap 2.
2. Fenstermacher JD, Johnson JA: Filtration and reflection coefficients of the rabbit blood-brain barrier. *Am J Physiol* 211:341, 1966.
3. Baethmann A, Maier-Hauff K, Kempski O, et al.: Mediators of brain edema and secondary brain damage. *Crit Care Med* 16:972, 1988.
4. Rosner MJ: Pseudotumor cerebri and sodium toxicity. In: Avezatt, et al. (eds): *Intracranial Pressure VIII.* Munich, Springer-Verlag. In press.
5. Rosner MJ: Pseudotumor cerebri: A disease of sodium toxicity? *J Neurosurg* 72:343A, 1990.
6. Levine JE, Povlishock JT, Becker DP: The morphological correlates of primate cerebrospinal fluid absorption. *Brain Res* 241:31, 1982.
7. Early CB, Fink LH: Some fundamental applications of the law of LaPlace in neurosurgery. *Surg Neurol* 6:185, 1976.
8. Foltz EL, Blanks JP, Yonemura K: CSF pulsatility in hydrocephalus: Respiratory effect on pulse wave slope as an indicator of intracranial compliance. *Neurol Res* 12:67, 1990.
9. Marmarou A, Shulman K, LaMorgese J: Compartmental analysis of compliance and outflow resistance of the cerebrospinal fluid system. *J Neurosurg* 43:523, 1975.
10. Kontos HA: Regulation of the cerebral circulation. *Annu Rev Physiol* 43:397, 1981.
11. Kontos HA, Wei EP, Navari RM, Levasseur JE, Rosenblum WI, Patterson JL Jr: Responses of cerebral arteries and arterioles to acute hypotension and hypertension. *Am J Physiol* 234:H371, 1978.
12. Dewey RC, Pieper HP, Hunter WE: Experimental cerebral hemodynamics. Vasomotor tone, critical closing pressure and vascular bed resistance. *J Neurosurg* 41:597, 1974.
13. Fein JM, Lipow K, Marmarou A: Cortical artery pressure in normotensive and hypertensive aneurysm patients. *J Neurosurg* 59:51, 1983.

14. Forbes HS: The cerebral circulation: I. Observation and measurement of pial vessels. *Arch Neurol Psychiatry* 19:751, 1928.
15. Kety SS: Circulation and metabolism of the human brain in health and disease. *Am J Med* 8:205, 1950.
16. Fieschi C, Battistini N, Beduschi A, Boselli L, Rossanda M: Regional cerrebral blood flow and intraventricular pressure in acute head injuries. *J Neurol Neurosurg Psychiatry* 37:1378, 1974.
17. Grubb RL Jr, Raichle ME, Phelps ME, Ratcheson RA: Effects of increased intracranial pressure on cererbral blood volume, blood flow and oxygen utilization in monkeys. *J Neurosurg* 43:385, 1975.
18. Magnaes B: Body position and cerebrospinal fluid pressure. Part I: Clinical studies on the effect of rapid postural changes. *J Neurosurg* 44:687, 1976.
19. Palvolgyi R: Regional cerebral blood flow in patients with intracranial tumors. *J Neurosurg* 31:149, 1969.
20. Enevoldsen EM, Jensen FT: Autoregulation and CO_2 responses of cerebral blood flow in patients with acute severe head injury. *J Neurosurg* 48:689, 1978.
21. Lewelt W, Jenkins LW, Miller JD: Autoregulation of cerebral blood flow after experimental fluid percussion injury of the brain. *J Neurosurg* 53:500, 1980.
22. Bouma GJ, Miuzelaar JP, Bandok K, Marmarou A: Blood pressure and intracranial pressure volume dynamics in severe head injury: Relationship with cerebral blood flow. *J Neurosurg* 77:15, 1992.
23. Muizelaar JP, van der Poel HG, Li ZC, et al.: Pial arteriolar vessel diameter and CO_2 reactivity during prolonged hyperventilation in the rabbit. *J Neurosurg* 69:923, 1988.
24. Sakaki T, Tsujimoto S, Nisshitani M, Ismida Y, Morimoto T: Perfusion pressure breakthrough threshold of cerebral autoregulation in chronically ischemic brain: An experimental study in cats. *J Neurosurg* 765:468, 1992.
25. Handa Y, Mayashi M, Takeuchi H, Kubota T, Vobazashi H, Kawano H: Time course of the impairment of autoregulation during chronic cerebral vasospasm after subarachnoid hemorrhage in primates. *J Neurosurg* 76:493, 1992.
26. DeWitt DS, Prough DS, Taylor CL, Whitley JM: Reduced cerebral blood flow, oxygen delivery and electroencephalographic activity after traumatic brain injury and mild hemorrhage in cats. *J Neurosurg* 76:812, 1992.
27. Gray WJ, Rosner MJ: Pressure-volume index: Part II. The effects of low cerebral perfusion pressure and autoregulation. *J Neurosurg* 67:377, 1987.
28. El Adawy Y, Rosner MJ: Cerebral perfusion pressure, autoregulation and the PVI reflection point: Pathological ICP. In: Hoff JT, et al. (eds): *Intracranial Pressure VII*, Munich, Springer-Verlag, 1988, pp 829–833.
29. Schrader H, Zwentnow NM, Morkrid L: Regional cerebral blood flow and CSF pressures during Cushing response induced by a supratentorial expanding mass. *Acta Neurol Scand* 71:453, 1985.
30. Marienne JP, Robert G, Bagnat E: Post-traumatic acute rise of ICP related to subclinical epileptic seizures. *Acta Neurochir* 28(Suppl):89, 1979.
31. Miller JD, Garibi J, Pickard JD: Induced changes of cerebrospinal fluid volume. Effects during continuous monitoring of ventricular fluid pressure. *Arch Neurol* 28:265, 1973.
32. Marmarou A, Shulman K, Rosende RM: A nonlinear analysis of the cerebrospinal fluid system and intracranial pressure dynamics. *J Neurosurg* 48:332, 1978.
33. Schrader H, Lofgren J, Zwetnow NM: Influence of blood pressure on tolerance to an intracranial expanding mass. *Acta Neurol Scand* 71:114, 1985.
34. Marmarou A, Maset AL, Ward JD, et al.: Contribution of CSF and vascular factors to elevation of ICP in severely head-injured patients. *J Neurosurg* 66:883, 1987.
35. Avezaat CJJ, van Eijndhoven JHM: The conflict between CSF pulse pressure response during plateau waves. In: Ishii S, Nagai H, Brock M (eds): *Intracranial Pressure V.* New York, Springer-Verlag, 1983, pp 326–332.
36. Gray WJ, Rosner MJ: Pressure-volume index as a function of cerebral perfusion pressure: Part I. The effects of cerebral perfusion pressure changes and anesthesia. *J Neurosurg* 67:376, 1987.
37. Obrist WD, Gennarelli TA, Segawa N, Dolinskas CA, Langfitt TW: Relation of cerebral blood flow to neurologic status and outcome in head-injured patients. *J Neurosurg* 51:292, 1979.
38. Obrist WD, Langfitt TW, Jaggi JL, Cruz J, Gennarelli TA: Cerebral blood flow and metabolism in comatose patients with acute head injury. *J Neurosurg* 61:241, 1984.
39. Overgaard J, Tweed WA: Cerebral circulation after head injury: Part 1. Cerebral blood flow and its regulation after closed head injury with emphasis on clinical correlations. *J Neurosurg* 41:531, 1974.
40. Miller JD, Garbi J, North JB, Teasdale GM: Effects of increased arterial pressure on blood flow in the damaged brain. *J Neurol Neurosurg Psychiatry* 38:657, 1975.
41. Miller JD, Stanek AE, Langfitt TW: Cerebral blood flow regulation during experimental brain compression. *J Neurosurg* 39:186, 1973.
42. Miller JD, Stanek AE, Langfitt TW: Effect of expanding intracranial lesions on cerebral blood flow. *Surg Forum* 22:422, 1971.
43. Weinstein JD, Langfitt TW, Kassell NF: Vasopressor response to increased intracranial pressure. *Neurology* 14:1118, 1964.

44. Langfitt TW, Weinstein JD, Kassell NF: Cerebral vasomotor paralysis produced by intracranial hypertension. *Neurology (NY)* 15:622, 1965.
45. Langfitt TW: Increased intracranial pressure. *Clin Neurosurg* 16:436, 1969.
46. Leech P, Miller JD: Intracranial volume-pressure relationships during experimental brain compression in primates. 2. Effect of induced changes in systemic arterial pressure and cerebral blood flow. *J Neurol Neurosurg Psychiatry* 37:1099, 1974.
47. Kuroda Y, Inglis FM, Miller JD, McCulloch J, Graham D, Bullock R: Transient glucose hypermetabolism after acute subdural hematoma in the rat. *J Neurosurg* 76:471, 1992.
48. Shirane R, Weinstein PR: Effect of mannitol on local cerebral blood flow after temporary complete cerebral ischemia in rats. *J Neurosurg* 76:486, 1992.
49. Merrill EW: Rheology of blood. *Physiol Rev* 49:863, 1969.
50. Mendelow AD, Teasdale GM, Russell T, Floof J, Patterson J, Murray GD: Effect of mannitol on cerebral blood flow and cerebral perfusion pressure in human head injury. *J Neurosurg* 63:43, 1985.
51. Muizelaar JP, Wei EP, Kontos HA, Becker DP: Mannitol causes compensatory cerebral vasoconstriction and vasodilation in response to blood viscosity changes. *J Neurosurg* 59:822, 1983.
52. Kontos HA, Wei EP, Raper AJ, Roseblum WI, Navari RM, Patterson JL Jr: Role of tissue hypoxia in local regulation of cerebral microcirculation. *Am J Physiol* 234:H582, 1978.
53. Johnston IH, Harper AM: The effect of mannitol on cerebral blood flow: An experimental study. *J Neurosurg* 38:461, 1973.
54. Muizelaar JP, Lutz HA, Becker DP: Effect of mannitol on ICP and CBF and correlation with pressure autoregulation in severely head-injured patients. *J Neurosurg* 61:700, 1984.
55. Brown FD, Johns L, Jafar JJ, Crockard HL, Mullan S: Detailed monitoring of the effects of mannitol following experimental head injury. *J Neurosurg* 50:423, 1979.
56. Muizelaar JP, Wei EP, Knotos HA, Becker DP: Cererbral blood flow is regulated by changes in blood pressure and in blood viscosity alike. *Stroke* 17:44, 1986.
57. Rosner MJ, Coley I: Mannitol and cerebral perfusion pressure. *Neurosurgery* 16:725, 1985.
58. Motomiya M, Nakagaura Y, Kinomoto H, Mabuchi S, Tsura M: Possible mechanism influencing decrease of intracranial pressure following arousal. In: Ishii S, Nagai H, Brock M (eds): *Intracranial Pressure V.* New York, Springer-Verlag, 1983, pp 352–357.
59. Katayama Y, Nakamura T, Becker DP, Hayes RL: Intracranial pressure variations associated with activation of the cholinoceptive pontine inhibitory area in the unanesthetized drug-free cat. *J Neurosurg* 61:713,
60. Gucer G, Viernstein LJ: Intracranial pressure in the normal monkey while awake and asleep. *J Neurosurg* 51:206, 1979.
61. Forsyth RP, Hoffbrand BI: Redistribution of cardiac output after sodium pentobarbital anesthesia in the monkey. *J Physiol* 218:214, 1970.
62. Lafferty JJ, Keykhah MM, Shapiro HM, et al.: Cerebral hypometabolism obtained with deep pentobarbital anesthesia and hypothermia (30 degree C). *Anesthesiology* 49:159, 1978.
63. Nakatani S, Hagiwara I, Ozaki K, et al.: Paradoxical effect of barbiturate on ICP acutely increased by cold-induced edema in cats. In: Ishii S, Nagai H, Brock M (eds): *Intracranial Pressure V.* New York: Springer-Verlag. 1983.
64. Jones JV, Fitch W, MacKenzie ET, et al.: Lower limit of cerebral blood flow autoregulation in experimental renovascular hypertension in the baboon. *Circ Res* 39:555, 1976.
65. Sheinberg M, Kanter MJ, Robertson SC, Contant CF, Narazan RK, Grossman RG: Continuous monitoring of jugular venous oxygen saturation in head-injured patients. *J Neurosurg* 76:212, 1992.
66. Burke AM, Quest DO, Chien S, Cerri C: The effects of mannitol on blood viscosity. *J Neurosurg* 55:550, 1981.
67. Takagi H, Saitoh T, Kitahara T, Morii S, Ohwada T, Yada K: The mechanism of ICP reducing effect of mannitol. In: Ishii S, Nagai H, Brock M (eds): *Intracranial Pressure V.* New York, Springer-Verlag, 1983, pp 729–733.
68. Roberts PA, Pollay M, Engles C, et al.: Effect on intracranial pressure of furosemide combined with varying doses and administration rates of mannitol. *J Neurosurg* 66:440, 1987.
69. Pollay M, Fullenwider CH, Roberts PA, Stevens FA: The effect of mannitol and furosemide on the blood-brain barrier osmotic gradient and intracranial pressure. *J Neurosurg* 59:945, 1983.
70. Jones MD Jr, Traystman RJ, Simmons MA, Molteni RA: Effects of changes in arterial O_2 content on cerebral blood flow in the lamb. *Am J Physiol* 240:H209, 1981.
71. Shapiro HM, Marshall LF: Intracranial pressure responses to PEEP in head-injured patients. *J Trauma* 18:254, 1978.
72. Frost EAM: Effects of positive end-expiratory pressure on intracranial pressure and complicance in brain-injured patients. *J Neurosurg* 47:195, 1977.
73. Durward QJ, Amacher AL, Del Maestro RF, et al.: Cerebral and cardiovascular responses to changes in head elevation in patients with intracranial hypertension. *J Neurosurg* 59:938, 1983.
74. Kenning JA, Toutant SM, Saunders RL: Upright pa-

tient positioning in the management of intracranial hypertension. *Surg Neurol* 15:148, 1981.

75. Magnaes B: Body position and cerebrospinal fluid pressure. Part 2. Clinical studies on orthostatic pressure and the hydrostatic indifferent point. *J Neurosurg* 44:698, 1976.
76. Ropper AH, O'Rourke D, Kennedy SK: Head position, intracranial pressure, and compliance. *Neurology* 32:1288, 1982.
77. Feldman Z, Kanter MJ, Robertson CS, et al.: Effect of head elevation on intracranial pressure, cerebral perfusion pressure, and cerebral blood flow in head-injured patients. *J Neurosurg* 76:207, 1992.
78. Rosner MJ, Coley I: Cerebral perfusion pressure, the ICP and head elevation. *J Neurosurg* 65:636, 1986.
79. Gauer OH, Thron HL: Postural changes in the circulation. In: Hamilton WR (ed): *Handbook of Physiology.* Baltimore: Williams & Wilkins, 1965, sec. 2, vol 3, pp 2409–2439.
80. Rosner MJ: Cerebral perfusion pressure: The link between the cerebral and systemic circulations. In: Wood JH (ed): *Cerebral Blood Flow: Physiologic and Clinical Aspects.* New York: McGraw-Hill, 1987, pp 425–448.
81. Fog M: Cerebral circulation. the reaction of the pial arteries to a fall in blood pressure. *Arch Neurol Psychiatry* 37:351, 1937.
82. Weinstein JD, Langfitt TW: Reponses of cortical vessels to brain compression: Observations through a transparent calvarium. *Surg Forum* 18:430, 1967.
83. Wolff HG, Forbes HS: The cererbral circulation: V. Observations of the pial circulation during changes in intracranial pressure. *Arch Neurol Psychiatry* 20:1035, 1928.
84. Clasen RA, Bezkorovainy A, Pandolfi S: Protein and electrolyte changes in experimental cerebral edema. *J Neuropathol Exp Neurol* 44:113, 1982.
85. Gazendam J, Go KG, van Zanten AK: Composition of isolated edema fluid in cold-induced brain edema. *J Neurosurg* 51:70, 1979.
86. Gaab M, Knoblich OE, Schupp J, Herrmann F, Fuhrmeister U, Pflughaupt KW: Effect of furosemide (Lasix) on acute severe experimental cerebral edema. *J Neurol* 220:185, 1979.
87. Tornheim PA, McLaurin RL, Sawaya R: Effect of furosemide on experimental traumatic cerebral edema. *Neurosurgery* 4:48, 1979.
88. Jennett B, Teasdale G, Fry J, et al.: Treatment for severe head injury. *J Neurol Neurosurg Psychiatry* 43:289, 1980.
89. Muizelaar JP, Marmarou A, Ward JD, et al.: Adverse effects of prolonged hyperventilation in patients with severe head injury: A randomized clinical trial. *J Neurosurg* 75:731, 1991.
90. Proctor HJ, Cairns C, Fillipo D, Palladino GW, Rosner MJ: Brain metabolism during increased intracranial pressure as assessed by niroscopy. *Surgery* 96:273, 1984.
91. Rosner MJ, Becker DP: Experimental brain injury: Successful therapy with the weak base, tromethamine (with a review of CNS acidosis). *J Neurosurg* 60:961, 1984.
92. Ward JD, Becker DP, Miller JD, et al.: Failure of prophylactic barbiturate coma in the treatment of severe head injury. *J Neurosurg* 62:383, 1985.
93. Eisenberg HM, Frankowski RF, Contant CF, et al.: High-dose barbiturate control of elevated intracranial pressure in patients with severe head injury. *J Neurosurg* 69:15, 1988.

CHAPTER 5
Radiographic Techniques

Mark E. Harris
Patricia A. Hudgins

INTRODUCTION

Radiology plays an important role in the management of the seriously ill neurosurgical patient, and although sophisticated imaging such as computed tomography (CT), magnetic resonance imaging (MRI), transcranial Doppler ultrasound, and cerebral angiography must be readily available, plain film radiographs, including the chest x-ray, abdominal films, and skull, facial, sinus, and spine films are the most commonly ordered examinations on the patient in the intensive care unit (ICU).

PLAIN FILM RADIOGRAPHY

Computed radiography (CR) has replaced the standard film/screen conventional systems in many hospitals. It acquires the image in digital form and can then be printed as hard copy or transmitted to distant sites electronically. This enables the clinician in the ICU to view the film immediately after it is processed. Additionally, the image can be viewed at multiple sites simultaneously. Image storage and retrieval are more secure and efficient than with the standard x-ray, and the clinician can recall the prior examinations without leaving the ICU.

COMPUTED TOMOGRAPHY

Technique

Computed tomography is readily available in most hospitals, is noninvasive, and can be acquired quickly, with most head scans obtained in less than 15 min and limited spine scans in less than 30 min. These advantages make it the most common method for evaluating many complications of the patient in the neurosurgical ICU. Life-support systems, including ventilators, intracranial monitors, and multiple intravascular lines can easily be accommodated in the CT suite and do not interfere with either the scan acquisition or the images.

Iodinated contrast, used to characterize central nervous system (CNS) lesions, is visualized when a breakdown in the normal integrity of the blood-brain barrier allows accumulation of contrast and results in high density on the CT. Systemic steroids will stabilize the blood-brain barrier and result in less enhancement in or around a lesion.[1] Intravenous contrast is contraindicated if there is a history of severe allergic reaction, or in the setting of renal failure. A creatinine of 1.8 to 2.0 mg/dL precludes its use, although the new lower osmolality agents may be safer in the patient with renal failure.[2] Fatal reaction to intravenous contrast agents occurs with a frequency of 1 in 40,000 to 66,500[3]; this low reaction rate has not definitively been shown to have decreased with the use of newer low osmolality agents.[4,5] Current available agents of lower osmolality have, however, been shown to decrease mild (nausea, urticaria, itching, heat sensation, vomiting) and severe (dyspnea, hypotension, loss of consciousness, cardiac arrest) adverse reactions.[2,4,6] A steroid pretreatment regimen of 32 mg of methylprednisolone given 12 and 2 h prior to contrast administration may reduce the incidence of adverse reactions.[7] Another potential complication of intravenous contrast is a seizure, which may occur in 6 to 19 percent of patients immediately after intravenous contrast is administered, especially when there is an underlying metastatic or primary brain tumor, or other seizure focus.[8,9] Although therapeutic levels of diphenylhydantoin reduce the incidence of seizures related to contrast, 5 mg intravenous diazepam has been shown to further reduce the incidence of contrast media–associated seizures.[9]

Computed Tomography of the Brain

A CT scan of the brain is the study of choice in assessing the etiology of acute neurologic change in the ICU patient, including the postoperative patient.[10] Most brain scans obtained on patients in the ICU are performed without iodinated intravenous contrast. Acute or subacute stroke and intracranial hemorrhage, especially subarachnoid and petechial parenchymal, may be obscured by contrast. Hydrocephalus or evidence of increased intracranial pressure (ICP), common complications of the seriously ill neurosurgical patient, are easily seen without contrast. The scan may be normal in the first 24 h following an ischemic event, but after that period nonhemorrhagic acute cerebral infarction is manifested by subtle low density, loss of the normal gray-white junction, and mass effect usually evidenced by flattening of cortical sulci. Acute parenchymal, subdural, or epidural blood is high density on CT and remains bright for approximately 72 h, after which time it gradually decreases in CT density (Fig. 5-1). Subarachnoid blood is usually visualized for up to a week and rapidly decreases in conspicuity after that time.[11] If there is only a small amount of subarachnoid blood, it may not be seen at all or only for several days. MRI will not routinely detect acute blood in the subarachnoid space.

The presence of hydrocephalus, another poten-

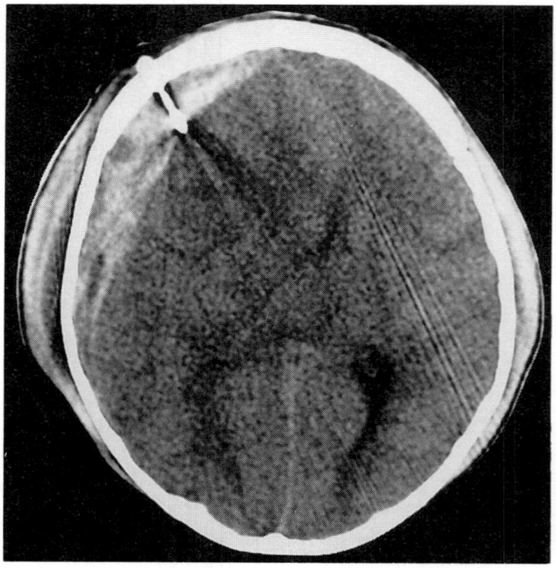

Figure 5-1 Two-year-old boy with closed head injury. Initial head CT was normal; now with increasing ICP. Axial nonenhanced CT obtained several hours after insertion of an ICP monitor reveals a new subdural hematoma at the site of monitor.

tial complication in the neurosurgical patient, is easily seen on noncontrast CT as dilatation of the ventricles. The earliest changes are seen in the temporal horns and anterior third ventricle, which become rounded; dilatation of the lateral and fourth ventricles are relatively late findings. The CT finding that best predicts increased ICP and is of prognostic importance is nonvisualization of the perimesencephalic and basal cisterns.[12–14] Absence of the cisterns correlates with an ICP of approximately 30 mmHg.

Computed tomography contrast material is recommended if infection, such as parenchymal abscess, cerebritis, ventriculitis, empyema, meningitis, or wound infection, is suspected. The various lesions occur in different compartments within the CNS, but the CT findings on contrast-enhanced studies are the same: abnormal enhancement due to breakdown of the blood-brain barrier. Sequential scans are useful to follow therapy; with successful treatment the abnormal enhancement should resolve.

Contrast-enhanced CT may also be used in the evaluation of a primary or metastatic brain tumor, although MRI with gadopentetate dimeglumine (Gd-DTPA) is preferable for the initial examination of these patients because of improved sensitivity for lesion detection and because the direct multiplanar acquisitions facilitate resection planning. In the early postoperative period, however, CT both without and with contrast is often obtained. Early postoperative hemorrhage is easily detected on noncontrast CT, although differentiation of residual tumor from postoperative changes on the contrast-enhanced scan remains problematic. Several studies suggest that benign nonneoplastic postoperative enhancement resulting from neovascularity within the surgical bed is not seen until 5 to 7 days following surgery.[15,16] Therefore, contrast-enhanced CT to detect residual disease should be performed within the first 3 to 4 days postoperatively, when enhancement on the initial follow-up scan is likely to represent residual neoplasm. Benign postoperative enhancement on CT may be seen along the dura and encephalotomy, is maximum at 2 to 4 weeks after surgery, and decreases thereafter but may persist for months.[15–17] Enhancement of the ependyma or leptomeninges remote from the resection site is uncommon, and when seen, infection or remote spread of neoplasm should be considered.

Computed Tomography of the Spine

The most common indication for CT of the spine in the ICU patient is to evaluate a spinal column fracture or injury. All spinal fractures, with or without neurologic deficit, should be fully assessed with CT. Other indications for spine CT include inability to adequately visualize the craniocervical or cervicothoracic junctions with plain radiographs. Plain films, including routine lateral, anteroposterior, and, in the cervical spine, odontoid and oblique films, should always be obtained prior to CT as the findings on the views will direct the levels to be scanned. The accuracy of CT in detecting and characterizing spinal fractures is directly related to slice thickness; 1.5 to 3 mm is optimal. The scan should extend from one vertebral level above the fracture, through the fracture, and include one vertebral level below the fracture, as coincidental fractures usually occur directly above or below the known fracture.[18] Sagittal and coronal reformations should always be performed and are of better quality when axial slices are thinner and when the patient remains still within the scanner. Thus, patient sedation may be necessary. Horizontal fractures that occur in the same plane as the axial slices, such as the type II dens fracture, may be missed without reformations. Subluxation and encroachment on the canal are often better appreciated on sagittal reformations.

At this time, CT-myelography (CTM) has limited indications and is usually reserved for patients who have a contraindication to MRI (such as a cardiac pacemaker or a ferromagnetic aneurysm clip). Nerve root avulsions or dural tears are most accurately detected with CTM. It is an excellent screening tool for spinal cord dural arteriovenous malformations and may be positive even when the MRI is normal.

Magnetic resonance imaging has largely replaced CT for evaluating other serious spinal lesions. Metastatic disease with cord compression, spinal infections (including discitis and epidural abscess), spinal cord tumors, and complications of trauma including epidural hematoma, traumatic herniated disc, cord contusion, or syringomyelia

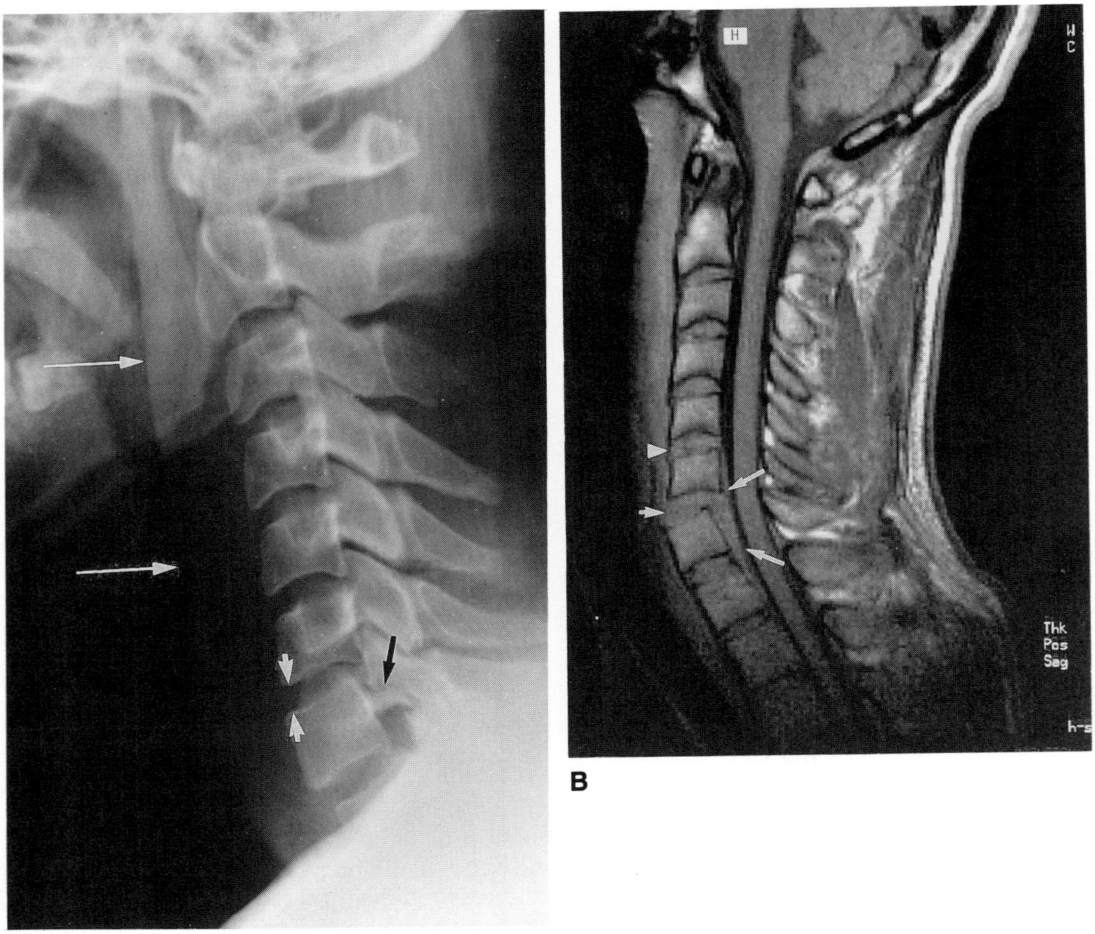

A

B

Figure 5-2 Twenty-year-old man with neck pain following motor vehicle accident. *A*. Lateral plain film reveals marked prevertebral soft tissue swelling (long white arrows), widening of the anterior C6–C7 disc space (short white arrows), and a fracture of the C7 pedicle (black arrow). *B*. T1-weighted sagittal MRI shows disruption of the anterior longitudinal ligament at C6–C7 (short white arrow), subluxation at that level, and a homogeneous ventral extradural soft tissue mass (long white arrows). Notice the normal and intact anterior longitudinal ligament at C5–C6 (white arrowhead).

or hematomyelia are indications for MRI (Fig. 5-2).

MAGNETIC RESONANCE IMAGING

Technique

Magnetic resonance imaging has had a significant impact on the practice of neurosurgery, as its spectacular soft tissue contrast allows visualization of structures and pathologic processes never before seen. Most hospitals now have MRI scanners readily available, and it has become an important aid in the care of the patient in the neurosurgical ICU.

Compared to CT, however, obtaining an MRI on the seriously ill patient is more complicated and requires careful planning. A routine MRI ex-

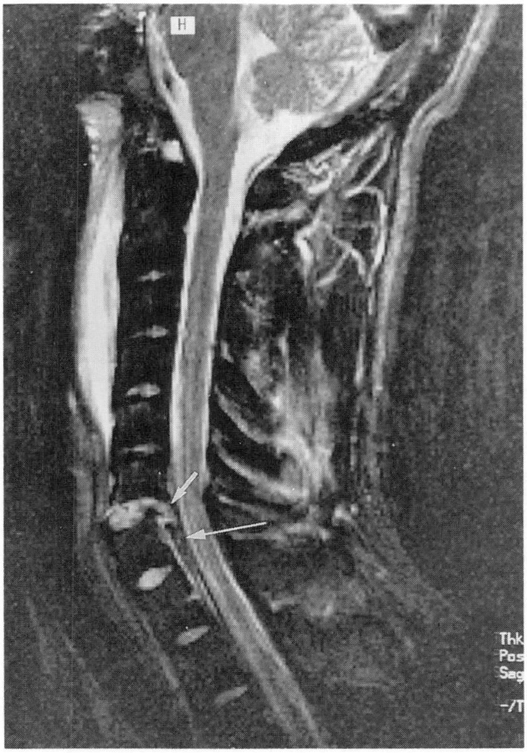

C

Figure 5-2 continued *C.* T2-weighted sagittal MRI shows prevertebral soft tissue swelling, high signal intensity at the C6–C7 disc space as well as a traumatic herniated nucleus pulposis (short white arrow), and low signal intensity soft tissue (long white arrow), presumably acute blood, tracking extradurally. This sequence was helpful in differentiating the HNP from the extradural acute blood.

amination of either the brain or the spinal cord typically takes from 30 to 60 min to obtain, which may be prohibitive in the seriously ill patient. Because even the subtlest patient motion degrades image quality on an MRI, it may be necessary to sedate the patient. Sedation may also be required for the 15 to 20 percent of patients who are too claustrophobic to remain in the small bore of the magnet. The MRI scanner itself is a magnet with strong magnetic fields surrounding the unit. Two potential complications must be considered. First, any life-support device, such as a ventilator or a monitoring instrument, brought into the MRI suite must be nonferromagnetic or sufficiently shielded from the strong magnetic fields. Second, the patient must be screened for any ferromagnetic biomedical substance on or near the body, including aneurysm clips, intravascular filters, stents, coils, or even bullet fragments.

Ventilators, monitors for temperature, O_2 and CO_2, spine braces, and skeletal traction systems are now modified and stripped of all ferrous materials to be MRI-compatible.[19–22] Any device that is not MRI-compatible can potentially damage the unit or cause image artifacts. If there is any concern about compatibility, a direct call to the manufacturer should answer the question.

Biomedical devices are more problematic. The risks of deflecting, heating, inducing an electric current, or malfunction, especially with cardiac pacemakers, are real. Aneurysm clips that have been tested for deflection and appear to be safe include the Sugita (Elgiloy), Yasargil (316 SS and Phynox), Heifetz (Elgiloy), and Vari-Angle McFadden (MP35N).[23–27] Magnetic resonance imaging is probably safe for most patients with permanent stainless steel carotid vascular clamps, except the Poppen-Blaylock clamp which deflects at 1.5 T.[28] Most currently used intraventricular shunts and connectors, including the Accu-Flow (Codman & Shurtleff) straight, right angle, and T-connector, are MRI-compatible, although the shunt connectors will cause a typical "signal-void" artifact (Fig. 5-3).[25,29] The Camino parenchymal ICP monitor (10-4B) and ventriculostomy (10-4H) (Camino Laboratories, San Diego) are both nonmagnetic and will cause an artifact but should not deflect in the MRI scanner (personal communication). Surgical wires, skin staples, and surgical clips will routinely cause a similar artifact, but no adverse experiences are reported.[29,30] Electroencephalogram electrodes and intracerebral depth electrodes are now available that are MRI-compatible.[31,32]

Any patient undergoing an MRI should be carefully screened for the presence of intraocular foreign bodies.[33] Patients who have worked previously as sheet metal workers should be screened with thin-section orbital CT to exclude ocular metallic fragments. If a fragment is found, the MRI should not be performed. MRI is contraindicated in patients with cochlear implants,[34] but other otologic implants such as ventilation tubes, stapes prostheses, and ossicular wires appear to be safe.[35]

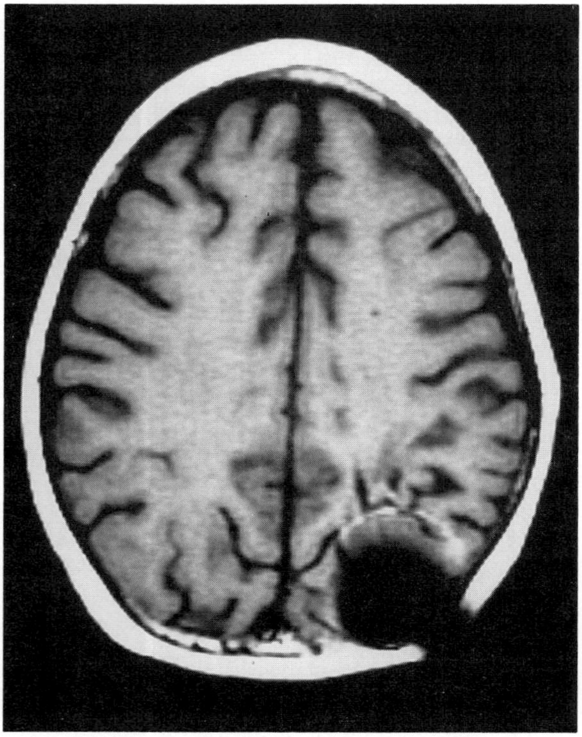

Figure 5-3 T1-weighted axial image shows typical "signal void" artifact from the shunt connector.

Metallic ballistic fragments pose potential risk by deflecting or torquing in soft tissue when they are perpendicular to the magnetic field, especially if located near important neurovascular structures. A variety of 21 metallic bullets and pellets were recently tested in a 1.5-T magnet; 4 of the 21 showed marked deflection and aligned within seconds in the magnetic field.[36] Three of these four were made outside of the United States, and the fourth was a bullet used during World War II. No pellets deflected, but BB's made by both Daisy and Crosman have been reported to deflect.[25,36] Commercial sporting ammunition is usually nonferromagnetic.[37] Other rifle or pistol bullets that are known to deflect include AK-47, .30-06 military, .375 hunting, 9-mm military pistol bullet, Geco .25 Auto, and WCC 42 .45 Auto.[37] Any patient with a ballistic fragment near the orbits or important neurovascular structure should be studied with caution, and if there is any question of potential for deflection, the MRI should not be performed.

Magnetic resonance imaging is far more complex than CT with many more variables controlled by the radiologist. Close consultation between the clinician and radiologist is important to assure the adequate examination is acquired. Most brain MRI examinations will include at the minimum sagittal T1-weighted and axial T2-weighted sequences. T1-weighted images are useful for depicting anatomy, while T2-weighted images are most sensitive to abnormalities within the parenchyma itself. The two sequences together are necessary to characterize tissue. For example, it is the different appearance on the two sequences that allows the detection of fat, acute, subacute, or chronic blood, or proteinaceous or cholesterol components that may be found in a variety of tumors or cysts. Other planes are often helpful and easily obtained, and the clinician should request specific sequences, such as the coronal or thin-section axial images, if deemed necessary for surgical planning or improved lesion visualization. The MRI contrast agent, Gd-DTPA, is not routinely used but is reserved for specific clinical situations. Like iodinated CT contrast, it reveals loss of integrity in the blood-brain barrier, usually signifying active lesions. It is most commonly used when imaging suspected primary or metastatic brain tumors, intracranial infections, leptomeningeal disease (including infection and CNS neoplasms metastatic to the leptomeninges), and acute stroke. It is extremely well-tolerated with few side effects and less than a dozen reported contrast-related anaphylactoid reactions worldwide.[38,39]

MRI of the Brain

The role of MRI in clinical practice is still evolving, especially with respect to the patient in the neurosurgical ICU. CT is often the first test obtained, as it is more convenient and the most common complications, especially those with surgical implications, are so easily assessed. To reiterate, CT is preferred over MRI for the following clinical situations: (1) the initial evaluation in any patient suspected of suffering severe head injury or harboring a life-threatening intracerebral hematoma, either parenchymal or extraaxial; (2) to detect a shunt malfunction; (3) suspected subarachnoid hemorrhage; (4) any spine fracture, with or without neurologic injury; (5) any patient who is clinically unstable and potentially unable to remain in the radiology department for the time required to perform an MRI. In many settings, MRI is complementary to CT and provides information not obtainable with CT.

Magnetic resonance imaging has been shown to be more sensitive than CT for a number of intracranial lesions, and perhaps its most useful role in the neurosurgical patient is when the clinical findings are out of proportion to the CT findings. Traumatic lesions better detected on MRI than CT include nonhemorrhagic axonal injuries or contusions (especially in the brainstem and corpus callosum) (Fig. 5-4), small extraaxial collections, and differentiating a chronic hygroma from chronic subdural hematoma.[40–43] Although small extraaxial collections may not be surgical lesions, the detection of a small subdural hematoma on MRI may be important in confirming the diagnosis of battered child syndrome. MRI with contrast is more sensitive for metastatic lesions than CT[44,45] and is indicated when a CT scan of a patient who is being considered for curative surgical resection shows a solitary lesion. Many surgeons prefer multiplanar MRI to axial CT for planning resection of a primary brain tumor, especially when the lesion is in the posterior fossa where streak artifact on CT limits lesion detection. As with CT, the differentiation of residual tumor from postsurgical nonneoplastic changes is diffi-

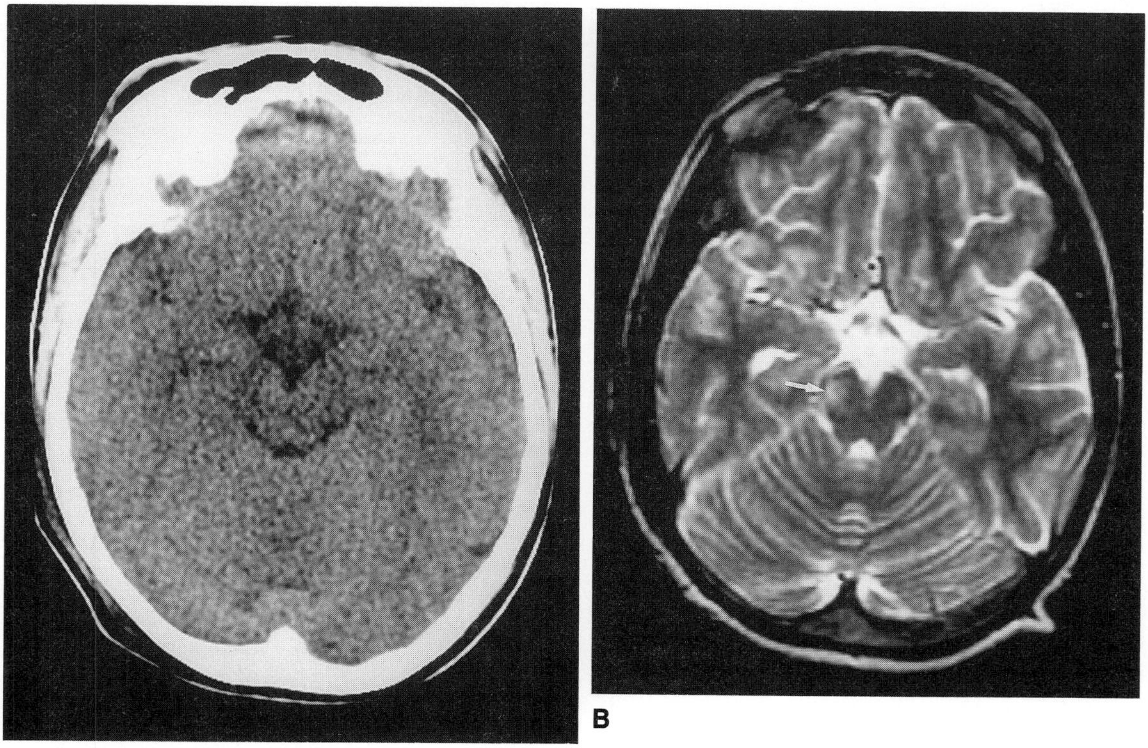

A B

Figure 5-4 Six-year-old boy in an MVA with left hemiparesis. *A*. Axial noncontrast CT at level of cerebral peduncles is normal. *B*. T2-weighted axial MRI at same level obtained within 3 days of CT shows focal nonhemorrhagic contusion in right cerebral peduncle (white arrow).

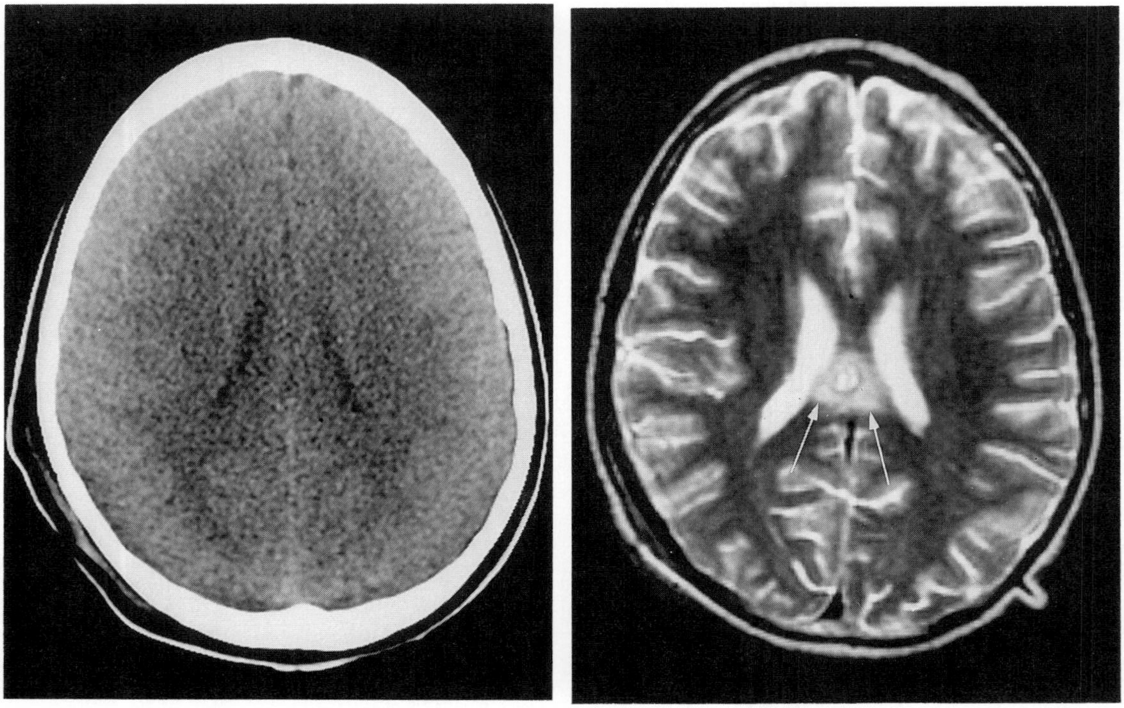

C D

Figure 5-4 continued *C*. CT scan at body of corpus callosum is normal. *D*. MRI reveals nonhemorrhagic contusion in body of corpus callosum (white arrows).

cult on MRI. However, an early baseline postoperative enhanced MRI is helpful for the follow-up of brain tumors.

Several studies have shown that MRI, especially following Gd-DTPA enhancement, is extremely sensitive in the detection of early stroke and may be positive when the CT is still normal.[46–49] Furthermore, the appearance of the stroke on MRI may have prognostic significance, as early (within 3 days of infarction) and/or intense parenchymal enhancement tends to be associated with minimal or reversible deficits.[46] Contrast-enhanced MRI is more sensitive than CT for detecting leptomeningeal disease, either infectious or neoplastic (Fig. 5-5). Small subdural or epidural empyemas may be seen on MRI when the CT is normal.[50] Subtle white matter or parenchymal lesions such as demyelinating plaques, vasculitis, or nonenhancing infiltrative infections such as HIV encephalitis or progressive multifocal leukoencephalopathy may be detected on MRI when the CT is normal.

Despite tremendous enthusiasm and high expectations for magnetic resonance angiography (MRA), conventional angiography remains the examination of choice for evaluating intracranial aneurysm, dural fistula, carotid-cavernous sinus fistula, and even for the initial workup of major arterial dissection. Early experience suggests inoperable vascular lesions, such as carotid aneurysms located at the skull base and dissections, can be followed with MRI and MRA, avoiding repeat angiography (Fig. 5-6).[51] Flow-sensitive MRI studies that do not require intravascular contrast have replaced angiography for the diagnosis of major venous occlusion such as superior sagittal sinus occlusion.[52–54]

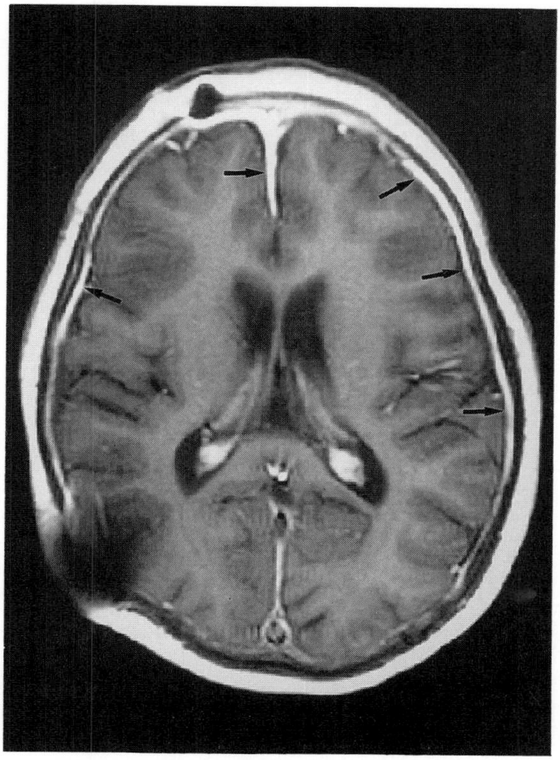

Figure 5-5 Gd-DTPA-enhanced T1-weighted axial image reveals diffuse, symmetric meningeal enhancement (black arrows) in this patient with viral meningitis. The contrast-enhanced CT scan at this time was normal. The meningeal enhancement resolved on follow-up MRI scans with resolution of the meningitis. The artifact is from a shunt connector.

MRI of the Spine

With the widespread availability of MRI-compatible traction systems and halos, MRI has become extremely important in the evaluation of the patient with spinal injury and neurologic deficit. Spinal cord transection, epidural hematoma, traumatic herniated disc (Fig. 5-2), spinal cord contusions or hematomas may be easily detected without a CTM.[55-57] The sequelae of the injured spinal cord, such as myelomalacia and syringomyelia, are better detected and differentiated on MRI than CTM.[58] CT is still necessary and more sensitive for detecting bony fractures, but the two tests provide complementary information.

CEREBRAL ANGIOGRAPHY

The role of cerebral angiography in the neurosurgical ICU patient is limited, as it has been replaced by CT and/or MRI. Angiography does play a vital role in evaluating the neurosurgical patient who develops a delayed neurologic deficit of vascular origin. The most common disorders seen in this setting are posttraumatic vascular disease, mycotic aneurysm, subarachnoid hemorrhage, vasospasm, and neurologic deterioration following surgery for arteriovenous malformation (AVM) or aneurysm.

Technique

The patient is moved to the angiography suite, which is typically large enough to accommodate ventilators and monitoring or support equipment. Most radiology departments have nurses who are experienced with the care of the critically ill patient and familiar with a variety of radiologic procedures. The examination begins with a standard catheterization procedure using the Seldinger technique for femoral arterial puncture and catheter introduction. Cerebral angiography is generally performed with an end-hole catheter introduced over a flexible-tip guide wire. Catheters with multiple holes are routinely used for aortic arch angiography. Fluoroscopy is used throughout the procedure to monitor the progress of the catheter–guide wire complex and to avoid inadvertent small-branch catheterization or subintimal dissection. The hazards of cerebral angiography have been markedly reduced by the use of heparin-coated guide wires and catheters of appropriate diameter for the patient. In the absence of significant aortic elongation or brachiocephalic tortuosity, most catheterizations can be performed with catheters that are 5 French in diameter.

When the patient is acutely ill and unstable, only the vessel of concern is studied. In the stable patient, the first injection acquired is an aortic arch study to exclude the possibility of significant extracranial disease and to identify any unusual anatomy of the proximal carotid and vertebral arteries. The arch study also serves as a "road map"

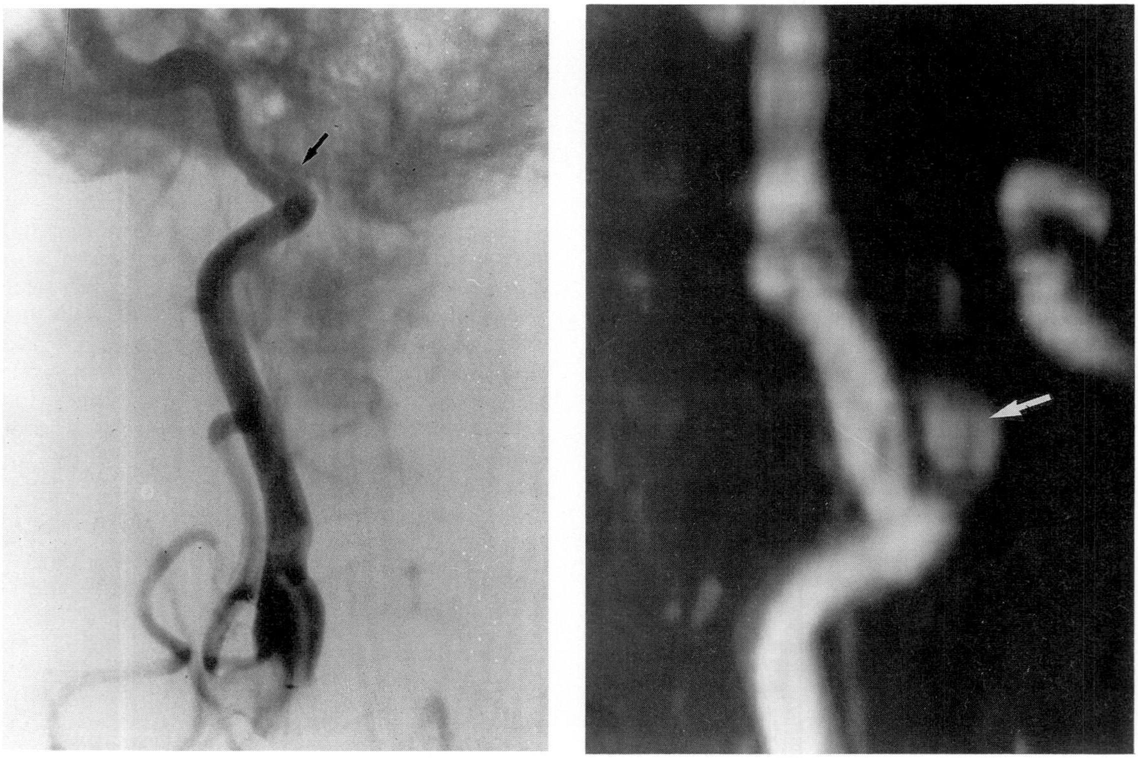

A B

Figure 5-6 Posttraumatic pseudoaneurysm. *A*. Right common carotid artery injection, lateral view, reveals a small pseudoaneurysm in the high cervical carotid artery (black arrow). *B*. MRA was obtained to follow aneurysm. Lateral projection obtained several weeks after angiogram reveals enlargement of aneurysm (white arrow).

in planning the remainder of the angiographic examination in patients with extremely tortuous vascular anatomy. The standard four-vessel cerebral angiogram is then performed.

Whether digital subtraction angiography (DSA) or conventional cut-film angiography is used depends on personal preference of the surgeon and radiologist. DSA, which uses digitalized fluoroscopy[59] to obtain high-quality angiographic images with low intraarterial iodine concentration, delivers less radiation to the patient and can be performed in less time than conventional angiography. DSA using a portable C-arm unit can be routinely performed by the radiologist in the operating room to assess placement of aneurysm clips or following resection of an AVM to check for residual abnormal vessels, retrograde thrombosis, or filling of normal vessels.

Complication rates have been reduced, largely due to the femoral artery approach replacing the direct carotid artery puncture and the development of smaller, more flexible catheters. Potential complications of cerebral angiography are categorized as neurologic (stroke, reversible neurologic deficit, seizure), allergic (mild, moderate, or severe contrast reactions, including cardiorespiratory arrest or death), or related to the femoral artery puncture (hematoma, pseudoaneurysm, or dissection). In one series comparing transfemoral catheter examinations to direct carotid puncture tech-

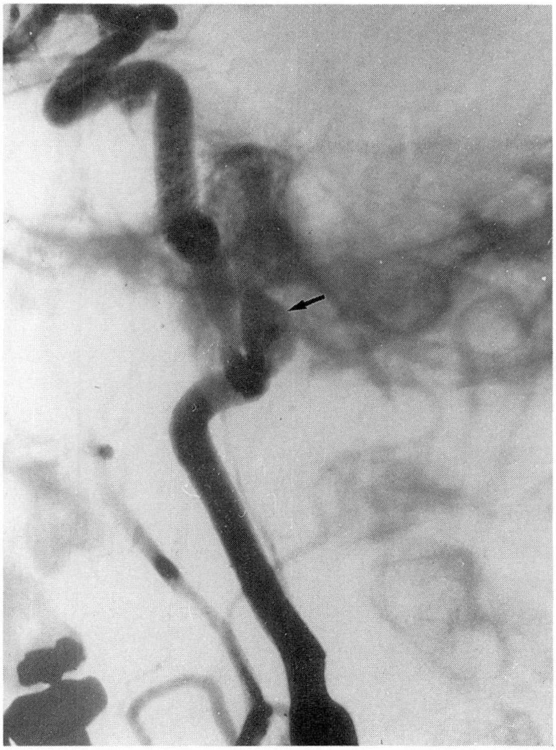

C

Figure 5-6 continued *C*. Right common carotid artery injection, lateral view, confirms interval enlargement of aneurysm (black arrow).

niques, the incidence of serious complications with the transfemoral technique was less than 0.5 percent and ranged from 0.18 to 0.28 percent.[60] Transient neurologic complications varied from 2.1 to 3.6 percent in these patients. Mani and coworkers reported 5000 cases performed with transfemoral catheterization only.[61] Permanent neurologic complications were 0.1 percent in both nontraining and training hospitals. Transient complications in the same series performed in hospitals training radiologists were 3.9 percent and in nontraining hospitals, 0.9 percent. Complications of 1.2 to 1.9 percent have been reported in patients examined for cerebral vascular disease, trauma, subarachnoid hemorrhage, and follow-up after neurosurgical procedures.[62] An incidence of less than 0.36 percent was found in patients with tumor, seizure, and headache. Variables that appear to affect complication rates include procedures lasting longer than 80 min, particularly in patients over 60 years of age with cerebral vascular disease or tumor, and the use of contrast agents containing sodium.[63] The number of arteries individually selected and injected did not appear to be an important factor affecting incidence of complications.

Indications for Cerebral Angiography

Direct and indirect vascular trauma results in a variety of arterial, capillary, and venous manifestations.[64] Three entities may warrant careful angiographic evaluation: cerebral aneurysms, extracranial dissection, and intracranial fistula.

The correct diagnosis of traumatic aneurysm depends upon a high index of suspicion. Although these lesions are rare, they have a definite association with delayed neurologic deterioration following head trauma. When a traumatic aneurysm is suspected, angiography is mandatory. Clinical settings in which a traumatic aneurysm is most likely to occur include patients with head injury severe enough to warrant early CT scanning, especially when there is a large intracranial hemorrhage; patients with penetrating head trauma secondary to stab wounds; or patients with remote history of trauma who present with new intracranial hemorrhage, recurrent epistaxis, progressive cranial nerve deficit, or an enlarging skull fracture.

Traumatic cerebral aneurysms may be due to penetrating or nonpenetrating trauma. Aneurysms secondary to nonpenetrating trauma are much more common and can be divided into skull base and peripheral (distal) lesions. Peripheral traumatic aneurysms commonly occur in the distal anterior cerebral artery due to trauma against the falcine edge or in distal cortical arteries associated with an overlying skull fracture (Fig. 5-7).

Several pertinent conclusions have been made concerning the angiographic appearance of traumatic intracranial aneurysms.[65] Traumatic intracranial aneurysms may appear on the angiogram as early as 2 h after the injury, but they have also been documented as late as months to years following injury. Twenty percent of traumatic intracranial aneurysms are multiple and may not nec-

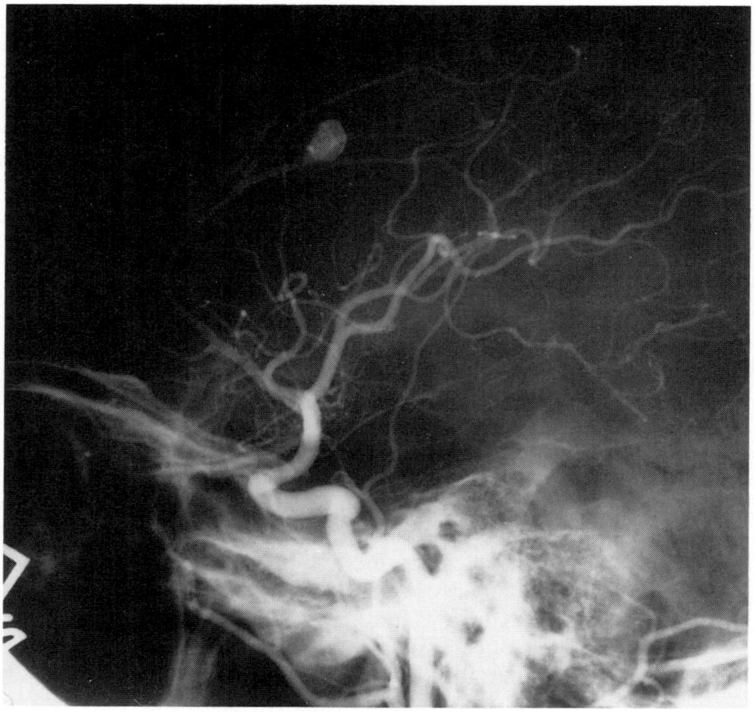

A

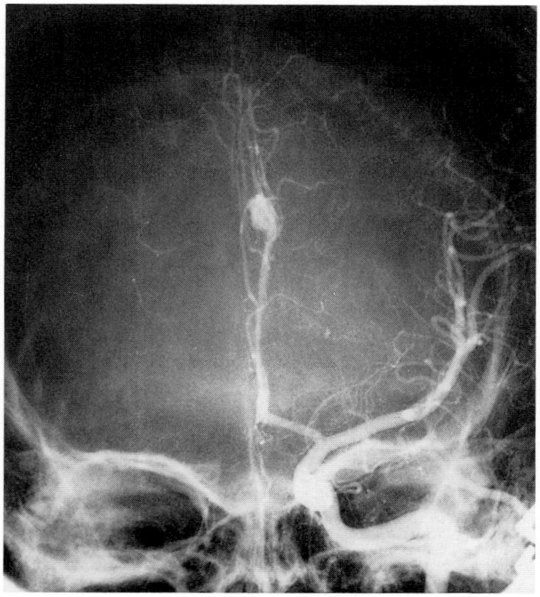

B

Figure 5-7 Young man with neurologic deterioration several days following closed head injury. *A*. Left common carotid artery injection, lateral view, shows post-traumatic lobular aneurysm arising from the pericallosal artery. *B*. Left common carotid artery injection, anterior-posterior projection, shows same pericallosal aneurysm.

essarily have the same latent period. These aneurysms occur more frequently on peripheral branches of the middle cerebral artery and less often on the posterior cerebral artery. They are associated with intracerebral hemorrhage in 80 percent of cases and with subdural hemorrhage in 26 percent of cases. These percentages are higher than those observed in penetrating head injuries not associated with traumatic intracranial aneurysms.

A history of trauma is not always obtained in patients with carotid dissections, while an identifiable traumatic episode is more commonly recalled for those with vertebral artery dissections. In both groups with a history of trauma, there is a rotary component to the traumatic event. The remaining cases are presumably spontaneous. Whether there is a specific inciting event or not, the angiographic findings are the same. Most carotid artery dissections occur in the high cervical area between C1 and C4, corresponding to a segment of the internal carotid artery beginning approximately 2 cm beyond the common carotid bifurcation. The intimal dissection can extend from the cervical to the supraclinoid carotid artery. The characteristic angiographic feature of the dissection is the delineation of an intimal flap, intimal disruption, or both. A subintimal hematoma frequently accompanies the intimal flap and on angiography is seen as an asymmetric subintimal filling defect.[66] The involved arterial segment often becomes tortuous, a state that resolves over time. Partial luminal narrowing can progress to total obstruction. No angiographic feature can be used to predict which vessels will proceed to complete thrombosis. In unilateral dissections, there is a high probability that the lumen of the involved vessel will be restored within a 6-week period. The major risk during this period is cerebral emboli, with the likelihood of stroke depending on the extent of collateral intracranial blood supply.

Vertebral artery dissection commonly occurs in the high cervical region as well but may develop more proximally when associated with a spinal fracture. The angiographic features of vertebral artery dissection are the same as those of cervical carotid artery dissection. There is also the possibility that cervical vertebral artery dissection can result in a vertebral artery-to-paravertebral venous fistula. This occurs because of the close anatomic association between the vertebral artery and radicular veins within the intervertebral foramina.

Cranial trauma, including iatrogenic trauma during surgery, can produce disruption of the carotid artery in its cavernous segment. Carotid-cavernous fistulas also occur spontaneously and are thought to be related to the rupture of cavernous carotid aneurysms. As opposed to a dural or arteriovenous fistula in the parasellar region, carotid-cavernous fistulas are considered high-volume, high-pressure fistulas.[67] They have no associated vascular network or matrix, but they do have marked arteriovenous shunting, the extent of which may preclude opacification of the intracranial circulation during angiography (Fig. 5-8). The venous drainage is into the cavernous sinus and subsequently into the inferior petrosal sinus and retrograde into the superior ophthalmic vein. The latter produces striking ophthalmic symptoms in-

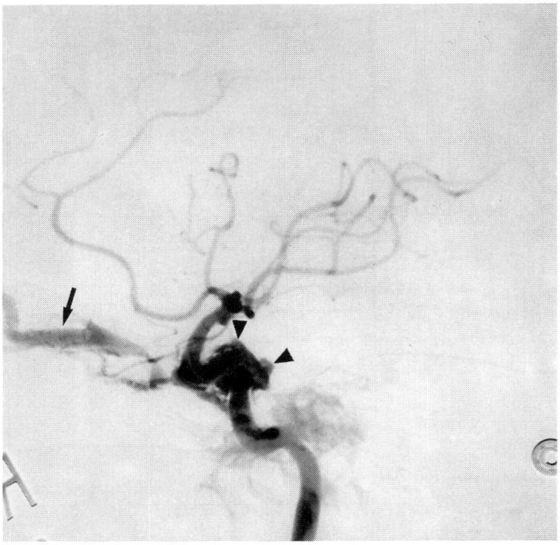

Figure 5-8 Middle-aged patient who presented with chemosis and proptosis following trauma. Right internal carotid artery injection, lateral view, early arterial phase, shows retrograde flow in the superior ophthalmic vein (black arrow) and opacification of the cavernous sinus (black arrowhead).

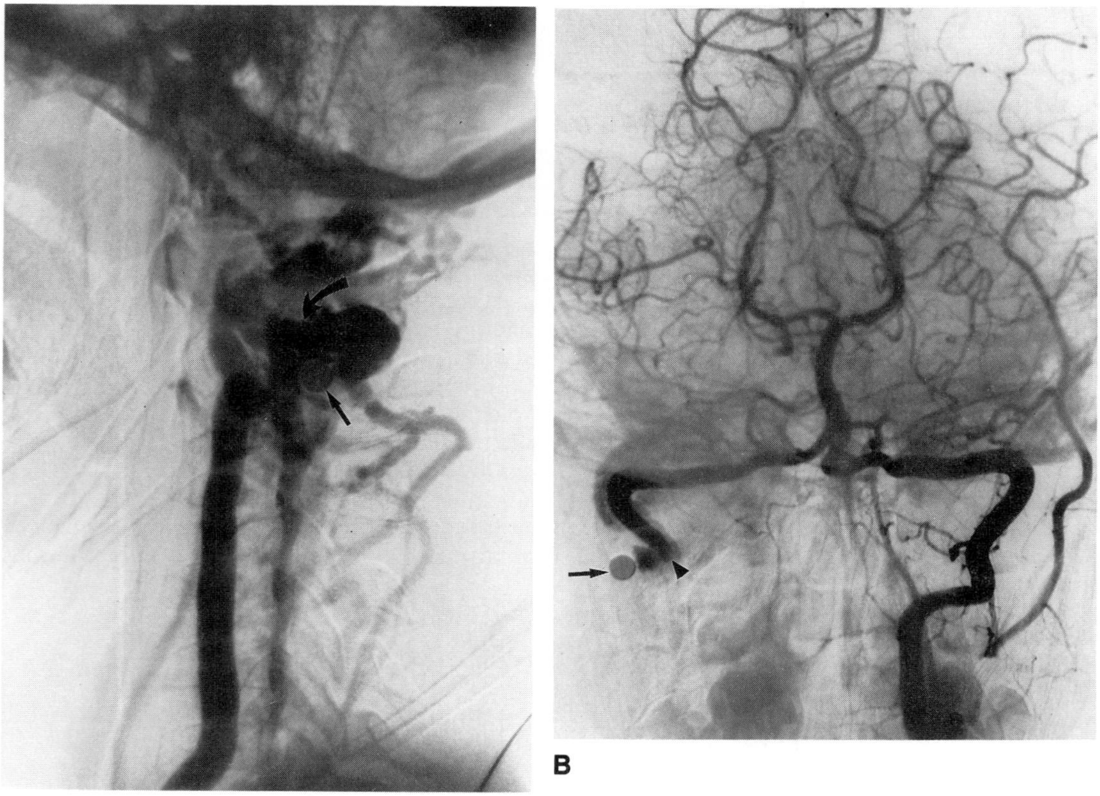

B

A

Figure 5-9 Young man who sustained a BB to the right neck. *A*. Right vertebral artery injection, lateral view, reveals opacification of the vertebral artery only to the level of C2. No filling of the basilar artery or intracranial circulation is seen. There is opacification of the paravertebral venous plexus (curved black arrow) at this level due to the vertebral artery – paravertebral venous fistula. Notice the BB (black arrow). *B*. Left vertebral artery injection, Towne projection, shows BB (black arrow) and site of right vertebral artery – paravertebral venous fistula (black arrowhead).

cluding chemosis, proptosis, and ocular cranial nerve deficits. The shunting can be sufficient to reflux into the contralateral cavernous sinus, thereby producing bilateral symptoms. The actual fistula is often difficult to see by carotid angiography but is evident when vertebral angiography is performed and the sump effect of the fistula fills the cavernous segment via retrograde opacification through the circle of Willis.[67] Similar fistulas can originate between the vertebral artery and the paravertebral veins (Fig. 5-9). They are invariably associated with penetrating injury. The angiographic features are similar to those of carotid-cavernous fistula.

Fracture of the skull can result in injury to the dural arteries. This most commonly involves the

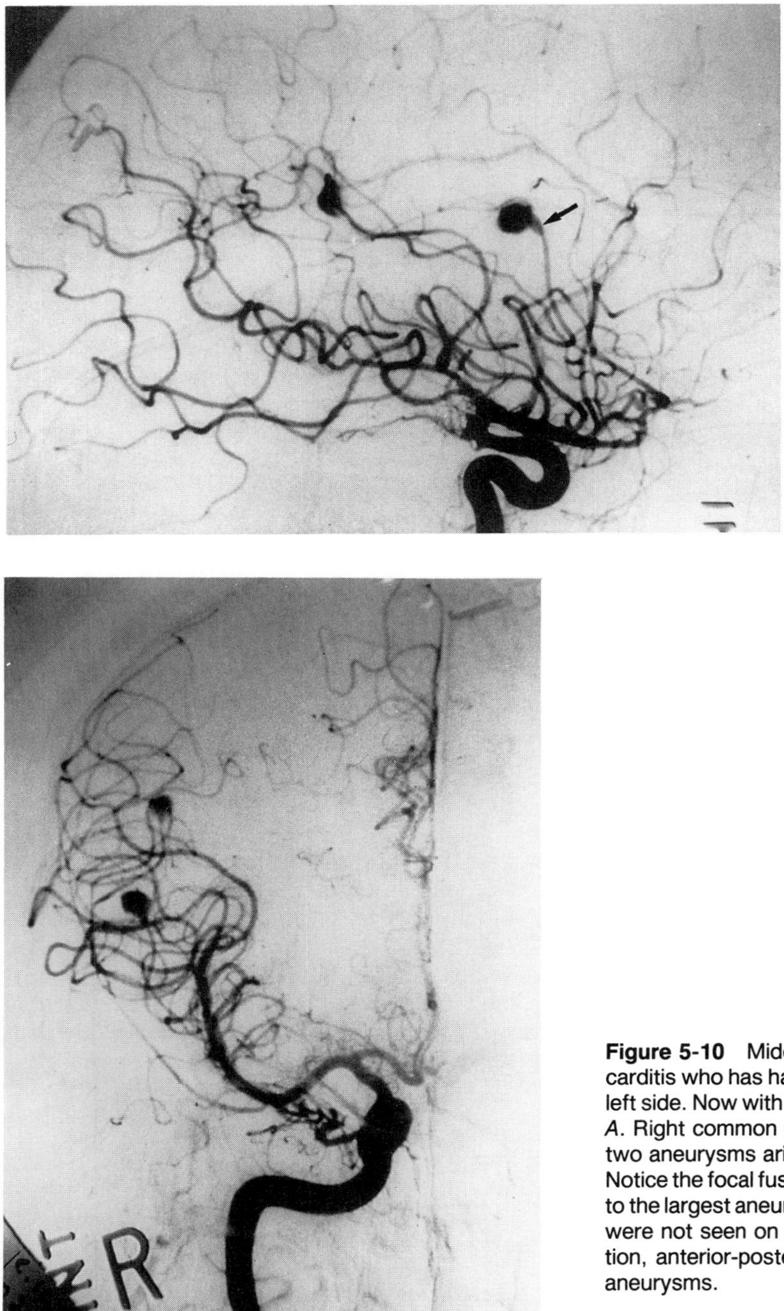

Figure 5-10 Middle-aged patient with bacterial endocarditis who has had a mycotic aneurysm clipped on the left side. Now with progressive neurologic deterioration. *A*. Right common carotid injection, lateral view, shows two aneurysms arising from the middle cerebral artery. Notice the focal fusiform dilatation of the vessel proximal to the largest aneurysm (black arrow). These aneurysms were not seen on the initial angiogram. *B*. Same injection, anterior-posterior view, again shows the mycotic aneurysms.

meningeal artery. When this vessel is injured within the meningeal groove, a fistula can form between the meningeal artery and meningeal veins. This has a characteristic "tram track" appearance, and the arteriovenous shunting is usually obvious.

Infectious intracranial aneurysms are uncommon. When they do occur, however, they are most often found in the setting of infective endocarditis with consequent septic embolization.[68] They generally appear on the anterior circulation, and they may be multiple.[69] Making the diagnosis without characteristic clinical findings of bacterial endocarditis requires a high index of suspicion, because the aneurysms are often not a consideration until they produce a devastating hemorrhage.[68-72]

Mycotic aneurysms arise in peripheral branch points of the middle and anterior cerebral arteries, and they appear least often in the posterior cerebral arteries (Fig. 5-10). They may be multiple, may change in size on subsequent angiograms, and often have a broad neck that blends with or incorporates part of the parent artery. When there is a focal abnormality of the contour of the parent artery adjacent to the aneurysm neck, the possibility of a mycotic aneurysm exists.[73] The status of the parent artery must be evaluated for symmetrical intimal irregularity, which is a possible indication of vasculitis. Intracranial bacterial aneurysms, which may be multiple about 20 percent of the time, occur in 4 to 15 percent of patients with bacterial endocarditis.[74-76]

Vasospasm is the primary cause of delayed neurologic deterioration in the patient following subarachnoid hemorrhage (SAH) due to rupture of an intracranial aneurysm. The vasospasm most frequently occurs between post-SAH day 3 and day 14,[77] although it has been documented up to several weeks following the hemorrhage. Early diagnosis is critical so that appropriate therapy can be initiated. The mortality and morbidity associated with vasospasm can be significantly reduced with early and aggressive medical therapy.[78,79] Transcranial Doppler ultrasound at the bedside is a simple and effective method of diagnosing vasospasm.[80,81] It is important to document with cerebral angiography the exact nature and location of arterial vasospasm, as this may significantly influence one's choice of therapy. Recently, balloon angioplasty has been used with some success in certain types of vasospasm such as that localized to major vessel disease.[82,83]

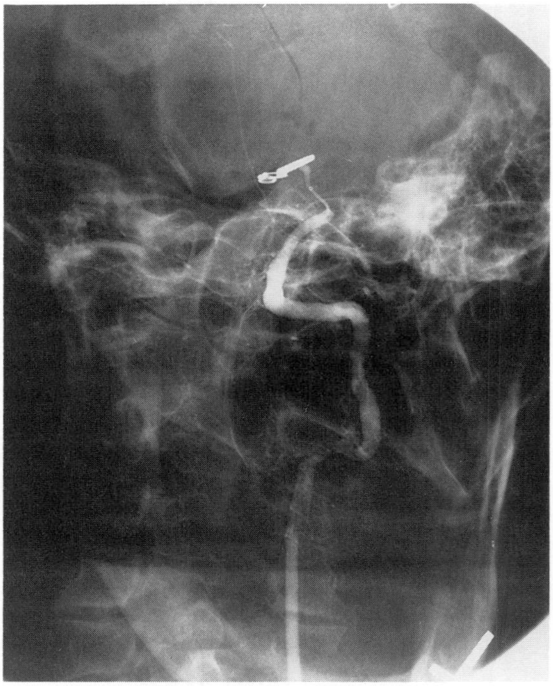

Figure 5-11 Fifty-year-old male 1 day postoperative, 4 days post-SAH with obtundation. Angiogram reveals severe vasospasm in mid and distal basilar artery.

Finally, any patient who has undergone surgery for intracranial aneurysm or AVM resection who develops new or fluctuating neurologic deficits should be evaluated with angiography. Potential causes for neurologic deterioration include poor placement of aneurysm clip, vasospasm (Fig. 5-11), or retrograde thrombosis.

REFERENCES

1. Marty R, Cain ML: Effects of corticosteroid (Dexamethasone) administration on the brain scan. *Radiology* 107:117, 1973.
2. McClennan BL: Low-osmolality contrast media: Premises and promises. *Radiology* 162:1, 1987.
3. Hayman LA, Hinck VC: Water-soluble iodinated contrast media for imaging the brain and spinal cord. In:

Latchaw RE (ed): *MR and CT Imaging of the Head, Neck, and Spine*, 2d ed. Baltimore, Mosby, chap 4, pp 65–93.
4. Katayama H, Yamaguchi K, Kozuka T, et al.: Adverse reactions to ionic and nonionic contrast media. *Radiology* 175:621, 1990.
5. Curry NS, Schabel SI, Reiheld CT, et al.: Fatal reactions to intravenous nonionic contrast material. *Radiology* 178:361, 1991.
6. Wolf GL, Arenson RL, Cross AP: A prospective trial of ionic vs nonionic contrast agents in routine clinical practice: Comparison of adverse effects. *AJR* 152:939, 1989.
7. Lasser EC, Berry CC, Talner LB, et al.: Pretreatment with corticosteroids to alleviate reactions to intravenous contrast material. *N Engl J Med* 317:845, 1987.
8. Scott WR: Seizures: A reaction to contrast media for computed tomography of the brain. *Radiology* 137:359, 1980.
9. Pagani JJ, Hayman LA, Bigelow RH, et al.: Diazepam prophylaxis of contrast media-induced seizures during computed tomography of patients with brain metastases. *AJNR* 4:67, 1983.
10. Lin JP, Pay N, Naidich TP, et al.: Computed tomography in the postoperative care of neurosurgical patients. *Neuroradiology* 12:185, 1977.
11. Scotti G, Ethier R, Melancon D, et al.: Computed tomography in the evaluation of intracranial aneurysms and subarachnoid hemorrhage. *Radiology* 123:85, 1977.
12. van Dongen KJ, Braakman R, Gelpke GJ: The prognostic value of computerized tomography in comatose head-injured patients. *J Neurosurg* 59:951, 1983.
13. Toutant SM, Klauber MR, Marshall LF, et al.: Absent or compressed basal cisterns on first CT scan: Ominous predictors of outcome in severe head injury. *J Neurosurg* 61:691, 1984.
14. Mizutani T, Manaka S, Tsutsumi H: Estimation of intracranial pressure using computed tomography scan findings in patients with severe head injury. *Surg Neurol* 33:178, 1990.
15. Jeffries BF, Kishore PRS, Singh KS, et al.: Contrast enhancement in the postoperative brain. *Radiology* 139:409, 1981.
16. Cairncross JG, Pexman JHW, Rathbone MP, DelMaestro RF: Postoperative contrast enhancement in patients with brain tumor. *Ann Neurol* 17:570, 1985.
17. Johnson DW, Lathchaw RE: Imaging of the brain following surgery, radiation therapy, and chemotherapy. In: Latchaw RE (ed): *MR and CT Imaging of the Head, Neck, and Spine*, 2d ed. Baltimore, Mosby, chap 21, pp 645–663.
18. Acheson MB, Livingston RR, Richardson ML, Stimac GK: High-resolution CT scanning in the evaluation of cervical spine fractures: Comparison with plain film examinations. *AJR* 148:1179, 1987.
19. Clayman DA, Murakami ME, Vines FS: Compatibility of cervical spine braces with MR imaging: A study of nine nonferrous devices. *AJNR* 11:385, 1990.
20. Mirvis SE, Borg U, Belzberg H: MR imaging of ventilator-dependent patients: Preliminary experience. *AJR* 149:845, 1987.
21. Brunberg JA, Papadopoulos SM: Technical note. Device to facilitate MR imaging of patients in skeletal traction. *AJNR* 12:746, 1991.
22. Dunn V, Coffman CE, McGowan JE, Ehrhardt JC: Mechanical ventilation during magnetic resonance imaging. *Magn Reson Imaging* 3:169, 1985.
23. Becker RL, Norfray JF, Teitelbaum GP, et al.: MR imaging in patients with intracranial aneurysm clips. *AJNR* 9:885, 1988.
24. Shellock FG: MR imaging of metallic implants and materials: A compilation of the literature. *AJR* 151:811, 1988.
25. Shellock FG, Curtis JS: MR imaging and biomedical implants, materials, and devices: An updated review. *Radiology* 180:541, 1991.
26. Holtas S, Olsson M, Romner B, et al.: Comparison of MR imaging and CT in patients with intracranial aneurysm clips. *AJNR* 9:891, 1988.
27. Dujovny M, Kossovsky N, Kossowsky R, et al.: Aneurysm clip motion during magnetic resonance imaging: In vivo experimental study with metallurgical factor analysis. *Neurosurgery* 17:543, 1985.
28. Teitelbaum, GP, Lin MCW, Watanabe AT, et al.: Ferromagnetism and MR imaging: Safety of carotid vascular clamps *AJNR* 11:267, 1990.
29. Laakman RW, Kaufman B, Han JS, et al.: MR imaging in patients with metallic implants. *Radiology* 157:711, 1985.
30. Davis PL, Crooks L, Arakawa M, et al.: Potential hazards in NMR imaging: Heating effects of changing magnetic fields and RF fields on small metallic implants. *AJR* 137:857, 1981.
31. Lufkin R, Jordan S, Lylyck P, Vinuela F: MR imaging with topographic EEG electrodes in place. *AJNR* 9:953, 1988.
32. Duckwiler GR, Levesque M, Wilson CL, et al.: Technical note: Imaging of MR-compatible intracerebral depth electrodes. *AJNR* 11:353, 1990.
33. Kelly WM, Paglen PG, Pearson JA, et al.: Ferromagnetism of intraocular foreign body causes unilateral blindness after MR study. *AJNR* 7:243, 1986.
34. Mattucci KF, Setzen M, Hyman R, Chaturvedi G: The effect of nuclear magnetic resonance imaging on metallic middle ear prostheses. *Otolaryngol Head Neck Surg* 94:441, 1986.
35. Shellock FG, Schatz CJ: Metallic otologic implants: In

vitro assessment of ferromagnetism at 1.5 T. *AJNR* 12:279, 1991.

36. Teitelbaum GP, Yee CA, Van Horn DD, et al.: Metallic ballistic fragments: MR imaging safety and artifacts. *Radiology* 175:855, 1990.
37. Gieszl R, Williams KD, Drayer BP, Keller PJ: Magnetic resonance imaging and ferromagnetic bullets. *Assoc Firearm Toolmark Examiner J* 21:595, 1989.
38. Goldstein HA, Kashanian FK, Blumetti RF, et al.: Safety assessment of gadopentetate dimeglumine in the U.S. clinical trials. *Radiology* 174:17, 1990.
39. Tisher S, Hoffman JC Jr: Anaphylactoid reactions to IV gadopentetate dimeglumine. *AJNR* 11:1167, 1990.
40. Snow RB, Zimmerman RD, Gandy SE, Deck MDF: Comparison of magnetic resonance imaging and computed tomography in the evaluation of head injury. *Neurosurgery* 18:45, 1986.
41. Hesselink JR, Dowd CF, Healy ME, et al.: MR imaging of brain contusions: A comparative study with CT. *AJNR* 9:269, 1988.
42. Gentry LR, Godersky JC, Thompson B, Dunn VD: Prospective comparative study of intermediate-field MR and CT in the evaluation of closed head trauma. *AJNR* 9:91, 1988.
43. Kelly AB, Zimmerman RD, Snow RB, et al.: Head trauma: Comparison of MR and CT—Experience in 100 patients. *AJNR* 9:699, 1988.
44. Sze G, Milano E, Johnson C, Heier L: Detection of brain mestastases: Comparison of contrast-enhanced MR with unenhanced MR and enhanced CT. *AJNR* 11:785, 1990.
45. Davis PC, Hudgins PA, Peterman SB, Hoffman JC Jr: Diagnosis of cerebral metastases: Double-dose delayed CT vs contrast-enhanced MR imaging. *AJNR* 12:293, 1991.
46. Crain MR, Yuh WTC, Greene GM, et al.: Cerebral ischemia: Evaluation with contrast-enhanced MR imaging. *AJNR* 12:631, 1991.
47. Yuh WTC, Crain MR, Loes DJ, et al.: MR imaging of cerebral ischemia: Findings in the first 24 hours. *AJNR* 12:621, 1991.
48. Bryan RN, Levy LM, Whitlow WD, et al.: Diagnosis of acute cerebral infarction: Comparison of CT and MR imaging. *AJNR* 12:611, 1991.
49. Sato A, Takahashi S, Soma Y, et al.: Cerebral infarction: Early detection by means of contrast-enhanced cerebral arteries at MR imaging. *Radiology* 178:433, 1991.
50. Weingarten K, Zimmerman RD, Becker RD, et al.: Subdural and epidural empyemas: MR imaging. *AJNR* 10:81, 1989.
51. Goldberg HI, Grossman RI, Gomori, JM, et al.: Cervical internal carotid artery dissecting hemorrhage: Diagnosis using MR. *Radiology* 158:157, 1986.
52. Sze G, Simmons B, Krol G, et al.: Dural sinus thrombosis: Verification with spin-echo techniques. *AJNR* 9:679, 1988.
53. Tsuruda JS, Shimakawa A, Pelc NJ, Saloner D: Dural sinus occlusion: Evaluation with phase-sensitive gradient-echo MR imaging. *AJNR* 12:481, 1991.
54. Spritzer CE, Sostman HD, Wilkes DC, Coleman RE: Deep venous thrombosis: Experience with gradient-echo MR imaging in 66 patients. *Radiology* 177:235, 1990.
55. Kalfas I, Wilberger J, Goldberg A, Prostko ER: Magnetic resonance imaging in acute spinal cord trauma. *Neurosurgery* 23:295, 1988.
56. Kulkarni MV, Bondurant FJ, Rose SL, Narayana PA: 1.5 tesla magnetic resonance imaging of acute spinal trauma. *Radiographics* 8:1059, 1988.
57. Mirvis SE, Geisler FH, Jelinek JJ, et al.: Acute cervical spine trauma: Evaluation with 1.5-T MR imaging. *Radiology* 166:807, 1988.
58. Quencer RM, Sheldon JJ, Post MJD, et al.: Magnetic resonance imaging of the chronically injured cervical spinal cord. *AJNR* 7:457, 1986.
59. Mistretta CA, Crummy AB, Strother CM: Digital angiography: A perspective. *Radiology* 139:273, 1981.
60. Huckman MS, Shenk GI, Neems RL, Tinor T: Transfemoral cerebral arteriography versus direct percutaneous carotid and brachial arteriography: A comparison of complication rates. *Radiology* 132:93, 1979.
61. Mani RL, Eisenberg RL, McDonald EJ, et al.: Complications of catheter cerebral arteriography: Analysis of 5,000 procedures. I. Criteria and incidence. *Am Roentgenol* 131:861, 1978.
62. Mani RL, Eisenberg RL: Complications of catheter cerebral arteriography: Analysis of 5,000 procedures. II. Relation of complication rates to clinical and arteriographic diagnosis. *Am Roentgenology* 131:867, 1978.
63. Mani RL, Eisenberg RL: Complications of catheter cerebral arteriography: Analysis of 5,000 procedures. III. Assessment of arteries injected, contrast medium used, duration of procedure, and age of patient. Am J Roentgenol 131:871, 1978.
64. Quisling R, Friedman W, Rhoton A Jr: Spontaneous regression of high cervical carotid artery dissection. *AJNR* 2:463, 1980.
65. Haddad FS, Haddad GF, Taha J: Traumatic intracranial aneurysms caused by missiles. Their presentation and management. *Neurosurgery* 28:1, 1991.
66. Friedman AH: Arterial dissections. In: Wikins RH, Rengachary SS (eds): *Neurosurgery*, 3d ed. New York, McGraw-Hill, chap 31, pp 1297–1300.
67. Harris ME, Barrow DL: Traumatic carotid-cavenous sinus fistulas. In: Barrow DLB (ed): *Complications and Sequelae of Head Injury*. Illinois, American Assoc. Neurological Surgeons, chap 2, pp 13–30.

68. Ojemann RG, New PFJ, Fleming TC: Intracranial aneurysms associated with bacterial meningitis. *Neurology* 16:1222, 1966.
69. Cantu RC, LeMay M, Wilkinson HA: The importance of repeated angiography in the treatment of mycotic-embolic intracranial aneurysms. *J Neurosurg* 25:189, 1966.
70. Molinari GF: Septic cerebral embolism. *Stroke* 3:117, 1972.
71. Roach MR, Drake CG: Ruptured cerebral aneurysms caused by microorganisms. *N Engl J Med* 273:240, 1965.
72. Sypert GW, Young HF: Ruptured mycotic pericallosal aneurysm with meningitis due to Neisseria Meningitidis infection. *J Neurosurg* 37:467, 1972.
73. Kaufman S, White R Jr, Harring D, et al.: Protean manifestations of mycotic aneurysms. *AJR* 13:1019, 1978.
74. Bohmfalk GL, Story JL, Wissinger JP, et al.: Bacterial intracranial aneurysm. *J Neurosurg* 48:369, 1978.
75. Barrow DL, Prats AR: Infectious intracranial aneurysms: Comparison of groups with and without endocarditis. *Neurosurgery* 27:562, 1990.
76. Venger BH, Aldama AE: Mycotic vasculitis with repeated intracranial aneurysmal hemorrhage. *J Neurosurg* 69:775, 1988.
77. Wilkins RH: Cerebral vasospasm. *Crit Rev Neurobiol* 6:51, 1990.
78. Jakobsen M, Overgard J, Marcussen E, et al.: Relationship between angiographic cerebral vasospasms and regional CBF in patients with SAH. *Acta Neurol Scand* 82:109, 1990.
79. Awad IA, Little JR: Perioperative management and outcome after surgical treatment of anterior cerebral artery aneurysms. *Can J Neurol Sci* 18:120, 1991.
80. Sloan MA, Haley EC, Kassel NF, et al.: Sensitivity and specificity of transcranial Doppler ultrasonography in the diagnosis of vasospasm following subarachnoid hemorrhage. *Neurology* 39:1514, 1989.
81. Fornezza U, Carraro R, Demo P, et al.: The transcranial Doppler ultrasonography in the evaluation of vasospasm and of intercranial hypertension after subarachnoid hemorrhage. *Aggressologie* 31:259, 1990.
82. Grimes CM: Cerebral balloon angioplasty for treatment of vasospasm after subarachnoid hemorrhage. *Heart Lung* 20:431, 1991.
83. Bracard S, Picard L, Marchal JC, et al.: Role of angioplasty in the treatment of symptomatic vascular spasm occurring in the post-operative course of intracranial ruptured aneurysms. *J Neuroradiol* 17:6, 1991.

CHAPTER 6

Fluid, Electrolyte, and Acid-Base Balance in Neurosurgical Intensive Care

Joseph M. Darby
Paul B. Nelson

GENERAL CONSIDERATIONS

The central nervous system (CNS) plays a vital role in fluid, electrolyte, and acid-base homeostasis. Critically ill neurosurgical patients are uniquely predisposed to perturbations in this homeostasis due to the combined effects of CNS injury and routine therapeutic interventions employed in the treatment of such injuries. Moreover, the potential consequences of such disturbances on brain function are profound. Altered consciousness, impaired autoregulation, the presence of brain edema, and intracranial hypertension are all factors that present unique challenges in management. Early recognition and appropriate management of fluid, electrolyte, and acid-base disorders should favorably affect secondary brain injury in the neurosurgical intensive care unit (ICU).

Body Compartments, Water, and Electrolyte Distributions

Normally, total body water (TBW) in the adult male is approximately 60 percent of body weight and varies with age and body leanness. Newborns and children have a higher body water content than adults, while women and the obese have a lower body water content due to the lower percentage of water in adipose tissue. Roughly two-thirds of TBW is intracellular fluid (ICF) with the remaining one-third distributed to the extracellular fluid (ECF). Approximately one-fourth of the ECF is in the intravascular compartment with the remaining three-fourths in the interstitial space. The *third-space* includes water formed by active transport of extracellular water across epithelial cells into such spaces as the gastrointestinal (GI) tract, cerebrospinal fluid (CSF), biliary tract, and lymphatics.[1] The term *third-space* is also commonly used to refer to fluid accumulating in tissue as a result of direct injury or inflammation that is functionally excluded from the ECF for a variable period of time.

Total body potassium (K^+) is approximately 50 mEq/kg, 98 percent of which is intracellular and 2 percent is extracellular. The intracellular [K^+] ranges from 140 to 150 mEq/L, while the extracellular concentration ranges from 3.5 to 5 mEq/L. The high intracellular to extracellular concentration gradient is maintained primarily by the Na^+, K^+-ATPase pump and is essential for the maintenance of a normal resting membrane potential. Total body sodium (Na^+) is approximately 40 mEq/kg with a concentration gradient that is similar to K^+ but in the opposite direction. Extracellular [Na^+] ranges from 138 to 142 mEq/L, while the intracellular concentration ranges from 5 to 15 mEq/L.

Osmolality and Tonicity

Osmolality is the sum total of particles in solution and is expressed as the *molal concentration* of all solutes in water (mOsm/kg). Although relative solute concentrations between the ICF and ECF differ, most cell membranes are freely permeable to water permitting osmotic equilibrium to occur. Thus, *osmolality is a major determinant of water distribution between the ICF and ECF.* Osmotic pressure is the force for water movement that is generated by differences in osmolality across membranes. Oncotic pressure is the osmotic pressure that is due solely to differences in protein concentration.

ECF osmolarity is determined principally by Na^+ and its associated anion, Cl^-, along with glucose and urea. Normal serum osmolality is 286 ± 4 mOsm/kg and can be estimated by the following equation[2]:

$$\text{Osmolality (mOsm/kg)} = 2 \times [Na^+] + [\text{glucose}]/18 + \text{BUN}/2.8$$

The measured osmolality is about 10 mOsm/kg greater than the calculated osmolality because of other minor solutes including calcium, magnesium, protein, and amino acids. This "osmolal gap" can be increased by unmeasured solutes such as alcohol and mannitol, or when there is pseudohyponatremia, secondary hyperlipidemia, or hyperproteinemia.

For the purposes of determining the relative state of hydration, the concept of *tonicity* or *effective osmolality* is useful, especially in regard to the CNS. Effective osmolality refers to osmolality as it relates to solutes that are capable of creating an osmotic gradient. Highly permeable solutes such as alcohol and urea generally do not contribute to the development of an osmotic gradient and, therefore, have little influence on the distribution of water between compartments.

$$\text{Effective osmolality (mOsm/kg)} = 2 \times [Na^+] + [\text{glucose}]/18$$

To this equation, the osmolal concentration of any other osmotically active solute (e.g., mannitol) can be added to calculate effective osmolality. As has been noted, urea is freely permeable to most cell membranes. However, it is only partially permeable to capillaries of the blood-brain barrier (BBB). Therefore, urea contributes to effective osmolality and water flux across the brain when plasma urea concentration is acutely changed, as in therapeutic administration of urea.

In the neurosurgical patient, hypo- or hyperosmolar states are common clinical problems caused mainly by disturbances in water balance [e.g., syndrome of inappropriate antidiuretic hormone (SIADH), diabetes insipidus] or by osmotherapy. Nonetheless, routine serum osmolality measurements are of limited value in the ICU for the evaluation of fluid and electrolyte disorders because effective osmolality can easily be estimated using plasma sodium and glucose. Monitoring serum osmolarity, however, may be of value in patients receiving mannitol for the control of brain swelling or intracranial hypertension to minimize the potential for exacerbation of brain edema[3] and the prevention of mannitol-induced renal failure,[4] especially when patients are receiving very high doses or prolonged therapy. The recommended upper limits of plasma osmolality during mannitol therapy have ranged from 320 to 350 mOsm/kg.[5,6] In this regard, it is probably wise to keep plasma osmolality < 340 mOsm/kg to minimize any effect of hyperosmolality on the sensorium. Calculation and monitoring of the osmolal gap is also useful during mannitol therapy, especially when there is coexistent hyponatremia. The osmolal gap will be an indirect measure of plasma mannitol concentration and should be kept <55 mOsm/kg to prevent renal failure.[4]

REGULATION OF BODY FLUIDS

Regulation of Body Water and Osmolality

The regulation of body water and tonicity is of extreme importance for proper cellular function, especially within the CNS. Hypo-osmolality and cellular swelling within the CNS not only has deleterious effects on cellular function but, when unchecked, may also increase brain volume and intracranial pressure (ICP). Hyperosmolality and cellular dehydration may also impair CNS function and cause intracranial hemorrhage.

In healthy adults, plasma Na^+ and osmolality are maintained within a markedly narrow range. This stability is achieved primarily by adjusting TBW to keep it in balance with sodium. Water balance is largely controlled by the posterior pituitary hormone, arginine vasopressin (AVP), or antidiuretic hormone. AVP is a small peptide made in the supraoptic and paraventricular nuclei of the anterior hypothalamus. It is carried down the hypothalamo-hypophyseal tract to the posterior lobe of the pituitary gland from which it is secreted. AVP acts on the collecting duct of the renal tubule, increasing water reabsorption. Osmoreceptors are located in the anterior hypothalamus in the area of the organum vasculosum laminae terminalis (OVLT), a structure that is excluded from the BBB. Changes in osmoreceptor cell volume as a consequence of changes in effective plasma osmolarity are the likely stimuli for osmotic AVP release.[7] The osmotic threshold for AVP release in humans is approximately 280 mOsm/kg, with AVP levels increasing linearly with osmolality.[8] Under maximal stimulation by AVP, the kidney can concentrate urine to achieve a urinary osmolality well over 1000 mOsm/kg, thereby conserving water. For example, if solute intake is 600 mOsm/kg, renal concentrating mechanisms can raise urine osmolality to 1200 mOsm/kg, necessitating a daily urine output of only 500 mL to eliminate the solute load:

$$\frac{600 \text{ mOsm/day}}{1200 \text{ mOsm/kg}} = 500 \text{ mL/day}$$

Under hyperosmolar conditions, thirst and drinking behavior also are important to the maintenance of water balance. Even in the absence of AVP, plasma osmolality can generally be maintained as long as water is available and the patient's level of consciousness permits thirst perception and drinking behavior.

Suppression of AVP release is the major mechanism controlling water balance under hypo-osmolar conditions, permitting the excretion of a maximally dilute urine (50 to 100 mOsm/kg). However, renal water excretion is not only dependent on circulating levels of AVP, but also dependent on solute intake. For example, if solute intake is 900 mOsm/kg and urine can be diluted to 50 mOsm/kg, 18 L of urine can be excreted:

$$\frac{900 \text{ mOsm/day}}{50 \text{ mOsm/kg}} = 18 \text{ L/day}$$

Conceptually, 3 L of this fluid is near isotonic and 15 L is solute free or *free water*. If solute intake decreases to 450 mOsm/day, maximum urinary water excretion is only 9 L and free water excretion is reduced to 7.5 L. In addition, it can be seen that if AVP levels are increased, thereby reducing urinary dilution, free water excretion will be further impaired. Thus, under conditions of reduced solute intake and/or increased AVP, water intake in excess of renal capacity to excrete a free water load will result in hyponatremia and hypo-osmolarity.

Although the main stimulus for AVP release is an increase in plasma osmolality, AVP can also be released by a variety of nonosmotic stimuli including drugs commonly used in neurointensive care, such as narcotics, barbiturates, and carbamazepine; nausea; and conditions associated with an increase in sympathetic tone, such as pain, hemorrhage, and hypovolemia.[8] One of the most potent nonosmotic stimuli to AVP release is hypovolemia. Baroreceptors in the atria, aortic arch, and carotid sinus are sensitive to decreases in pressure resulting in AVP release. Hypovolemia is such a potent stimulus to AVP release that AVP will continue to be released even in the presence of plasma hypo-osmolality.[9] Renal diluting capacity, therefore, can be impaired under hypovolemic conditions and may, in part, explain the development of hyponatremia and excess circulating AVP in some postoperative patients who are receiving hypotonic fluids.[10,11] Intracranial hypertension has been shown in animal studies to result in nonsuppressible increases in AVP and increases in both plasma and CSF AVP in humans.[12–14] These findings may partially explain why hyponatremia occurs commonly in the neurosurgical population. It has been suggested that AVP release under such circumstances may be an adaptive response to maintain brain perfusion under ischemic or near ischemic conditions.

Regulation of Intracellular Volume

Many cells have been shown to possess mechanisms for control of cellular volume that balance changes in plasma osmolality with changes in intracellular solute concentration. These adaptive solute changes are operative in the CNS and appear to be important in controlling brain volume under both hypo-osmolar or hyperosmolar conditions.[15–19] Under hypo-osmolar conditions, intracellular solute concentration decreases by a variety of mechanisms including increased intracellular binding and extrusion of Na^+, K^+, and Cl^-, preventing cellular swelling. Under hyperosmolar conditions, intracellular solute content increases by an influx of electrolytes, decreased intracellular binding, and increases in amino acid concentration, preventing cellular dehydration.

Transcapillary Water Flux

Although water movement between the extracellular and intracellular space is driven mainly by osmotic forces, water flux from the intravascular to the interstitial space is more complex and is of concern in the critically ill patient, especially as it relates to the formation of fluid in the lung and brain. The forces operative in the bulk transport of water across the capillary membrane are hydrostatic and osmotic. The Starling equation generally describes the factors determining the transcapillary filtration rate (Q_f).

$$Q_f = K_f[(P_c - P_i) - \delta(\pi_c - \pi_i)]$$

K_f is the hydraulic conductivity or filtration coefficient of the membrane and is a measure of the relative permeability of the membrane to water under osmotic or hydrostatic stress. P_c is the capillary hydrostatic pressure and P_i is the interstitial hydrostatic pressure. The relative permeability of a given solute to the membrane is given by its reflection coefficient (δ) and is a measure of its osmotic effectiveness. The higher the reflection coefficient, the more impermeable the solute. π_c is plasma capillary osmotic pressure and π_i the interstitial osmotic pressure. Because most capillaries are relatively permeable to salts (e.g., Na^+) and impermeable to proteins, osmotic pressure is determined by oncotic pressure in the steady state. Differences in oncotic pressure between plasma and the interstitium result in a net force favoring fluid movement from the interstitium to the vascular compartment, while hydrostatic pressure forces favor fluid movement out of the vascular space. The net effect in most capillary beds is a slight positive fluid movement out of the vascular space into the interstitium. The lymphatics remove interstitial fluid until their capacity is exceeded, at which point, edema occurs.

Unlike most other organ systems, the CNS does not have a lymphatic system nor is there a wide margin of safety in regard to the accumulation of edema fluid since it is rigidly encased. CNS capillaries, with their tight junctions, are well adapted to prevent and buffer water movement across the capillary membrane and are an integral component of the BBB.[20,21] Capillaries within the CNS have a very low hydraulic conductivity for water, resulting in relatively less water flux for a given hydrostatic or osmotic gradient. Furthermore, the BBB has very high reflection coefficients for almost all solutes, including Na^+. Consequently, any water flux across the intact BBB into the brain interstitium tends to be solute free, setting up an opposing osmotic gradient and buffering further water flux. Under normal conditions, these membrane characteristics minimize water flux between the plasma and brain interstitium. When the BBB is disrupted, hydraulic conductivity and solute permeability increase, resulting in an increase in water flux across the capillary membrane via hydrostatic forces (vasogenic edema); by reducing the normally high osmotic buffering capacity, salts become freely permeable and proteins leak into the brain interstitium. Excess interstitial fluid may be accommodated in the brain via the Virchow-Robin spaces or by bulk flow through white matter to the ventricular CSF.

Regulation of Body Sodium

Sodium salts are the predominant osmotically active solutes in the ECF and thus are important in determining ECF volume. Body Na^+ balance is controlled by a variety of mechanisms affecting renal Na^+ excretion, which have been described in detail elsewhere.[22,23] Briefly, the relative fullness of the ECF is detected by receptors located in low, or intrathoracic, and high, or intraarterial, pressure areas of the cardiovascular system. Once changes in ECF volume are detected, renal, neural, and hormonal mechanisms modulate renal Na^+ excretion, decreasing renal Na^+ and water excretion when absolute or relative ECF volume is low and increasing excretion when ECF volume is high. One of the principal renal mechanisms influencing Na^+ excretion in response to changes in ECF volume are physical factors in the peritubular capillary environment, i.e., hydrostatic and oncotic pressure. Accordingly, when renal perfusion pressure is decreased or oncotic pressure is increased in the peritubular capillary, the balance of Starling forces will favor net Na^+ and water reabsorption in the proximal tubule. Similarly, increases in hydrostatic pressure in the peritubular capillary will favor Na^+ excretion. Independent of changes in renal perfusion pressure or oncotic pressure, changes in the resistance of the glomerular afferent or efferent arteriole can also affect renal Na^+ reabsorption. Vasodilation with low-dose dopamine, for example, will tend to increase capillary hydrostatic pressure and renal Na^+ excretion, while vasoconstriction (e.g., heart failure) reduces hydrostatic pressure and Na^+ excretion. Adrenergic nerve fibers innervate the renal tubules and can influence renal Na^+ excretion independent of changes in renal hemodynamics. Adrenergic stimulation enhances renal Na^+ reabsorption, while denervation reduces reabsorption of Na^+.

The main hormonal mechanism influencing renal Na^+ excretion is the renin-angiotensin-aldosterone system. Reductions in effective blood volume are detected by the juxtaglomerular apparatus increasing renin release from the kidney, ultimately increasing angiotensin II and aldosterone levels. Aldosterone increases distal tubular Na^+ reabsorption and K^+ excretion. In addition to increasing adrenal aldosterone release, angiotensin also increases systemic vascular resistance and proximal Na^+ reabsorption by increasing resistance in the efferent arteriole.

Another recently discovered hormone, atrial natriuretic peptide (ANP), also is important in body Na^+ regulation. ANP is produced both in atrial myocytes and within the CNS.[24,25] Its overall actions generally oppose those of AVP and angiotensin and thus appear to play an important role in the regulation of systemic fluid, electrolyte balance, and hemodynamics. Furthermore, evidence is accumulating that ANP may also be intimately involved with local control of brain volume and water and electrolyte content as well.[26,27]

ANP is released into the systemic circulation from the atria under conditions of increased intravascular volume, increased atrial pressure independent of intravascular volume, and under salt loading conditions. In addition to causing a decrease in renal vascular resistance, an increase in glomerular filtration rate, natriuresis, and diuresis, it also is an inhibitor of the renin-angiotensin-aldosterone axis. ANP also reduces systemic vascular resistance and blood pressure.

ANP found in the CNS is of lower molecular weight than the 28-amino-acid peptide that circulates in the periphery. ANP containing cell bodies and receptor sites are widely distributed throughout the CNS with their locations and physiologic effects suggesting an important role in cardiovascular and endocrine homeostasis.[25,28–30] ANP containing neurons are concentrated in the anteroventral-periventricular region of the third ventricle, the lateral hypothalamus, and visceral centers in the brainstem. Projections of these neurons and ANP receptors are found in such areas as the median eminence, hypothalamus, spinal cord, mesencephalon, and choroid plexus. In concert with its systemic actions, ANP released locally in the CNS does appear to inhibit AVP release and block angiotensin II–mediated increases in blood pressure and dipsogenesis. Angiotensin II also appears to be locally produced in the brain with binding sites or local effects in regions that are involved in the control of fluid balance and hemodynamics (e.g., OVLT, subfornical area, nucleus tractus solitarius, and area postrema).[29,31,32]

ANP locally released in the CNS also appears to play an important role in the control of intracellular volume of the brain.[33-36] ANP opposes AVP-mediated increases in brain capillary permeability, reduces brain water after ischemic insult, and prevents water accumulation under systemic hypo-osmolar conditions. These protective effects may occur through ANP-mediated alterations in capillary permeability for both Na^+ and water. ANP has also been reported to decrease CSF production and, therefore, may be important in overall volume homeostasis of the brain as well.[26,27]

FLUID MANAGEMENT

Fluid and electrolyte therapy is an essential but often complicated therapeutic intervention in the critically ill patient. Its complexity derives from a variety of neurohumoral responses to critical illness; variable degrees of organ system dysfunction; and commonly used therapeutic interventions such as mechanical ventilation, diuretics, and parenteral nutrition; all of which may affect fluid and electrolyte balance. While proper water and Na^+ balance are essential in preventing or minimizing brain edema, the restoration and maintenance of an adequate circulating blood volume and tissue oxygenation is essential to prevent multisystem organ failure (MSOF) and secondary ischemic neuronal injury in the neurosurgical patient.

Fluid and Electrolyte Shifts

Fluid and electrolyte changes associated with acute critical illness, such as hypovolemia, hemorrhage, or surgical stress, are characterized by salt and water retention and are briefly summarized here. Under such conditions, neurohumoral and renal mechanisms act in concert with compensatory cardiovascular reflexes to preserve intravascular volume and maintain vital organ perfusion. Reduced renal perfusion results in enhanced proximal tubular reabsorption of Na, while reductions in effective circulating blood volume activate the renin-angiotension-aldosterone system, reducing renal Na^+ excretion further. Water accompanies retained sodium and baroreceptor-mediated AVP release decreases renal free water excretion, promoting further water retention. Another mechanism acting to preserve intravascular volume in patients with hemorrhage involves the translocation of interstitial fluid to the intravascular compartment.[37]

As a consequence of changes in salt and water balance, critically ill patients often become edematous, gain weight, and occasionally develop hyponatremia with fluid resuscitation. Increases in vascular permeability associated with sepsis or severe third-space fluid losses with multiple trauma further increase fluid requirements and aggravate fluid retention and weight gain. Sodium and water retention are usually maximal during the first several days after insult but may last longer, especially if the patient remains on positive-pressure ventilation, which may cause continued AVP release.[38] Resolution is heralded by mobilization of retained salt and water with a spontaneous diuresis and weight loss. Mobilization of retained fluid into the intravascular space can be associated with the development of pulmonary vascular congestion and edema, especially in patients with impaired cardiac function. Tissue trauma or prolonged impaired tissue perfusion causes cellular K^+ release and a transient increase in plasma K^+. If renal function is intact, increased filtered and excreted K^+ combined with elevated aldosterone levels may cause depletion of total body K^+, predisposing to hypokalemia.

Assessment of Requirements

Among variables to be considered in the daily assessment of fluid and electrolyte requirements are body weight, prior fluid intake and output, serum electrolytes, arterial blood gases, hemodynamics, renal function, and the radiographic appearance of the lungs. Time-related changes in the distribution of fluids as a result of injury, sepsis, or prior fluid resuscitation must also be anticipated and taken into consideration. Fluid administration is continually reevaluated in the clinical context using basic principles to restore and maintain normal water and electrolyte balance and tissue oxygenation while avoiding complications of therapy.

Fluid requirements can be broken down into

three basic components: maintenance needs, ongoing losses, and deficits. Maintenance water requirements in the uncomplicated surgical patient average 30 to 35 mL/kg/day to balance a urinary loss of 800 to 1500 mL/day, a GI loss of 0 to 250 mL/day, and insensible losses through the lungs and skin of 600 to 900 mL/day. Fever increases insensible water loss by approximately 250 to 300 mL/day per °C. In the critically ill patient, maintenance water requirements may be reduced variably. For example, patients receiving mechanical ventilation will have insensible water loss through the lung reduced to near zero as a result of breathing fully warmed and saturated gas. In addition, water normally produced via the oxidation of food (100 to 200 mL/day) can be increased to as much as 1000 mL/day in highly stressed patients as a result of tissue catabolism.[1] These factors, combined with increased circulating levels of AVP occurring in response to hemorrhage, hypovolemia, and intracranial disease, may notably reduce maintenance water requirements, perhaps to as low as 20 to 25 mL/kg per day in some patients. Minimum maintenance electrolyte requirements are approximately 75 mEq Na and 40 mEq K^+.

Until the patient resumes a normal dietary intake or nutritional support is instituted, routine maintenance intravenous fluids are generally given as 5% dextrose in 0.21 to 0.45% saline solutions with supplemental K^+, unless intravascular volume deficits or ongoing losses dictate the need to use fluids with better intravascular retention [e.g., 0.9% saline or Ringer's lactate (RL)]. The choice of maintenance fluids becomes problematic in the neurosurgical patient given their unique predisposition to impaired water excretion and the potential consequences of hyponatremia. Cerebral or spinal cord autoregulation may also be impaired early after injury, necessitating the maintenance of intravascular volumes higher than would normally be necessary in the routine postoperative patient. Furthermore, clinical studies in patients early after stroke,[39-41] cardiac arrest,[42] and head injury[43-46] have suggested that hyperglycemia is associated with a poor outcome. In clinical studies, glucose levels >200 to 250 mg/dL appear in the range where adverse outcomes increase. Hyperglycemia has also been shown to adversely impact outcome in experimental spinal cord injury.[47] Although hyperglycemia may simply be a reflection of injury severity, increased glucose may provide substrate to marginally perfused tissue resulting in anaerobic metabolism, lactic acidosis, and cellular injury. With these considerations in mind, early maintenance fluid therapy in critically ill neurosurgical patients at risk for further brain ischemia or edema should be isotonic to plasma (0.9% saline) and dextrose free for at least the first 24 h after insult. Beyond the early phase of insult, maintenance fluid and electrolytes are tailored after reassessing the clinical condition, fluid and electrolyte balance, and response to therapy. Nutritional support is usually instituted within 48 to 72 h when possible to meet energy and protein requirements and minimize catabolism (reviewed in Chap. 7).

Ongoing fluid and electrolyte losses in the neurosurgical patient commonly occur as a result of nasogastric suction, diarrhea, osmotic diuretic use, and third-space fluid losses in those that are multiply traumatized. Accurate replacement requires measurement of the electrolyte composition and volume of lost fluids. Ongoing third-space fluid losses cannot be directly measured but are usually manifest by evidence of volume contraction, hemodynamic instability, or impaired organ perfusion. These losses are usually replaced with isotonic crystalloids with or without supplemental colloid.

Volume Resuscitation

Intravascular volume deficits and volume resuscitation are discussed below and separately from common water and electrolyte deficits. Absolute deficits in intravascular volume are usually the result of hemorrhage, third-space losses from trauma or sepsis, or overaggressive diuretic use. Relative deficits may occur in patients who are receiving positive-pressure ventilation or in those who are vasodilated from sepsis or spinal cord injury. Typically, hypovolemia is manifest by one or more signs including hypotension, tachycardia, oliguria, and/or lactic acidosis. In such patients, the indications and therapeutic endpoints for volume resuscitation will usually be clear. Often, however, clinical estimates of volume status may be inaccurate because of coexisting organ dysfunction, inexperience, or misinterpretation of available data.[48-51] In addition, the volume status and appropriate hemodynamic endpoints in neurosurgical patients may be uncertain or require a therapeutic trial to optimize cerebral or spinal cord O_2 delivery under conditions in which autoregulation may be impaired.

Empiric volume resuscitation using crystalloid, colloid, and/or blood are appropriate in acute shock or when there is obvious hypovolemia. Invasive hemodynamic monitoring using either central venous or pulmonary artery catheterization should be considered when empiric volume resuscitation fails to work as anticipated or when hemodynamic status remains in question. As is reviewed in Chap. 13, reductions in circulating blood volume probably occur more commonly than appreciated in patients after subarachnoid hemorrhage and may increase the risk of delayed cerebral ischemia from vasospasm.[52–55] Benefit from volume expansion in these patients may derive from improvement in cerebral O_2 delivery by augmentation of low cardiac output or blood pressure, or by independent mechanisms such as hemodilution and improved microcirculatory flow. Patients at risk for vasospasm should, at a minimum, have CVP monitored. Pulmonary artery catheterization will provide the best guide to therapy in those who develop clinical vasospasm.

Multiply traumatized patients with head or spinal cord injury, or other neurosurgical patients, particularly those requiring high-dose barbiturate therapy, should also be strongly considered for invasive hemodynamic monitoring for appropriate volume resuscitation. In the multiply traumatized patient with head injury, volume resuscitation may need to be titrated to provide a hyperdynamic circulation, as systemic O_2 consumption may be markedly increased.[56] Mean arterial pressure should be restored and maintained at at least 80 to 90 mmHg to minimize the risk of secondary ischemia through underperfusion.[57] When there are problems with intracranial hypertension, maintaining a cerebral perfusion pressure of at least 70 to 80 mmHg may be of value in preventing sudden rises, or plateau waves, in ICP.[58,59] Patients with acute spinal cord injury and spinal shock should be volume resuscitated to normotensive blood pressure ranges with the goal of minimizing secondary ischemic injury.[60] Caution should be exercised, however, as they are at risk for fluid overload and pulmonary edema due in part to impaired ventricular function, especially when pulmonary capillary wedge pressure (PCWP) exceeds 18 mmHg.[61] Volume resuscitation in other neurosurgical patients with septic shock, ARDS, or preexisting cardiopulmonary disease may also be most appropriately guided using the pulmonary artery catheter.

Titration of volume resuscitation to absolute central pressure values (CVP and PCWP) may unreliably reflect cardiac filling volumes when there is coexisting cardiac or lung disease or when high amounts of PEEP are required for oxygenation. Under such conditions, timed fluid boluses guided by baseline pressures and their response to the fluid challenge may be helpful in assessing the limits of volume resuscitation (Table 6-1).[62]

Resuscitation Fluids Once the need for volume resuscitation or expansion has been established, the type of fluid employed (i.e., crystalloid versus colloid) must be chosen. Characteristics of commonly available crystalloids and colloids are shown in Table 6-2. Isotonic crystalloid solutions such as RL and 0.9% NaCL are the least expensive and most commonly used fluids for acute volume resuscitation. Under normal conditions, isotonic crystalloids are evenly distributed to the ECF, with only one-fourth or less of the administered volume remaining in the intravascular space in critically ill patients.[63,64] Volumetric replacement of acute blood losses with crystalloid therefore requires at least 3 to 4 times the estimated blood loss and is associated with an expansion of the interstitial space.

Colloid volume expanders are solutions of high molecular weight compounds with low vascular permeability. They have longer intravascular retention resulting in a rapid and more sustained volume expanding effect compared to crystalloids.[64,65] Intravascular retention times of the available colloids are variably quoted, with albumin preparations having relatively shorter intravascular retention than other available colloids. Hyperoncotic colloids, such as hydroxyethyl starch (HES) and dextran 70, may result in an acute expansion of the intravascular space that transiently exceeds the administered volume. In addition to their added expense, all colloids share common problems including the potential for vol-

Table 6-1 Fluid Challenge Protocol

	Pressures (mmHg) CVP	PCWP	Volume challenge (mL/10 min)
Baseline observations	<6		
		<12	200
	<10	<16	100
	≥10	≥16	50
Increase during infusion	>4	>7	Stop
Increase after infusion	≤2	≤3	Continue infusion
	>2 <4	>3 <7	Wait 10 min
Increase after 10-min wait	>2	>3	Stop Challenge
	≤2	≤3	Repeat Challenge

Source: Modified from Weil.[62]

ume overload, dilutional coagulopathy, anaphylactoid reactions, and interstitial edema when capillary permeability is increased.[66] Human albumin has a molecular weight of approximately 69,000 and is available in hyperoncotic (25 percent) and iso-oncotic (5 percent) preparations. Five percent purified protein fraction (PPF), containing 83 to 90 percent albumin, is also available. However, it has no physiologic advantage over 5 percent albumin and has occasionally been reported to cause hypotension related to impurities. Human albumin has been a favored colloid in neurosurgical

Table 6-2 Characteristics of Commonly Available Crystalloids and Colloids

Type	[Na⁺] (mEq/L)	Osmolality (mOsm/kg)	Oncotic pressure (mmHg)
Crystalloids			
Hypotonic			
0.21% NaCl	34	68	—
0.45% NaCl	77	154	—
Isotonic			
0.9% NaCl	154	308	—
Ringer's lactate	130	273	—
Hypertonic			
3% NaCl	513	1026	—
5% NaCl	856	1712	—
7.5% NaCl	1280	2560	—
Colloids			
5% albumin	130–160	300	
5% PPF	130–160	290	20
6% HES	154	310	30
6% dextran 70	154	310	40–60

Note: PPF-purified protein fraction, HES-hydroxyethylstarch.

practice because of early reports suggesting that albumin might have a favorable effect on brain edema and ICP[67–70] and by recent reports suggesting a beneficial effect on microcirculatory flow.[71] Although there are no prospective controlled trials assessing efficacy of albumin as a volume expander in neurosurgical patients, a recent review of randomized studies comparing crystalloid to albumin has suggested that crystalloids are as effective as albumin when titrated to hemodynamic stabilization.[72] When colloids are chosen for volume expansion in the neurosurgical patient, albumin is probably the safest of those presently available in regard to the potential for bleeding complications.

Dextrans are polymers of glucose that are available as low molecular weight (dextran 40) and high molecular weight (dextran 70 and dextran 75) preparations. The higher molecular weight dextrans have been preferred to the lower molecular weight preparations because of better vascular retention. The total dosage is limited to 20 mL/kg within the first 24 h of use. Interference with platelet function and resultant coagulopathy limits the utility of dextrans in the neurosurgical population.

HES is a synthetic starch polymer composed mainly of amylopectin with an average molecular weight of 450,000. Similar to dextrans, infusion volumes have been limited to no greater than 20 to 30 mL/kg because of interference with platelet function. Reports of bleeding problems in neurosurgical patients argue strongly against its use as a volume expander if there is any risk of intracranial hemorrhage.[73,74]

Colloids versus Crystalloids The choice of crystalloids over colloids in acute fluid resuscitation has been a subject of long-standing controversy in critical care medicine. Until recently, attention has focused on the effect of the type of resuscitation fluid on the development or exacerbation of pulmonary edema. Although this issue is not entirely resolved, several recent studies have suggested that differences in the degree of pulmonary dysfunction are difficult to discern.[75–77] Recent summaries evaluating the results of available randomized trials suggest that colloids are no better in regard to survival and are less cost effective than crystalloids.[78,79] Although there are other aspects to this controversy (e.g., wound healing, gut edema), the effects of fluid type on intracranial dynamics are germane.

It is well recognized that volume expansion with hypo-osmolal crystalloids promotes brain edema in both the normal and injured brain. Hemodilution by high-volume isotonic crystalloid resuscitation has been of concern with regard to the potential for generation or exacerbation of brain edema and intracranial hypertension due to lowered oncotic pressure. Although controlled clinical data are lacking, isovolemic hemodilution studies in uninjured animals suggest that crystalloids increase brain water and ICP only when they result in hypo-osmolality.[80,81] Furthermore, studies in animals with cryogenic brain injury and hemorrhagic shock with and without epidural brain compression have shown no important benefit of colloidal solutions over isotonic crystalloids with regard to ICP and brain water or cerebral hemodynamics.[82–85] In a recent study, ICP and electrical function were worse in animals receiving 0.9% saline compared to 6% HES after cryogenic brain injury.[86] However, this study was heavily criticized on both methodologic and statistical grounds.[87]

In summary, the available data suggest that any detrimental effects of fluid resuscitation on brain edema or ICP are dependent on changes in osmolality rather than oncotic pressure. Thus, high-volume resuscitation with iso-osmolal crystalloids appears to be safe. Although it has been difficult to show clear benefits of colloids over isotonic crystalloids in regard to brain edema or ICP, colloids do provide a measure of greater effectiveness in the rapidity and duration of hemodynamic response and should be considered when these effects are desirable. When large-volume resuscitations are required in neurosurgical patients, combined use of isotonic crystalloid and colloid in a proportion of 3 to 4 : 1 may provide a cost effective regimen. It should be noted that RL, a common isotonic crystalloid used in acute volume resuscitation, has a measured osmolality that is less than its calculated osmolality. A random sampling of the RL available at our institution showed a measured osmolality of approximately 244 mOsm/kg, which was lower than the labeled calculated osmolality of 273 mOsm/kg. Therefore, large-volume crystalloid resuscitations in neurosurgical patients should employ 0.9% saline rather than RL to minimize the potential for the production of hypo-osmolality.

Recently, as reviewed in Chap. 12 in more detail, a great deal of interest in the use of hypertonic saline resuscitation, especially in head-injured patients, has arisen because of experimental studies[82,88-90] and clinical reports[91] indicating a beneficial effect on ICP and brain edema. Indeed, a recent randomized study suggested improved outcome in hypotensive head-injured patients given a combination of 7.5% saline/dextran in the prehospital phase of care, although differences in survival were not statistically significant.[92] Whereas hypertonic saline resuscitation may be useful in the prehospital setting, the development of hypernatremia and hyperosmolarity restricts the volume of fluid that can be administered, limiting its routine use as a volume expander in the ICU.

Red Cell Transfusion Red blood cell transfusion, reviewed more fully in Chap. 12, is indicated in volume resuscitation when there are ongoing blood losses due to hemorrhage or when serial laboratory studies show a reduction in hematocrit. Although the maintenance of a hematocrit in the range of 30 to 35 percent has been advocated as being optimal for the maintenance of systemic and brain O_2 delivery,[93,94] a recent evaluation of cerebral blood flow studies in humans has suggested that the hematocrit that maximizes cerebral O_2 delivery in the normal brain is in the range of 40 percent and possibly even higher in patients with focal ischemia[95] (Fig. 6-1). In patients with intracranial hypertension, excessive hemodilution might also increase ICP as autoregulatory changes compensate for the reduced cerebral O_2 delivery. Transfusion to maintain hematocrit in the range of 35 to 40 percent would, therefore, seem reasonable in patients at risk for ischemia or exacerbation of intracranial hypertension.

DISORDERS OF WATER AND ELECTROLYTE BALANCE

Hyponatremia and Hypo-osmolality

Hyponatremia (plasma $Na^+ < 135$ mEq/L) is frequently seen in neurosurgical patients and is of particular importance since the osmotic buffering capacity of the brain may be impaired after primary brain injuries. In such cases, even small decreases in osmolality may cause cellular swelling, impairing brain function or promoting edema formation or raised ICP.

Hyponatremia occurs in association with various states of body fluid tonicity. Hyponatremia with hyperosmolality is seen with hyperglycemia or mannitol use, while pseudohyponatremia due to hyperlipidemia or hyperproteinemia is associated with normal plasma osmolality. Hyponatremia acquired in the neurosurgical ICU is usually associated with hypo-osmolality and is generally thought to represent the SIADH.[96-100] ICU patients with subarachnoid hemorrhage and closed head injury are most likely to develop this complication. The reported incidence of hyponatremia after aneurysmal subarachnoid hemorrhage has been variable, with most studies indicating an incidence of approximately 30 to 35 percent.[97,101-103] Despite these figures, the International Cooperative Study, involving over 3500 patients, reported an incidence of only 3.6 percent.[104] Patients at increased risk for hyponatremia include those with anterior communicating artery aneurysms[105,106] or those that develop third ventricular enlargement.[107] The onset of hyponatremia appears to coincide closely with the time of greatest risk of vasospasm and is associated with an increased incidence of ischemia and infarction.[101,103] In head-injured adults, the incidence of hyponatremia is reported in 5 to 12 percent and as high as 25 percent in pediatric patients.[100,108-110] The risk of hyponatremia appears to be greater in those with more severe head injuries and those with chronic subdural hematoma and basilar skull fracture.[100,109] Patients with chronic spinal cord injury have been reported to have a prevalence of hyponatremia of 10 to 15 percent that is related to both renal factors and postural AVP release.[111-114] Deterioration in level of consciousness, new focal deficits, myoclonus, seizures, or increasing ICP should raise the suspicion of hyponatremia and hypo-osmolality in the acutely brain-injured patient.

The evaluation of hyponatremia with hypo-osmolality has classically been approached by clinical assessment of volume status and urinary indices (Table 6-3). In many cases, the clinical

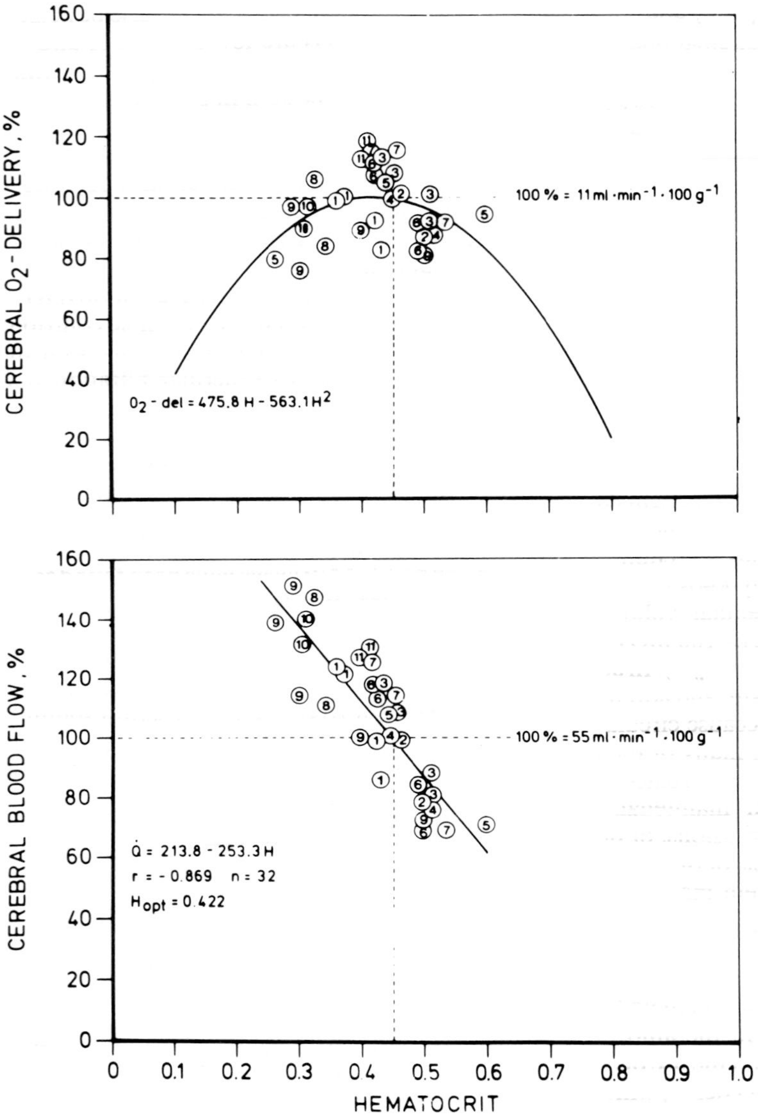

Figure 6-1 Summary of human data on the relationship between hematocrit and cerebral O_2 delivery (top) and cerebral blood flow (bottom). The hematocrit optimizing O_2 delivery is approximately 42 percent. From Gaehtgens.[95] Used by permission.

evaluation of volume status is relatively straightforward. Urinary Na^+ measurement is used adjunctively to differentiate salt-retaining states such as hyponatremic dehydration, heart failure, and cirrhosis from those conditions associated with urinary salt loss. Almost all cases of hyponatremia encountered in the neurosurgical ICU will be associated with a urinary osmolality > 100 mOsm/kg.

Syndrome of Inappropriate ADH Secretion As has been noted, hypo-osmolal hyponatremia occurring in neurosurgical patients has typ-

Table 6-3 Extracellular Volume (ECV) and Urinary Sodium (UNa^+) in Hyponatremia and Hypo-osmolality

Diagnosis	ECV	UNa^+ (mEq/L)
Dehydration	Decreased	<10
Congestive heart failure, cirrhosis	Increased	<10
Renal disease, adrenal insufficiency, diuretics, cerebral salt wasting	Decreased	>25
SIADH	Normal or increased	>25

ically been ascribed to SIADH. Increased AVP (ADH) levels have been found in such patients in plasma, CSF, and urine.[102,110,115–117] The syndrome is defined as the continuous secretion of AVP, despite hyponatremia and hypo-osmolality and normal or expanded extracellular volume. Urine is less than maximally dilute (> 100 mOsm) and urinary Na^+ is high (> 25 to 30 mEq/L). In addition, renal disease, hypothyroidism, and adrenal insufficiency must be excluded. Because circulating levels of AVP are increased in many of these patients, the hyponatremia may be exacerbated by increased free water intake with maintenance fluids, parenteral nutrition, drug infusions, or decreased solute intake. The diagnosis of SIADH in the critically ill neurosurgical patient may be obscured because volume status may be difficult to assess clinically, especially when on positive-pressure ventilation, and may require invasive evaluation. Extracellular volume may also fluctuate because of blood losses, variability in the amount and type of fluid administration, and the use of diuretics. The presence of peripheral edema, which normally suggests an expanded extracellular volume, may also be present with a markedly decreased effective intravascular volume (e.g., sepsis, multiple trauma, on hypoalbuminemia). Similarly, urinary Na^+ measurements are affected by the frequent use of osmotic and nonosmotic diuretics in this patient population. Although more sophisticated testing can be done, the diagnosis can be presumptively confirmed in the ICU when simple restriction of fluids results in reduction of urinary Na^+ losses and correction of hyponatremia. Measurement of uric acid may also be helpful since uric acid levels are low in SIADH and increased in hypovolemia. A clinical picture similar to SIADH can also be seen in patients with hypopituitarism.[118] AVP levels are increased but the hyponatremia in these patients is responsive to glucocorticoids. Given the nature of this population, hypopituitarism should be considered in the differential diagnosis of hyponatremia in the neurosurgical patient.

The presence of high urinary Na^+ in SIADH is not yet clearly understood. The possible contributors to the natriuresis characteristically seen include (a) an increased glomerular filtration rate with an increased filtered load of sodium, (b) decreased aldosterone secretion, and (c) decreased reabsorption of sodium in the kidney secondary to atrial natriuretic peptide. Several recent studies have focused on the question of the possible role of ANP in the natriuresis seen in this syndrome. Plasma and CSF ANP levels have been found to be elevated in both eunatremic and hyponatremic patients with subarachnoid hemorrhage and non aneurysmal intracranial hemorrhage.[102,119–123] Thus far, there has been no clearly defined relationship between ANP levels and serum sodium, osmolality, urinary sodium, or indices of volume status in these patients. In those with subarachnoid hemorrhage (SAH), plasma ANP levels appear to be higher in patients with suprasellar and intraventricular blood.[123] CSF ANP levels have also been found to be significantly increased in SAH patients with increased ICP.[120] Taken together, these findings may suggest that elevated ANP levels in these patients may just be a reflection of injury to regions of the brain involved in neurohumoral regulation of body fluids and electrolytes. Despite these findings, water loading studies in other patients with SIADH and in normal volunteers administered AVP have shown that plasma ANP and urinary Na^+ excretion increase in patients with SIADH, indicating that ANP does play a role in the natriuresis seen in the syndrome and may be an appropriate response in the regulation of extracellular volume.[124]

Cerebral Salt Wasting Syndrome The "cerebral salt wasting syndrome," originally described in the 1950s,[125,126] presents laboratory findings similar to SIADH, but ultimately results in a negative salt balance and volume contraction.[125,126] Persistent urinary Na^+ losses should be demonstrable during restricted fluid intake since it appears that urinary salt loss persists in SIADH only when fluid intake is liberal. Recent reports in patients with head injury[117,127] and studies of plasma volume and salt balance in patients with subarachnoid hemorrhage[53,55,127a] have suggested that many cases thought to be SIADH may in fact be the cerebral salt wasting syndrome with consequent treatment implications. Experimental studies in monkeys with SAH lend support to these clinical reports in that natriuresis and hyponatremia can occur without increases in AVP[128] and may be related to the unregulated release of ANP.

Treatment of Hyponatremia Treatment of critically ill neurosurgical patients with hyponatremia and hypo-osmolarity may be complicated because the etiology of the hyponatremia may be multifactorial and/or the overall treatment goals of maintaining an expanded intravascular volume for perfusion pressure may be in conflict with the need to restrict fluids to correct hyponatremia. In mild, asymptomatic cases of hyponatremia with obvious signs of hypovolemia ($UNa^+ < 25$ mEq/L or > 25 mEq/L with diuretic therapy or cerebral salt wasting syndrome), isotonic saline is administered and titrated to restore circulating blood volume and normalize serum Na^+. When urinary Na^+ is high and volume status is judged to be normal or increased as in SIADH, standard treatment of uncomplicated cases consists of fluid restriction of approximately 800 mL/day. For patients receiving enteral feedings, Na^+ intake may need to be supplemented since most standard enteric feeds contain only 25 to 45 mEq/L of Na^+. In patients at risk for vasospasm or patients with acute head injury, fluids should not be restricted. Rather, plasma volume should be maintained with volume expanders, while a negative water balance can be effected by employing loop diuretics such as furosemide to correct hyponatremia. Any antibiotics or drug infusions should be administered in saline to minimize free water intake. This approach requires the use of invasive monitoring and frequent titration of fluids to maintain appropriate volume status.

The rate at which severe symptomatic hyponatremia (<120 mEq/L) is corrected has been of considerable concern and controversy. Rapid correction of hyponatremia has been linked to the development of neurologic complications such as central pontine myelinolysis or more generally, the osmotic demyelination syndrome.[129–131] Experimental studies[132] and a review of clinical studies[133] suggest that neurologic complications resulting from correction of severe hyponatremia depend not only on the rate of correction but also on the rate of development of hyponatremia. Cellular adaptation over time to hypo-osmolar conditions with the associated loss of intracellular electrolytes probably predisposes to cellular dehydration and injury when challenged by an acute hyperosmolar stress, as would occur when slowly developing hyponatremia is rapidly corrected. It appears that patients who develop hyponatremia at the chronic rate of <0.5 mEq/L/h are more prone to develop neurologic complications when their rate of correction is >0.5 mEq/L/h. On the other hand, patients developing hyponatremia at a faster rate can be safely corrected to mildly hyponatremic levels (130 to 134 mEq/L) at rates of correction ranging from 1 to 2 mEq/L/h. Most neurosurgical patients developing severe hyponatremia in the ICU will fall into this acute category and should be rapidly corrected when there are seizures, an abrupt deterioration in level of consciousness, or evidence of progressive brain swelling or intracranial hypertension.

Rapid correction of severe hyponatremia is usually accomplished with hypertonic saline and a loop diuretic such as furosemide. It should be remembered that in SIADH, the primary problem is usually not salt depletion, but an excess in TBW. Therefore, treatment is aimed at the reduction of body water with the goal of restoring osmolality to normal. The main effect of hypertonic saline is to facilitate a solute diuresis rather than raise serum Na^+, primarily since most of the administered salt is excreted in the urine in SIADH. The use of a loop diuretic enhances free water excretion and contracts intravascular volume, ultimately reducing renal Na^+ loss. In most cases, 3% saline at an infusion rate of 1 to 2 mL/kg per h is sufficient to result in a serum Na^+ increase of 1 to 2 mEq/h.[134] Hypertonic saline is discontinued when signs or symptoms have resolved or when mildly hyponatremic levels have been achieved. In patients with intracranial hypertension or mass effect from brain edema, bolus mannitol (12.5 to 25 g) or urea (40 to 80 g) as a 30% solution infused over 6 to 8 h[135,136] in combination with isotonic saline to maintain intravascular volume may be preferred to furosemide, since both agents will lower ICP and cause a negative water balance. Following symptomatic correction, serum Na^+ is restored to normal more slowly using simple fluid restriction or, when fluid restriction is not possible, with intermittent doses of furosemide. Demeclocycline HCl (1200 mg/day in divided doses) can be used in treating the patient with chronic SIADH but has little value in the rapid correction of hyponatremia.[137,138] Demeclocycline should be used cautiously in patients with impaired renal function. Patients with refractory salt wasting and hyponatremia may respond with high salt intakes and fludrocortisone 0.1 to 0.4 mg/day.[117]

Hypernatremia and Hyperosmolality

Hyperosmolar states in the neurosurgical patient are usually caused by hypernatremia ($Na^+ > 145$ mEq/L). Severe hyperglycemia occasionally contributes to hyperosmolality in the ICU in states of insulin resistance, e.g., sepsis, or as a result of inadequate insulin administration with parenteral nutrition. As has been noted, hyperosmolality without hypertonicity can occur with alcohol intoxication or renal failure.

In general, hypernatremia can be caused by excessive salt administration (e.g., hypertonic saline resuscitation, $NaHCO_3$) or more commonly, by excessive water losses. Causes of mild hypernatremia and hyperosmolality in the neurosurgical ICU include excess free water losses secondary to osmotic diuretics, episodic diaphoresis in patients with fever or hypothalamic dysfunction, and high solute loads administered to fluid-restricted patients receiving enteral feedings. Excessive free water losses may also occur in spontaneously breathing patients who are hyperventilating unhumidified air. More profound degrees of hypernatremia are, however, usually seen in patients with diabetes insipidus.

Clinical signs of isolated hypernatremia and hyperosmolality are generally seen when serum Na^+ exceeds 160 mEq/L and osmolality is greater than 320 to 340 mOsm/kg. In a group of unstratified but severely head-injured patients, a serum Na^+ > 155 mEq/L and osmolality of > 340 mOsm/kg was associated with a high mortality.[139] Symptoms are generally referable to the CNS. A graded impairment of consciousness that depends on the severity of hyperosmolality is the main manifestation of hypernatremia.[140] Seizures are reported but may be related to rapid correction of hypernatremia.[141] Acute hypernatremia may cause severe brain dehydration and result in subdural, subarachnoid, and intraparenchymal hemorrhage. Venous thrombosis and venous infarction may also occur. The development of intracranial hypotension may predispose to the development of subdural hygromas. When hypernatremia occurs over a more prolonged period, an adaptive increase in intracellular electrolytes and solute occurs, predisposing the patient to the development of cerebral edema when hypernatremia is corrected rapidly.

In cases of simple dehydration, the free water deficit is calculated using the following formula.

$$\text{Free water deficit} = [0.6 \times \text{wt(kg)}] \times \text{current Na}^+/140 - 1$$

For example, a patient weighing 70 kg, with a plasma sodium of 165 mEq/L, would have an estimated free water deficit of approximately 7.5 L.

$$\text{Free water deficit} = (0.6 \times 70\text{ kg})\ (165/140 - 1) = 7.5\text{ kg (L) water}$$

In general, half the free water deficit can be replaced acutely with the remainder replaced over the next 24 to 36 h.[142] In patients receiving osmotic diuretics or in those with prolonged hyperglycemia, hypernatremia may be accompanied by solute loss and depletion of intravascular volume. In such cases, intravascular volume should be repleted with volume expanders followed by correction of free water deficits.

Diabetes Insipidus Diabetes insipidus (DI) is a disorder of excessive renal loss of water which is usually due to a deficiency in secretion of AVP (central DI) and occurs most commonly in the neurosurgical population as a whole. Patients with tumors of pituitary origin as well as head-injured patients account for most of the cases.[143,144] Overall, the incidence of DI in critically ill neurosurgical patients is relatively small and dependent on overall case mix. One study found only a 6.7 percent incidence of DI in postcraniotomy patients, the majority of whom were operated on for brain tumors.[145] All cases occurred in patients who had undergone treatment for pituitary tumor. The incidence of DI in patients undergoing aneurysm surgery has been reported at approximately 4 percent and at 2 percent[105,146] in patients with severe head injury. Head-injured patients with temporal-parietal injuries and those with fractures that involve the skull base and sella turcica appear to be at increased risk for DI.[147–149] Diabetes insipidus can be expected with high frequency in patients who develop brain death while receiving somatic life support.[150,151]

In most cases encountered in the ICU, the onset of DI will be heralded by the onset of polyuria (urine output >30 mL/kg per h), hypernatremia, and plasma hyperosmolality as early as 12 to 24 h after trauma or in surgical patients, 1 to 3 days postoperatively.[152,153] If damage is limited to the pituitary or lower pituitary stalk, DI may only be transient. High stalk lesions or injury to the hypothalamus usually results in permanent DI. After complete stalk section, a triphasic response may be seen.[154] Polyuria and hypernatremia occur during the first phase which may last for 2 to 5 days. A second phase of antidiuresis with decreased urinary output and a lower serum Na^+ may last for 5 to 14 days and is eventually followed by permanent diabetes insipidus. Because of associated hypopituarism, head-injured patients developing DI should have formal endocrine workup once the patient's clinical condition has stabilized.[148]

Patients with complete DI usually have urinary volumes of 10 to 15 L/day or more, with low urinary osmolality (50 to 200 mOsm/kg) and specific gravity (1.001 to 1.005). Characteristically, these patients do not increase urinary osmolality when fluid is restricted, but they remain sensitive to exogenous vasopressin. Since most critically ill neurosurgical patients will not be able to control their own water intake, hemodynamic instability with hypotension is likely in patients with untreated complete DI. Patients with partial DI have urinary volumes well below those with complete DI. Urinary osmolality is in the range of 290 to 600 mOsm/kg and increases with exogenous vasopressin.[155] Several other causes of polyuria must be considered in the neurosurgical patient and include osmotic diuretics, such as mannitol or iodinated contrast, severe hyperglycemia, and fluid overload. In contrast to DI, a solute diuresis is usually associated with a higher specific gravity (1.009 to 1.0035) with urinary osmolality usually between 250 to 320 mOsm/kg.[153] In most cases, the diagnosis of DI will be obvious when a patient at risk begins to excrete dilute urine in volumes that exceed fluid intake. Plasma Na^+ and osmolality may be normal at the onset of polyuria; however, the patient will eventually develop hypernatremia and hyperosmolality on repeated measurements. The diagnosis can be confirmed when the administration of vasopressin or the synthetic analog DDAVP causes urine output to decrease and osmolality to increase. When there are confounding factors such as overhydration or a solute diuresis, examination of the relationship of plasma to urine osmolality may be helpful in evaluating the cause of polyuria (Fig. 6-2). Patients who have received excessive fluid resuscitations will concentrate their urine and maintain normonatremia when fluids are limited, while patients with DI will develop hypernatremia and hyperosmolality. A solute diuresis will usually be evident by the history, by measurements of plasma and urinary glucose, and by examining the relationship between plasma and urinary osmolality.

Fluid balance is usually in flux during the first few days of ICU admission, complicating management of patients who develop DI. Nonetheless, once the diagnosis is considered, fluid intake, urinary output, and specific gravity must be monitored at least every 1 to 2 h until the patient has been adequately fluid resuscitated, electrolytes corrected, and a stable regimen of vasopressin established. Standard regimens for acute management have included the use of aqueous vasopressin administered subcutaneously or intramuscularly in doses of 5 to 10 units every 4 to 6 h. Preexisting expansion of the extracellular volume with resultant edema may result in variable and unpredictable absorption when these routes are

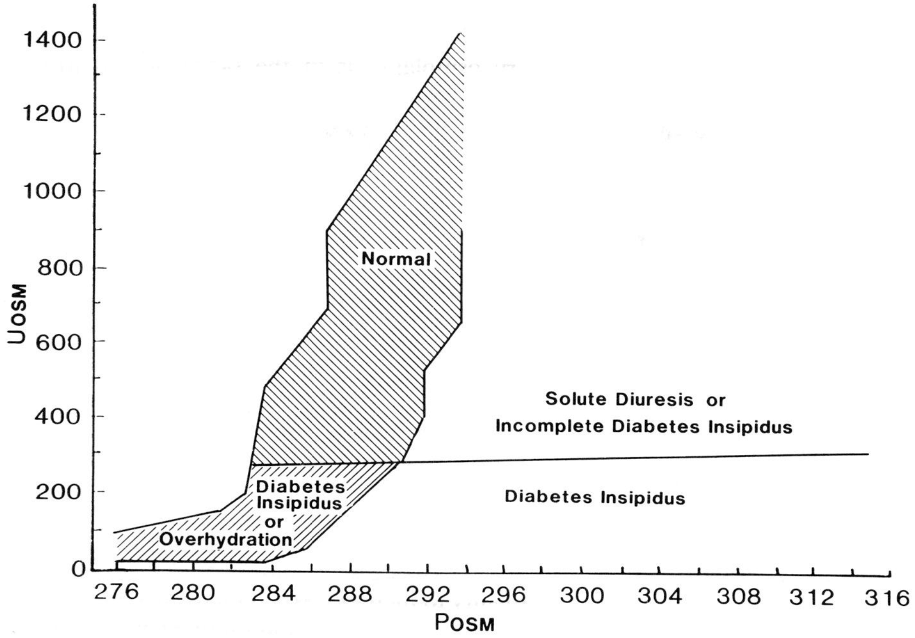

Figure 6-2 Relationship of plasma to urinary osmolality under normal and polyuric conditions. Adapted from Moses.[155] Used by permission.

used, creating unnecessary difficulty in management. Aqueous vasopressin can be administered intravenously. However, it has a very short half-life and when used should be given as a continuous infusion starting at 2.5 units/h and titrated to a urine output of approximately 100 mL/h.[156] A simpler approach is to use intermittent doses of DDAVP intravenously in amounts of 0.5 to 2 μg. The duration of effect is dose-dependent and usually ranges from 8 to 12 h. Overtreatment can be problematic in patients who have a triphasic response or who develop only transient DI. Therefore, the risk of hyponatremia and brain swelling can be minimized in the ICU phase of care by initiating therapy at lower doses and by redosing when breakthrough polyuria and urinary hypo-osmolality occur. Concomitant with the initiation of vasopressin therapy, the existing free water deficit is estimated and corrected with 5 percent dextrose in water. Similarly, ongoing excess urinary water losses (e.g., $>$100 mL/h) are replaced intravenously on an hourly basis until polyuria is controlled with vasopressin or DDAVP. Although saline solutions are not recommended for urinary replacement because of associated water loss,[153] salt-containing volume expanders should not be withheld in critically ill patients who are hypotensive and severely volume depleted as a result of DI or associated injuries.

Once the patient has stabilized and has left the ICU, a formal dehydration test can be carried out if there is any question of whether the patient has partial or complete DI.[157] Patients with complete DI can be transitioned to intranasal DDAVP, while those with incomplete DI may respond to one of several oral agents including carbemazepine (200 to 600 mg/day), chlorpropamide (100 to 500 mg/day), or clofibrate (500 mg every 6 h).[158]

Other Electrolyte Disorders

Hypokalemia Hypokalemia ($K^+ < 3.5$ mEq/L) is probably the most commonly recognized and treated electrolyte abnormality in the ICU. As is the case in many other electrolyte disturbances, to be discussed later, hypokalemia generally occurs as a result of decreased dietary intake, excessive renal or GI losses, or intracellular shift from the extracellular space. In most critically ill patients, hypokalemia is likely to be multifactorial in origin and associated with some deficit in total body K^+. Although there are few systematic studies in the neurosurgical population, hypokalemia has been reported to occur in the majority of severely head-injured patients on initial presentation[159] and in approximately 26 percent of patients within 48 h of subarachnoid hemorrhage.[160] Although supportive data is limited, the critically ill neurosurgical population is obviously at high risk for hypokalemia. For example, excessive renal losses of K^+ occur as a result of diagnostic and therapeutic use of osmotic diuretics; DI, high doses of glucocorticoids, such as methylprednisolone for spinal cord injury, catabolic losses in trauma; and high aldosterone levels in hypovolemic patients. Excessive renal K^+ loss can also be expected in the presence of alkalemia and hypomagnesemia. GI K^+ losses frequently are the result of vomiting, nasogastric suction, and diarrhea. Intracellular shift of K^+ occurs through a variety of mechanisms. Respiratory or metabolic alkalosis, exogenous insulin, or increased insulin stimulated by glucose infusion can all cause intracellular K^+ shift. Adrenergic stimulation by endogenous or exogenous catecholamines also causes intracellular K^+ shift and may be the principal mechanism for hypokalemia seen early after severe head injury.[159]

Clinical manifestations of hypokalemia may include ventricular and supraventricular arrhythmias, enhancement of digitalis toxicity, reduced gastric and intestinal motility, and impaired renal water conservation resulting in polyuria when hypokalemia is severe and prolonged. Neuromuscular manifestations include hyporeflexia, weakness, and even paralysis when K^+ depletion is severe.

Treatment of hypokalemia is generally initiated when $K^+ < 3.5$ mEq/L. Although there is a linear relationship between serum K^+ and total body K^+ in uncomplicated cases of hypokalemia,[161] acid-base disturbances and other causes of intracellular K^+ shift make estimates of total body K^+ difficult to predict in the critically ill patient. Therefore, K^+ therapy must be monitored by frequent determinations of serum K^+, especially when hypokalemia is severe, large doses of K^+ are administered, or there are acid-base disturbances or renal insufficiency. Mild asymptomatic hypokalemia is usually treated with 10 to 20 mEq of KCl administered in saline over 1 h into a large peripheral vein or the central circulation and repeated as necessary. Larger doses of 30 to 40 mEq/h can be safely infused in critically ill patients with moderate degrees of hypokalemia.[162] The maximum increase in K^+ after such infusions usually occurs at the end of the 1 h infusion. Profound, symptomatic hypokalemia ($K^+ \leq 2$ mEq/L) can be treated with higher doses of KCl. In fact, doses as high as 80 to 100 mEq/h have been given.[163] When doses larger than 20 mEq/h are administered, the total dose should be split and administered in aliquots to minimize the risk of inadvertent rapid infusion of a large dose. On the very rare occasion when >40 mEq/h is necessary, the dose should be split and administered through separate sites, preferably in large veins away from central veins entering the heart, to avoid local cardiac hyperkalemia. Persistent K^+ deficits can be treated by adding KCl or potassium phosphate in phosphate-deficient patients, to maintenance intravenous fluids in a concentration no greater than 40 mEq/L. Alternatively, K^+ can be supplemented via the enteric route if nasogastric suction is not being employed. A serum magnesium level should be measured in patients with refractory hypokalemia, as both electrolyte disturbances often occur together. Hypokalemia will be difficult to correct without correction of hypomagnesemia. Finally, hypokalemia protects against tetany related to hypocalcemia. Therefore, hypocalcemia should be corrected before or concomitant with correction of hypokalemia.

Hypocalcemia Hypocalcemia occurs with a frequency of up to 70 percent in critically ill surgical and medical patients.[160a,164,165] Systematic evaluations of hypocalcemia in critically ill neurosurgical patients are not available. Despite this high frequency, hypocalcemia is only clinically important when the physiologically active, ionized fraction (40 percent of total) is reduced. The remainder is bound to albumin (50 percent) or chelated (10 percent). While hypoalbuminemia can lower total calcium, ionized calcium can be reduced by a variety of factors including alkalosis, high circulating free fatty acids as in sepsis or pancreatitis, and by agents that chelate calcium such as with albumin infusions, bicarbonate administration, and high citrate loads administered with massive transfusion.[166] Although citrate received with massive transfusion will lower ionized calcium, this effect is usually transient unless there is a concomitant impairment in citrate metabolism as may occur in patients with hepatic and renal failure or hypothermia. Ionized hypocalcemia occurs in up to 15 to 20 percent of critically ill patients,[167] but cannot be predicted by either total calcium measurements or calculations of ionized calcium corrected for pH and serum albumin concentration.[164]

Common etiologies of hypocalcemia that might be expected to occur in the neurosurgical patient include hypomagnesemia, respiratory alkalosis, sepsis, or, in the multiply traumatized patient, rhabdomyolysis. Hypomagnesemia impairs both parathyroid hormone (PTH) release and action. Alkalosis increases protein binding of calcium. Thus, patients with marginal calcium levels may develop evidence of frank hypocalcemia when therapeutic hyperventilation is employed. Patients with sepsis or critically ill patients with unexplained ionized hypocalcemia may be vitamin D deficient, have an impairment in vitamin D metabolism or action, or may have impaired release of PTH.[164,168,169] Hyperphosphatemia in severe rhabdomyolysis causes hypocalcemia by calcium precipitation or impaired vitamin D metabolism. Patients with renal insufficiency may also develop hypocalcemia secondary to impaired vitamin D metabolism.

Clinical manifestations of ionized hypocalcemia are generally not evident until ionized calcium is <0.7 mmol/L. The normal range is 1 to 1.25 mmol/L. Manifestations include hypotension, impaired ventricular function, bradycardia, bronchospasm, and laryngospasm. Neuromuscular manifestations have been described mainly in patients with hypoparathyroidism and include weakness, tetany, paresthesias, hyperreflexia, agitation, confusion, and seizures.[170-172] The response to catecholamines and digoxin may also be impaired in patients with hypocalcemia.

Before specific treatment for hypocalcemia is initiated, hypomagnesemia should be excluded since hypomagnesemic patients respond poorly to calcium without correction of magnesium deficiency. Severe symptomatic hypocalcemia is treated with intravenous calcium chloride or calcium gluconate as a bolus of 100 to 200 mg of elemental calcium over 10 min (1 g calcium chloride equals 272 mg Ca^{2+}, and 1 g calcium gluconate equals 93 mg Ca^{2+}). Subsequently, a continuous infusion of 1 to 2 mg/kg per h is initiated and titrated to normalize calcium.[166] Correction usually requires 6 to 12 h with this regimen. Calcium administration in hyperphosphatemic patients should be done cautiously and concomitant with attempts to lower phosphate to minimize the risk of calcium precipitation in tissues. Rapid infusions of calcium may cause hypertension, bradycardia, and arterioventricular nodal blockade, and may precipitate digitalis toxicity. Thus, patients must be monitored closely during infusion. Emergent treatment with intravenous calcium is generally unnecessary in asymptomatic patients with ionized calcium levels >0.8 mmol/L. In such cases, calcium supplementation in parenteral nutrition or by the enteric route should be sufficient. Unexplained and persistent hypocalcemia should be further evaluated to exclude hypoparathyroidism and vitamin D deficiency.

Hypophosphatemia Hypophosphatemia is defined as a serum phosphate level <2.7 mg/dL. Clinical manifestations of hypophosphatemia, however, are usually not seen unless levels are severely reduced (<1 mg/dL). Overall, severe hypophosphatemia occurs in <0.5 percent of all hospitalized patients.[173-175] However, a much higher frequency can be expected in critically ill patients, those with multiple trauma,[176] and in brain-injured patients who are being hyperventilated.[177] In general, patients who are malnourished, alcoholic, or septic, or those with diabetic ketoacidosis, are at increased risk for the development of severe hypophosphatemia. Decreased dietary intake, transcellular shift, or excessive losses through the GI tract or kidney are the main mechanisms by which hypophosphatemia occurs. Transcellular shift of phosphate from the extracellular to the intracellular space occurs by insulin-mediated intracellular transport of phosphate with glucose when carbohydrates are administered parenterally or enterally and has been referred to as the "refeeding syndrome."[178,179] Respiratory alkalosis causes intracellular shift of phosphate by stimulating glycolysis and intracellular phosphate trapping. Hypophosphatemia caused by transcellular shift is associated with hypophosphaturia and the maintenance of normal body stores of phosphate. Drugs such as phosphate-binding antacids, diuretics, and steroids are also commonly implicated as causing or contributing to the development of severe hypophosphatemia. Hypokalemia and hypomagnesemia may promote hypophosphatemia by impairing renal phosphate reabsorption.[180,181]

A number of complications of severe hypophosphatemia are relevant to the ICU population, including diaphragmatic weakness,[182,183] ventricular dysfunction,[184,185] impaired white cell function,[186] and increased affinity of Hb for O_2 as a result of decreased red cell 2,3-DPG.[187] Neurologic manifestations of hypophosphatemia have been reported to include confusion, seizures, and coma.[188-190] However, a direct causal relationship is not clearly established. Other reported complications include hemolytic anemia, impaired platelet function, and rhabdomyolysis.

Treatment of severe hypophosphatemia has been an issue of some debate. Since most patients developing complications of severe hypophosphatemia have had preexisting illness, alcoholism, or malnutrition, and were likely to have severe total body phosphate depletion,[191] aggressive treatment in previously healthy but acutely ill patients may not be indicated, especially when the hypophosphatemia is related to transient intracellular shifts such as occur with acute hypocapnia. Nonetheless, patients with severe hypophosphatemia who appear to be at risk for complications and those with impaired organ function (e.g., respiratory or cardiac failure) should probably be treated with intravenous phosphate salts when serum phosphate is <1 mg/dL. Infusion of 10 to 15 mmol of phosphate over 4 h successfully and safely raises serum phosphate over 1 mg/dL in critically ill patients.[192] Potential complications associated with intravenous phosphate administration include hypocalcemia and hypotension. Patients without severe hypophosphatemia can be supplemented with a variety of enteric preparations or by adding phosphate to standard TPN formulations as necessary.

Hypomagnesemia Hypomagnesemia is a common electrolyte disorder noted in the critically ill.[193-195] There are no available data in neurosurgical ICU populations. However, in critically ill general surgical patients, the frequency of hypomagnesemia (<1.5 mg/dL) has been reported to be as high as 61 percent and is associated with increased mortality.[195] Similar to hypophosphatemia, decreased dietary intake, excessive renal or GI losses, and transcellular shift are general causes of hypomagnesemia, and it is also commonly seen in alcoholic and malnourished patients. Detailed reviews of the pathophysiology and specific etiologies of hypomagnesemia are presented elsewhere.[196,197] Common etiologies to be expected in the neurosurgical patient include osmotic and nonosmotic diuretic use, diabetes insipidus, respiratory alkalosis, sepsis, and the use of drugs such as aminoglycosides.

The clinical diagnosis of magnesium depletion is difficult because only 1 percent of total body magnesium is represented in plasma and because total plasma magnesium does not accurately reflect the ionized fraction (55 percent of the total), which is the physiologically active form.[194] The remaining plasma magnesium is bound to protein (33 percent) or is chelated. Although methods are available for estimating magnesium stores, they are neither practical nor routinely available for clinical use in the ICU. Measurement of ionized magnesium is not available, but measurement of the fraction unbound to protein shows promise for routine estimation of ionized magnesium.[194] Despite its limitations, total plasma magnesium levels <1 mEq/L are associated with hypokalemia and increased mortality and serve as a practical threshold for initiating aggressive therapy.

A variety of complications of hypomagnesemia have been described. They include hypocalcemia, refractory hypokalemia, peripheral and diaphragmatic muscle weakness, tetany, cardiac arrhythmias, and enhancement of digitalis-induced arrhythmias. Neurologic manifestations include tremor, hyperreflexia, agitation, confusion, and seizures.[198,199] Some of these clinical manifestations may be related to hypocalcemia which is commonly associated with hypomagnesemia.[200] Interesting but limited investigations have suggested that magnesium may play an important role in the pathophysiology of vasospasm after subarachnoid hemorrhage[201] and warrants further investigation.

Severe hypomagnesemia is treated with intravenous magnesium salts.[202,203] Patients with normal renal function can excrete at least half of the administered dose so that large doses of magnesium can be given to deficient patients without causing hypermagnesemia.[204] Symptomatic hypomagnesemia (e.g., refractory cardiac arrhythmias or seizures) can be treated with 2 to 3 g of 10 to 25% magnesium sulfate (1 g equals 8 mEq Mg^{2+}) administered slowly over 2 to 3 min while arterial blood pressure and heart rhythm are monitored. Following the initial bolus, a continuous infusion of 2 g/h for 5 h followed by 1 g/h for 10 h has been successfully employed.[202] For patients with asymptomatic but severe hypomagnesemia, 6 g of $MgSO_4$ is administered over 3 h followed by 10 g administered continuously over the remainder of the day. Additional doses of 6 g/day for the next 2 to 5 days can be given as necessary to correct residual deficits. Less severe degrees of hypomagnesemia can be treated as indicated by supplements added to total TPN or by enteric administration of magnesium oxide.

ACID-BASE DISORDERS

Acid-base disorders occurring in the critically ill are usually acute, commonly mixed, may cause or contribute to electrolyte imbalance, and may adversely affect organ function, including the CNS. In-depth reviews of the evaluation and treatment of acid-base disorders is presented elsewhere.[205,206] The following discussion will focus on disorders that can be expected to occur in the neurosurgical ICU with emphasis on their effect on the CNS.

Respiratory Disorders

Of all common acid-base disorders, acute respiratory disturbances most profoundly affect CNS function. As a consequence of rapid CO_2 diffusion across the blood-brain barrier and limited acute buffering capacity, brain extracellular and intracellular pH tracks systemic pH in acute respiratory alkalosis or acidosis.[207-209] Functional disturbances that occur may be related to both changes in intracellular pH or cerebral blood flow (CBF). CBF decreases approximately 3 to 4 percent per millimeter of mercury (mmHg) decrease in $PaCO_2$, with an associated 1 percent reduction in cerebral blood volume. Similar changes in the opposite direction occur under hypercapnic conditions. Changes in perivascular pH caused by changes in Pa_{CO_2} modulate changes in CBF. Compensatory mechanisms do exist that return CSF and brain pH toward normal in a matter of hours by increased lactate production, decreased bicarbonate in the case of respiratory alkalosis, or the generation of bicarbonate in the case of respiratory acidosis. These compensatory mechanisms help explain, in part, why CBF returns to near normal values in as few as 4 to 6 h after acute hyperventilation-induced hypocapnia and why chronic hypercarbia may be tolerated with minimal symptoms unless there is coexistent hypoxia.

Respiratory Alkalosis Respiratory alkalosis ($Pa_{CO_2} < 35$ mmHg) is present with or without alkalemia (pH > 7.44) in many neurosurgical patients as a result of the primary brain insult,[210] associated pulmonary complications (e.g., pneumonia, aspiration),[211] fever, pulmonary embolism, inappropriate ventilator settings, and when therapeutic hyperventilation is being employed to control ICP. Systemic pH may be normal or lower than expected when there is superimposed metabolic acidosis or it may be inappropriately high when treatments such as diuretics, nasogastric suction, or corticosteroids are being employed simultaneously. Acute hypocapnia may cause paresthesias, altered sensorium, and seizures.[212,213] Extreme degrees of hypocapnia can also impair brain tissue oxygenation,[214-217] either by a reduction in CBF or as a result of increased affinity of Hb for O_2 or the Bohr effect. Acute respiratory alkalosis also predisposes to a variety of electrolyte disorders, myocardial ischemia, and a reduction in cardiac output in patients on mechanical ventilation. Other potentially detrimental effects of respiratory alkalosis include increases in plasma lactic acid concentrations and diminished lactate clearance.[217a]

Severe hypocapnia ($Pa_{CO_2} < 20$ to 25 mmHg) and alkalemia (pH < 7.55) should generally be avoided. Treatment is directed at the underlying cause or by adjusting minute ventilation downward in mechanically ventilated patients. Changing the mode of mechanical ventilation (e.g., from assist control to IMV) in patients with driven respiration, as in cases of sepsis or brain injury, does not usually affect blood gas abnormalities. Therefore, judicious use of narcotics to suppress respiratory drive or the addition of dead space to the ventilator circuit is often required to correct the alkalosis. Narcotics are preferred in order to minimize ventilatory work. If extreme degrees of hypocapnia are being used to control ICP, consideration should be given to measuring CBF or sampling venous blood from the jugular bulb to ensure adequate CBF and brain oxygenation.

Respiratory Acidosis Respiratory acidosis ($Pa_{CO_2} > 45$ mmHg) with acidemia (pH < 7.36) is an early complication in some neurologic patients after acute intracranial insults as a result of airway obstruction and/or hypoventilation. Patients with high cervical spine injury are also at risk for hypoventilation and hypercapnia as a result of loss of motor control over the muscles of respiration and because of inadequate ventilatory reserve, retained secretions, and impaired coughing.[218] In the brain-injured patient, hypercapnia may increase ICP and contribute to secondary brain ischemia and poor outcome.[219,220] While in the ICU, metabolic alkalosis, inadequate ventilation, or excessive use of sedatives may also cause or contribute to hypoventilation and hypercapnia. Superimposed metabolic acid-base disorders may cause arterial pH to be greater or less than what would be expected for a simple respiratory acidosis. In addition to its effect on the CNS, severe respiratory acidosis may impair cardiac function and result in hypotension.

Treatment of respiratory acidosis is usually straightforward and requires definitive airway control and mechanical ventilation adjusted to normalize systemic pH. Withholding or reversal of narcotic sedatives and correction of metabolic alkalosis is indicated when they may be contributory. Patients with intracranial hypertension or nonintubated patients with spinal cord injury should be monitored closely for hypercapnia with frequent blood gases or by capnography.

Metabolic Disorders

Isolated acute metabolic alkalosis and acidosis have little effect on CNS acid-base balance or function because of the relative impermeability of H^+ and HCO_3^- to the blood-brain barrier. Paradoxically, CSF pH can shift in a direction opposite to systemic pH when respiratory compensation for these acute disorders results either in hyperventilation in the case of metabolic acidosis or hypoventilation in the case of metabolic alkalosis. Acute administration of bicarbonate or inorganic acids can also produce paradoxic shifts in CSF pH when arterial Pa_{CO_2} is not held constant.[208]

Metabolic Alkalosis Metabolic alkalosis (serum HCO_3^- or total $CO_2 > 30$ mEq/L) is the most common acid-base disturbance noted in hospitalized patients.[221,222] Metabolic alkaloses are divided into chloride-responsive and chloride-resistant types.[223,224] In chloride-responsive alkaloses, chloride loss stimulates renal HCO_3^- reabsorption. In the neurosurgical patient, common causes of chloride-responsive alkaloses include vomiting, nasogastric suction, and diuretics. Chloride-responsive alkaloses are commonly associated with volume contraction which may compound the alkalosis as the kidney responds by increasing reabsorption of HCO_3^- and secretion of acid. There are a variety of causes for chloride-resistant alkaloses; however, in the neurosurgical patient, the use of glucocorticoids with mineralocorticoid activity (e.g., hydrocortisone, methylprednisolone) is likely to be the most common cause. The mineralocorticoids cause sodium retention and renal H^+ and K^+ loss. Hypokalemia can perpetuate or contribute to metabolic alkalosis by increasing renal tubular acid secretion.

The main complications of metabolic alkalosis that are of concern include hypokalemia, hypoventilation, and the possibility of impaired O_2 delivery due to increased affinity of Hb for O_2 under alkalemic conditions. Neurologic manifestations of severe metabolic alkalosis have been reported to include altered sensorium and seizures[225,226] but are difficult to separate from associated electrolyte and blood gas abnormalities.

Treatment of metabolic alkalosis is generally directed at the underlying cause when possible. The chloride-responsive alkaloses respond to the administration of saline and K^+. In patients with large volumes of nasogastric drainage, H_2-blockers can be used to minimize chloride loss. Glucocorticoid-related alkalosis are treated by either discontinuing the offending drug and/or by repleting K^+. Acetazolamide administration of 250 to 1000 mg/day in divided doses has been used in selected patients with diuretic-induced alkaloses or in hypercapnic patients to correct metabolic alkalosis. However, this agent should not be used in neurosurgical patients with elevated ICP, as it may cause acute cerebral acidosis and increased CBF and volume. Although seldom required in the neurosurgical patient, patients with severe metabolic alkaloses in whom saline therapy is contraindicated can be corrected using intravenous HCl administered through a central vein.[224]

Metabolic Acidosis Metabolic acidoses (HCO_3^- <25 mEq/L) are divided into anion-gap and non-anion-gap types. The anion gap ($Na^+ - [Cl^- + HCO_3^-]$) represents the sum of all unmeasured anions in plasma including negatively charged albumin, sulfate, phosphate, and organic anions. The anion gap is normally 10 to 14 mEq/L. In critically ill patients it must be further recognized that the anion gap can be artifactually lowered when there is coexistent hypoalbuminemia. Lactic acidosis as a result of impaired systemic tissue perfusion or secondary to respiratory alkalosis can be expected to be the most common cause of an increased anion gap in the neurosurgical ICU patient. Less common causes of an increased anion gap in these patients include diabetic ketoacidosis and inorganic acidoses due to acute renal failure. The nonanion gap acidoses are characterized by an increased chloride concentration and a normal anion gap. Hyperchloremic acidoses are commonly seen in neurosurgical patients after prolonged hypocapnia. Other potential causes in this population include large volume saline administration, diarrhea, and the administration of chloride salts of amino acids used in TPN formulations. Hyperchloremic and anion-gap acidoses can coexist or be found in association with other acid-base disorders and are suggested when the serum bicarbonate is decreased or increased to a greater degree than would be expected by the calculated anion gap.

Treatment of metabolic acidoses is, as is the case with other disorders, first directed at the underlying pathophysiology. Patients with severe systemic acidemia (pH<7.1 to 7.2) are at risk for myocardial depression and hypotension and should be given $NaHCO_3$ when lactic acidosis is present.[227,228] When bicarbonate is used to treat severe lactic acidosis, the immediate goal is to raise systemic pH to non-life-threatening levels (7.25 to 7.3) which may minimize the risk of overcorrection, paradoxic CSF acidosis, and alkali-related electrolyte problems such as hypokalemia, hypocalcemia, hypernatremia, and hyperosmolality. Estimation of bicarbonate requirements by classical formulas may either overestimate or underestimate bicarbonate requirements. A simple formula that appears to raise pH to acceptable ranges while avoiding overcorrection is[229]:

$$\text{Dose(mEq)}: = (\tfrac{1}{2}\ Pa_{CO_2} - [HCO_3^-]) \times 0.5\ (\text{wt in kg})$$

Treatment is subsequently modified according to repeated measurements of arterial blood gases. Posthypocapnic hyperchloremic acidosis requires no specific therapy as renal mechanisms will normalize bicarbonate concentration in 12 to 36 h. TPN-associated hyperchloremic acidosis can be corrected by discontinuation of administration or minimized by using Na^+ or K^+ acetate as electrolyte supplements rather than the usual chloride salts.

REFERENCES

1. Shoemaker WC: Fluids and electrolytes in the acutely ill adult. In: Shoemaker WC, Ayres S, Grenvik A, Holbrook PR, Thompson WL (eds): *Textbook of Critical Care*, 2d ed. Philadelphia, Saunders, pp 1128–1152, 1989.
2. Gennari FJ: Current concepts: Serum osmolality, uses and limitations. *N Engl J Med* 310:102, 1984.
3. Stuart FP, Torres E, Fletcher R, et al: Effects of single, repeated and massive mannitol infusion in the dog: Structural and functional changes in kidney and brain. *Ann Surg* 172:190, 1970.
4. Dorman HR, Sondheimer JH, Cadnapaphornchai P: Mannitol-induced acute renal failure. *Medicine* 69:153, 1990.
5. Marsh ML, Marshall LF, Shapiro HM: Neurosurgical intensive care. *Anesthesiology* 47:149, 1977.
6. Grotta JC: Current medical and surgical therapy for cerebrovascular diseases. *N Engl J Med* 317:1505, 1987.
7. Robertson GL: Thirst and vasopressin function in

normal and disordered states of water balance. *J Lab Clin Med* 101:351, 1983
8. Schrier RW, Berl T, Anderson RH: Osmotic and nonosmotic control of vasopressin release. *Am J Physiol* 236(4):F321, 1979.
9. Gauer OH: Osmocontrol versus volume control. *Fed Proc* 27:1132, 1968.
10. Arieff AI: Hyponatremia, convulsions, respiratory arrest, and permanent brain damage after elective surgery in healthy women. *N Engl J Med* 314:1529, 1986
11. Chung HM, Kluge R, Schrier RW, Anderson RJ: Postoperative hyponatremia: A prospective study. *Arch Intern Med* 146:333, 1986.
12. Gaufin L, Skowsky WR, Goodman SJ: Release of antidiuretic hormone during mass-induced elevation of intracranial pressure. *J Neurosurg* 46:627, 1977.
13. Sorensen PS: Studies of vasopressin in the human cerebrospinal fluid. *Acta Neurol Scand* 74:81, 1986.
14. Sorensen PS, Gjerris F, Hammer M: Cerebrospinal fluid and plasma vasopressin during short-term induced intracranial hypertension. *Acta Neurochir* 77:46, 1985.
15. Cserr HF, dePasquale M, Patlak CS: Volume regulatory influx of electrolytes from plasma to brain during acute hyperosmolality. *Am J Physiol* 253:F530, 1987.
16. Thurston JH, Hauhart RE: Brain amino acids decrease in chronic hyponatremia and rapid correction causes brain dehydration: Possible clinical significance. *Life Sci* 40:2539, 1987.
17. Solis JM, Herranz AS, Herreras O, et al: Does taurine act as an osmoregulatory substance in the rat brain? *Neurosci Lett* 91:53, 1988.
18. Wade JV, Olson JP, Samson FE, et al: A possible role for taurine in osmoregulation within the brain. *J Neurochem* 51:740, 1988.
19. Thurston HG, Sherman WR, Hauhart RE, Kloepper RF: Myoinositol: A newly identified nonnitrogenous osmoregulatory molecule in mammalian brain. *Pediatr Res* 26:482, 1989.
20. Fenstermacher JD: Volume regulation of the central nervous system. In: Staub NC, Taylor AE (eds): *Edema*. New York, Raven, 1984, pp 383–403.
21. Rapoport SI: A Model for brain edema. In: Inaba Y, Klatzo I, Spatz M (eds): *Brain Edema*, Berlin, Springer-Verlag, 1984.
22. Schrier RW, Anderson RJ: Renal sodium excretion, edematous disorders, and diuretic use. In: Schrier RW (ed): *Renal and Electrolyte Disorders*, 2d ed. Boston, Little Brown, 1980, pp 65–114.
23. Raymond KH, Reineck HJ, Stein JH: Sodium metabolism and maintenance of extracellular fluid volume. In: Arieff AI, DeFronzo RA (eds): *Fluid Electrolyte and Acid-Base Disorders*, New York, Churchill Livingstone, 1985, pp 39–76.
24. Needleman P, Greenwald JE: Atriopeptin: A cardiac hormone intimately involved in fluid, electrolyte, and blood-pressure homeostasis. *N Engl J Med* 314:828, 1986.
25. Samson WK: Atrial natriuretic factor and the central nervous system. *Endocrinol Metab Clin North Am* 16:145, 1987.
26. Steardo L, Nathanson JA: Brain barrier tissues: End organs for atriopeptins. *Science* 235:470, 1987.
27. Szczepanska-Sadowska EWA: Mechanisms subserving brain water electrolyte homeostasis. *Acta Physiol Pol* 40:301, 1989.
28. Itoh H, Nakao K, Yamada T, et al: Brain renin-angiostensin, central control of secretion of atrial and natriuretic factor from the heart. *Hypertension* 11:157, 1988.
29. Unger T, Gohlke P, Kotrba M, et al: Angiotensin II and atrial natriuretic peptide in the brain: Effects on volume and Na^+ balance. *Resuscitation* 18:309, 1989.
30. Bahner U, Geiger H, Palkovits M, et al: Atrial natriuretic peptides in brain nuclei of rats with inherited diabetes insipidus (Brattleboro rats). *Neuroendocrinology* 51:721, 1990.
31. Rettig R, Ganten D, Lange RE, Unger T: Brain angiotensin II: Localization and possible functions. *Adv Biochem Psychopharmacol* 43:129, 1987.
32. Harding JW, Jensen LL, Quirk WS, et al: Brain angiotensin: Critical role in the ongoing regulation of body fluid homeostasis and cardiovascular function. *Peptides* 10:261, 1989.
33. Doczi T, Joo F, Szerdahelyi P, Bodosi M: Regulation of brain water and electrolyte content: The possible involvement of central atrial natriuretic factor. *Neurosurgery* 21:454, 1987.
34. Doczi T, Joo F, Szerdahelyi P, Bodosi M: Regulation of brain water and electrolyte contents: The opposite actions of central vasopressin and atrial natriuretic factor. *Acta Neurochir* 43(suppl):186, 1988.
35. Doczi T, Joo F, Bodosi M: Central neuroendocrine control of the brain water, electrolyte, and volume homeostasis. *Acta Neurochir* 47(suppl):122, 1990.
36. Nakao N, Itakura T, Yokote H, et al: Effect of atrial natriuretic peptide on ischemic brain edema: Changes in brain water and electrolytes. *Neurosurgery* 27:39, 1990.
37. Zollinger RM, Skillman JJ, Moore FD: Alterations in water, colloid, and electrolyte distribution after hemorrhage. In: Fox CL, Nahas GG (eds): *Body Fluid Replacement in the Surgical Patient*, New York, Grune & Stratton, 1969, pp 2–9
38. Sladen A, Laver MB, Pontoppidan H: Pulmonary

complications and water retention in prolonged mechanical ventilation. *N Engl J Med* 279:448, 1968.
39. Candelise L, Landi G, Orazio EN, Boccardi E: Prognostic significance of hyperglycemia in acute stroke. *Arch Neurol* 42:661, 1985.
40. Berger L, Hakim AM: The association of hyperglycemia with cerebral edema in stroke. *Stroke* 17:865, 1986.
41. Helgason C: Blood glucose and stroke. *Stroke* 19:1049, 1988.
42. Longstreth WT Jr, Inui TS: High blood glucose level in hospital admission and poor neurologic recovery after cardiac arrest. *Ann Neurol* 15:59, 1984.
43. Young B, Ott L, Dempsy R, et al: Relationship between admission hyperglycemia and neurologic outcome of severely brain-injured patients. *Ann Surg* 210:466, 1989.
44. Lam AM, Winn HR, Cullen BF, Sundling N: Hyperglycemia and neurological outcome in patients with head injury. *J Neurosurg* 75:545, 1991.
45. Michaud LJ, Rivara FP, Longstreth WT, Grady MS: Elevated initial blood glucose levels and poor outcome following severe brain injuries in children. *J Trauma* 31:1355, 1991.
46. Robertson CS, Goodman JC, Narayan RK, et al: The effect of glucose administration on carbohydrate metabolism after head injury. *J Neurosurg* 74:43, 1991.
47. Drummond JC, Moore SS: The influence of dextrose administration on neurologic outcome after temporary spinal cord ischemia in the rabbit. *Anesthesiology* 70:64, 1989.
48. Connors AF, McCaffree DR, Gray BA: Evaluation of right heart catheterization in the critically ill patient without acute myocardial infarction. *N Engl J Med* 308:263, 1983.
49. Eisenberg PR, Joffe AS, Schuster DP: Clinical evaluation compared to pulmonary artery catheterization in the hemodynamic assessment of critically ill patients. *Crit Care Med* 12:549, 1984.
50. Connors AF, Dawson NV, McCaffree R, et al: Assessing hemodynamic status in critically ill patients: Do physicians use clinical information optimally? *J Crit Care* 2:174, 1987.
51. Tuchschmidt J, Sharma OP: Impact of hemodynamic monitoring in a medical intensive care unit. *Crit Care Med* 15:840, 1987.
52. Kudo T, Suzuki S, Iawbuchi T: Importance of monitoring the circulating blood volume in patients with cerebral vasospasm after subarachnoid hemorrhage. *Neurosurgery* 9:514, 1981.
53. Nelson PB, Seif SM, Maroon JC, Robinson AG: Hyponatremia in intracranial disease: Perhaps not the syndrome of inappropriate secretion of antidiuretic hormone (SIADH). *J Neurosurg* 55:938, 1981.
54. Solomon RA, Post KD, McMurty JG: Depression of circulating blood volume in patients after subarachnoid hemorrhage: Implications for the management of symptomatic vasospasm. *Neurosurgery* 15:354, 1984.
55. Wijdicks EFM, Vermeulen M, ten Haff JA, et al: Volume depletion and natriuresis in patients with a ruptured intracranial aneurysm. *Ann Neurol* 18:211, 1985.
56. Shoemaker WC, Appel PL, Kram HB: Prospective trial of supranormal values of survivors and therapeutic goals in high risk surgical patients. *Chest* 94:1176, 1988.
57. Marmarou A, Anderson RL, Ward JD, et al: Impact of ICP instability and hypotension on outcome in patients with severe head trauma. *J Neurosurg* 75:S59, 1991.
58. Rosner MJ, Becker DP: Origin and evolution of plateau waves. *J Neurosurg* 60:312, 1984.
59. Rosner MJ, Coley IB: Cerebral perfusion pressure, intracranial pressure, and head elevation. *J Neurosurg* 65:636, 1986.
60. Tator CH, Fehlings MG: Review of the secondary injury theory of acute spinal cord trauma with emphasis on vascular mechanisms. *J Neurosurg* 75:15, 1991.
61. Mackenzie CF, Shin B, Krishnaprasad D, et al: Assessment of cardiac and respiratory function during surgery on patients with acute quadriplegia. *J Neurosurg* 62:843, 1985.
62. Weil MH: Patient evaluation, "vital signs," and initial care. Critical care: State of the art. *Soc Crit Care Med* 1(A):1, 1980.
63. Hauser CJ, Shoemaker WC, Turpin I, et al: Oxygen transport responses to colloids and crystalloids in critically ill surgical patients. *Surg Gynecol Oncol* 150:811, 1980.
64. Hankeln K, Radel C, Beez M, et al: Comparison of hydroxyethyl starch and lactated Ringer's solution on hemodynamics and oxygen transport of critically ill patients in prospective crossover studies. *Crit Care Med* 17:133, 1989.
65. Shoemaker WC, Schluchter M, Hopkins JA, et al: Comparison of the relative effectiveness of colloids and crystalloids in emergency resuscitation. *Am J Surg* 142:73, 1981.
66. Nearman HS, Herman ML: Toxic effects of colloids in the intensive care unit. In: Carlson RW, Geheb MA, Blumer JL, Bond GR (eds): *Critical Care Clinics*, Philadelphia, Saunders, 1991, pp 713–723.
67. Hughes J, Mudd S, Strecker EA: Reduction of increased intracranial pressure by concentrated solutions of human lyophile serum. *Arch Neurol Psychiatry* 39:1277, 1938.

68. Wright D, Bond D, Hughes J: Reduction of cerebrospinal fluid pressure by concentrated lyophile serum. Further observations. *Arch Neurol Psychiatry* 39: 1288, 1938.
69. Turner JWA: Concentrated serum in head injuries. *Lancet* 2:557, 1941.
70. Gates EM, Graig WM: The use of serum albumin in cases of cerebral edema: Preliminary report. *Mayo Clin Proc* 23:89, 1948.
71. Little JR, Lugg RM, Latchaw JP, Lesser RP: Treatment of acute focal cerebral ischemia with concentrated albumin. *Neurosurgery* 9:552, 1981.
72. Erstad BL, Gaels BL, Rappaport WD: The use of albumin in clinical practice. *Arch Intern Med* 151:901, 1991.
73. Cully MD, Larson CP, Silverberg GD: Hetastarch coagulopathy in a neurosurgical patient. *Anesthesiology* 66:706, 1987.
74. Symington BE: Hetastarch and bleeding complications. *Ann Intern Med* 105:627, 1986.
75. Lowe RJ, Moss GS, Jilek J, Levine HD: Crystalloid versus colloid in the etiology of pulmonary failure after trauma—a randomized trial in man. *Crit Care Med* 7:107, 1979.
76. Virgilio RW, Rice CL, Smith DE, et al: Crystalloid versus colloid resuscitation: Is one better? *Surgery* 85:129, 1979.
77. Moss GS, Lowe RJ, Tilek J, Levine HD: Colloid or crystalloid in the resuscitation of hemorrhagic shock: A controlled clinical trial. *Surgery* 89:434, 1981.
78. Velanovich V: Crystalloid versus colloid fluid resuscitation: A meta-analysis of mortality. *Surgery* 105:65, 1989.
79. Bisonni RS, Holtgrave DR, Lawler F, Marley DS: Colloids versus crystalloids in fluid resuscitation: An analysis of randomized controlled trials. *J Fam Pract* 32:387, 1991.
80. Zornow MH, Todd MM, Moore SS: The acute cerebral effects of changes in plasma osmolality and oncotic pressure. *Anesthesiology* 67:936, 1987.
81. Tommasino C, Moore S, Todd MM: Cerebral effects of isovolemic hemodilution with crystalloid or colloid solutions. *Crit Care Med* 16:862, 1988.
82. Gunnar W, Jonasson O, Merlotti G, et al: Head injury and hemorrhagic shock: Studies of the blood brain barrier and intracranial pressure after resuscitation with normal saline solution, 3% saline solution, and dextran-40. *Surgery* 103:398, 1988.
83. Zornow MH, Scheller MS, Todd MM, Moore SS: Acute cerebral effects of isotonic crystalloid and colloid solutions following cryogenic brain injury in the rabbit. *Anesthesiology* 69:185, 1988.
84. Kaieda R, Todd MM, Cook LN, Warner DS: Acute effects of changing plasma osmolality and colloid oncotic pressure on the formation of brain edema after cryogenic injury. *Neurosurgery* 24:671, 1989.
85. Poole GV, Prough DS, Johnson JC, et al: Effects of resuscitation from hemorrhagic shock on cerebral hemodynamics in the presence of an intracranial mass. *J Trauma* 27:18, 1987.
86. Tranmer BI, Iacobacci RI, Kindt GW: Effects of crystalloid and colloid infusions on intracranial pressure and computerized electroencephalographic data in dogs with vasogenic brain edema. *Neurosurgery* 25:173, 1989.
87. Todd M, Zornow MH: Effects of crystalloid and colloid infusions on intracranial pressure. *Neurosurgery* 26:546, 1990.
88. Prough DS, Johnson JC, Stump DS, et al: Effects of hypertonic saline versus lactated Ringer's solution on cerebral oxygen transport during resuscitation from hemorrhagic shock. *J Neurosurg* 64:627, 1986.
89. Todd MM, Tommasino C, Moore S: Cerebral effects of isovolemic hemodilution with a hypertonic saline solution. *J Neurosurg* 63:944, 1985.
90. Zornow MH, Scheller MS, Hackford SR: Effect of hypertonic lactated Ringer's solution on intracranial pressure and cerebral water content in a model of traumatic brain injury. *J Trauma* 29:484, 1989.
91. Worthley LIG, Cooper DJ, Jones N: Treatment of resistant intracranial hypertension with hypertonic saline. *J Neurosurg* 68:478, 1988.
92. Vassar MJ, Perry CA, Gannaway WL, Holcroft JW: 7.5% sodium chloride/dextran for resuscitation of trauma patients undergoing helicopter transport. *Arch Surg* 126:1065, 1991.
93. Hint H: The pharmacology of dextran and the physiological background for the clinical use of rheomacrodex and macrodex. *Acta Anesthesiol Belg* 19:119, 1968.
94. Czer LSC, Shoemaker WC: Optimal hematocrit value in critically ill postoperative patients. *Surg Gynecol Obstet* 147:363, 1978.
95. Gaehtgens P, Marx P: Hemorrheological aspects of the pathophysiology of cerebral ischemia. *J Cereb Blood Flow Metab* 7:259, 1987.
96. Goldberg M, Handler JS: Hyponatremia and renal wasting of sodium in patients with malfunction of the central nervous system. *N Engl J Med* 263:1037, 1960.
97. Fox JL, Falik JL, Shalhoub RJ: Neurosurgical hyponatremia: The role of inappropriate antidiuresis. *J Neurosurg* 34:506, 1971.
98. Hantman D, Rossier B, Zohlman R, Schrier R: Rapid correction hyponatremia in the syndrome of inappropriate secretion of antidiuretic hormone. *Ann Intern Med* 78:870, 1973.

99. Hayes RM: Antidiuretic hormone. *N Engl J Med* 295:659, 1976.
100. Steinbok P, Thompson GB: Metabolic disturbances after head injury: Abnormalities of sodium and water balance with special reference to the effects of alcohol intoxication. *Neurosurgery* 3(1):9, 1978.
101. Widjicks EFM, Vermeulen M, Hijdra A, Van Gijn J: Hyponatremia and cerebral infarction in patients with ruptured intracranial aneurysms: Is fluid restriction harmful? *Ann Neurol* 17:137, 1985.
102. Shimoda M, Yamada S, Yamamoto I, et al: Atrial natriuretic polypeptide in patients with subarachnoid hemorrhage due to aneurysmal rupture. Correlation to hyponatremia. *Acta Neurochir* 97:53, 1989.
103. Hasan D, Wijdicks EF, Vermeulen M: Hyponatremia is associated with cerebral ischemia in patients with aneurysmal subarachnoid hemorrhage. *Ann Neurol* 27:106, 1990.
104. Kassell NF, Torner JC, Haely EC, et al: The international cooperative study on the timing of aneurysm surgery. *J Neurosurg* 73:18, 1990.
105. Landolt AM, Yasargil MG, Krayenbuhl H: Disturbances of the serum electrolytes after surgery of intracranial arterial aneurysms. *J Neurosurg* 37:210, 1972.
106. Takaku A, Shindo K, Tanaka S, et al: Fluid and electrolyte disturbances in patients with intracranial aneurysms. *Surg Neurol* 11:349, 1979.
107. Wijdicks EFM, Van Dongen KJ, Vangijn J, et al: Enlargement of the third ventricle and hyponatraemia in aneurysmal subarachnoid hemorrhage. *J Neurol Neurosurg Psychiatry* 51:516, 1988.
108. Epstein M, Ward JD, Becker DP: Medical complications of head injury. In: Cooper PR (ed): *Head injury*, 2d ed. Boston, Williams & Wilkins, 1987, pp 390–421.
109. Doczi T, Tarjanyi J, Huszka E, Kiss J: Syndrome of inappropriate secretion of antidiuretic hormone (SIADH) after head injury. *Neurosurgery* 10:685, 1982.
110. Padilla G, Leake JA, Castro R, et al: Vasopressin levels and pediatric head trauma. *Pediatrics* 83:700, 1989.
111. Leehey DJ, Picache AA, Robertson GL. Hyponatremia in quadriplegic patients. *Clin Sci* 75:441, 1988.
112. Sica D, Zawada E, Midha M, et al: Hyponatremia in the cord injured patient—a neglected phenomenon. *Kidney Int* 24:137, 1984.
113. Sica DA, Culpepper RM: Case report: Severe hyponatremia in spinal cord injury. *Am J Med Sci* 298(5):331, 1989.
114. Williams HH, Wall BM, Horan JM, et al: Nonosmotic stimuli alter osmoregulation in patients with spinal cord injury. *J Clin Endocrinol Metab* 71:1536, 1990.
115. Mather H, Ang V, Jenkins JS: Vasopressin in plasma and CSF of patients with subarachnoid hemorrhage. *J Neurol Neurosurg Psychiatry* 44:216, 1981.
116. Sorensen PS: Studies of vasopressin in the human cerebrospinal fluid. *Acta Neurol Scand* 74:81, 1986.
117. Ishikawa SE, Saito T, Aneko K, et al: Hyponatremia responsive to fludrocortisone acetate in elderly patients after head injury. *Ann Intern Med* 106:187, 1987.
118. Oelkers W: Hyponatremia and inappropriate secretion of vasopressin (antidiuretic hormone) in patients with hypopituitarism. *N Engl J Med* 321:492, 1989.
119. Diringer M, Ladenson PW, Stern B, et al: Plasma atrial natriuretic factor and subarachnoid hemorrhage. *Stroke* 19:1119, 1988.
120. Doczi T, Joo F, Vecsernyes M, Bodosi M: Increased concentration of atrial natriuretic factor in the cerebrospinal fluid of patients with aneurysmal subarachnoid hemorrhage and raised intracranial pressure. *Neurosurgery* 23:16, 1988.
121. Rosenfeld JV, Barnett GH, Sila CA, et al: The effect of subarachnoid hemorrhage on blood and CSF atrial natriuretic factor. *J Neurosurg* 71:32, 1989.
122. Diringer MN, Kirsch JR, Ladenson PW, et al: Cerebrospinal fluid atrial natriuretic factor in intracranial disease. *Stroke* 21:1550, 1990.
123. Diringer MN, Lim JS, Kirsch JR, Hanley DF: Suprasellar and intraventricular blood predict elevated plasma atrial natriuretic factor in subarachnoid hemorrhage. *Stroke* 22:577, 1991.
124. Cogan E, Debieve MF, Pepersack T, Abramow M: Natriuresis and atrial natriuretic factor secretion during inappropriate antidiuresis. *Am J Med* 84:409, 1988.
125. Peters JP, Welt LG, Sims EAH, et al: A salt wasting syndrome associated with cerebral disease. *Trans Assoc Am Physicians* 63:57, 1950.
126. Cort JH: Cerebral salt wasting. *Lancet* 1:752, 1954.
127. Vingerhoets F, De Tribolet N: Hyponatremia hypo-osmolarity in neurosurgical patients. "Appropriate secretion of ADH" and "Cerebral salt wasting syndrome." *Acta Neurochir* 91:50, 1988.
127a. Wijdicks EFM, Ropper AH, Hunnicutt EJ, et al: Atrial natriuretic factor and salt wasting after aneurysmal subarachnoid hemorrhage. *Stroke* 22:1519, 1991.
128. Nelson PB, Seif S, Gutai J, Robinson AG: Hyponatremia and natriuresis following subarachnoid hemorrhage in a monkey model. *J Neurosurg* 60:233, 1984.
129. Messert B, Orrison WW, Hawkins MJ, Cuaglieri CE: Central pontine myelinolysis: Considerations of eti-

ology, diagnosis and treatment. *Neurology* 29:147, 1979.

130. Norenberg MD, Leslie KO, Robertson AS: Association between rise in serum sodium and central pontine myelinolysis. *Ann Neurol* 11:128, 1982.
131. Sterns RH, Riggs JE, Schochet SS: Osmotic demyelination syndrome following correction of hyponatremia. *N Engl J Med* 314:1535, 1986.
132. Sterns RH, Darbbie JD, Herndon RM: Brain dehydration and neurologic deterioration after rapid correction of hyponatremia. *Kidney Int* 35:69, 1989.
133. Cluitmans FHM, Meinders AE: Management of severe hyponatremia: Rapid or slow correction. *Am J Med* 88:161, 1990.
134. Sterns RH: The management of hyponatremic emergencies. In Carlson RW, Geheb MA, Zaloga GP (eds): *Critical Care Clinics*, Philadelphia, Saunders, 1991, pp 127–142.
135. Decaux G, Unger J, Brimioulle S, Mockel J: Hyponatremia in the syndrome of inappropriate secretion of antidiuretic hormone. Rapid correction with urea, sodium chloride and water restriction therapy. *JAMA* 247(4):471, 1982.
136. Reeder RF, Harbaugh RE: Administration of intravenous urea and normal saline for the treatment of hyponatremia in neurosurgical patients. *J Neurosurg* 70:201, 1989.
137. De Troyer A: Demeclocycline. *JAMA* 237:2723, 1977.
138. Forrest JN, Cox M, Hong C, et al: Superiority of demeclocycline over lithium in the treatment of chronic syndrome of inappropriate secretion of antidiuretic hormone. *N Engl J Med* 298:173, 1978.
139. Bingham WF: The limits of cerebral dehydration in the treatment of head injury. *Surg Neurol* 25:340, 1986.
140. Ross EJ, Christie SBM: Hypernatremia. *Medicine* 48:441, 1969.
141. Kahn A, Brachet E, Blum D: Controlled fall in natremia and risk of seizures in hypertonic dehydration. *Intensive Care Med* 5:27, 1979.
142. Geheb MA: Clinical approach to the hyperosmolar patient. In: Geheb M, Carlson R (eds): *Critical Care Clinics*, Philadelphia, Saunders, 1987, pp 797–815.
143. Coculescu M, Dumitrescu C: Etiology of cranial diabetes insipidus in 164 adults. *Endocrinologie* 22:135, 1984.
144. Moses M: Clinical and laboratory observations in the adult with diabetes insipidus. *Front Horm Res* 13:156, 1985.
145. Balestrieri FJ, Chernow B, Rainey TG: Postcraniotomy diabetes insipidus: Who's at risk? *Crit Care Med* 10:108, 1982.
146. Shibata S, Mori K, Teramoto S: Diabetes insipidus after surgery of intracranial arterial aneurysms. *No Shinkei Geka* 6:795, 1978.
147. Crompton MR: Hypothalamic lesions following closed head injury. *Brain* 94:165, 1971.
148. Edwards OM, Clark JDA: Post-traumatic hypopituitarism. *Medicine* 65:281, 1986.
149. Defoer F, Mahler C, Dua G, Appel B: Post-traumatic diabetes insipidus. *Acta Anaesthesiol Belg* 38:297, 1987.
150. Outwater KM, Rockoff MA: Diabetes insipidus accompanying brain death in children. *Neurology* 34:1243, 1984.
151. Fiser DH, Jimenez JF, Wrape V, Woddy R: Diabetes insipidus in children with brain death. *Crit Care Med* 15:551, 1987.
152. Notman DD, Mortek MA, Moses AM: Permanent diabetes insipidus following head trauma: Observations on ten patients and an approach to diagnosis. *J Trauma* 20:599, 1980.
153. Shucart WA, Jackson I: Management of diabetes insipidus in neurosurgical patients. *J Neurosurg* 44:65, 1976.
154. Sharkey PC, Perry JH, Ehni G: Diabetes insipidus following section of hypophyseal stalk. *J Neurosurg* 18:445, 1961.
155. Moses AM, Blumenthal SA, Streeten DH: Acid-base and electrolyte disorders associated with endocrine disease: Pituitary and thyroid. In: Arief AI, Defronzo RA (eds): *Fluid Electrolyte and Acid-Base Disorders*. New York, Churchill Livingstone, 1985, pp 851–892.
156. Levitt MA, Fleischer AS, Meislin HW: Acute post-traumatic diabetes insipidus: Treatment with continuous intravenous vasopressin. *J Trauma* 24:532, 1984.
157. Miller M, Dalakos T, Moses AM: Recognition of partial defects in antidiuretic hormone secretion. *Ann Intern Med* 73:721, 1970.
158. Robinson AG, Verbalis JG: Treatment of central diabetes insipidus. *Front Horm Res* 13:292, 1985.
159. Pomeranz S, Constantini S, Rappaport ZH: Hypokalemia in severe head trauma. *Acta Neurochir* 97:62, 1989.
160. Andreoli A, di Pasquale G, Pinelli G, et al: Subarachnoid hemorrhage: Frequency and severity of cardiac arrhythmias. *Stroke* 18:558, 1987.
160a. Zaloga GP, Chernow B: Hypocalcemia in critical illness. *JAMA* 256(14):1924, 1986.
161. Sterns R, Cox M, Feig P: Internal potassium balance and the control of the plasma potassium concentration. *Medicine* 60:339, 1981.
162. Hamill RJ, Robinson LM, Wexler HR, Moote C: Efficacy and safety of potassium infusion therapy in hy-

pokalemic critically ill patients. *Crit Care Med* 19(5):694, 1991.
163. DeFronzo RA, Bia M: Intravenous potassium chloride therapy. *JAMA* 245:2446, 1981.
164. Zaloga GP, Chernow B, Cook D: Assessment of calcium homeostasis in the critically ill patient: The diagnostic pitfalls of the Mclean Hastings nomogram. *Ann Surg* 202:587, 1985.
165. Desai TK, Carlson RW, Gehab MA: Prevalence and clinical implications of hypocalcemia in acutely ill patients in a medical intensive care setting. *Am J Med* 84:209, 1988.
166. Zaloga GP, Chernow B: Hypocalcemia in critical illness. *JAMA* 256(14):1924, 1986.
167. Zaloga GP: Hypocalcemic Crisis. *Crit Care Clinics* 7:191, 1991.
168. Desai TK, Carlson RW, Gehab MA: Parathyroid-vitamin D axis in critically ill patients with unexplained hypocalcemia. *Kidney Int* 32(22):S225, 1987.
169. Zaloga GP, Chernow B, Cook D, et al: Assessment of calcium homeostasis in the critically ill surgical patient. *Crit Care Med* 12:236, 1984.
170. Gotta H: Tetany and epilepsy. *Arch Neurol Psychiatry* 66:714, 1951.
171. Sugar O: Central neurological manifestations of hypoparathyroidism. *Arch Neurol Psychiatry* 70:86, 1953.
172. Fonseca OA, Calverly JR: Neurological manifestations of hypoparathyroidism. *Arch Intern Med* 120:202, 1967.
173. King AL, Sica DA, Miller G, Pierpaoli S: Severe hypophosphatemia in a general hospital population. *South Med J* 80:831, 1987.
174. Halevy J, Bulvik S: Severe hypophosphatemia in hospitalized patients. *Arch Intern Med* 148:153, 1988.
175. Camp MA, Allon M: Severe hypophosphatemia in hospitalized patients. *Miner Electrolyte Metab* 16:365, 1990.
176. Daily WH, Tonnesen A, Allen SA: Hypophosphatemia incidence, etiology, and prevention in the trauma patient. *Crit Care Med* 18:1210, 1990.
177. Gadisseux P, Sica DA, Ward JD, Becker DP: Severe hypophosphatemia after head injury. *Neurosurgery* 17:35, 1985
178. Hayek ME, Eisenberg PG: Severe hypophosphatemia following the institution of enteral feedings. *Arch Surg* 124:1325, 1989.
179. Solomon SM, Kirby DF: The refeeding syndrome: A review. *J Parenteral Enteral Nutrition* 14:90, 1990.
180. Vianna MJ: Severe hypophosphatemia due to hypokalemia. *JAMA* 215:1497, 1971.
181. Whang R, Oei TO, Aikawa JK, et al: Predictors of clinical hypomagnesia: Hypokalemia, hypophosphatemia, hyponatremia and hypocalcemia. *Arch Intern Med* 144:1794, 1984.
182. Aubier M, Murcian D, Lecocguic Y, et al: Effect of hypophosphatemia on diaphragmatic contractility in patients with acute respiratory failure. *N Engl J Med* 313:420, 1985.
183. Gravelyn TR, Brophy N, Siegart C: Hypophosphatemia-associated respiratory muscle weakness in a general inpatient population. *Am J Med* 84:870, 1988.
184. O'Connor LR, Wheeler WS, Bethune JE: Effect of hypophosphatemia on myocardial performance in man. *N Engl J Med* 297:901, 1977.
185. Davis SV, Olichwier KK, Chakko SC: Reversible depression of myocardial performance in hypophosphatemia. *Am J Med Sci* 295(3):183, 1988.
186. Craddock PR, Yawata Y, Vansanten L: Acquired phagocyte dysfunction: A complication of the hypophosphatemia of parenteral hyperalimentation. *N Engl J Med* 290(25):1403, 1974.
187. Lichtman MA, Miller DR, Cohen J: Reduced red cell glycolysis, 2,3-diphosphoglycerate and adenosine triphosphate concentration, and increased hemoglobin-oxygen affinity by hypophosphatemia. *Ann Intern Med* 74:562, 1971.
188. Silvis SE, Paragas PD: Paresthesias, weakness, seizures, and hypophosphatemia in patients receiving hyperalimentation. *Gastroenterology* 62:513, 1972.
189. Lee JL, Sibbald WJ, Holliday RL, Linton AL: Hypophosphatemia associated with coma. *Can Med Assoc J* 119:143, 1978.
190. Young GB, Amacher AL, Paulseth JE, et al: Hypophosphatemia versus brain death. *Lancet* 1(1):617, 1982.
191. Knochel JP: The clinical status of hypophosphatemia. *N Engl J Med* 313:447, 1985.
192. Kingston M, Al-Siba MB: Treatment of severe hypophosphatemia. *Crit Care Med* 13:16, 1985.
193. Ryzen E, Wagners PW, Singer FR: Magnesium deficiency in a medical ICU population. *Crit Care Med* 13:19, 1985.
194. Zaloga GP, Wilkens R, Tourville J, et al: A simple method for determining physiology active calcium and magnesium concentrations in critically ill patients. *Crit Care Med* 15(9):813, 1987.
195. Chernow B, Bamberger S, Stoiko M, et al: Hypomagnesemia in patients in postoperative intensive care. *Chest* 95:391, 1989.
196. Rude RK, Singer FR: Magnesium deficiency and excess. *Ann Rev Med* 32:245, 1981.
197. Chernow B, Smith J, Rainey TG, Finto C: Hypomagnesemia: Implications for the critical care specialist. *Crit Care Med* 10(3):193, 1982.
198. Fishman RA: Neurological aspects of magnesium metabolism. *Arch Neurol* 12:562, 1965.

199. Shils ME: Experimental human magnesium depletion. *Medicine* 48:61–85, 1969.
200. Kingston ME, Al-siba MB, Skooge WC: Clinical manifestations of hypomagnesemia. *Crit Care Med* 14:950, 1986.
201. Ram Z, Sadeh M, Shacked I, et al: Magnesium sulfate reverses experimental delayed cerebral vasospasm after subarachnoid hemmorrhage in rats. *Stroke* 22:922, 1991.
202. Boriss MN, Papa L: Magnesium: A discussion of its role in the treatment of ventricular dysrhythmia. *Crit Care Med* 16(3):292, 1988.
203. Salem M, Munoz R, Chernow B: Hypomagnesemia in critical illness: A common and clinically important problem. *Crit Care Clin* 7(1):191, 1991.
204. Flink EB: Therapy of magnesium deficiency. *Ann NY Acad Sci* 162:901, 1969.
205. Narins RG, Emmett M: Simple and mixed acid-base disorders: A practical approach. *Medicine* 59(3):161, 1980.
206. Fencl V, Rossing TH: Acid-base disorders in critical care medicine. *Ann Rev Med* 40:17, 1989.
207. Severinghaus JW, Lassen N: Step hypocapnia to separate arterial from tissue P_{CO2} in the regulation of cerebral blood flow. *Circ Res* 20:272, 1967.
208. Katzman R, Pappius HM: *Brain Electrolytes and Fluid Metabolism.* Baltimore, Williams & Wilkins, 1973.
209. Arieff AI, Kerian A, Massry SG, DeLima J: Intracellular pH of brain: Alterations in acute respiratory acidosis and alkalosis. *Am J Physiol* 230(3):804, 1976.
210. North JB, Jennett S: Abnormal breathing patterns associated with acute brain damage. *Arch Neurol* 31:338, 1974.
211. Frost EAM: The physiopathology of respiration in neurosurgical patients. *J Neurosurg* 50:699, 1979.
212. Kilburn KH: Shock, seizures and coma with alkalosis during mechanical ventilation. *Arch Intern Med* 65:977, 1966.
213. Froman C: Adverse effects of low carbon dioxide tensions during mechanical over-ventilation of patients with combined head and chest injuries. *Br J Anaesth* 40:383, 1968.
214. Alexander SC, Smith TC, Strobel G, et al: Cerebral carbohydrate metabolism of man during respiratory and metabolic alkalosis. *J Appl Physiol* 24(1):66, 1968.
215. Kennealy JA, McLennan JE, Loudon RG, McLaurin RL: Hyperventilation-induced cerebral hypoxia. *Am Rev Respir Dis* 122:407, 1980.
216. Obrist WD, Langfitt TW, Jaggi JL, et al: Cerebral blood flow and metabolism in comatose patients with acute head injury: Relationship to intracranial hypertension. *J Neurosurg* 61:241, 1984.
217. Proctor HJ, Carins C, Fillipo D, et al: Brain metabolism during increased intracranial pressure as assessed by niroscopy. *Surgery* 96(2):273, 1984.
217a. Druml W, Grimm G, Laggner AN, et al: Lactic acid kinetics in respiratory alkalosis. *Crit Care Med* 19:1120, 1991.
218. Myllynen P, Kivioja A, Rokkanen P, Wilppula E: Cervical spinal cord injury: The correlations of initial clinical features and blood gas analyses with early prognosis. *Paraplegia* 27:19, 1989.
219. Becker DP, Miller JD, Ward JD: The outcome from severe head injury with early diagnosis and intensive management. *J Neurosurg* 47:491, 1977.
220. Miller JD, Butterworth JF, Gudeman SK: Further experience in the management of severe head injury. *J Neurosurg* 54:289, 1981.
221. Wilson RF, Gibson D, Percinel AK: Severe alkalosis in critically ill surgical patients. *Arch Surg* 105:197, 1972.
222. Hodgkin JE, Soeprono EF, Chan DM: Incidence of metabolic alkalemia in hospitalized patients. *Intensive Care Med* 8:725, 1980.
223. Rimmer JM, Gennari FJ: Metabolic alkalosis. *J Intensive Care Med* 2:137, 1987.
224. Friedman BS, Lumb PD: Prevention and management of metabolic alkalosis. *J Intensive Care Med* 5(suppl)S22, 1990.
225. Grace WJ, Barr DP: Complications of alkalosis. *Am J Med* 4:331, 1948.
226. Lubash GD, Coehn BD, Young CW: Severe metabolic alkalosis with neurologic abnormalities. *N Engl J Med* 258:1050, 1958.
227. Darby TD, Aldinger EE, Gadsden RH: Effects of metabolic acidosis on ventricular isometric systolic tension and the response to epinephrine and levarterenol. *Circ Res* 8:1242, 1960.
228. Wildenthal K, Mierzwiak DS, Myers RW: Effects of acute lactic acidosis of left ventricular performance. *Am J Physiol* 214:1352, 1968.
229. Hazard PB, Griffin JP: Calculation of sodium bicarbonate requirement in metabolic acidosis. *Am J Med Sci* 283(1):18, 1982.

CHAPTER 7
Metabolic and Nutritional Management

Linda Ott
Byron Young

Modulating the detrimental metabolic responses to critical illness could decrease patient convalescence time and improve patient outcome. In patients with severe head injury, adverse metabolic effects include hypermetabolism, hypercatabolism (increased urinary nitrogen excretion, altered plasma amino acid profiles, increased skeletal muscle efflux of amino acids), hyperglycemia, immunosuppression, altered vascular permeability, the acute-phase response (fever, increased positive acute-phase proteins, and decreased negative acute-phase proteins), and altered gastric function.[1-25] The metabolic response to severe head injury has been related to infection rate, muscle weakness, and delay in wound healing and tissue repair.

Nutrient administration alone cannot override the metabolic response to head injury.[2,24] Despite adequate caloric administration, severe head injury is followed by negative nitrogen balance, weight loss, depression of immune status, and depression of plasma protein levels. Wilmore has suggested some strategies for modulating the stress response while providing adequate nutrient administration; these include altering the stress response, providing specific fuels, and administering growth factors.[26]

This chapter describes the metabolic response to head injury, reviews studies evaluating the effects of nutrient administration on patient outcome following head injury, details the current state of debate concerning parenteral and enteral nutrition, describes methods of nutritionally assessing the patient with severe head injury, and discusses the current state of affairs for modulating the metabolic response to head injury.

The Metabolic Response to Severe Head Injury

Increased Measured Energy Expenditure (MEE) Patients sustaining severe head injury must overcome two insults: the direct injury to the

Table 7-1 Overview of Consequence, Current Therapy, and Future Therapy of Metabolic Response to Head Injury

Metabolic response	Consequence	Current therapy	Possible future therapy
↑ Caloric expenditure	Weight loss Muscle weakness	↑ Calorie intake	Growth factors Anticytokine and hormone agents
↑ Nitrogen loss	Body wasting	↑ Nitrogen intake Physical therapy	Nutrient modification Growth factors Anticytokine and hormone agents
↑ ICP*	Secondary brain injury	Control ICP*	Alteration of stress response Neurotropic factors
Immune dysfunction	Infection	Antibiotics	IL-2 Antiprostaglandin agents
Hyperglycemia	Secondary neural damage	Insulin Withhold glucose	Growth factors Nutrient modification
Amino acid abnormalities	Body wasting	Give unique amino acid formula	Growth factors Antihormone agents
Altered gastric emptying	Intolerance to gastric feeding	Parenteral nutrition Duodenal or jejunal feedings	Antiopioid, cytokine, corticotropin-releasing ↓ ICP*
Altered vascular permeability	Albumin depression Lung injury Exacerbation of cerebral edema Multiple system organ failure	Albumin	Anticytokine agents Antiendotoxin agents

*Intracranial pressure.

brain and the indirect systemic effects. One of these systemic insults is hypermetabolism, which has been correlated to severity of brain injury (Table 7-1). More than 15 investigators have measured energy expenditure following head injury.[2-10,18,20,24,27-29] A general increase of 40 percent above normal MEE levels has been found in these patients for approximately three weeks postinjury. Some observed MEE variations have been attributed to drug therapy and clinical condition.[3,4] These studies have found that patients in barbiturate coma or otherwise sedated by medication have the lowest energy expenditure, whereas those with decerebrate and decorticate activity have the highest energy expenditures.[5,6,18,24,27,28] The few long-term studies of MEE suggest that the response becomes normal by three months postinjury.[24] Haider et al., however, suggest that the alterations in these patients' metabolic responses may persist for up to 1 year postinjury.[7] Nutrient administration, steroid administration, incidence of infection, and other variables have been suggested as factors contributing to the increase in metabolic rate observed in these patients, but most studies indicate that these variables play only a minor role, if any, in the metabolic rate increase. Fruin et al. and Robertson et al. found no relationship between nutrient intake and metabolic rate increase.[15,18] Studies show no significant difference in metabolic rate between steroid- and nonsteroid-treated patients.[30,31] Greenblatt et al. showed higher MEE levels in head injury patients receiving steroids; however, the large variation in levels rendered any statistical comparisons insignificant.[31] No one has yet explained the mediators causing MEE increase in these patients and exactly how this increase affects patient outcome. Bucci et al. found a strong correlation between increased intracranial pressure (ICP) and increased MEE in these patients.[32] Whether this is a direct or an indirect effect is unknown. Hormonal surge, cytokine increase, or brain inflammation could be mediating the increase in MEE.[33–37] The consequences of this increased metabolic rate are weight loss and muscular fatigue. This metabolic rate increase might also serve some useful physiologic function, such as an increased demand for adenosine triphosphate necessary to support tissue and organ work.[38] Currently, this increased metabolic rate is managed by providing nutrients in amounts equal to those expended so that positive caloric balance can be achieved. Clifton et al. developed a nomogram for estimation of caloric expenditure during the first two weeks after head injury; the most potent predicting factors are Glasgow Coma Scale (GCS) score and number of days since injury.[39] Many hospitals have indirect calorimetry units. Since patient response is variable, measurement of energy expenditure might be useful in certain patients. Measuring metabolic rate more than twice per week is unnecessary unless a unique change in clinical condition occurs. Future management might center on modulating the response or providing anabolic agents. Studies have shown that insulin-like growth factor 1 decreases metabolic rate and weight loss in rats with burn injury.[40] Clinical trials are currently being performed with this agent. Some of the mediators which have been suggested to play a role include hormones, cytokines, and increased ICP. Future studies should be able to determine which mediator is specifically responsible for the increase in metabolic rate. Subsequent studies will then determine which agent or agents are most effective in reducing metabolic rate while still providing adequate nutrition for vital organ processes.

Increased Protein Turnover Protein turnover has been speculated to increase in these patients secondary to observed biochemical and physiologic changes (weight loss, muscle wasting, plasma protein level depression). Urinary nitrogen excretion is increased in these patients, plasma amino acid levels are decreased, and skeletal efflux of amino acids is increased.

Increased Urinary Nitrogen Excretion Many investigators have found increased urinary nitrogen excretion in patients with severe head injury.[1–4,6–9,14,15,17–19,22,24,41,42] Factors such as immobility, steroid therapy, and nutrient administration may play a role in causing this increase in urinary nitrogen excretion.[3,4] Complete immobilization with casts causes negative nitrogen balance and increased urinary nitrogen excretion in healthy young men after a period of 5 to 6 days.[43,44] The immediate increase in nitrogen excretion after all types of trauma, including head injury, suggests that immobilization does not play an important role in the period immediately after injury. The patient with head injury who displays some movement or posturing would not fit into the immobilization theory, however, the patient who is flaccid or paralyzed might. Four investigators have found that head injury patients administered steroids have significantly higher fasting urinary nitrogen output, unique plasma amino acid protein levels, increased urinary 3-methylhistidine excretion, altered lactate/pyruvate ratios, and increased blood glucose levels.[4,30,31,42] Zagara et al., however, found no difference in weight, blood glucose, serum albumin, creatinine, or urinary urea nitrogen excretion in patients with severe head injury randomized to receive steroids in a prospective randomized trial.[45] Patients with head injury have decreased nitrogen efficiency; this is evidenced by increased output despite adequate nitrogen intake.[46] Clifton et al. found that the level of calorie and protein intake influences nitrogen excretion more strongly than any other variable.[39] At 140 percent above predicted energy expenditure, an average of 50 percent of administered nitrogen is excreted. Nitrogen balance cannot be achieved in head injury patients for approximately 2 to 3 weeks postinjury. A decrease in urinary nitrogen excretion may require further modulation of the types of nutrients administered or the administration of pharmacologic and physiologic agents such as anabolic drugs.

Amino Acids Five groups of researchers have studied plasma amino acids. Head injury patients exhibit depressions in the levels of almost all amino acids except threonine, glutamate, aspartate, glycine, citrulline, valine, methionine, tyrosine, phenylalanine, ornithine, and arginine.[3,15,17,21,45] A similar pattern is found in burn and multiple-injury patients.[47] Depressed plasma amino acid levels are speculated to occur secondary to increased tissue requirements. Levels of plasma amino acids seem to be more altered in those patients who have received steroid therapy. Arterial venous amino acid flux to the forearm was studied in eight nonsteroid-treated patients with severe head injury to observe the net flux of amino acids from the skeletal muscle. There was a significant relationship between the degree of metabolic rate increase and glutamine flux. Nitrogen balance was significantly correlated to leucine and isoleucine flux. Most patients experienced a negative flux of overall amino acids. These preliminary data suggest that these patients have increased skeletal muscle efflux of amino acids correlating to metabolic variables of hypermetabolism and hypercatabolism.

Some of the consequences of increased nitrogen excretion and altered amino acid metabolism are muscular atrophy and weakness. Several investigators have suggested that these patients should be put in a decreased metabolic state with drugs such as barbiturates and propranolol to decrease metabolic rate and nutrient need during the first 2 weeks after injury. Current research is directed toward anabolic hormone administration.[18,48] In critically ill, burn-, and multiple-injury patients, growth hormone administration has been able to decrease urinary nitrogen and weight loss.[49,50] In severe head injury and spinal cord injury patients, Behrman et al. found that growth hormone administration significantly decreased serum C-reactive protein levels, improved serum transferrin and insulin growth factor 1 levels, and significantly elevated serum glucose.[51] Although growth hormone administration has positive effects, negative effects such as hyperglycemia and enhanced fluid and sodium retention also occur.[52,53] Many of the beneficial effects of growth hormone are caused by an increased production of insulin-like growth factor 1. Insulin-like growth factor is now recognized to stimulate many of the cellular effects originally attributed to the action of growth hormone.

In addition, patients with head injury may have a relative deficiency of insulin-like growth factor 1 levels. Postmortem studies of head injury patients have revealed pituitary and hypothalamic damage.[54,55] Edwards, and Clark and King et al. found an absence or alteration of growth hormone response in patients with head injury.[56,57] Gottardis et al. reported that, after growth hormone-releasing factor administration, serum growth hormone levels were significantly higher in head injury patients who survived than in those who died.[50] Most important, insulin-like growth factor 1 could not be stimulated by growth hormone-releasing factor, although basal values were significantly higher in patients who survived. Current clinical trials will determine whether or not insulin-like growth factor 1 can decrease urinary nitrogen excretion and weight loss and improve amino acid metabolism in these patients.

Other metabolic mediators which may play a role in causing negative nitrogen balance and altered amino acid metabolism include hormones, cytokines, and prostaglandins.[26] Chiolero et al. found that isolated head injury induced a full response in the secretion of urinary adrenaline, noradrenaline, and such counterregulatory hormones as serum glucagon, insulin, and cortisol.[41] Furthermore, negative nitrogen balance was significantly related to the levels of these hormones. The cytokines interleukin-1 (IL-1) and interleukin-6 (IL-6) are elevated in the serum and ventricular fluid of these patients.[10,12] Goodman et al. found significantly elevated tumor necrosis factor levels in the serum of head injury patients during the first week post-injury.[59] This group found no relationship between tumor necrosis level and urinary nitrogen excretion. Prostaglandins have been suggested to play a role in muscle proteolysis. Some investigators have reported that cyclooxygenase inhibitors may decrease protein catabolism in vitro or in vivo.[60] Although researchers have extensively studied the cause of protein turnover and the optimal method of decreasing urinary nitrogen excretion and plasma amino acid alterations, more work is necessary to determine the optimal mode of decreasing body erosion in these patients.

Hyperglycemia Severe brain injury associated with cerebral edema and increased ICP results in secondary and ongoing cerebral ischemia/infarction. Increased tissue pressure decreases blood perfusion, which leads to ischemia and the release of toxic by-products of cellular injury. These cause vasoconstriction and a cycle of further ischemic neuronal injury and edema. Factors other than the primary brain injury, such as systemic hyperglycemia, may secondarily influence the extent of brain injury.[61] Hyperglycemia, a component of both the acute-phase and stress responses, almost always follows isolated brain injury.[62] Blood glucose levels are inversely related to GCS score and outcome. The deleterious effects of hyperglycemia prior to and during brain ischemic insult have been repeatedly well demonstrated in animal and clinical studies. Hypoxic areas of injured brain metabolize glucose by anaerobic pathways. Lactate rather than pyruvate is the end product of anaerobic glycolysis. Elevated levels of lactate and the consequent acidosis cause further secondary injury to neurons. In general, most studies show that hyperglycemia causes a detrimental effect on cell survival. Insulin, whether by lowering blood glucose or by a mechanism independent of its effect on hyperglycemia, decreased cerebral infarction in two studies.[63,64] The roles of glucose and lactate in ischemia are complex, however; some studies suggest a protective effect of lactate, which is the sole source of nutrients during the ischemic period in the reperfusion model.[65] While the exact cause of the observed hyperglycemia is unknown, researchers speculate that it is related to an increase in hormone or cytokine level. Triple hormone infusion (glucagon, cortisol, and epinephrine) in healthy humans causes elevated blood glucose levels.[66] Some researchers suggest that cytokines such as tumor necrosis factor alter glucose metabolism by affecting pancreatic cell function. It is unclear whether glucose infusion affects glucose metabolism and outcome, or whether the hyperglycemia observed is a stress response alone. Robertson et al. randomized 21 patients with severe head injury to receive intravenous alimentation with or without glucose.[67] Patients were assigned to receive either saline and amino acids or 5% glucose with amino acids. Patients who received saline had increased brain oxidation of ketone bodies and decreased oxidation of glucose. Because oxidation of glucose during ischemic periods may be detrimental, this increased oxidation of ketone bodies may be a protective alimentation method for these patients. Cerebral lactate production and CSF lactate concentration were indeed lower in the saline group. Based on these studies, these investigators suggest that alimentation with 3% amino acid solution and saline during days 1 to 5 postinjury may provide sufficient calories and nitrogen without producing hyperglycemia. This group also suggests that supplementation of 25% glucose rather than 5% glucose may have raised blood glucose concentration. These findings need further study. The results of this study do not justify this method as the optimal nutrient regimen. Future studies must evaluate the detrimental or positive effects of each alimentation solution in a large number of patients before absolute guidelines can be generated. Instead of not providing adequate nutrients, it may be equally efficacious to provide an anabolic hormone such as insulin-like growth factor 1, which can assist in nitrogen balance and also enhance glucose uptake in cells and reduce blood glucose levels.[68] This can be done without depriving the patient of needed nutritional supplementation.

Immunosuppression Patients with head injury have decreased immune responsiveness. A high percentage of these patients have bacterial infections.[69,71] Trauma to the brain results in the release of a number of immunosuppressive neurally derived substances such as cortisol, catecholamines, and β-endorphin.[72] In contrast to the patient with thermal injury, the immune status of the head injury patient has not been well studied. Anergy to the common skin antigens has been detected up to 3 weeks following head injury.[73] Quattrochi et al. found that lymphocyte phenotype expression and blastogenesis were severely impaired following head injury.[71] Hoyt et al. observed decreased lymphocyte proliferation evidenced by a dysfunction in early T-cell activation of helper cells after incubation with phytohemagglutinin, ConA, and pokeweed mitogens.[74] We found that patients with severe head injury who developed infections had, on admission, lower serum IL-2 levels, lower numbers of total T-lymphocytes (CD3+), and lower helper T-cell levels (CD4+) than patients without infections. The proliferative response of B and T cells to mitogens in our study indicated that a relationship might exist between depressed responses and morbidity and mortality. What mediates the immunosuppression observed after head injury remains unresolved. Cytokine depression, nutrient deficiencies, and hormonal release are all speculated to play a role.[74-77] In burn injury patients, Grbic et al. found that: prostaglandin E_2 has a role in the suppression of immunity after burn injury and exerts its suppressive effect principally by inhibition of lymphocyte IL-2 production; endotoxin mimics the effects of injury on prostaglandin E_2 production, T-cell activation, and IL-2 production; and administration of cyclooxygenase inhibitors is likely to be essential for the success of clinical regimens designed to correct the immune suppression that follows major injury.[78] Future studies should determine what specific mediators cause the immune response observed in the patient with head injury and whether immunomodulation can improve the immune status and decrease infection rate.

Altered Vascular Permeability Hypoalbuminemia is commonly observed after head injury. Albumin plays an important role in a number of physiologic processes such as drug transport, maintenance of oncotic pressure, and enteral feeding tolerance.[11,79,80] Studies from our group with in vitro endothelial studies have shown that a semipurified monokine preparation having IL-1 activity and human recombinant IL-1 causes an endothelial leak of albumin.[11] Tumor necrosis factor exposure results in a dose-dependent increase in transendothelial passage of albumin.[81] In addition, tumor necrosis injection in rabbits causes significant hypoalbuminemia. In other studies, Fleck and coworkers demonstrated transcapillary escape of radioiodinated albumin in patients undergoing cardiac surgery and patients in septic shock.[82] We suggest that hypoalbuminemia following head injury may occur in two stages. Initially, cytokines such as IL-1, other cytokines, and other mediators cause an increase in endothelial loss of albumin. Subsequently, a decrease in albumin production occurs because of the known depressive effect of IL-1 for the messenger RNA for albumin. Studies from our research group have shown that human recombinant IL-1 and tumor necrosis factor initiate pulmonary vascular endothelial injury and pulmonary edema in experimental animals.[83] Thus, we speculate that these cytokines may not only cause hypoalbuminemia via an endothelial leak, but may also play an important role in the adult respiratory distress syndrome and cerebral edema seen in severely head-injured patients.

Studies in other critically injured patients have suggested that serum albumin levels can be elevated by albumin supplementation, but whether this improves patient morbidity and mortality is unclear.[79,84,85] Modulation of the stress response causing altered vascular permeability, depression of serum albumin synthesis, and altered vascular permeability may improve outcome. Growth factor administration and specific nutrient administration may also be a possible avenue for improving albumin level and decreasing vascular permeability.

The Acute-Phase Response The acute-phase response occurs after head injury and is manifested by hypozincemia, hyperzincuria, hypercupria, fever without infection, depression of negative acute-phase proteins, and elevation of positive acute-phase proteins.[13,22] Some of these physiologic responses probably serve a useful biologic purpose, while others may increase morbidity and mortality. In patients with severe head injury, hypoalbuminemia correlates negative to severity of injury and patient prognosis.[11] Increased tissue utilization of zinc may necessitate administration of this mineral.[13] However, changes in plasma protein concentrations after injury have been postulated to serve as a protective zone around tissue destruction.[22] Alpha-1-antitrypsin and alpha-2-macroglobulin levels, which are increased during the acute-phase response, inhibit leukocytes and lysosomes that are released from destroyed cells. An increase in fibrinogen may be necessary for formation of fibrin and blood coagulation at the wound site. C-reactive protein increase may play a positive role in immune status.

Cytokines play a major role in the initiation of the acute-phase response. IL-6 is the major initiator and exhibits a dose- and time-dependent regulation on albumin depression and the synthesis of serum alpha-2-macroglobulin, fibrinogen, cysteine proteinase inhibitor, C-reactive protein, and alpha-1-acid glycoprotein.[86] Future work will determine how to alter the negative acute-phase response variables while maintaining those which are essential for bodily function.

Gastrointestinal Function Patients with severe head injury have altered gastric motility including delayed, rapid, and biphasic responses of liquid gastric emptying.[16] The biphasic response often observed in these patients is similar to that observed after pyloroplasty or vagotomy. This suggests that head injury may cause suppression of the vagal influence. The consequence of this altered gastric function is unknown, but it may play a role in increased bacterial translocation. We correlated gastric enteral feeding intolerance with delayed gastric emptying. Whether altered gastric emptying has any effect on enteral small bowel feeding tolerance is unknown, as is the cause of altered gastric emptying in these patients. Increased ICP and increased cytokine, opioid, and corticotropin-releasing factor levels may all contribute.

EFFECT OF NUTRITION ON OUTCOME FROM SEVERE HEAD INJURY

Six studies have correlated nutrient administration with patient outcome after severe head injury. Three of these have been prospective, randomized clinical trials, and three were retrospective associations. The study by Rapp et al. performed in the early 1980s is probably the most well known.[73] These investigators randomize 38 patients with severe head injury to receive either parenteral or enteral nutrition. The groups were then followed for a 1-year period. Intolerance to enteral feeding rendered the enteral group relatively starved; these patients received a mean of only 685 kcal and 4 g nitrogen per day, whereas the parenteral group received 1750 kcal and 10.2 g nitrogen daily over the 18-day study period. Eight deaths occurred in the enteral group within 18 days of injury, whereas no patient in the parenteral group died within this period ($p < 0.0001$). Young et al., in a prospective trial, randomized 51 patients with severe head injury to receive parenteral or enteral nutrition.[69] Improved enteral feeding techniques decreased the difference in nutrient administration between the enteral and parenteral groups. Nitrogen balance and cumulative caloric balance were significantly more positive in the parenteral group than in the enteral group. The parenteral group's neurologic recovery proceeded faster than did that of the enteral group. The change over time in GCS score was significantly higher in the parenterally fed group than in the enteral group over the 18-day study period. At 3 months, the parenterally fed group exhibited a higher percentage of favorable outcomes than did the enterally fed group. The trend continued for a 1-year period, although significance was observed only at 3 months. Hadley et al. prospectively randomized 45 patients with severe head injury to receive parenteral or enteral nutrition.[87] The parenteral group received significantly more nitrogen than the enteral group, but caloric intake was not significantly different. This group found no differences in morbidity and mortality between groups. Kaufman et al. studied the relationship between outcome and nutrient intake in 76 patients with closed head injury.[88] They could not find a significant relationship between nutrient intake and outcome and suggested that outcome was determined by the patients' initial neurologic status. In a study of 10 patients with head injury, Waters et al. found that a caloric deficit of less than 8000 cal was related to a better neurologic outcome than those patients with caloric deficits of more than 11,000 cal.[89] Finally, Balzola, in a study of patients with head injury, cerebral neoplasm, and cerebrovascular pathology, found that the recovery period was shorter among patients who received higher intakes of nutrients within 10 days of cerebral damage compared to a control group whose diet was administered more gradually or following a longer period of time.[90]

Sublethally damaged nerve cells are capable of repair and regeneration.[91] Future nutrition studies may center on providing an optimal environment so that injured neural cells may repair and regenerate and prevent secondary injury. Vigorous nutritional support seems to affect mortality favorably and speed recovery from head injury, but future work is necessary for specifically delineating the effects of nutrient deficiency on outcome from severe head injury.

PARENTERAL VERSUS ENTERAL NUTRITION

A current issue undergoing lively debate is whether parenteral or enteral nutrition should be administered in the immediate postinjury period. The design and inclusion criteria of studies performed make comparisons difficult to interpret.

Clearly, the enteral route is the route of choice since research indicates that this less expensive, more physiologic feeding mode may play a role in improved immunity and attenuation of the stress response.[92–94] Unlike patients with burns or multiple injuries who do not seem to exhibit a problem with gastric function or enteral tolerance immediately after injury, the patient with head injury seems to have unique problems that may inhibit early enteral tolerance. These patients often exhibit delayed and altered biphasic responses to liquid gastric emptying. In addition, there is often fear that enteral feeding may cause aspiration pneumonitis in an individual without a gag reflex who is often lying flat. Other investigators suggest that enteral feeding can be administered to these patients via the small bowel with meticulous intensive care.[95]

In 1983, Rapp et al. showed that patients with severe head injury often do not tolerate adequate gastric enteral feedings through the nasogastric route.[73] Patients with severe head injury who are fed gastrically are prone to aspiration pneumonitis. We found that patients fed enterally had a threefold higher rate of aspiration pneumonitis than did a parenterally fed group.[69] Olivares et al., in a study of autopsy examinations, found a significant correlation between the use of a nasogastric tube and the postmortem finding of aspiration and concluded that gastric tube feeding increased the risk of aspiration by six times.[96] Hunt et al., Twyman et al., and Clifton et al. showed that, although a majority of patients could tolerate enteral feedings by week 1 postinjury, 35 to 50 percent could not.[97–99]

In 1989, Grahm et al. found that nasojejunal feeding tubes put in place with fluoroscopy (if they did not migrate by themselves) could adequately nourish patients with severe head injury.[100] By the third day postinjury, a mean of 2499 cal and 15.7 g of nitrogen could be tolerated through the nasojejunal route. This group did not document aspiration of feedings into the pharynx, endotracheal tube, or stomach. Feedings were not withheld for gastric outputs or diarrhea. The feeding tube was not dislodged in any patient. These investigators had a 100 percent success rate with early enteral feeding.

Other investigators have not been as successful with small bowel feedings in these patients. Strong et al. prospectively randomized patients with similar GCS scores to have either percutaneous endoscopic gastrojejunostomy (PEJ) or percutaneous endoscopic gastrostomy (PEG). They found no difference in aspiration risk.[101] Kirby et al. found that PEG or PEJ could improve feeding tolerance in these patients but suggested that tolerance was not observed in those patients who were in a barbiturate coma.[102] This group also did not achieve the high level of calorie and protein administration observed by Grahm et al.

The precise role of early enteral nutrition in the patient with head injury is not firmly established. Clearly, theoretical advantages exist for administering enteral feeding to these patients. Future studies may improve the techniques of early feeding administration and may also be directed toward blocking the mediators of delayed gastric emptying and improving feeding administration through that mode.

The safety of parenteral nutrition in head-injured patients is also being debated. Lutz et al., in an early study, suggested that these patients did not tolerate parenteral nutrition.[103] In 1986, Waters et al. administered parenteral nutrition to cold-injured cats and suggested that vasogenic edema was increased by a parenteral mixture composed of 35% dextrose and 3.5% amino acids and by a 40% mannitol solution.[104] Combs et al. investigated the long-term effects of total parenteral nutrition infusion on vasogenic edema development in rats.[105] Total parenteral nutrition was found to cause significant hyperglycemia and hyperosmolarity in cold-injured rats after both 4 and 26 h, but it did not enhance edema development in any of five brain regions studied as measured by specific gravity. Young et al. randomized 96 patients with severe head injury to receive parenteral or enteral nutrition.[106] A significant difference was observed in calorie and protein intake between groups: the parenteral group received markedly more calories and nutrients over the first 12 days after injury. Serum glucose levels and calculated serum osmolality were not significantly different between the two groups, although the parenteral group tended to have higher serum osmolality levels for the first 5 days after injury and higher serum glucose levels for the first 13 days after injury. The patients were not significantly different with respect to daily ICP peak levels or number of days that ICP monitoring was required. These authors concluded that parenteral nutrition can be safely administered in these patients.

NUTRITIONAL MONITORING AND ASSESSMENT

Nutritional assessment parameters have been devised to represent body compartment measurements.[107] Alterations in body composition should correspond to alterations in these measurements. Persons sustaining head injury are usually well-nourished young adults. The goal of nutritional assessment for these patients is to prevent the development of malnutrition. During the acute period of head injury, however, traditional nutritional assessment parameters such as serum albumin, delayed hypersensitivity, and total lymphocyte count are not useful in assessing the nutritional status of these patients.[22] Serum albumin and many of the visceral proteins which have been suggested to represent body protein loss are negative or positive acute-phase reactants that are affected for approximately 2 weeks after injury. Anthropometric measurements such as triceps skin fold and midarm circumference, suggested to represent body protein and fat stores, are difficult to perform in this patient population due to the patient's inability to cooperate. These parameters are also slow to change. Body weights can give an overall estimation of body erosion; however, they must be measured at the same time of the day with a euvolemic patient.[24] Delayed hypersensitivity would be a useful measure of immunocompetence. However, it is depressed immediately postinjury and shows no consistent pattern but usually becomes normal by rehabilitation.[69] Urinary nitrogen excretion can give an estimation of protein turnover. Increased levels have long been used as an indicator of increased protein turnover.[107] Urinary nitrogen loss is related to severity of injury and reflects the mobilization and utilization of amino acids from muscle to meet the increased demands for tissue fuel or liver protein synthesis. Although it has been suggested that urinary nitrogen loss in patients with severe head injury is associated with poor neurologic status, no statistical correlation has been observed.[88] Perhaps the most useful measurements in the acute period are nitrogen and caloric balance. Nitrogen balance is calculated by subtracting nitrogen output (using urinary nitrogen excretion) from nitrogen intake. Caloric balance can be estimated by subtracting caloric output from caloric intake. Caloric output can be estimated by a formula which estimates resting energy expenditure and multiplies it by a stress factor, which is an estimation of percentage increase in energy expenditure caused by the type of stress. A better estimation of energy expenditure is calculated by indirect calorimetry, which estimates energy expenditure through measurement of O_2 consumption.

When nutritional assessment parameters are followed in a serial fashion from hospital admission through rehabilitation, they can serve as a guideline for measuring patient progress. Nutrient administration affects these parameters; however, many other nonnutritive factors also play a role, limiting their clinical utility as indicators of adequate nutritional support. We suggest that indirect calorimetry, nutritional history obtained from the patient's family, subjective global assessment, urinary urea nitrogen or total nitrogen excretion, nitrogen balance, and body weights be used to assess the patient's nutritional status and nutrient requirements.[107] These should be assessed biweekly until the patient's metabolic status returns to normal.

STATUS OF MEDICAL THERAPEUTIC INTERVENTION IN HEAD INJURY

Patients with head injury sustain a metabolic response that has certain negative effects. Nutrient administration alone cannot override the metabolic response to stress. In the next section, the current status of other methods which may decrease the negative effects of the metabolic response to stress and improve the environmental milieu for nerve cell regeneration will be delineated.

Alteration of the Stress Response

As in other types of injury, a simple explanation for the metabolic response does not occur in the patient with head injury. Mediators suggested to play a role include hormones, cytokines, and lipid mediators.[26] In the patient with head injury, investigators have observed increases in hormones and cytokines, but lipid mediators such as platelet-activation factor, thromboxane A_2, leukotriene B_4, or prostaglandin E_2 have not been well studied. One factor that has limited studies has been the lack of an adequate animal model.

In other types of injury, antibodies that block the effects of endotoxin and cytokines have been studied. Blocking of endotoxin in patients with infection decreases the stress response.[108] In studies with baboons, Tracey and coworkers found that pretreatment with a monoclonal antibody to tumor necrosis factor prevented mortality and markedly attenuated the pathophysiologic responses to a lethal infusion of gram-negative organisms.[109] Blocking cyclooxygenase in normal individuals receiving endotoxin decreased some of the negative effects observed after endotoxin administration. Blocking cyclooxygenase in patients with burns also seems to play a major role in reversing immunodeficiency.[78] Thus, it seems that studies in other types of patients illustrate that alterations in the stress response can occur to the patient's benefit. In head injury patients, any number of combinations of drugs that alter the systemic or secondary detrimental responses can be used to improve outcome of head injury. In animals with cold injury, indomethacin and ibuprofen given 6 to 24 h after the lesions occurred increased local cerebral glucose utilization and inhibited prostaglandin formation.[110,111]

Neurologic recovery by grip test showed a dose-related improvement with attenuation of synthesis of vasoactive arachidonic acid metabolites and oxygen free radical–induced lipid peroxidation. Rosner et al. found that TRIS infusion, which counteracts lactic acidosis, improved survival in a cat head injury model.[42] Certainly, more studies will be performed in the next decade to further delineate how we can alter the stress response of patients with head injury and improve outcome.

Nutritional Modification

In head injury patients, unique amino acid solutions and zinc supplementation have been studied as specific nutrient modification agents.

Alterations in plasma amino acids were described earlier. The ramifications of these plasma alterations in patients with head injury include effects on overall nitrogen retention, availability of excitatory amino acids and other amino acids to the brain, and gut atrophy. Correction or improvement in branched chain amino acid (leucine, isoleucine, valine) levels may improve nitrogen balance in patients. Branched chain amino acids are oxidized primarily by skeletal muscle. Infusion of these amino acids that supply the skeletal muscle with nutrients may decrease catabolism. Rowlands et al. randomized 23 patients with severe head injury to receive either a branched chain–enriched regimen or a standard regimen for 2 weeks postinjury.[113] Nitrogen balance was significantly less negative, and urinary urea nitrogen excretion was significantly less in the group that received the intravenous or enteral product enriched with branched chain amino acids. Our group randomized 20 patients with severe head injury to one of two standard formulas, one of which had a higher composition of branched chain amino acids than did the other.[15] Overall mean urinary urea nitrogen excretion and nitrogen balance were significantly improved in the group receiving the branched chain–enriched formula.

Robertson et al. reported that stress-induced changes in plasma amino acids may effect the cerebral flux of amino acids needed for repairing damaged neural cells and for cell nourishment.[114] Glutamic acid, an excitatory amino acid associated with cell necrosis observed in neural tissue culture and animal brain subjected to ischemia, was elevated in the arterial plasma; these levels correlated to net cerebral influx of glutamic acid. The net cerebral influx of glutamic acid may contribute to excitotoxic cell death occurring as a delayed sequela of head injury, particularly if it is compounded by hypoxic-ischemic conditions.[115] Thus, alterations of plasma amino acid levels may affect what substrates are available to the brain.

Glutamine also plays an important role in bacterial translocation.[116,117] Increased gut permeability, lack of oral intake, diminished host defenses, and bacterial overgrowth following injury cause bacterial translocation.[93,94] Bacterial products released as a result of this translocation may enhance the metabolic response to stress through cytokine synthesis and release.[94] In addition, glutamine is avidly consumed by various organs during stress, thus causing a relative deficiency of this amino acid.[116,117] Attempts have been made to prevent or ameliorate bacterial translocation by maintaining gut integrity through use of specialized enteral formulas enriched with glutamine, the major energy source for the small intestine. This theory has not been tested in the patient with severe head injury.

Other nutrients such as arginine have not yet been tested in the patient with head injury. In patients with cancer, it has been suggested that supplementation of this nutrient can enhance the immune system.[118] The administration of omega-3 fatty acids may also modify the immune response by competing as a substrate for the cyclooxygenase and lipoxygenase pathways and decreasing the synthesis of cytokines.[26]

Zinc alterations are observed in the patient with head injury. Research has not yet firmly established whether the depression of serum zinc levels or increase in urinary zinc loss indicates that a deficiency in zinc is occurring, or whether supplementation will improve outcome. We performed a prospective randomized study of zinc supplementation and found that the patients who received zinc had a faster improvement in neurologic recovery than patients who received placebo. Whether variables will show improvement in these patients secondary to zinc supplementation remains to be tested.

Growth Factors

One area undergoing intensive study is the possible positive effects of growth factor supplementation in trauma patients. The recent development of recombinant growth factors has made possible the administration of these agents for study. Growth hormone has many beneficial effects such as stimulation of DNA and RNA synthesis; enhancement of nitrogen and mineral retention; stimulation of lipolysis, protein synthesis, and insulin and insulin-like growth hormone-1 release; antagonization of insulin's effects on glucose homeostasis; and regulation of immune function.[49–53] Current research suggests that many of the effects of growth hormone are secondary to insulin-like growth hormone-1 elevation.[51,119] In addition, insulin-like growth hormone-1 is a potent neurotropic factor.[120] Thus, trials are currently being conducted to assess the role of this growth factor in the metabolic response to head injury.

SUMMARY

The patient with severe head injury sustains a systemic response to stress that may cause a secondary injury to the brain and may increase morbidity and mortality. Nutrient administration alone cannot completely counteract these responses. Future studies will determine the combinations of modalities necessary for decreasing the systemic response in these patients, will provide an optimal environment for nerve cell regeneration, and should improve patient outcome. Nutritional assessment of these patients in the early period of injury is very difficult because many of the variables used are affected by the stress state rather than by a nutrient deficiency. Adequate nutrient replacement can be achieved by calculating nitrogen and caloric balance. Specific fuels such as glutamine, branched chain amino acids, and zinc may become commonplace supplementation in future medical therapy of these patients. The route of providing nutrients to these patients (parenteral versus enteral nutrition) is debatable and improvement in enteral feeding technique is a future goal. The next decade should determine the best medical treatment for improving outcome in these patients.

REFERENCES

1. Boop FA, Andrassy RJ, Brown WE, et al: Excessive nitrogen losses in severe brain injury (abstract). *Neurosurgery* 16:725, 1985.
2. Clifton GL, Robertson CS, Grossman RG, et al: The metabolic response to severe head injury. *J Neurosurg* 60:687, 1984.
3. Deutschman CS, Konstantinides FN, Raup S, et al: Physiological and metabolic response to isolated closed-head injury. Part 1: Basal metabolic state: Correlations of metabolic and physiological parameters with fasting and stressed controls. *J Neurosurg* 64:89, 1986.
4. Deutschman CS, Konstantinides FN, Raup S, et al: Physiological and metabolic response to isolated closed-head injury. Part 2: Effects of steroids on metabolism. Potentiation of protein wasting and abnor-

malities of substrate utilization. *J Neurosurg* 66:388, 1987.
5. Fruin AH, Taylor C, Pettis S: Caloric requirements in patients with severe head injuries. *Surg Neurol* 25:25, 1986.
6. Gadisseux P, Ward JD, Young HF, et al: Nutrition and the neurosurgical patient. *J Neurosurg* 60:219, 1984.
7. Haider W, Lackner F, Schlick W, et al: Metabolic changes in the course of severe acute brain damage. *Eur J Intensive Care Med* 1:91, 1975.
8. Kahn RC, Koslow M, Butcher S: Metabolic studies in head injured patients (abstract). *J Parenteral Enteral Nutrition* 11:9S, 1987.
9. Long CL, Schaffel N, Geiger JW, et al: Metabolic response to injury and illness: Estimation of energy and protein needs from indirect calorimetry and nitrogen balance. *J Parenter Ent Nutr* 3:452, 1979.
10. McClain CJ, Cohen D, Ott L, et al: Ventricular fluid interleukin-1 activity in patients with head injury. *J Lab Clin Med* 110:48, 1987.
11. McClain CJ, Hennig B, Ott L, et al: Mechanisms and implications of hypoalbuminemia in head injured patients. *J Neurosurg* 69:386, 1988.
12. McClain CJ, Cohen D, Phillips R, et al: Increased plasma and ventricular fluid interleukin-6 levels in head injury patients. *J Lab Clin Med* 118:225, 1991.
13. McClain CJ, Twyman D, Ott L, et al: Serum and urine zinc response in head injured patients. *J Neurosurg* 64:224, 1986.
14. Miller SL: The metabolic response to head injury. *S Afr Med J* 65:90, 1984.
15. Ott L, Schmidt J, Young B, et al: Comparison of administration of two standard intravenous amino acid formulas to severely brain-injured patients. *Drug Intell Clin Pharm* 22:763, 1988.
16. Ott L, Phillips R, Young B, et al: Altered gastric emptying after head injury and its relationship to feeding intolerance. *J Neurosurg* 74:738, 1991.
17. Piek J, Lumenta CH, Bock WJ: Amino acid metabolism in patients with severe head injury. *Acta Neurochir* 68:165, 1983.
18. Robertson CS, Clifton GL, Grossman RG: Oxygen utilization and cardiovascular function in head injured patients. *Neurosurgery* 15:307, 1984.
19. Schiller WR, Long CL, Blackemore WS: Creatinine and nitrogen excretion in seriously ill and injured patients. *Surg Gynecol Obstet* 149:561, 1979.
20. Touho H, Karasawa J, Nakagawara J, et al: Measurement of energy expenditure in the acute stage of head injury (Part 1). *No To Shinkei* 39:739, 1987.
21. Twyman D, Young AB, Ott L, et al: Plasma amino acid profiles in nonsteroid-treated head injury patients (abstract). *J Parenteral Enteral Nutrition* 9:121, 1985.
22. Young B, Ott L, Beard D, et al: The acute-phase response of the brain-injured patient. *J Neurosurg* 69:375, 1988.
23. Young B, Ott L, Dempsey R, et al: Relationship between admission hyperglycemia and neurological outcome of severe brain-injured patients. *Ann Surg* 210:466, 1989.
24. Young B, Ott L, Norton J, et al: Metabolic and nutritional sequelae in the nonsteroid-treated head injury patient. *Neurosurgery* 17:784, 1985.
25. Young AB, Ott LG, Thompson JS, et al: The cellular immune depression of nonsteroid-treated severely head-injured patients (abstract). *Neurosurgery* 16:725, 1985.
26. Wilmore DW: Catabolic illness. *N Engl J Med* 325:10:695, 1991.
27. Dempsey DT, Guenter P, Mullen JL, et al: Energy expenditure in acute trauma to the head with and without barbiturate therapy. *Surg Gynecol Obstet* 160:128, 1985.
28. Gerold K, Frankenfield D, Turney S, et al: Energy expenditure in acute severe head injury (abstract). *J Parenteral Enteral Nutrition* 13:20S, 1989.
29. Moore R, Najarian P, Konvolinka C: Measured energy expenditure in severe head trauma. *J Trauma* 29:1633, 1989.
30. Robertson CS, Clifton GL, Goodman JS: Steroid administration and nitrogen excretion in the head injured patient. *J Neurosurg* 63:714, 1985.
31. Greenblatt SH, Long CL, Blakemore RS, et al: Catabolic effect of dexamethasone in patients with major head injuries. *J Parenteral Enteral Nutrition* 13:372, 1989.
32. Bucci MN, Dechert RE, Arnoldi DK, et al: Elevated intracranial pressure associated with hypermetabolism in isolated head trauma. *Acta Neurochir* 93:133, 1988.
33. Boraschi D, Tagliabue A: Structure-function relationship of interleukin-1 giving new insights for its therapeutic potential. *Biotherapy* 1:377–398, 1989.
34. Damask MC, Schwarz Y, Weissman C: Energy measurements and requirements of critically ill patients. *Crit Care Clin* 3:71, 1987.
35. Dinarello CA, Neta R: An overview of interleukin-1 as a therapeutic agent. *Biotherapy* 1:245, 1989.
36. Klasing KC: Nutritional aspects of leukocytic cytokines. *J Nutr* 118:1436, 1988.
37. Wilmore DW: The practice of clinical nutrition: How to prepare for the future. *J Parenteral Enteral Nutrition* 13:337, 1989.
38. Popp MB, Brennan MF: Metabolic response to trauma and infection. In: Fischer JE (ed): *Surgical Nutrition*. Boston, Little, Brown, 1983, pp 479–514.
39. Clifton GL, Robertson CS, Choi SC: Assessment of

nutritional requirements of head-injured patients. *J Neurosurg* 64:895, 1986.
40. Strock LL, Singh H, Abdullah A, et al: The effect on insulin-like growth factor I on postburn hypermetabolism. *Surgery* 108:161, 1990.
41. Chiolero R, Schutz Y, Lemerchand T, et al: Hormonal and metabolic changes following severe head injury and noncranial injury. *J Parenteral Enteral Nutrition* 13:5, 1989.
42. Hausmann D, Mosebach O, Caspari R, et al: Effects of steroid on nitrogen loss and plasma amino acid profiles after head injury. *J Parenteral Enteral Nutrition* 11:10S, 1987.
43. Deitrick JE, Whedon GD, Shorr E: Effects of immobilization upon various metabolic and physiologic functions of normal men. *Am J Med* 4:3, 1948.
44. Schonheyder F, Heilskov NSC, Olesen K: Isotopic studies on the mechanism of negative nitrogen balance produced by immobilization. *Scand J Clin Lab Invest* 6:178, 1954.
45. Zagara G, Scaravilli R, Bellucci CM, et al: Effect of dexamethasone on nitrogen metabolism in brain-injured patients. *J Neurosurg Sci* 31:207, 1987.
46. McLaurin RL, King L, Tutor FT, et al: Metabolic response to intracranial surgery. *Surg Forum* 10:770, 1959.
47. Alexander JW, Macmillan BG, Stinnett JD, et al: Beneficial effects of aggressive protein feeding in severely burned children. *Ann Surg* 192:505, 1980.
48. Fried R, Dempsey D, Guenter P, et al: Barbiturates improve nitrogen balance in patients with severe head trauma (abstract). *J Parenteral Enteral Nutrition* 8:86, 1984.
49. Jiang ZM, He GZ, Zhang SY, et al: Low dose growth hormone and hypocaloric nutrition attenuate the protein-catabolic response after major operation. *Ann Surg* 210:513, 1989.
50. Herndon DN, Barrow RE, Kunkle KR, et al: Effects of recombinant human growth hormone on donor-site healing in severely burned children. *Ann Surg* 212:424, 1990.
51. Behrman SW, Wojtysiak S, Brown RO, et al: The effect of growth hormone on nutritional markers in enterally fed, immobilized trauma patients. *Surg Forum* 41:20, 1990.
52. Manson JM, Wilmore DW: Positive nitrogen balance with human growth hormone and hypocaloric intravenous feedings. *Surgery* 100:188, 1986.
53. Ziegler TR, Young LS, Manson JM, et al: Metabolic effects of recombinant human growth hormone in patients receiving parenteral nutrition. *Ann Surgery* 208:6, 1988.
54. Crompton MR: Hypothalamic lesions following closed head injury. *Brain* 94:165, 1971.
55. Treip CS: Hypothalamic and pituitary injury. *J Clin Path* (Suppl 4):178, 1970.
56. Edwards OM, Clark JDA: Post-traumatic hypopituitarism. *Medicine* 65:281, 1986.
57. King LR, Knowles HC, McLaurin RL, et al: Pituitary hormone response to head injury. *Neurosurgery* 9:229, 1981.
58. Gottardis M, Nigitsch C, Schmutzhard E, et al: The secretion of human growth hormone stimulated by human growth hormone releasing factor following severe cranio-cerebral trauma. *Intensive Care Med* 16:163, 1990.
59. Goodman JC, Robertson CS, Grossman RG, et al: Increased tumor necrosis factor after head injury. *J Neuroimmunol* 30:213, 1990.
60. Goldberg AL: Factors affecting protein balance in skeletal muscle in normal and pathological stages. In: Blackburn GL, Grant JP, Young VR (eds): *Amino Acids Metabolism and Medical Application.* Boston, John Wright PSG, 1983, pp 201–211.
61. Marie C, Bralet J: Blood glucose level and morphological brain damage following cerebral ischemia. *Cerebrovasc Brain Metab Rev* 3:29, 1991.
62. Merguerian P, Perel A, Wald U, et al: Persistent nonketotic hyperglycemia as a grave prognostic sign in head-injured patients. *Crit Care Med* 9:838, 1981.
63. Voll CL, Auer RN: The effect of post-ischemic blood glucose levels on ischemic brain damage in the rat. *Ann Neurol* 24:638, 1988.
64. Voll CL, Whishaw IQ, Auer RN: Post-ischemic insulin reduces spatial learning deficit transient forebrain ischemia in rats. *Stroke* 20:646, 1989.
65. Schurr A, Rigor BM: Cerebral ischemia revisited: New insights as revealed using in vitro brain slice preparations. *Experientia* 45:684, 1989.
66. Bessey PQ, Walters JM, Aoki TT, et al: Combined hormonal infusion stimulates the metabolic response to injury. *Ann Surg* 200:264, 1984.
67. Robertson CS, Goodman JC, Narayan RK, et al: The effect of glucose administration on carbohydrate metabolism after head injury. *J Neurosurg* 74:43, 1991.
68. Jacobs R, Barrett E, Plewe G, et al: Acute effects of insulin-like growth factor 1 on glucose and amino acid metabolism in the awake fasted rat. *J Clin Invest* 83:1717, 1989.
69. Young B, Ott L, Twyman D, et al: The effect of nutritional support on outcome from severe injury. *J Neurosurg* 67:668, 1987.
70. Helling RS, Evans LL, Gowler DL, et al: Infectious complications in patients with severe head injury. *J Trauma* 28:1575, 1988.
71. Quattrocchi KB, Frank EH, Miller CH, et al: Suppression of cellular immune activity following severe head injury. *J Neurotrauma* 7(2):77, 1990.

72. Ader R, Felten DL, Cohen W: *Psychoneuroimmunology*, 2d ed. San Diego, Academic, 1991.
73. Rapp R, Young R, Twyman D, et al: The favorable effect of early parenteral feeding on survival in head-injured patients. *J Neurosurg* 58:906, 1983.
74. Hoyt DB, Ozkan AN, Hansbrough JF, et al: Head injury: An immunological deficit in T-cell activation (abstract). *J Trauma* 49(7):1031, 1989.
75. Crabtree GR, Gillis S, Smith KA, et al: Glucocorticoids and immune responses. *Arthr Rheum* 22:1246, 1979.
76. Gross RL, Newberne PM: Nutrition and immunologic function. *Physiol Rev* 60:188, 1980.
77. Roderick ML, Wood JJ, Grbic JT, et al: Defective IL-2 production in patients with severe burns and sepsis. *Lymphokine Res* 5:575, 1986.
78. Grbic JT, Mannick JA, Gough DB, et al: The role of prostaglandin E2 in immune suppression following injury. *Ann Surg* 214:253, 1991.
79. Ford EF, Jennings LM, Andrassey R: Serum albumin (oncotic pressure) correlates with enteral feeding tolerance in the pediatric surgical patients. *J Pediatr Surg* 22:597, 1987.
80. Boosalis MG, Ott L, Levine AB, et al: The relationship of visceral proteins to nutritional status in chronic and acute stress. *Crit Care Med* 17:741, 1989.
81. Hennig B, Honchel R, Goldblum SE, et al: Tumor necrosis factor-mediated hypoalbuminemia in rabbits. *J Nutr* 118:1586, 1988.
82. Fleck A, Raines G, Hawker F, et al: Increased vascular permeability: A major cause of hypoalbuminemia in disease and injury. *Lancet* 1:781, 1985.
83. Goldblum SE, Cohen DA, Gillepsie MN, et al: Interleukin-1-induced granulocytopenia and pulmonary leukostasis in rabbits. *J Appl Physiol* 62:122, 1987.
84. Brown RO, Bradley JE, Bekemeyer WB, et al: Effect of albumin supplementation during parenteral nutrition on hospital morbidity. *Crit Care Med* 16:1177, 1988.
85. Foley EF, Borlase BC, Dzik WH: Albumin supplementation in the critically ill. *Arch Surg* 125:739, 1990.
86. Castell JV, Andus T, Kunz D, et al: Interleukin-6. The major regulator of acute-phase protein synthesis in man and rat. *Ann NY Acad Sci* 557:87, 1988.
87. Hadley MN, Grahm TW, Harrington T, et al: Nutritional support and neurotrauma: A critical review of early nutrition in forty-five acute head injury patients. *Neurosurgery* 19:367, 1986.
88. Kaufman HH, Bretaudiere JP, Rowlands BJ, et al: General metabolism in head injury. *Neurosurgery* 20:254, 1987.
89. Waters DC, Dechert R, Bartlett R: Metabolic studies in head injury patients: A. Preliminary report. *Surgery* 100:531, 1986.
90. Balzola F, Boggio BD, Solerio A, et al: Dietetic treatment with hypercaloric and hyperproteic intake in patients following severe brain injury. *J Neurosurg Sci* 24:131, 1980.
91. Davis JN: Neuronal rearrangements after brain injury: A proposed classification. In: Becker DP, Povlishock JT (eds): *Central Nervous System Trauma Status Report*, National Institute of Neurological and Communicative Disorders and Stroke, 1985, pp 491–502.
92. Heymsfield SB, Bethel RA, Ansley JD, et al: Enteral hyperalimentation: An alternative to central venous hyperalimentation. *Ann Intern Med* 90:63, 1979.
93. Meyer J, Yurt RW, Duhaney R, et al: Differential neutrophil activation before and after endotoxin infusion in enterally versus parenterally fed volunteers. *Surg Gynecol Obstet* 167:501, 1988.
94. Mochizuki H, Trocki O, Dominioni L, et al: Mechanism of prevention of postburn hypermetabolism and catabolism by early enteral feeding. *Ann Surg* 200:297, 1984.
95. Turner W: Nutritional considerations in the patient with disabling brain disease. *Neurosurgery* 16:707, 1985.
96. Olivares L, Segovia A, Revuelta R: Tube feeding and lethal aspiration in neurological patients: A review of 720 autopsy cases. *Stroke* 5:654, 1974.
97. Hunt D, Rowlands B, Allen S: The inadequacy of enteral nutritional support in head injury patients during the early post-injury period (abstract). *J Parenteral Enteral Nutrition* 9:121, 1985.
98. Twyman D, Young B, Ott L, et al: High protein enteral feedings: A means of achieving positive nitrogen balance in head-injured patients. *J Parenteral Enteral Nutrition* 9:679, 1985.
99. Clifton GL, Robertson CS, Contant CF: Enteral hyperalimentation in head injury. *J Neurosurg* 62:186, 1985.
100. Grahm TW, Zadrozny DB, Harrington T: The benefits of early jejunal hyperalimentation in the head-injured patient. *Neurosurgery* 25:729, 1989.
101. Strong RM, Namihas N, Matsuyama R, et al: Random, prospective assessment of aspiration risk for percutaneous endoscopic gastrojejunostomy and percutaneous endoscopic gastrostomy (abstract). *J Parenteral Enteral Nutrition* 14:18S, 1990.
102. Kirby D, Turner J, Barrett J, et al: Early enteral feeding with PEG/J's in severe head injury. *J Parenteral Enteral Nutrition* 15:298, 1991.
103. Lutz H, Peter K, Van Ackern K: Total parenteral alimentation in neurosurgical and neurological patients. In: *Total Parenteral Alimentation*, Amsterdam, Excerpta Medica, 1976, pp 214–217.
104. Waters DC, Hoff JT, Black KL: Effect of parenteral nutrition on cold-induced vasogenic edema in cats. *J Neurosurg* 64:460, 1986.

105. Combs DJ, Ott L, McAninch PS, et al: The effect of total parenteral nutrition on vasogenic edema development following cold injury in rats. *J Neurosurg* 70:623, 1989.
106. Young B, Ott L, Haack D, et al: Effect of total parenteral nutrition upon intracranial pressure in severe head injury. *J Neurosurg* 67:76, 1987.
107. Smith LC, Mullen JL: Nutritional assessment and indications for nutritional support. *Surg Clin North Am* 71(3):449, 1991.
108. Ziegler EJ, Fischer CJ Jr, Sprung CL, et al: Treatment of gram-negative bacteremia and septic shock with HA-1A monoclonal antibody against endotoxin: A randomized, double-blind, placebo-controlled trial. *N Engl J Med* 324:429, 1991.
109. Tracey KJ, Fong Y, Hesse DG, et al: Anti-cachectin/TNF monoclonal antibodies prevent septic shock during lethal bacteraemia. *Nature* 330:662, 1987.
110. Hall ED: Beneficial effects of acute intravenous ibuprofen on neurologic recovery of head-injured mice: Comparison of cyclooxygenase inhibition with inhibition of thromboxane A2 synthetase of 5-liopxygenase. *Cent Nerv Syst Trauma* 2:75, 1985.
111. Pappius HM, Wolfe LS: Effects of indomethacin and ibuprofen on cerebral metabolism and blood flow in traumatized brain. *J Cereb Blood Flow Metab* 3:448, 1983.
112. Rosner MJ, Becker DP: Experimental brain injury: Successful therapy with the weak base, tromethamine. *J Neurosurg* 60:961, 1984.
113. Rowlands B, Hunt D, Roughneen P, et al: Intravenous and enteral nutrition with branched chain amino acid enriched products following multiple trauma with closed head injury (abstract). *J Parenteral Enteral Nutrition* 10:4S, 1986.
114. Robertson C, Clifton GL, Grossman RG, et al: Alterations in cerebral availability of metabolic substrate after severe head injury. *J Trauma* 28:1523, 1988.
115. Faden AL, Demediuk P, Panter SS, et al: The role of excitatory amino acids and NMDA receptors in traumatic brain injury. *Science* 244:798, 1989.
116. Hartmann F, Plauth M: Intestinal glutamine metabolism. *Metabolism* 38:18, 1989.
117. Souba WW, Smith RJ, Wilmore DW: Glutamine metabolism by the intestinal tract. *J Parenteral Enteral Nutrition* 9:608, 1985.
118. Daly JM, Reynolds J, Thom A, et al: Immune and metabolic effects of arginine in the surgical patient. *Ann Surg* 208:512, 1988.
119. Guler HP, Zapf J, Foresch ER: Short-term metabolic effects of recombinant human insulin-like growth factor I in healthy adults. *N Engl J Med* 317:137, 1987.
120. Skottner A, Arrhenius-Nyberg V, Kanje M, et al: Anabolic and tissue repair functions of recombinant insulin-like growth factor 1. *Acta Paediatr Scand* 367 (Suppl):63, 1990.

CHAPTER 8
Neuroendocrine Physiology and Management

Mark E. Harris
Daniel L. Barrow

INTRODUCTION

Essential elements of what is now the discipline of neuroendocrinology were recognized in ancient times. Before the concept of a nervous system or glandular function had been formulated, primitive herdsmen recognized the seasonal breeding of domestic animals and the differences in behavior between male and female creatures.

As a discipline, neuroendocrinology has progressed rapidly over the past decade. As is true for many areas of medicine, advances in basic research have outpaced subsequent application to clinical problems. Nevertheless, the use of bromocriptine in the management of hyperprolactinemia or the infusion of intrathecal opiates for the management of pain syndromes are just two examples of the application of basic neuroendocrinology to clinical practice.

Neuroendocrinology has traditionally been defined as the study of the interrelationship between the nervous and endocrine systems. These two systems interact and regulate most of the metabolic and homeostatic activities of the organism. Every hormone has potential influence on the central nervous system, and the secretion of virtually every hormone is regulated either directly or indirectly by the brain. The basic functional unit of the endocrine system is the secretory cell, which provides its regulatory influence through the circulating blood. The basic functional unit of the nervous system is the neuron, which provides an organized network of point-to-point connections. Specificity within the endocrine system is conveyed by the appearance of specialized receptors on target cells, and within the central nervous system by neurotransmitter specificity, receptor specificity, and by point-to-point hard-wiring. Importantly, the particular site at which neuropeptides and neurotransmitters are found determines their functional role, although not their mechanisms of action.

Secretory cells can be classified into three types:

exocrine, such as sweat and salivary glands, which secrete into a hollow lumen that communicates with the exterior of the body; *endocrine*, such as the adrenal and thyroid glands, which secrete into the circulation; and *neurosecretory*, which can secrete into the circulating blood (neurohormonal) or at synaptic contacts (neurotransmitter, neuromodulators). All secretory cells are regulated directly or indirectly by neural impulses. Exocrine glands are regulated mainly by secretomotor nerve fibers through the release of a neurotransmitter at a receptor site. The classical endocrine system is regulated by the pituitary gland which, in turn, is regulated by neurosecretory cells of the hypothalamus. Neurons are regulated by neurotransmitters. In addition to neuroregulation, virtually all glands are influenced by circulating hormones and metabolic factors.

THE HYPOTHALAMUS AND PITUITARY GLAND

The neuroendocrine system employs the pituitary gland to regulate the function of selected visceral organs (kidney, uterus, and breast), to regulate growth, and to trophically support and regulate the function of specific target organs of internal secretion — thyroid gland, adrenal gland, and gonads. Through the pituitary gland, the brain affects the growth and development of the organism, maintains its internal milieu, regulates its metabolism, and assures its reproduction.

The pituitary gland, or *hypophysis cerebri*, is composed of glandular and neural tissue and hence is divided into two lobes, the anterior or adenohypophysis and the posterior or neurohypophysis. The glandular cells that make up the adenohypophysis may be viewed as the effector cells of the neuroendocrine system.

The hypophysis develops in close association with the hypothalamus from the embryonic diencephalon (Fig. 8-1). The neurohypophysis develops as a downward evagination of the diencephalon called the infundibulum. By contrast, the adenohypophysis (anterior lobe) has a nonneural origin, developing from an ectodermal diverticulum of the primitive oral cavity called Rathke's pouch. This diverticulum elongates dorsally to contact the downgrowing infundibulum from which it ultimately fuses, losing contact with the oral cavity. Cells from the adenohypophysis subsequently extend along and around the pituitary stalk to form the pars tuberalis. Thus, the neurohypophysis is in neural communication with the overlying hypothalamus, from which it developed as a downgrowth. The adenohypophysis, conversely, has no direct neural contact with the hypothalamus. Instead a rich, vascular communication between the two develops, which is called the portal system. It is by this means that anterior pituitary secretion is controlled via humoral contact by the hypothalamus.[37,39,84]

The finding that some hypothalamic neurons are capable of synthesizing corticotropin and melanocyte-stimulating hormone (MSH), hormones that are also synthesized in the adenohypophysial cells, suggests that at least some adenohypophysial cells migrate from the brain to the adenohypophysis.[70,90] Although these two lobes have different embryologic origins, they become intimately related during embryonic life and remain that way.

Adenohypophysis

The adenohypophysis is divided into three regions: the pars tuberalis, pars intermedia, and pars distalis (Fig. 8-2). The pars distalis forms the bulk of the adenohypophysis and is the primary site of production of the classical anterior pituitary hormones, thyrotropin [thyroid-stimulating hormone (TSH)], corticotropin (ACTH), growth hormone or somatotropin (GH), prolactin (PRL), luteinizing hormone (LH), follicle-stimulating hormone (FSH), MSH, and beta-endorphin (End). The pars distalis contains no axon terminals.

The pars intermedia is applied to the lower part of the infundibular stem and the infundibular process — caudal regions of the neurohypophysis. Dopaminergic nerves are found in the pars intermedia and terminate near glandular cells. The pars intermedia is present in the human fetus and in the pregnant adult female but is vestigial in adult human males and in nonpregnant females. This region of the adenohypophysis has limited endocrinologic function.

The pars tuberalis is applied to the surface of the median eminence and the upper infundibular stem — rostral regions of the neurohypophysis. It is made up of epithelial cells, fenestrated capillaries, and stromal cells. Like the pars distalis, no nerve terminals are present in the pars tuberalis.

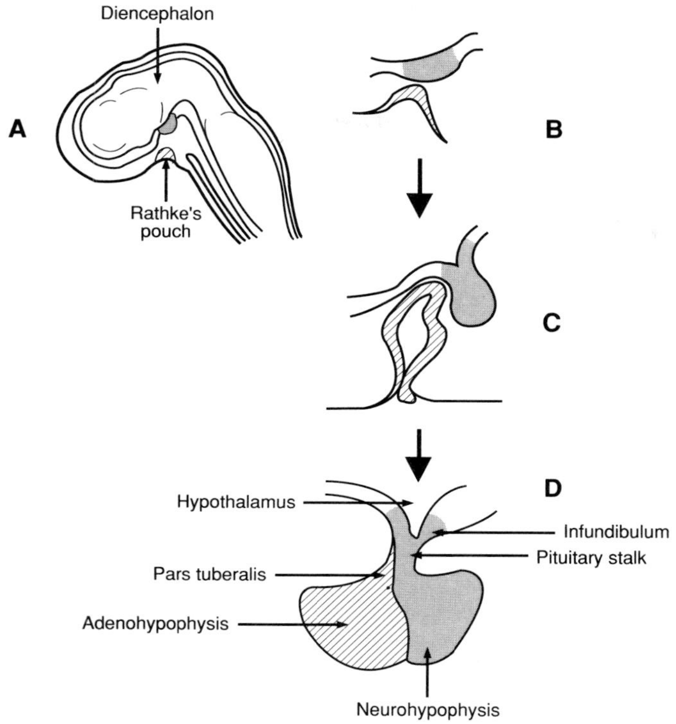

Figure 8-1 Development of the pituitary gland. The neurohypophysis is derived from a downward evagination of the diencephalon, the infundibulum (A,B). The adenohypophysis develops from an ectodermal diverticulum of the primitive oral cavity, Rathke's pouch (A,B). The two elements ultimately fuse (C,D) and contact with the oral cavity is lost.

The epithelial cells have been histochemically identified as thyrotropes and gonadotropes.

Neurohypophysis

The neurohypophysis is a diverticulum of brain, which appears early in human fetal life[1] and regulates the function of the adenohypophysis. The neurohypophysis contains no neuronal cell bodies, only axons and axon terminals. Axons terminate in the perivascular space of fenestrated capillaries, not on neurons or their processes. The neurohypophysis lacks a blood-brain barrier.[44,97]

The neurohypophysis is subdivided into three regions on the basis of regional and morphologic specializations: (1) the median eminence, (2) the infundibular stem, and (3) the neural lobe.[77] The median eminence with the paired lateral eminences make up the tuber cinereum, which is a visible structure on the inferior surface of the brain, lying caudal to the optic chiasm and rostral to the paired mamillary bodies.[65] The infundibular stem is the neural portion of the pituitary stalk. The neural lobe is the caudal region of the neurohypophysis. The classification of the neurohypophysis into the median eminence, infundibular stem, and neural lobe stresses the observation that the neural portion of the pituitary gland is a diverticulum of brain but is distinct from the hypothalamus with which it is contiguous.

The supraopticohypophysial and paraventriculohypophysial nerve tracts originate in the hypothalamus and terminate in the neurohypophysis after passing through the infundibulum (median eminence).[14] The hormones arginine vasopressin [AVP, or antidiuretic hormone (ADH)] and oxy-

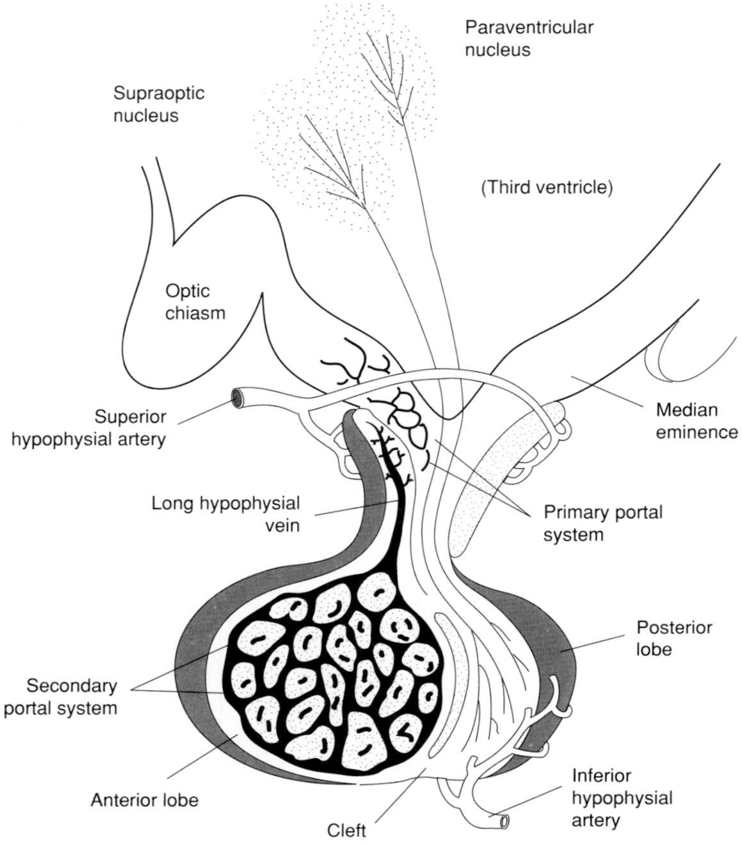

Figure 8-2 Sagittal diagram of pituitary and some of its anatomic features.

tocin are released from the nerve terminals into the perivascular space of the fenestrated capillaries of the neurohypophysis (neural lobe).[18,32,47,71,79,80] Oxytocin and AVP are found both in the supraoptic and paraventricular nuclei but are found in different cells within those nuclei. The paraventricular nuclei secrete the largest amount of oxytocin, while the supraoptic nuclei secrete predominantly AVP.

Pituitary Stalk

The pituitary gland and hypothalamus are connected by a stalk composed of glandular, vascular, and neural elements. The glandular portion of the stalk is made up of the pars tuberalis. The vascular component consists of nutrient arteries, the portal venous system, and capillary network. The paired hypophysial arteries form the main arterial supply to the median eminence, pituitary gland, and stalk. These arteries arise from the intracranial internal carotid artery, the proximal A1 segments of the anterior cerebral arteries, and the posterior communicating arteries. The neural lobe is supplied separately by the inferior hypophysial arteries. The adenohypophysis does not receive a direct arterial supply. Blood entering the adenohypophysis first passes through the neurohypophysis. The arteries divide into capillary tufts that come into contact with the nerve endings of the hypothalamic peptidergic neurons that synthesize the releasing hormones. The capillary tufts are drained by portal veins and are distributed to the sinusoids of the adenohypophysis. This vascular component is thus crucial for the transport of the hypothalamic hormones to the adenohypophysis.[2,9,35] The neural portion of the pituitary stalk is composed of the supraopticohypophysial and the paraventriculohypophysial nerve tracts (infundibular stem).

Hypothalamus

The hypothalamus is at the center of neuroendocrine, autonomic, and homeostatic regulation. Its outflow is directed in such a way as to influence the endocrine system (via the neurohypophysial and adenohypophysial neurosecretory systems), the autonomic nervous system (via projections to preganglionic cell groups in the brainstem and spinal cord), and behavioral responses to physiologic and environmental cues (via its interaction with limbic and somatomotor systems).

The hypothalamus and pituitary gland function as a unit that includes two systems, the hypothalamic-adenohypophysial system and the hypothalamic-neurohypophysial system (Fig. 8-3).

The hypothalamic-adenohypophysial system

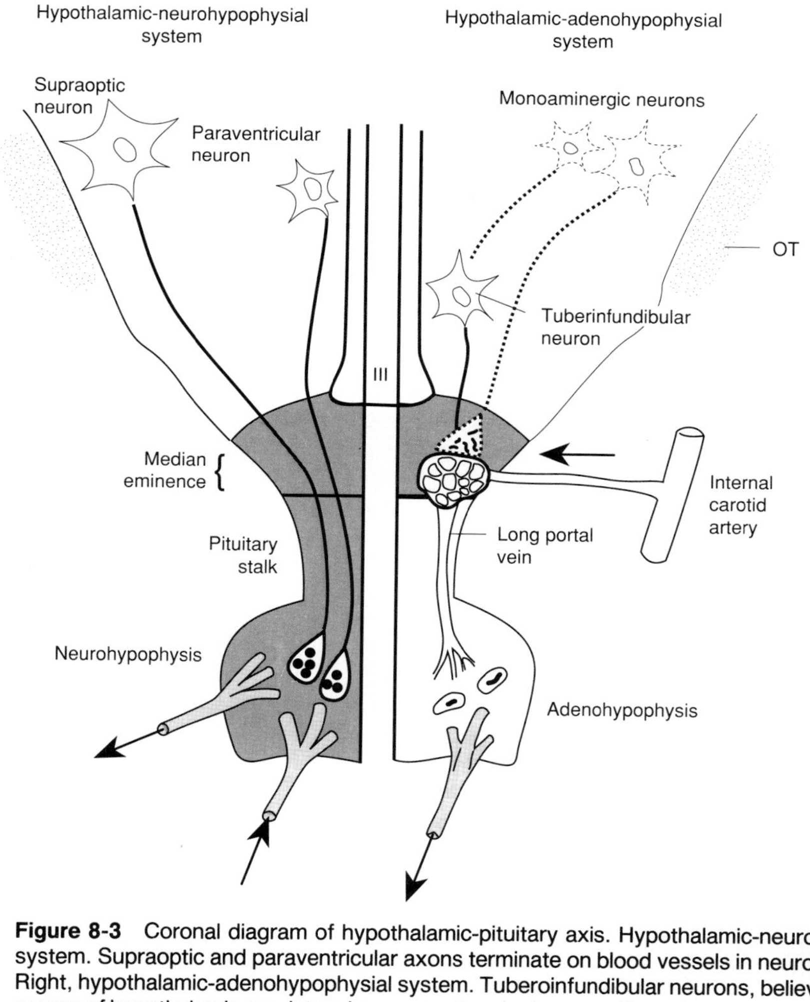

Figure 8-3 Coronal diagram of hypothalamic-pituitary axis. Hypothalamic-neurohypophysial system. Supraoptic and paraventricular axons terminate on blood vessels in neurohypophysis. Right, hypothalamic-adenohypophysial system. Tuberoinfundibular neurons, believed to be the source of hypothalamic regulatory hormones, terminate on capillary plexus in median eminence. Pituitary portal system is derived from branches of internal carotid artery, which forms primary capillary bed in median eminence. Portal veins drain capillary plexus into sinusoids of anterior pituitary.

includes the tuberoinfundibular neurons, all nerve cells (parvocellular) in the lower portion of the hypothalamus that produce anterior pituitary regulating (hypophysiotropic) hormones. Most of the cell bodies of the tuberoinfundibular neurons are located in the medial preoptic area, the anterior paraventricular nucleus, the medioparvocellular paraventricular nucleus, and the arcuate nucleus.[24,88] The following hypothalamic hormones have now been identified in these neurons: gonadotropin-releasing hormone (GnRH), corticotropin-releasing hormone (CRH), thyrotropin-releasing hormone (TRH), somatostatin (growth hormone release–inhibiting factor, SS), growth hormone–releasing hormone (GH-RH), neurotensin (NT), Met- and Leu-enkephalin, dinorphin, beta-endorphin, galanin, peptide HI (PHI) and the related vasoactive intestinal polypeptide (VIP), gamma-aminobutyric acid (GABA), and dopamine.[89] This incomplete list will probably enlarge considerably in the future as new biologically active peptides are discovered. Fibers from these cells travel to the median eminence of the neurohypophysis and the neural stalk. Their axons terminate on the primary capillary network of the pituitary portal system, which empties into the sinusoids of the anterior pituitary gland. Thus, a neurovascular link exists between the hypothalamus and the adenohypophysis.[49] The hypothalamic-hypophysiotropic hormones interact with specific receptors on the cell surface of target pituitary epithelial cells to modify the production of intracellular cyclic adenosine monophosphate (cAMP) and alter protein kinase activity. The brain causes a specific pituitary response by the release of specific hypothalamic stimulating and inhibiting hormones, which interact with specific receptors on pituitary target cells (Table 8-1). These hypothalamic hormones regulate adenohypophysial hormone secretion through the second messenger system.[46] There is accumulating evidence that the releasing hormones (GnRH and TRH) stimulate intracellular cAMP production in gonadotrophs and thyrotrophs and the inhibiting hormones (somatostatin and dopamine) inhibit cAMP production in somatotrophs and lactotrophs.[79]

The hypothalamic-neurohypophysial system is made up of magnocellular neurons located in the paired supraoptic nuclei situated above the optic tract and paraventricular nuclei immediately beneath the ependyma of the third ventricle.[3,69] The unmyelinated nerve fibers from these large cells descend through the infundibulum and neural stalk to end in the neural lobe of the pituitary gland, forming the supraopticohypophysial and the paraventriculohypophysial tracts.[75] Cells in this system contain oxytocin and AVP and their associated neurophysins (1 and 2, respectively).

Table 8-1 Major Hypothalamic Neuropeptides and Their Actions

Hypothalamic regulatory factor	Anterior pituitary hormone
TRH	↑TSH, PRL (GH)
GnRH	↑LH, FSH (GH)
SS	↓GH, TSH (PRL)
CRF	↑Corticotropin (GH)
GRF	↑GH (PRL)
DA	↓PRL
ADH	↑ACTH
Motilin	↑GH

*United effect on hormones in parentheses.

The secretion of hypothalamic-hypophysiotropic releasing factors and catecholamines into median eminence capillaries and their transport via portal vessels to the pars distalis is not the only mechanism by which the brain can control anterior pituitary function. The neural lobe hormone, AVP, released from peptidergic terminals in the median eminence can be carried by portal routes to the pars distalis to play a role in the regulation of corticotropin released by corticotrophs.[94] AVP and oxytocin can be transported by vascular (capillary) routes from the neural lobe to the pars distalis to participate in the regulation of MSH and PRL release by melanotrophs and lactotrophs, respectively.[7] The entire neurohypophysis appears to participate in controlling adenohypophysial function.

Physiology of the Adenohypophysial Hormones and End Organs

The anterior pituitary secretes hormones in pulses, the frequency and magnitude of which determine the peripheral levels of these hormones. The anterior pituitary produces, releases, and secretes at least six well-characterized trophic hormones: corticotropin, TSH, LH, FSH, GH, and PRL. The first four hormones listed stimulate the synthesis and release of hormones by target organs: the adrenal cortex, thyroid, ovary, and testes (LH and FSH), respectively. In discussing disorders of the pituitary-target organ systems, we will limit our review to those hormonal systems and disease processes most pertinent to the ICU patient.

PITUITARY-THYROID DISEASE

Thyrotropin is a glycoprotein hormone that increases the growth and activity of thyroid cells; its secretion is inhibited by rising levels of circulating thyroid hormones, thyroxine (T_4) and 3,5,3′-triiodothyronine (T_3) (Fig. 8-4). Like many other hormones, TSH appears to stimulate its target cells by activating adenyl cyclase in the cell membrane. The hypothalamic control of TSH is mediated primarily by TRH. TRH probably stimulates release of TSH by increasing the intracellular calcium of

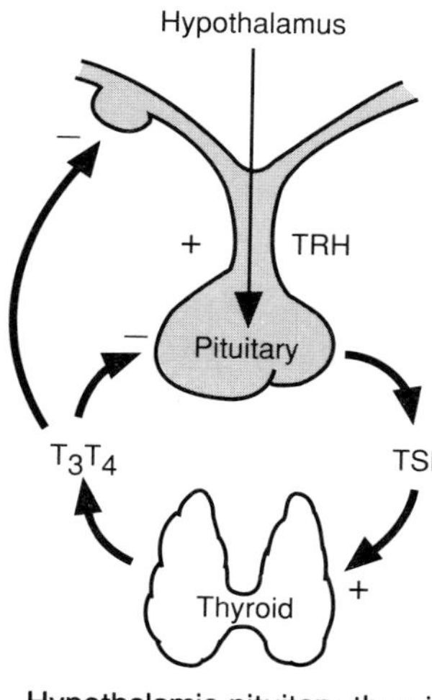

Figure 8-4 Hypothalamic-pituitary-thyroidal axis. Secretion of thyroid-stimulating hormone (TSH) by the anterior pituitary is inhibited by the negative feedback effects of thyroid gland secretions T_3 and T_4, which have a direct effect on the pituitary. The secretion of TSH is stimulated by the hypothalamic tripeptide, TRH.

the thyrotroph cells.[21] The measurement of TSH levels in plasma is an accurate indicator of the condition of the thyroid gland. Hypothyroidism due to target gland insufficiency results in increased secretion of TSH and eventually in hypertrophy and hyperplasia of the thyrotroph cells. On the other hand, primary thyroid activity leads to inhibition of these cells and reduces the circulating TSH to undetectable levels. The thyroid hormones (T_3 and T_4) exert marked effects on a variety of metabolic processes. Thyroid hormones significantly increase calorigenesis, made apparent by increased heart rate, increased temperature, and increased oxygen consumption. The increase in calorigenesis is due to a marked increase in protein synthesis and carbohydrate and lipid metabolism.[12,37,45,92]

Myxedema Coma

Myxedema coma represents a severe form of hypothyroidism characterized by coma or stupor, hypothermia, hypotension, hypoventilation, and hypoglycemia. This condition, although somewhat rare, represents a medical emergency and is associated with a 50 percent or greater mortality.[83] Most commonly, the disease develops in individuals with a long history of hypothyroidism; in fact, the presence of a scar on the neck from a prior thyroidectomy may serve as an aid in diagnosis.

Pathophysiology A deficiency of thyroid hormones causes a defect in thermogenesis. In the course of long-standing hypothyroidism, several physiologic adaptations occur to ensure the maintenance of body temperature. These efforts at heat conservation consist of peripheral vasoconstriction, bradycardia, and decreased cardiac output and result in a decrease in blood volume (up to 1 L) due to decreased circulating aldosterone concentrations.[69] These changes affect virtually every organ system and render the hypothyroid patient unable to maintain homeostasis in the face of precipitating stresses such as surgery, trauma, or infection.

Clinical and Laboratory Findings Recognition of myxedema coma on physical examination is important because therapy is best started early without waiting for the results of thyroid hormone determinations. The disease garners its name from the generalized edematous appearance of the patient. This edema is due to the accumulation of hyaluronic acid that complexes with water in the dermis. Unlike the edema of congestive heart failure, it is nonpitting and is especially noticeable periorbitally and on the dorsum of the hands and feet.

The cardiovascular changes in myxedema are secondary to the organism's efforts to ensure heat and to a decrease sensitivity to adrenergic stimuli. These changes are manifested by reduced cardiac stroke volume, bradycardia, and reduced cardiac output. There is also increased peripheral vascular resistance and decreased blood volume.

Respiratory changes in hypothyroidism are often implicated as one of the most important factors in decompensation of the patient and development of coma. In patients with myxedema, there is a state of hypoventilation, with associated hypercapnia and hypoxia being characteristic findings. The chest wall may function abnormally secondary to myxedematous infiltration of striated muscle.[13] Finally, there is evidence that these patients have a decreased central respiratory rate.[55]

Therapy The cornerstone of therapy for myxedema is early replacement of thyroid hormone along with careful attention to cardiovascular and respiratory support. Myxedematous patients may be treated with an initial intravenous dose of 100 to 500 μg of T_4 (with dosage based on cardiac function) followed by a daily maintenance dose of T_4 of 50 μg intravenously. Patients with myxedema have a decreased peripheral conversion of T_4 to T_3. Although T_3 has a more rapid onset of action and can penetrate the cerebrospinal fluid more rapidly and completely than does T_4, injectable T_3 is not as readily available. Improvement in body temperature, heart rate, blood pressure, and mental status may occur as early as 24 h following institution of therapy. Patients with myxedema coma have an impaired glucocorticoid response to stress, or frank adrenal insufficiency, and should receive hydrocortisone, 100 to 300 mg/day in divided doses every 8 h. Frequently, these patients also require ventilatory and cardiovascular support measures.

Altered function of respiratory centers results in defective hypoxic and hypercapnic drives. This depression is exacerbated by the use of sedatives, narcotics, and general anesthesia. Weaning from the ventilator may be extremely difficult until a euthyroid state is achieved.

Thyroid hormone directly affects myocardial contractility and beta-adrenergic receptor action. Therefore, a poor response to beta-adrenergic agonists can be expected. The sodium-potassium ATPase pump is thyroid hormone–dependent, and there is increased sensitivity to digitalis drugs during hypothyroidism. Digitalis and catecholamines must be administered cautiously and with continuous monitoring to hypothyroid patients, especially during thyroid hormone replacement therapy. Alpha-adrenergic agents should be avoided in patients with myxedema since these patients are already vasoconstricted. The combination of adrenergic agents and thyroid hormone can cause life-threatening arrhythmias.

Myxedematous patients usually have a diminished plasma volume and frequently require volume expansion therapy. Anemia, hypoglycemia, and electrolyte abnormalities are also seen and should be treated appropriately. Intravenous fluids should be administered cautiously because hypothyroid patients have diminished free water clearance. Temperatures as low as 24°C (75°F) have been recorded in myxedema coma.[86] Active rewarming is not recommended in hypothermic patients because these individuals have decreased plasma volume and intense peripheral vasoconstriction. Rapid peripheral vasodilatation may precipitate shock. Passive rewarming combined with thyroid hormone administration will correct the hypothermic state.

Euthyroid-Sick Syndrome

Patients experience rapid changes in hormonal function with the onset of critical illness.[22] The most common abnormality of thyroid function seen in critically ill patients is the euthyroid-sick syndrome, which results from the slowing of peripheral thyroid hormone metabolism. This syndrome is characterized by low serum levels of T_4 and T_3 and increased levels of 3,3′,5′-triiodothyronine (rT_3) (the physiologically inactive metabolite of T_4). This biochemical abnormality is due to the inhibition of thyroid hormone binding to protein and diminished metabolic enzyme activity. Therefore, T_4 is preferentially shunted to the rT_3 pathway in critical illness. In acutely ill hospitalized patients, the frequency of reduced serum T_3 concentration can be as high as 70 percent.[40] These patients are clinically euthyroid and have normal serum TSH concentrations.

The euthyroid-sick syndrome appears to be an adaptive phenomenon in states of critical illness. The decreased T_3 production limits the utilization of protein and oxygen and decreases the metabolic demand on the heart.[93,99] The combination of reduced T_3 and T_4 concentrations is found in patients with more severe illnesses and indicates a poor prognosis.[40,85] The frequency of this condition among patients admitted to a medical ICU is 30 to 50 percent.[41,85] The magnitude of the decrease in T_4 concentrations and patient outcome are correlated. In patients with a T_4 value less than 3.0 μg/dL, mortality is 68 to 84 percent.[40,41,85] Administration of thyroid hormone replacement is not beneficial and may be deleterious in these patients.[19,33,40,85] It is therefore important to distinguish the euthyroid-sick syndrome, which does not respond to thyroid replacement, from hypothyroidism, which does require treatment.

The serum TSH concentration may be misleading in critical illness. Serum TSH concentrations have not been found to be increased in response to decreased levels of circulating T_4 and T_3 in about 50 percent of patients with normal thyroid illness.[56] More reliable means of determining thyroid function in critical illness is to measure the free thyroxine index or to perform a TRH stimulation test. The TRH stimulation test is a simple bedside maneuver in which 250 to 500 μg of TRH is administered intravenously and TSH concentration is measured 30 min later. Serum TSH doubles or triples in patients with euthyroid-sick syndrome, whereas hypothyroid patients will exhibit an exaggerated response of 6 to 8 times normal.

PITUITARY-ADRENAL DISEASE

Corticotropin regulates growth and function of the adrenal cortex. It is especially important in the control of cortisol secretion. The production of aldosterone by the zona glomerulosa is largely controlled by the renin-angiotensin system and is much less dependent on corticotropin stimulation. The release of corticotropin appears to be governed by at least three independent mechanisms: negative feedback, diurnal rhythm, and a stress-activated mechanism.

Hypothalamic CRH stimulates the production and secretion of corticotropin, and circulating cortisol inhibits its release by negative feedback (Fig. 8-5). Glucocorticoids may also act directly on the brain to inhibit CRH release.

Corticotropin-releasing hormone levels fluctuate in relationship to a circadian rhythm linked to the light-dark cycle. In humans, adrenal activation is maximal in the early morning hours beginning with a 4 A.M. surge of corticotropin activity under the control of CRH. After 8 A.M. there is a gradual fall in corticotropin release and consequent cortisol secretion, so the plasma cortisol levels in the afternoon are only about half the 8 A.M. value. The diurnal rhythm is abolished by certain central ner-

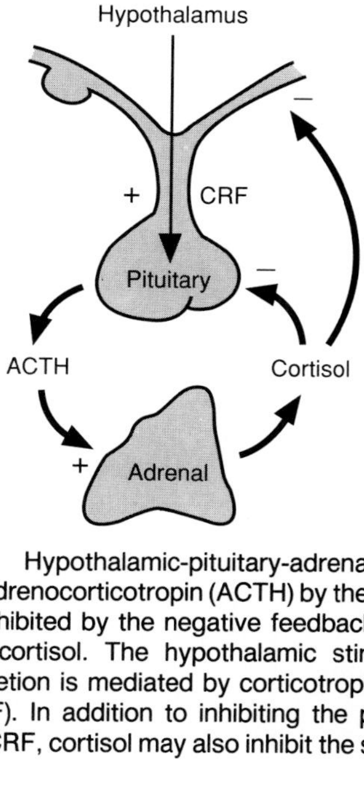

Figure 8-5 Hypothalamic-pituitary-adrenal axis. Secretion of adrenocorticotropin (ACTH) by the anterior pituitary is inhibited by the negative feedback effects of circulating cortisol. The hypothalamic stimulation of ACTH secretion is mediated by corticotropin-releasing factor (CRF). In addition to inhibiting the pituitary response to CRF, cortisol may also inhibit the secretion of CRF itself.

vous system lesions as well as alterations in the sleep pattern, such as occurs in a night worker.

Stressful stimuli, such as major operative trauma, hypoglycemia, or infection increase the delivery of CRH to the adenohypophysis via the portal circulation. This stress mechanism stimulates the corticotrophs and overrides the previously described control systems at any time. The greater the stress, the more corticotropin that is secreted.

Action of Adrenal Steroids

Adrenal steroids may be divided into two general categories, glucocorticoids and mineralocorticoids. Glucocorticoids is a term applied to steroid hormones that have primary effects on carbohydrate metabolism, particularly the promotion of gluconeogenesis, increased liver glycogen deposition, and elevation of blood glucose concentrations. The most common and potent is cortisol. Mineralocorticoids are steroid hormones that affect ion transport by the epithelial cells, resulting in sodium conservation and loss of potassium. The most potent and commonly occurring is aldosterone.

Glucocorticoids, when used in supranormal doses, have well-documented therapeutic effects, primarily through their anti-inflammatory response. It has been shown that glucocorticoids stabilize lysosomal membranes, inhibit the migration of white blood cells, inhibit granuloma formation, and cause a reduction in the number of circulating lymphocytes.

Adrenal Insufficiency (Addisonian Crisis)

Pathophysiology Adrenal insufficiency may result from adrenal gland failure (primary adrenal insufficiency), from pituitary corticotropin deficiency (secondary adrenal insufficiency), or from hypothalamic (CRH) deficiency (tertiary adrenal insufficiency). Causes of primary adrenal insufficiency include autoimmune, infectious, hemorrhagic, neoplastic, and surgical etiologies. Autoimmune disorders are the leading cause of adrenal insufficiency today. Bilateral adrenal hemorrhage may cause rapid and total adrenal destruction, leading to an acute loss of both glucocorticoid and mineralocorticoid secretion. This syndrome is seen in patients with overwhelming sepsis (i.e., meningococcemia, *Pseudomonas* infections, cytomegalovirus).[57]

Secondary or tertiary adrenal insufficiency may result from pituitary failure (due to tumor or infection) or hypothalamic insufficiency. The most common cause of secondary adrenal insufficiency is withdrawal of exogenous glucocorticoids. If glucocorticoids have been administered to a patient for more than 1 to 2 weeks, the drug should be slowly tapered to allow for recovery of normal adrenal function. Basal secretion of glucocorticoids may be adequate, but the patient may be unable to mount an appropriate stress response. It may take 6 to 12 months for the adrenal glands to fully recover after prolonged use of exogenous glucocorticoids. Patients with primary adrenal insufficiency have deficits of both glucocorticoid and mineralocorticoid secretion, whereas those with secondary adrenal insufficiency lose only glucocorticoid activity.

Clinical Manifestations and Diagnosis Clinical manifestations of adrenal insufficiency are related to glucocorticoid and/or mineralocorticoid deficiency. When adrenal destruction or insufficiency is gradual, there is a period characterized by normal basal steroid secretion but inability to respond to stress. The patient may be asymptomatic, but an adrenal crisis may be precipitated by surgery, trauma, or infection.

The diagnosis of adrenal insufficiency rests on the demonstration of decreased cortisol production. This should always be considered in the differential diagnosis of shock that is unresponsive to volume expansion or vasopressor agents. Weakness, fatigability, weight loss, anorexia, hypotension, and hyperpigmentation are seen in virtually all patients with adrenal insufficiency. The hyperpigmentation is most pronounced in skin creases, on extensor surfaces, and on old scars. Nausea and vomiting are seen in about one-half of patients.

The diagnosis of adrenal insufficiency should be considered in postoperative patients with acute decompensation when other causes are not evident. The key laboratory findings suggestive of acute adrenal insufficiency are serum sodium to potassium ratio less than 30 and a total blood eosinophil count greater than 300 cells per cubic millimeter.[29] A serum cortisol level of less than 20 μg/dL in a critically ill patient suggests the diagnosis. The ability of the adrenal glands to secrete glucocorticoids can be determined by a corticotropin stimulation test. To perform this test, serum cortisol measurements are obtained 30 and 60 min following the intravenous administration of 250 μg cosyntropin. A normal response is a rise in serum cortisol above 20 μg/dL. In patients without a rise, additional testing is required to locate the site of disease (primary or secondary). A normal response to a corticotropin bolus excludes primary adrenal insufficiency but does not exclude secondary adrenal insufficiency. Failure of cortisol or corticotropin to rise in response to stress, hypoglycemia, or metyrapone suggests secondary glandular failure.

Therapy The treatment of the patient in Addisonian crisis has three principal objectives: (1) repletion of glucocorticoids, (2) repletion of sodium and water deficits, and (3) correction of hypoglycemia. Therapy should be started immediately while awaiting results of testing in a critically ill patient with suspected adrenal insufficiency. Dexamethasone, 1 mg every 6 h, may be given as an initial glucocorticoid replacement, since it does not cross-react with cortisol measured in the plasma cortisol assessment by radioimmunoassay.

Initially, hydrocortisone hemisuccinate, 100 to 200 mg, should be administered intravenously as a slow bolus. Volume resuscitation should begin immediately in the form of isotonic normal saline, containing 5% dextrose. The first liter should be given over 30 min and then at 1 L/h until the patient is clinically euvolemic. Vasopressors may be required to sustain adequate blood pressure in the initial stages of therapy. If hypotension exists initially, vasopressor agents such as norepinephrine should be avoided as tissue perfusion is already compromised, and inotropes such as dopamine or dobutamine should be used instead. Hydrocortisone, 50 to 100 mg every 6 h, should be administered intravenously for the first 24 h of treatment. Glucocorticoid therapy may be switched to oral supplementation on day 2 if the patient is well stabilized. Mineralocorticoids are not required during initial therapy since large doses of hydrocortisone provide sufficient glucocorticoid and mineralocorticoid activity. When the dose of hydrocortisone decreases below 100 mg/day, the patient with primary adrenal insufficiency may require supplemental mineralocorticoids (i.e., 9 α-fludrocortisone, 0.05 to 0.1 mg/day).

Hyperkalemia is rarely in excess of 7 mEq/L and usually responds to glucocorticoid replacement, glucose administration, and rehydration. However, if the serum potassium level is greater than 6.5 mEq/L in the presence of cardiac arrhythmias, administration of one ampule of 50% dextrose and regular insulin should be given intravenously every 3 to 4 h as needed. Sodium bicarbonate is also used when the patient has severe hyperkalemia.

DISORDERS OF THE NEUROHYPOPHYSIS

Normally, neural, hormonal, hemodynamic, and renal mechanisms all function in a highly integrated manner to preserve sodium and water homeostasis. There are two major objectives. The first is to keep the concentration of sodium in the extracellular fluid (ECF) within very tight limits. Together with its associated anions, sodium constitutes more than 90 percent of the total solute in the ECF, and it controls the distribution of water between the cells and the extracellular space. Large deviations in ECF sodium concentration from normal cause the cells to shrink or swell. This can have disastrous effects, particularly on brain function. The body protects the sodium concentration constantly by finely adjusting the water content of the ECF. This is achieved through the secretion and action of AVP to control water loss from the kidney. The thirst mechanism helps by controlling the fluid intake to some extent. The second objective is to keep the total sodium *content* of the ECF within normal confines and thereby to maintain a normal ECF volume. Given that sodium is the major cation of the ECF and that the body adjusts the water around it to maintain a normal sodium concentration, the total number of sodium ions in the ECF will determine the ECF volume. Large deviations from normal in the ECF sodium content cause fluctuations in the circulating blood volume. Both volume contraction and expansion can have disastrous consequences on brain function, particularly in the presence of preexisting brain damage.[4] Normally, ECF sodium is regulated by many closely coordinated mechanisms that adjust the amount of sodium lost through the kidneys. Minor alterations in renal tubule reabsorption can have a profound effect on sodium balance since the filtered load of sodium is enormous in relation to the amount excreted.[48]

Fluid balance disturbances are common among patients with neurologic disorders and are frequently multifactorial in origin. It is essential to consider all aspects of sodium and water homeostasis in order to identify individual factors contributing to a disturbance before appropriate therapy can be initiated. Hyponatremia in neurosurgical patients has often been attributed to a cerebral salt-wasting state or to inappropriate secretion of antidiuretic hormone (SIADH). While these disorders undoubtedly occur,[25,50] recent reports have questioned the accuracy of these diagnoses in some patients[14,66] and suggest that hyponatremia is often iatrogenic.

Regulation of AVP Secretion

AVP is the major mammalian antidiuretic hormone. Its primary function is to regulate water balance by promoting reabsorption of water from the renal collecting ducts as they pass through the hyperosmolar gradient in the medulla of the kidney. At least four physiologic stimuli release AVP into the bloodstream by independent mechanisms in humans:[98] osmotic, hemodynamic (hypotension and/or hypovolemia), nausea and emesis, and hypoglycemia.[38,59,62,63,76,78] Of these, osmotic stimulation is normally the most important for fine control of secretion and maintenance of water balance.

Osmoregulation Changes in plasma osmotic pressure are sensed by osmosensitive cells in the brain, which relay impulses to AVP-producing cells in the supraoptic and paraventricular nuclei of the hypothalamus. These osmoreceptors probably lie outside the blood-brain barrier, perhaps in the region anterior and ventral to the third ventricle.[52] An increase in the ECF concentration of sodium ions, which are effectively excluded by the cell membranes, causes dehydration of the osmoreceptor cells. This stimulus is transmitted to the supraoptic and the paraventricular nuclei and triggers the release of AVP from the pituitary. Other solutes that are impermeable to cell membranes, for example mannitol, also stimulate the osmoreceptors. Solutes such as urea and glucose, which readily enter cells and do not therefore produce an osmotic gradient, have little or no effect. Osmoregulation is normally extraordinarily sensitive. For every unit rise in plasma osmolality, plasma AVP rises an average of 0.63 pmol/L, and a change in plasma osmolality of only 1 percent alters AVP by 1.8 pmol/L.[98] A threshold of the osmostat below which AVP secretion is suppressed is a plasma osmolality of around 280 to 284 mmol/kg water. Above this threshold, plasma AVP starts to increase, and maximum urinary concentration is achieved at a plasma osmolality of around 295 mmol/kg water. The threshold for stimulation of the thirst sensation is around 299 mmol/kg but varies widely.[98]

Hemodynamic Regulation Cardiovascular regulation is mediated by high-pressure receptors (baroreceptors) in the carotid body and the aortic arch, which respond to arterial blood pressure, and by low-pressure receptors in the atria of the heart, which respond to changes in blood volume. The afferents travel via the ninth and tenth cranial nerves.[52] Relatively large stimuli are required in healthy adults to increase plasma AVP: a fall in mean arterial pressure exceeding 5 percent or of blood volume of 10 to 20 percent.[28] Both high- and low-pressure receptors are stimulated if hypotension accompanies vasodilation, as in syncope. Once the stimulatory threshold is reached, there is a geometric rise in plasma AVP[81] to concentrations much higher than those achieved with maximal osmotic stimulation, and this overrides the normal suppression response to hypotonicity. Under conditions of hypotension or hypovolemia, the threshold of the osmoreceptors is lowered.

Nausea, Emesis, and Hypoglycemia Nausea and emesis lead to large increases in plasma AVP by an unknown mechanism. Insulin-induced hypoglycemia leads to a two- to fourfold increase in humans, but the physiologic significance of this is uncertain. The widely held belief that pain and other noxious stimuli stimulate AVP release has been questioned.[98] Other nonphysiologic stimuli may be important in neurosurgical patients, for example, a sudden increase in intracranial pressure.[74]

Drugs Of anesthetic agents in common use, halothane and chloralose produce modest increases and trichloroethylene more marked increases of AVP in rats. Phenobarbitone and althesin (alphaxalone/alphadolone) were without effect. Morphine in high doses[5] and positive-pressure ventilation increases release,[36] while atropine, reserpine, phenytoin, and chlorpromazine inhibit AVP release. Chlorpropamide and carbamazepine potentiate, and lithium and demethylchlortetracycline inhibit its peripheral action (Table 8-2).[31]

Diabetes Insipidus

Diabetes insipidus (DI) is characterized by excessive renal water loss due to an inability to generate a concentrated urine and conserve solute free water in the face of appropriate stimuli. This disorder is due either to a failure of the pituitary gland to secrete adequate amounts of AVP (central DI) or to a lack of renal tubule responsiveness, either congenital or acquired, to the antidiuretic actions of AVP (nephrogenic DI).[82] The cardinal features of the disease are polyuria, polydipsia, intense thirst, and tendency toward hyperosmolar plasma.[64]

Etiology The common causes of central DI are shown in Table 8-3 and include

1. *Neoplastic or infiltrating lesions of the hypothalamus or pituitary*, such as craniopharyngioma, pituitary adenoma, metastatic lesions, sarcoidosis, histiocytosis, leukemia, and lymphoma. Presence of DI is the single most important feature in differentiating a metastatic pituitary lesion from a benign pituitary adenoma.[53] In one series, 14 percent of patients with DI had pituitary gland metastases.[43] Lung and breast cancer are the most common primary tumors to metastasize to the pituitary gland.[43,53,91]

2. *Head trauma*, usually severe enough to cause skull or facial fractures,[15,34] may cause DI, although cases of DI have been reported from minor head trauma.[43] The pathophysiology is thought to be shearing trauma to the pituitary stalk. The time of onset for posttraumatic DI is variable, but it generally manifests 5 to 10 days after trauma.[42,72]

3. *Postoperative DI following surgery on the pituitary or hypothalamus*. This disorder is most common following surgery for posteriorly located pituitary adenomas or craniopharyngiomas, but may follow any manipulation of the pituitary stalk as may occur during surgery on large aneurysms of the ophthalmic segment of the internal carotid artery.[6]

4. *Idiopathic DI*. One must be careful to exclude occult cancer in patients in whom a diagnosis of idiopathic DI is suggested. An apparently normal CT of the brain should be followed carefully to identify a possible expanding pituitary lesion.[27]

5. *Nephrogenic DI*, either congenital or acquired.

Table 8-2 Drugs Effecting AVP Release

AVP stimulators	AVP inhibitors
Nicotine	Chlorpromazine
Morphine	Reserpine
Barbiturates	Diphenylhydantoin (Dilantin)
Vincristine	Ethanol
Cyclophosphamide	
Tricyclic antidepressants	
Certain anticonvulsants	

Table 8-3 Principal Causes of Diabetes Insipidus

Primary diabetes insipidus
Idiopathic
Familial or congenital
Secondary diabetes insipidus
Posttraumatic—head injury (e.g., basal skull fractures), neurosurgery
Neoplasm
Infections and granulomatous lesions—sarcoidosis, tuberculosis, cryptococcosis, meningovascular syphilis, pyrogenic meningitis
Histiocytosis X
Vascular lesions

Pathophysiology The defect in central DI may exist in the osmoreceptors, the cells of the supraoptic or paraventricular nuclei or other axons, the posterior pituitary storage site, or the site of AVP action on the renal collecting tubule. DI following surgery or trauma is presumably due to hemorrhage, trauma, or edema in the area of the neurohypophysis. Patients undergoing ablative pituitary surgery classically exhibit a triphasic vasopressin response[53] in the immediate postoperative period. Initially they exhibit polyuria with a fall in urine osmolality and a rise in urine volume. This phase is followed by 5 to 7 days of decreased urine output and a rise in urine osmolality. This so-called interphase is presumably due to vasopressin leakage from damaged and degenerating neurons. The final stage is characterized by frank DI, with a loss of urinary concentrating ability. This sequence is important for the critical care specialist because hypotonic fluids begun during the initial polyuric phase may lead to water overload and cerebral edema if continued in the interphase.

Removal or damage of the posterior pituitary alone does not necessarily cause DI.[20] Rather, injury may be sufficiently high in the pituitary stalk to damage the supraopticohypophysial and paraventriculohypophysial tracts and cause retrograde degeneration of the neurons in the supraoptic and paraventricular nuclei.[30] In patients undergoing surgery in the area of the hypothalamus and pituitary, it is always important to closely monitor urine output and serum sodium postoperatively.

Clinical and Laboratory Findings The classic clinical picture of DI includes polyuria, intense thirst for cold fluids, and nocturia. Patients with a complete loss of AVP secretion may urinate every 30 min and have a total daily urine volume of up to 18 L, equal to the total filtrate volume reaching the renal collecting ducts. Those with partial ability to synthesize and secrete AVP may lose lesser amounts of fluid. If denied access to water, the patient may develop striking symptomatology, including stupor, lethargy, and coma.

Laboratory studies in patients with DI show persistently hypotonic urine, with urine osmolality less than 200 mmol/kg, serum hypernatremia, and a normal glomerular filtration rate. Urine specific gravity is generally less than 1.005. Urine osmolality is not necessarily below that of plasma. In mild cases, the urine osmolality may be 300 to 600 mmol/kg, and the disease manifests only when the patient is denied access to water. Under those circumstances, the ability to concentrate urine beyond a certain level causes excessive free water loss, plasma hypertonicity, and thirst. DI is important to recognize in the unconscious patient without an intact thirst mechanism or ability to intake fluids, since hypertonicity can develop rapidly when water is lost in excess of solute. Isotonic saline administration in large volumes is particularly dangerous unless adequate volume of solute free water is also administered.

Diagnosis The diagnosis of DI is made by establishing that the kidney is unable to produce maximally concentrated urine in the presence of osmotic stimuli, such as dehydration or hypertonic saline infusion. Radioimmunoassay of plasma AVP is available but is seldom necessary to establish a diagnosis. The easiest and safest test to confirm the diagnosis is the dehydration or water deprivation test. The principle of this test is to determine whether the patient can respond to an osmotic stimulus by elaboration of a concentrated urine and then to assess the effect of exogenous AVP on urine osmolality.

AVP increases the permeability of the collecting tubules to water, allowing the flow of water down the osmotic gradient between the lumen and the medullary interstitium. The ability to concentrate urine, therefore, is dependent upon both the medullary interstitial tonicity and the presence of AVP. The medullary tonicity is affected by previous water diuresis[16] and illness such as pyelonephritis, so it is not relevant to define an absolute minimum value for normal maximal concentrating ability. One study showed a maximum urine osmolality in randomly selected hospital patients of 764 mmol/kg and a value of 1067 mmol/kg in normal volunteers.[58]

To perform the water deprivation test, water intake is restricted and changes in urine volume and plasma concentration are measured for 6 to 8 h. In normal individuals, water deprivation causes a dehydration that produces a fall in urine volume and rise in urine osmolality. After 6 to 8 h of fluid deprivation, the urine flow will be reduced to less than 0.5 mL/min, urine osmolality plateaus between 700 and 1100 mmol/kg, and plasma osmolality rises to the range of 288 to 291 mmol/kg. The subcutaneous administration of 5 units of aqueous AVP will not cause a further increase in urine osmolality, indicating that the kidneys have reached their maximum ability to concentrate urine.

Patients with severe central DI are unable to concentrate urine above plasma osmolality when challenged by dehydration. Urine will be concentrated to only 200 mmol/kg, and plasma osmolality may rise as high as 320 to 330 mmol/kg. Furthermore, they demonstrate a greater than 50 percent increase in urine osmolality when administered exogenous AVP.[16] Patients with milder DI are able to produce urine that is hyperosmolar relative to plasma. When given exogenous AVP, they show a greater than 10 percent rise in urine osmolality.[16] This finding implies that the endogenous levels of AVP are insufficient to maximally stimulate the collecting tubules to reabsorb water. If patients with partial DI are dehydrated for longer periods of time, they eventually show a paradoxical fall in urine osmolality, implying exhaustion of a limited AVP reserve. Normal patients and patients with primary polydipsia are able to concentrate their urine beyond plasma levels and do not increase their urine osmolality more than 10 percent with exogenous AVP. Patients with nephrogenic DI or polyuria from potassium depletion show little rise in plasma osmolality with dehydration and do not respond to exogenous AVP.

The diagnosis of polyuria in the critically ill patient is frequently encountered. The physician must distinguish between excessive water intake (primary polydipsia, central thirst center disorder), central DI, nephrogenic DI (congenital, lithium intake, hypokalemia, hypocalcemia, chronic renal disease), and osmotic diuresis (glycosuria, mannitol, diuretics). Patients with primary polydipsia have a urinary concentrating defect due to a diluted medullary interstitium caused by long-standing polyuria. They can be distinguished from those with DI by the dehydration test. Urine should be examined for the presence of glucose, and a history of mannitol or other diuretic use should be elicited. Causes of renal resistance to AVP, particularly hypokalemia, hypercalcemia, drug use, and renal disease should be sought.

Therapy The primary goals of the treatment of DI are to decrease urine output and restore normal plasma tonicity. Those patients with urine output of under 5 L/day may not require specific therapy. Patients with mild DI who have an intact thirst mechanism and a readily available supply of water are usually safe. The associated polyuria and polydipsia can be annoying, often interfere with sleep, and may need to be treated for convenience and comfort. In clinical practice, varying degrees of DI will be encountered and treatment must be tailored to the individual patient (Table 8-4).

Desmopressin [1-(3-mercaptopropionic acid)-8-D-arginine-vasopressin] (DDAVP) may be administered intravenously, intranasally, or subcutaneously. It is similar in structure to AVP; the modifications result in a molecule with a high antidiuretic activity and an increased duration of action (12 to 24 h) compared with arginine AVP.[23] Because of its long duration of action, its availability as an intranasal spray, its paucity of side effects, and its potent antidiuretic activity, desmopressin has become the drug of choice for managing and controlling daytime polyuria.[23] Rarely, patients may exhibit tolerance to the drug.[23]

Desmopressin also temporarily increases factor VIII:C and von Willebrand factor and is useful in augmenting hemostasis.[11,51,72] It should not be used in patients with factor VIII activities less than 5 percent, patients with factor IX deficiency, or patients with type II:B von Willebrand's disease.[54] The dosage used is 0.3 μg/kg in 50 mL normal saline infused intravenously over 15 to 30 min. This dosage can be used daily, but administration more often than every 2 to 3 days diminishes the response.

Injectable AVP is available in an aqueous solution or as Pitressin tannate in oil. The short duration of action of aqueous AVP is advantageous in treating postoperative neurosurgical or trauma patients receiving intravenous fluids, especially unconscious patients, because it carries a low risk of producing water intoxication. In patients with an altered level of consciousness and DI, aqueous vasopressin is administered intramuscularly or subcutaneously in doses of 5 to 10 U. Pitressin tannate in oil has a longer duration of action and may be used in similar dosage for more chronic treatment of DI in such patients.

Table 8-4 Agents Used to Treat Diabetes Insipidus*

Agent	Usual dose	Duration of action, h	Clinical indication
Hormone replacement			
8-Lysine vasopressin (Lypressin) (5-mL bottle, 50 U/mL)	10–20 U IN	4–6	Severe, transient, or permanent DI
1-Deamino-8-D-arginine vasopressin (DDAVP IV) (3.5-mL bottle, 200 μg/mL)	10–20 μg IN	12–24	Severe, transient, or permanent DI
Aqueous vasopressin (5 U/mL ampule)	5–10 U SC	3–6	DI in unconscious patient
Parenteral vasopressin (20 U/mL)	1–3 U/h IV	1–2	Severe DI in ICU
Vasopressin tannate in oil (5 U/mL ampule)	5 U IM	24–72	Severe idiopathic DI
Nonhormonal agents			
Chlorpropamide (100- and 200-mg tablets)	200–500 mg/day	24	Some residual AVP function
Clofibrate (500-mg capsules)	500 mg QID	24	Some residual AVP function
Thiazide diuretics			
Hydrochlorothiazide	50–100 mg/day	24	Nephrogenic DI

*IV = intravenous; IN = intranasal; IM = intramuscular; SC = subcutaneous; QID = 4 times daily; AVP = antidiuretic hormone.

Source: Adapted from A. M. Moses.[60]

Other drugs used in the management of DI include chlorpropamide, clofibrate, carbamazepine, and thiazide diuretics. Chlorpropamide acts by potentiating the effect of AVP at the renal tubules.[61] It is useful in patients who have some ability to produce AVP. Dosages of 250 to 750 mg/day are usually sufficient to effect antidiuresis in 50 to 80 percent of patients. Clofibrate, given in doses of 400 to 600 mg/day, stimulates AVP release and produces an antidiuresis.[60] The combination of clofibrate and chlorpropamide is also effective.[96] Thiazide diuretics are useful in both central and nephrogenic DI. They paradoxically reduce polyuria by producing a state of relative volume depletion and reducing glomerular filtration rate. Proximal solute reabsorption is increased and the delivery of filtrate to the diluting segment is reduced, therefore interfering with the ability of the kidneys to generate dilute urine. The usual dose is 50 to 100 mg hydrochlorothiazide daily.[26] It is effective only in conjunction with salt restriction.

Syndrome of Inappropriate Secretion of Antidiuretic Hormone

This syndrome was initially proposed to explain the occurrence of renal salt loss in hyponatremic patients having neither renal nor adrenal disease. The basis of the syndrome is an expanded ECF volume resulting from an abnormal and thus inappropriate secretion of AVP. The primary features of SIADH include (1) hyponatremia with corresponding hypo-osmolality of the serum and ECF, (2) continued renal excretion of sodium (> 25 nmol/L), (3) absence of fluid volume depletion [serum creatinine and blood urea nitrogen (BUN) are usually low], (4) greater osmolality of the urine than is appropriate for the osmolality of the plasma, (5) normal renal and normal adrenal function, and (6) absence of peripheral edema.[65]

In the broadest classification, SIADH is a form of dilutional hyponatremia, the sine qua non of which is increased ECF volume. Under these conditions, the hypothalamic neurons should be inhibited from secreting AVP. In SIADH, however, AVP excess induces water retention by the kidneys to the point of hyponatremic expansion of the ECF volume and a secondary natriuresis. The size of the increase in ECF volume is usually 3 to 4 L, so peripheral edema is not present. Because of the expanded ECF volume, the glomerular filtration rate is increased and the renin-angiotensin-aldosterone mechanism is suppressed, leading to a decrease in the renal absorption of sodium. SIADH can occur in a wide variety of CNS disorders, including encephalitis, stroke, head trauma, and brain tumors. It also has been described in pulmonary disorders such as fungal, viral, and bacterial pneumonia (Table 8-5).

Table 8-5 Causes of Inappropriate Antidiuretic Hormone (AVP) Secretion

Central hypersecretion of ADH
Hypothalamic disorders
Trauma
Surgery
Metabolic encephalopathy
Acute intermittent porphyria
Myxedema
Subarachnoid hemorrhage
Vascular lesions
Suprahypothalamic disorders
Cerebral infarcts
Subdural hematoma
Infections, meningitis (tuberculosis)
Peripheral hypersecretion
Excessive stimulation in recumbant posture (coma)
Excessive production from nonhypothalamic sites (ectopic ADH)
Pulmonary infections: TB, etc.
Tumors: lung, etc.
Drugs
Vincristine
Chlorpromazine
Chlorothiazide
Cyclophosphamide
Carbamazepine
Clofibrate

Vasopressin secreted from the neurohypophysis is no longer under its normal regulatory influences. Whether there is an alteration of the osmoreceptor function or inappropriate information being transmitted centrally from peripheral volume receptors, or whether some other situation prevails, is uncertain. In some instances, SIADH may result from the ectopic production of AVP from tumors such as oat cell carcinoma of the bronchus. Since surgical stress, morphine, barbiturates, and anesthetics may stimulate AVP secretion, a transient form of SIADH may occur in the immediate postoperative period.

Clinical Manifestations The clinical manifestations of SIADH are related to the resulting water retention and depend to some extent on the degree of associated hyponatremia and the rapidity with which it develops. SIADH associated with a slow drop in serum sodium usually causes no symptoms until the serum sodium concentration falls below 120 nmol/L. However, if there is a progressive retention of water with rapid reduction in serum sodium, significant symptoms can appear with a higher serum sodium concentration. Symptoms are often nonspecific and include anorexia, nausea, irritability, and accentuation of focal neurologic deficits if there is underlying structural brain damage. If serum sodium concentration drops to less than 110 nmol/L, neurologic dysfunction due to brain edema may occur with areflexia, diffuse muscle weakness, seizures, stupor, or coma.

Diagnosis and Management SIADH must be differentiated from other causes of hyponatremia such as sodium depletion from prolonged vomiting, adrenal insufficiency, or cerebral salt-wasting syndrome. Each of these disorders requires distinctly different treatment. The laboratory criteria for SIADH are (1) a serum sodium $\leq$ 135 nmol/L, (2) urinary sodium $\geq$ 25 nmol/L, (3) serum osmolality $\leq$ 280 nmol/kg, and (4) urine osmolality inappropriately concentrated compared to serum osmolality.[8] For the diagnosis of SIADH to be made, the patient must be in a normal state of hydration and have normal renal, adrenal, and thyroid function.

The treatment of SIADH is determined by the

severity of the symptoms. The basis of all treatment is the elimination of excess water and treatment of the underlying disease. In patients with minor symptoms, restriction of fluid intake to about 500 mL/day is adequate. A weight loss of 5 to 10 lb is generally required before serum sodium returns to normal. In senile patients or those with behavioral disorders in whom it is difficult to control oral fluid intake, the use of demeclocycline (600 to 1200 mg/day) or lithium carbonate (600 to 900 mg/day), both of which block the renal tubular response to AVP, can be helpful. Furosemide, a loop diuretic that facilitates free water clearance, may also be useful at 40 to 60 mg/day.

If symptoms are acute and severe, the patient's serum osmolality should rise quickly. Hypertonic saline infusions and the use of diuretics may be necessary to expedite the water loss. In this situation, 1000 mL of 3% sodium chloride is given over 6 to 8 h, with plasma sodium levels measured every 2 to 3 h. Furosemide, 40 to 60 mg, is given intravenously at the beginning of the infusion and may be repeated in 3 to 4 h. Mannitol infusion can also be used to accelerate the water loss. Too rapid a correction of serum sodium has been associated with the development of central pontine myelinolysis.[95] This disorder occurs in up to 60 percent of individuals when correction rates exceed 2.5 nmol/L per 1 h or 20 nmol/L per 24 h.[10,87]

Differentiation of SIADH from the hyponatremia seen in salt depletion is straightforward; none of the signs of hypovolemia such as decreased blood pressure, decreased tissue turgor, and elevated BUN are present in SIADH. The clinical picture most often confused with SIADH is that of a patient with isotonic fluid loss, usually due to the administration of diuretics, who is treated with hypotonic fluid replacement. In that case, the body will sacrifice the maintenance of tonicity for the sake of preserving volume, really a form of hypotonic dehydration. Once again, it should be stressed that the absence of an increase of ECF volume precludes a diagnosis of SIADH.

Cerebral Salt-Wasting Syndrome

In 1981, Nelson and coworkers described 12 patients with intracranial disease who fulfilled the laboratory criteria for SIADH.[66] In 10 of these patients, however, significant decreases in red blood cell mass and in plasma and total blood volume were detected. Renal loss of sodium and free water, rather than SIADH, was suggested as the mechanism for hyponatremia in these patients. In follow-up, Nelson and coworkers reported the occurrence of natriuresis and hyponatremia in 7 of 10 monkeys after experimental subarachnoid hemorrhage.[67] During the period of natriuresis, there was no significant change in measured AVP levels, and plasma volume was slightly decreased. Four of the affected monkeys showed normal regulation of AVP in response to challenge with both water and hypertonic saline. These results provided additional support for the role of primary renal loss of sodium and water in the development of hyponatremia in neurosurgical patients. Since the initial report by Nelson and coworkers, there have been several papers that have supported the early data.[17,68,73] Production of a brain natriuretic factor and alteration in neural control of the kidney have been proposed as possible causes of this renal dysfunction.

Patients who develop hyponatremia after CNS damage or surgery must not be assumed to have SIADH. Their volume status must be assessed; if weight loss and dehydration are evident and other conditions capable of producing hyponatremia are absent, a diagnosis of cerebral salt-wasting and treatment with volume and electrolyte replacement must be considered.[1] This also suggests that in neurosurgical patients with hyponatremia, fluid restriction could, in fact, be deleterious.[89]

REFERENCES

1. Andrews BT, Fitzgerald PA, et al.: Cerebral salt wasting after pituitary exploration and biopsy: Case report. *Neurosurgery* 18:4, 469, 1986.
2. Antunes JL, Murwzko K: The vascular supply of the hypothalamus-pituitary axis. *Acta Neurochir Suppl* 47:42, 1990.
3. Atwell WJ: The development of the hypophysis cerebri in man, with special reference to the pars tuberalis. *Am J Anat* 37:159, 1926.
4. Aubry RH, Nankin HR, et al.: Measurement of the osmotic threshold for vasopressin release in human subjects, and its modification by cortisol. *J Clin Endocrinol Metab* 25:1481, 1965.
5. Aziz LA, Forsling ML: Anaesthesia and vasopressin release in the rat. *J Endocrinol* 81:123, 1979.

6. Balesterieri F, Chernow B, et al.: Post-craniotomy diabetes insipidus—Who's at risk? *Crit Care Med* 10:108, 1982.
7. Barry J, Hoffman GE: LHRH-containing systems. In: Bjorklund A, Hokfelt T (eds): *Handbook of Chemical Neuroanatomy*, vol 4. Amsterdam, Elsevier, 1985.
8. Bartter FC, Schwartz WB: The syndrome of inappropriate secretion of antidiuretic hormone. *Am J Med* 42:790, 1967.
9. Bergland RM, Davis SL, et al.: Pituitary secretes to brain (experiment in sheep). *Lancet* 2:276, 1977.
10. Berl T: Treating hyponatremia: What is all the controversy about? *Ann Intern Med* 113:417, 1990.
11. Bighet DC, Razi M, et al.: Hemodynamic and coagulation responses to 1-desamino (8-D-arginine) vasopressin in patients with congenital nephrogenic diabetes insipidus. *N Engl J Med* 381:881, 1988.
12. Biron R, Burger A, et al.: Thyroid hormones and the energetics of active sodium-potassium transport in mammalian skeletal muscles. *J Physiol* 297:47, 1979.
13. Blum M: Myxedema coma. *Am J Med Sci* 264:432, 1972.
14. Bouzarth WF, Shenkin HA, et al.: Is cerebral hyponatraemia iatrogenic? *Lancet* 1:1061, 1982.
15. Bowerman J, Heslop I: Diabetes insipidus associated with maxillofacial injury. *Br J Oral Surg* 8:197, 1921.
16. Bray G: Freezing point depression of rat kidney slices during water diuresis and antidiuresis. *Am J Physiol* 199:915, 1960.
17. Brent GA, Heshman JM: Thyroxine therapy in patients with severe nonthyroidal illness and low serum thyroxin concentration. *J Clin Endocrinol Metab* 63:1, 1986.
18. Brownstein MJ, Russell JT, et al.: Synthesis, transport, and release of posterior pituitary hormones. *Science* 207:373, 1980.
19. Burman KD, Wartofsky L, et al.: The effect of T3 and reverse T3 administration on muscle protein catabolism during fasting as measured by 3-methyl-histidine excretion. *Metabolism* 28:805, 1979.
20. Camus J, Roussy G: Experimental researches on the pituitary body. *Endocrinology* 4:502, 1920.
21. Chernow B, Anderson DM: Endocrine responses to critical illness. *Semin Respir Med* 7:1, 1985.
22. Chernow B, Alexander HR, et al.: Hormonal responses to graded surgical stress. *Arch Intern Med* 147:1273, 1987.
23. Cobb W, Spare S, et al.: Neurogenic diabetes insipidus: management of DAVP. *Ann Intern Med* 88:183, 1978.
24. Conrad LCA, Pfaff DW: Efferents from the medial basal forebrain and hypothalamus in the rat. I. An autoradiographic study of the medial preoptic area. *J Comp Neurol* 169:185, 1976.
25. Cort JH, Yale MD, et al.: Cerebral salt wasting. *Lancet* 1:752, 1954.
26. Crawford J, Kennedy G: Clinical results of treatment of diabetes insipidus with drugs of the chlorothiazide series. *N Engl J Med* 262:737, 1960.
27. Dietemann J, Banneville J, et al.: The need for repeated CT examinations in hypothalamic-pituitary pathology. *J Neuroradiol* 12:113, 1985.
28. Edwards CRW: Vasopressin. In: Martin L, Besser GM (eds): *Clinical Neuroendocrinology*. New York, Academic Press, 1977, pp 527–567.
29. Faloon W, Reynold R, et al.: The use of the direct eosinophil count in the diagnosis and treatment of Waterhouse-Friederichsen syndrome. *N Engl J Med* 242:441, 1950.
30. Fisher C, Ingram W, et al.: Relation of hypothalamico-hypophysio system to diabetes insipidus. *Arch Neurol Psychiat* 34:124, 1935.
31. Fox JL, Falik JL, et al.: Neurosurgical hyponatremia: the role of inappropriate antidiuresis. *J Neurosurg* 34:506, 1971.
32. Gainer H: Biosynthesis of vasopressin and neurophysin. In: Reichlin S (ed): *The Neurohypophysis: Physiological and Clinical Aspects*. New York, Plenum, 1984. pp 35–50.
33. Gardner DF, Kaplan MM, et al.: The effect of the triiodothyronine replacement on the metabolic and pituitary responses to starvation. *N Engl J Med* 300:579, 1979.
34. Goldman K, Jacobs A: Anterior and posterior pituitary failure after head injury. *Br Med J* 2:1924, 1960.
35. Gorczycn W, Hardy J: Arterial supply of the human anterior pituitary gland. *Neurosurgery* 20:369, 1987.
36. Haas M, Glick SM: Radioimmunoassayable plasma vasopressin associated with surgery. *Arch Surg* 113:597, 1978.
37. Hamilton WJ, Mossman HW: *Human Embryology*, 4th ed. Cambridge, Heffer, 1982, pp 437–535.
38. Hayward JN: Functional and morphological aspects of hypothalamic neurons. *Physiol Rev* 57:574, 1977.
39. Heimer L: *The Human Brain and Spinal Cord*. Springer, New York, 1983.
40. Kaplan MM, Larsen PR, et al.: Prevalence of abnormal thyroid function test results in patients with acute medical illnesses. *Am J Med* 72:9, 1982.
41. Kaptein EM, Weiner JM, et al.: Relationship of altered thyroid hormone indices to survival in nonthyroidal illnesses. *Clin Endocrinol* 16:565, 1982.
42. Kern K, Meislin H: Diabetes insipidus: Occurrence after minor head trauma. *J Trauma* 24:69, 1984.
43. Kimmel D, O'Neill B: Systemic cancer presenting as diabetes insipidus. *Cancer* 52:2355, 1983.
44. Knigge KM, Scott DE: Structure and function of the median eminence. *Am J Anat* 129:223, 1970.
45. Ingbar SH, Woeber KA: The thyroid gland. In: Williams RH (ed): *Textbook of Endocrinology*, 6th ed. Philadelphia, WB Saunders, 1981, pp 117–247.

46. Labrie F, Godbout M, et al.: Mechanism of action of hypothalamic hormones and interaction with peripheral hormones at the pituitary level. In: Motta M (ed): *The Endocrine Functions of the Brain (Comprehensive Endocrinology)*. New York: Raven Press, 1980, pp 207–231.
47. Land HI, Schultz G, et al.: Nucleotide sequence of cloned cDNA encoding bovine arginine vasopressin-neurophysin 11 precursor. *Nature* 295:299, 1983.
48. Leader M: Atrial natriuretic peptide. *Lancet* II:371, 1986.
49. Lechan RM, Nestler JL, et al.: The tuberoinfundibular system of the rat as demonstrated by immunocytochemical localization of retrogradely transported wheat germ agglutinin from the median eminence. *Brain Res* 245:1, 1982.
50. Lester MC, Nelson PB: Neurological aspects of vasopressin release and the syndrome of inappropriate secretion of antidiuretic hormone. *Neurosurgery* 8:735, 1981.
51. Liddle C: Pathogenesis of glucocorticoid disorders. *Am J Med* 53:638, 1972.
52. Lightman SL, Everitt BJ: Water excretion. In: Lightman SL, Everitt BJ (eds): *Neuroendocrinology*. Oxford, Blackwell Scientific Publications, 1986, pp 197–206.
53. Lipsett M, MacLean J, et al.: An analysis of the polyuria induced by hypophysectomy in man. *J Clin Endocrinol Metab* 16:183, 1956.
54. Mannacci PM, Cancaini MT, et al.: Response of factor VIII/von Willebrand factor to dDAVP in healthy subjects and patients with haemophilia and von Willebrand's disease. *Br J Haematol* 47:283, 1981.
55. Massumi R, Winnacker J: Severe depression of the respiratory center in myxedema. *Am J Med* 36:876, 1964.
56. Maturo SJ, Rosenbaum RL, et al.: Variable thyrotropin response to thyrotropin releasing hormone after small decreases in plasma free thyroid hormone concentrations in patients with nonthyroidal disease. *J Clin Invest* 66:451, 1980.
57. Migeon C, Kenny F, et al.: Study of adrenal function in children with meningitis. *Pediatrics* 40:163, 1967.
58. Miller M, Dalakos T, et al.: Recognition of partial defects in antidiuretic hormone secretion. *Ann Intern Med* 73:721, 1970.
59. Miller M, Moses AM: Clinical states due to alteration of ADH release and action. In: Moses AM, Share L (eds): *Neurohypophysis*. Basel, S Karger, 1977, pp 153–161.
60. Moses A, Howanitz J, et al.: Clofibrate-induced antidiuresis. *J Clin Invest* 52:533, 1973.
61. Moses A., Numan P, et al.: Mechanism for chlorpropamide-induced antidiuresis in man. Evidence for release of ADH and enhancement of peripheral action. *Metabolism* 22:59, 1973.
62. Moses AM: Diabetes insipidus and ADH regulation. In: Krieger DT, Hughes JC (eds): *Neuroendocrinology*. Sunderland, Mass., 1980, Sindaver Assoc., p 141.
63. Moses AM: Clinical and laboratory features of central and nephrogenic diabetes insipidus and primary polydipsia. In: Reichlin S (ed): *The Neurohypophysis: Physiological and Clinical Aspects*. New York, Plenum, 1984, pp 115–138.
64. Moses A: Frontiers of hormone research. In: Czunichow P, Robinson A (eds): *Diabetes Insipidus in Man*, vol 13. Basel, Kayer, 1985.
65. Nauta WJH, Haymaker W: Hypothalamic nuclei and fiber connections. In: Haymaker W, Anderson E, Nauta WJH (eds): *The Hypothalamus*. Springfield, Ill., Charles C Thomas, 1960, pp 136–209.
66. Nelson PB, Seif SM, Maroon JC, et al.: Hyponatremia in intracranial disease: Perhaps not the syndrome of inappropriate secretion of antidiuretic hormone (SIADH). *J Neurosurg* 55:938, 1981.
67. Nelson PB, Seif SM, et al.: Hyponatremia and natriuresis following subarachnoid hemorrhage in a monkey model. *J Neurosurg* 60:233, 1984.
68. Nelson RJ: Blood volume measurement following subarachnoid haemorrhage. *Acta Neurochir Suppl* 47:114, 1990.
69. Nicoloff J: Myxedema coma and thyroid storm. *Med Clin North Am*, Sept. 1985, pp 111–116.
70. Nilaver G: Chemical anatomy of the hypothalamus. In: Zimmerman EA, Abrams GM (eds): *Neuroendocrinology and Brain Peptides*. Philadelphia, W.B. Saunders, 1986, pp 701–720.
71. Palkovits M: Neuropeptides in the median eminence: Their sources and destinations. *Peptides* 3:299, 1982.
72. Porter R, Miller R: Diabetes insipidus following closed-head injury. *J Neurol Neurosurg Psychiat* 11:258, 1948.
73. Poon WS, Mendelow AD, et al.: Secretion of antidiuretic hormone in neurosurgical patients: Appropriate or inappropriate? *Aust N Z J Surg* 53:173, 1989.
74. Rap ZM, Chwalbinska-Moneta J: Vasopressin concentration in blood during acute short-term intracranial hypertension in cats. *Adv Neurol* 20:381, 1978.
75. Reichlin S: Anatomical and physiological basis of hypothalamic-pituitary regulation. In: Post KD, Jackson IMD, Reichlin S (eds): *The Pituitary Adenoma*. New York, Plenum, 1980, pp 3–28.
76. Reichlin SS: The neurohypophysis: Historical overview. In: Reichlin S (ed): *The Neurohypophysis: Physiological and Clinical Aspects*. New York: Plenum, 1984, pp 1–4.
77. Rioch DM, Wislocki GB, et al.: A precis of preoptic, hypothalamic and hypophyseal terminology with atlas. *Res Publ Assoc Res Nerv Ment Dis* 20:3, 1939.
78. Robertson GL: The regulation of vasopressin function in health and disease. *Recent Prog Horm Res* 33:333, 1977.

79. Robinson AG: Neurophysins. In: Martini L, Besser GM (eds): *Clinical Neuroendocrinology*. New York: Academic, 1977, pp 585–602.
80. Robinson AG: The contribution of measured secretion of neurophysins to our understanding of neurohypophyseal function. In: Reichlin S (ed): *The Neurohypophysis: Physiological and Clinical Aspects*. New York: Plenum, 1984, pp 65–94.
81. Sawchenko PA, Swanson LW: The organization of noradrenergic pathways from the brainstem to the paraventricular and supraoptic nuclei in the rat. *Brain Res Rev* 4:275, 1982.
82. Schrier RW: Disorders in water metabolism. In: Schrier RW (ed): *Renal and Electrolyte Disorders*, 2d ed. Boston, Little, Brown, 1980, pp 1–64.
83. Sibbald W, Short A, et al.: Variations in adrenocortical responsiveness during severe bacterial infections. *Ann Surg* 186:29, 1977.
84. Sidman RL, Rakic P: Development of the human central nervous system. In: Haymaker W, Adams RD (eds): *Histology and Histopathology of the Nervous System*. Springfield, Ill., Charles C Thomas, 1982, pp 3–145.
85. Slag MF, Morley JE, et al.: Hypothyroxinenemia in critically ill patients as a predictor of high mortality. *JAMA* 245:43, 1981.
86. Smith JJ, Edelman FS: The role of sodium transport in thyroid thermogenesis. *Federal Proceedings* 38:2150, 1979.
87. Sterns RH: The treatment of hyponatremia: First, do no harm. *Am J Med* 88:557, 1990.
88. Swanson LW: An autoradiographic study of the efferent connections of the preoptic region in the rat. *J Comp Neurol* 167:227, 1976.
89. Swanson LW, Kuypers HGJM: The paraventricular nucleus of the hypothalamus. *J Comp Neurol* 194:555, 1980.
90. Takor TT, Pearse AGE: Neuroectodermal origin of avian hypothalamo-hypophyseal complex: The role of the ventral neural ridge. *J Embryol Exp Morphol* 34:311, 1975.
91. Teears R, Silverman E: Clinicopathologic review of 88 cases of carcinoma metastatic to the pituitary gland. *Cancer* 36:216, 1975.
92. Tobin R, Berdanier CD, et al.: Effects of thyroxine treatment on the hepatic membrane ATPase activity in rats. *J Environ Pathol Toxicol Oncol* 2:1235, 1979.
93. Utiger RD: Decreased extrathyroidal triiodothyronine production in nonthyroidal illness: Benefit or harm? *Am J Med* 69:807, 1980.
94. Van den Pol A: The magnocellular and parvocellular nucleus of rat: Intrinsic organization. *J Comp Neurol* 206:317, 1982.
95. Weissman JD, Weissman BM: Pontine myelinolysis and delayed encephalopathy following the rapid correction of acute hyponatremia. *Arch Neurol* 46:926, 1989.
96. Weitzman R, Kleeman C: The clinical physiology of water metabolism. Part II: renal mechanisms for urinary concentration: Diabetes insipidus. *West J Med* 131:486, 1979.
97. Wislocki GB, King LS: The permeability of the hypophysis and hypothalamus to vital dyes, with a study of the hypophyseal vascular supply. *Am J Anat* 58:421, 1936.
98. Zerbe RL, Baylis PH, et al.: Vasopressin function in clinical disorders of water balance. In: Beardwell C, Robertson (eds): *Butterworth International Medical Reviews, Clinical Endocrinology. I. The Pituitary*. London, Butterworth, 1981, pp 297–329.
99. Zucker A, Chernow B, et al.: Thyroid function in critically ill children. *J Pediatr* 107:552, 1985.

CHAPTER 9
Infectious Disease in Neurosurgical Intensive Care

L.D. Dickinson
J.T. Hoff

THE HOST DEFENSE SYSTEM AND MICROBIAL INVASION

Complex interactions between pathogenic microorganisms and the human host determine if an infection will develop. The ability of an organism to infect a host depends on the susceptibility of the host. Some pathogens can initiate disease in healthy individuals, whereas other, less virulent organisms cause disease only when the host defense system is compromised. An understanding of the host defense system is necessary to appreciate the possible methods of irradicating infection.

The first component of the host defense system is the epithelial barriers. Epidermis, respiratory epithelium, and gastrointestinal epithelium have evolved special mechanisms of impeding bacterial invasion. Virulent organisms have developed methods of adhering to human epithelial surface receptors and of breaching this barrier; some bacteria secrete exotoxins that damage mucosal integrity, while some viruses are selectively endocytosed by mucosal epithelium.

Once the epithelium is breached, organisms must evade a second line of host defense in the interstitial space. Compliment proteins and antibodies bind to microbes and stimulate the liberation of modulators that induce vasodilatation, stimulate leukocyte chemotaxis, and promote phagocytosis. This nonspecific inflammatory reaction is dependent on macrophages and neutrophils for microbial elimination. These cells nonspecifically phagocytose foreign particles and secrete enzymes, reactive oxygen species, and lipid-derived mediators that serve to kill microbes and may injure normal tissues in the immediate vicinity. Microbes, however, have developed complex mechanisms of evading these cellular defenses. The capsules of *Streptococcus pneumoniae* and *Hemophilus influenzae* inhibit phagocytosis. Exotoxins produced by *Streptococcus pyogenes*, *Streptococcus aureus*, and *Clostridia* kill neutrophils. Viruses and *Mycobacterium* species produce lysosomal inhibition proteins that allow them to survive in the macrophage after phagocytosis. When neutrophil populations are depressed in the host, opportunistic infections by fungi and fulminant infections by *Pseudomonas aeruginosa* become a significant problem.

Tissue macrophages, including brain microglia, are particularly critical in extenuating the inflammatory response. They produce cytokines that promote the recruitment of neutrophils to the inflammatory site, promote the growth of fibroblasts and endothelium that initiate the repair process, and activate lymphocytes that initiate the microbe-specific immune responses.

The specific immune response to an invading microbe is dependent on the host lymphocyte population, the only cells that recognize specific microbial antigens. Distinct subsets of lymphocytes perform different functions in the immune response. The helper T-lymphocyte subset, containing the CD4 surface receptor, coordinates the immune system response to infection. Signaled by macrophages through cytokines and surface presentation of microbial antigens, the CD4 T-cells secrete cytokines that activate macrophages and the cytolytic subset of T-lymphocytes to initiate the cell-mediated immune response, selectively lysing both the invading organism and infected host cells. Compromise of cell-mediated immunity is common in steroid therapy, myeloproliferative disease, transplantation, and acquired immunodeficiency syndrome (AIDS), causing difficulty in coping with intracellular pathogens like *Listeria monocytogenes*, *Cryptococcus*, *Toxoplasma*, *Aspergillus*, *Nocardia*, and *Mycobacterium* species. CD4 T-cells also initiate the humoral immune response by secreting cytokines that activate B-lymphocytes to produce microbe-specific antibodies. Deficiency in humoral immunity is frequently encountered after chemotherapy, and such patients are at risk for infections with *S. pneumoniae* and *H. influenzae*.

The importance of cytokines in inflammatory responses and immunologic function cannot be overemphasized. Table 9-1 summarizes specific effects of the well-characterized cytokines. Not all aspects of the host response to infection are beneficial to the host organism. The host defense system may be responsible for a majority of the pathology encountered in some CNS infections. Significant improvements in morbidity and mortality of CNS infections were made with the advent of antimicrobial drugs; however, greater strides may be de-

Table 9-1 A Partial List of Major Cytokines Involved in the Host Defense System

Cytokine	Source	Effects
Alpha interferon	Macrophages	Inhibits viral proliferation, activates natural killer (NK) cells
Tumor necrosis factor (TNF)	Macrophages	Stimulates the release of acute-phase reactants; stimulates the production of IL-1; induces fever, neutrophil chemotaxis, and muscle catabolism
Interleukin 1 (IL-1)	Macrophages	Activates T-cells; promotes lymphokine synthesis; induces fever, neutrophil chemotaxis
Interleukin 6 (IL-6)	Macrophages and T-cells	Stimulates growth of B- and T-cells; activates mature B-cells
Interleukin 2 (IL-2)	T-cells	Stimulates growth and activation of lymphocytes
Interleukin 4 (IL-4)	CD4 T-cells	Stimulates activation and growth of lymphocytes and macrophages
Gamma interferon	T-cells	Activates macrophages, and NK-cells
Interleukin 5 (IL-5)	T-cells	Activates eosinophils and B-cells

pendent on discovering agents that modify the nonspecific inflammatory responses or the immune responses. The pharmacology of modulators of inflammation and cytokines is a rapidly growing specialty that shows promise in improving the outcome in CNS infections.[63,100]

SYSTEMIC INFECTIONS IN NEUROINTENSIVE CARE

Pathogenesis and Prevention of Systemic Infection in Critically Ill Patients

The demands of caring for critically ill neurosurgical patients have led to the development of ICUs, functionally concentrating high-risk patients in small geographic areas. The concentration of these patients with frequent nursing intervention contributes to the spread of organisms from patient to patient. Current infection control theory considers cross infection by nurses, physicians, and other staff to be the major medium for nosocomial bacterial spread. Hands play the main role in cross infection and hand washing is "the single most important procedure for preventing nosocomial infection."[47] Unfortunately, hand washing discipline among nurses and physicians is poor.[4] Although the use of protective gowns still seems wise, other hygienic policies and practices such as the use of masks, cap, shoe covers, nebulizing disinfectants, ultraviolet lighting, sticky floor mats, fomite bacteriologic monitoring, and laminar air flow systems are now considered obsolete.[92]

All components of the host defense system can be compromised in ICU patients. Epithelial barriers are injured in multiple ways; the epidermis can be violated by trauma or surgical procedures, and mucosa can be injured by endotracheal tubes, nasogastric tubes, and urethral catheters. Due to the severity of underlying illness, indwelling vascular catheters are often necessary in ICU management and carry the risk of microbial invasion. The duration of peripheral line placement at one site and the care with which it is placed are directly related to the chance of sepsis.[106] Lines are often placed under emergency conditions. Such catheters should be replaced under more controlled, aseptic conditions as soon as it is feasible. The Center for Disease Control recommends that intravenous fluids be changed daily, that peripheral intravenous catheters and tubing be changed every 2 to 3 days, and that arterial catheters be changed every 4 days to prevent sepsis.[124] Another prophylactic measure is changing ventilator circuits every 2 days.[92] The increased use of triple-lumen central venous catheters has brought with it an increase in sepsis. A temporal relationship between the time a catheter is placed, the onset of catheter colonization, and the onset of patient sepsis has been documented, and changing centrally placed intravascular lines every 7 days decreases line-related sepsis.[139]

Critically ill patients have seriously impaired protective mechanisms for maintaining microbial homeostasis in the oropharynx. Normally, the oropharynx is colonized by nonpathogenic anaerobic bacteria (resident microflora) and occasionally low numbers of *Staphylococcus*, *Streptococcus*, and *Haemophilus* species. The growth of newly ingested pathogenic bacteria, viruses, and yeast is suppressed by the hostile environment created by this microflora and by the normal oropharyngeal reflexes of salivation and swallowing.[140] Frequently used antimicrobial agents, especially penicillins, kill the anaerobic resident microflora impairing this important defense mechanism. Neurosurgical patients frequently have impaired salivation and swallowing because of depressed consciousness. It has been shown that the acquisition of nearly all ICU nosocomial infections is dependent on antecedent colonization of the oropharnx with the infecting bacteria.

Trauma and postsurgical patients frequently develop ileus and it has been shown that peristalsis helps to limit colonization of the GI tract with pathogenic microbes. Commonly used in comatose patients to decrease stomach acidity for ulcer prophylaxis, antacids and H_2 antagonists have been shown to contribute to the colonization of the stomach with pathogenic gram-negative bacteria.[135] Colonization is common in ICU patients 24 to 48 h after admission and usually precedes oropharyngeal colonization. Recent studies have shown that raising the pH to greater than 4 with antacids and H_2 antagonists has no detectable benefit on ulcer formation.[112] With the advent of effective gastric protective agents like sucralafate, it has been suggested that the routine use of antacids and H_2 antagonists for ulcer prophylaxis should be discontinued.[135]

The gag and cough reflexes help preserve asepsis in the bronchopulmonary system. These defense mechanisms are frequently depressed or absent in neurosurgical patients, promoting aspiration. Procedures such as nasogastric tub placement and airway intubation can also introduce pathogenic oropharyngeal microbes into the pulmonary system. It has been hypothesized that nosocomial infections in ICU patients can be prevented by suppressing colonization of the oropharynx with pathogenic bacteria and fungi. Studies investigating selective flora suppression have demonstrated reductions in gram-negative colonization and systemic nosocomial infections in several prospective, controlled studies.[3,56,67,77,133] The incidence of nosocomial pneumonia in critically ill, intubated patients decreased from 18 to 59 percent to 3 to 8 percent with local application of tobramycin, polymixin E, and amphotericin B as a paste to the oropharynx and as an aqueous solution down the gastric tube. Less dramatic, but significant decreases have also been reported in the incidence of urinary tract infections and bacteremia with this regimen. There have been no reports of the development of resistant gram-negative bacillary strains to these nonabsorbed enteral antimicrobials. Certainly, this therapy would be appropriate in a subpopulation of neurosurgical ICU patients that classically have prolonged intubation such as severe traumatic brain injury patients and poor grade SAH patients.

In summary, approaches to infection prophylaxis in the ICU include minimizing risk, preventing cross-infection, ensuring optimum aseptic technique, and instituting prompt therapy when infection develops.

Pneumonia

As previously mentioned, depressed levels of consciousness coupled with the need for endotracheal intubation predispose critically ill neurosurgical patients to the development of nosocomial pulmonary infection. Fever, rales, peripheral leukocytosis, and increasing hypoxemia are the usual presenting signs. Chest roentgenograms may show a new infiltrate, but other underlying pulmonary processes may make x-ray interpretation difficult. A good sputum Gram stain with few contaminating squamous epithelial cells is essential; the presence of a large number of neutrophils supports the diagnosis of pneumonia, and a predominant organism can usually be seen.

Treatment of pneumonia should be guided by sputum culture results. Pending culture results, knowledge of local epidemiology is often useful in selecting initial therapy. Often a particular organism will "circulate" in an ICU; awareness of its expected antimicrobial susceptibility should guide early therapy. If no predominant organism is encountered in a particular ICU, a common approach is to treat empirically for the most difficult possible organism, *P. aeruginosa*, pending culture results. An antipseudomonal penicillin in combination with an aminoglycoside, or monotherapy with ceftazidime, is recommended. *S. aureus* can be encountered as a cause of pulmonary infection and the presence of organisms morphologically compatible with staphylococcus required adding a penicillinase-resistant, beta-lactam antibiotic or vancomycin.

Vigorous pulmonary toilet and adequate hydration are important adjuvant measures, although hydration may be contraindicated in some neurosurgical patients. The use of oscillating beds has been shown to be beneficial in prophylaxis of pneumonia in blunt trauma patients and we have found it to be a useful adjuvant treatment once pulmonary infection develops.[40] Despite aggressive therapy, mortality remains high for nosocomial pneumonia.

Sinusitis

Sinusitis can be difficult to diagnose in critically ill patients unable to complain of pain or tenderness. Nosocomial sinusitis should be considered in patients with unexplained fever and leukocytosis.[24] Major risk factors include nasogastric and nasotracheal tubes, especially if intubation is prolonged.[35] Skull fractures and nasal packing can be contributing factors. The traditional upper respiratory pathogens *H. influenzae* and *S. pneumoniae* can be involved, but nosocomial gram-negative pathogens are common. Sinusitis requires prompt therapy since intracranial complications, including osteomyelitis, subdural empyema, meningitis, and brain abscess, have an approximate 4 percent incidence.[29]

Genitourinary Infections

Infections of the urinary tract are common in the ICU setting and are frequently the focus for secondary bacteremia. Bladder catheterization is primarily responsible for the development of bacteriuria. The risk of infection is correlated with the duration of bladder catheterization and lack of maintenance of a closed urinary drainage system.[71] Every effort should be made to minimize the duration of catheterization and to use aseptic technique when collecting specimens. The use of prophylactic antimicrobials and antibiotics is not effective for maintaining sterility of indwelling catheters. Urinalysis and cultures remain the cornerstones of diagnosis. The most common infecting pathogens are the enteric gram-negative rods, *P. aeruginosa* and *Streptococcus faecalis.*

Bacteremia

Bacteremia in the severely ill patient is most often secondary to a focus in the urinary tract, skin, soft tissue, or lungs. When no obvious focus can be identified, an infected intravascular device should be suspected and semiquantitative culturing of catheter tips performed.[85] Organisms such as *Staphylococcus epidermidis, S. aureus*, and *Candida* species are the common pathogens; however, gram-negative bacilli must always be taken into account. One approach to presumptive therapy for suspected bacteremia due to an intravascular device combines vancomycin with a third generation cephalosporin, the former agent to provide activity for *S. epidermidis*, as well as the increasingly important methicillin-resistant *S. aureus* isolates encountered in many hospitals. Therapy is then adjusted when culture and sensitivity results are available.

BACTERIAL INFECTIONS OF THE CENTRAL NERVOUS SYSTEM

Subgaleal Abscess

Subgaleal abscess is a localized infection between the galea of the scalp and the pericranium. The process is usually initiated by contamination of a scalp wound by staphylococci, streptococci, or anaerobic organisms. Localized scalp tenderness and swelling are signs of abscess formation. Fever, lymphadenopathy, and facial swelling suggests regional and systemic spread of the infection. Infection rarely extends intracranially unless the skull has been penetrated. Osteomyelitis of the skull occasionally occurs secondarily. Treatment includes open drainage and debridement coupled with systemic antibiotics.

Osteomyelitis

Osteomyelitis of the skull may develop from extension of a local infection, such as sinusitis or mastoiditis, from direct contamination of the skull at operation or after trauma, or rarely, by hematogenous spread from a distant source such as the respiratory or urinary tract. An established skull infection may extend inward to produce an epidural abscess or outward into the subgaleal space.[134] The usual pathogens are staphylococci and anaerobic streptococci. Occasionally, gram-negative organisms and fungi are responsible. Treatment consists of drainage, debridement of infected bone, and appropriate antibiotics for at least 6 weeks. Erythrocyte sedimentation rate and skull x-rays are valuable in following the response to therapy.

Osteomyelitis of the spine usually presents with pain and is acute in children and more insidious in adults. Myelopathy or radiculopathy are presenting symptoms in approximately 50 percent of patients. Magnetic resonance imaging (MRI) is extremely valuable in detecting spinal cord compression in patients with neurologic deficit. Surgical intervention is indicated for all patients with neurologic deficit and biopsy is often necessary to confirm the diagnosis and identify the causative organism. *S. aureus* is the most common pathogen; however, gram-negative infections made up 16.7 percent of cases in a recent series.[103] Successful treatment depends on isolating the causative organism and requires at least 6 to 8 weeks of intravenous antibiotics combined with immobilization (bedrest and rigid orthosis) for pain reduction.[23,103] Again, serial sedimentation rates and spine films are valuable for following response to therapy.

Epidural Abscess

Isolated intracranial infection of the epidural space is a rare complication of traumatic or operative contamination of epidural tissue. More commonly, it results from extension of adjacent osteomyelitis. If the dura is intact, infection rarely extends transdurally. Treatment consists of drainage, debridement, and systemic antibiotics.

Spinal epidural abscess is more common and is usually a surgical emergency. It is characterized by fever, local spinal tenderness, and the rapid progression of neurologic deficits. Radicular pain and myelopathy often occur within a few days of the initial symptoms. Most epidural abscesses are caused by local extension of vertebral osteomyelitis and rarely by hematogenous spread from a distant infection. The CSF shows markedly elevated protein levels and mild pleocytosis. A myelogram or MRI defines the extent of the epidural mass. The most common causative organism is *S. aureus* and, occasionally, *Streptococcus* species.[65] Gram-negative bacilli are commonly isolated in intravenous drug abusers. *Mycobacterium tuberculosis* is still a principal cause of epidural abscess in many parts of the world. Treatment includes urgent laminectomy and abscess drainage followed by prolonged specific antibiotic therapy. Recovery of neurologic function is directly related to the duration and severity of impairment prior to surgery.[65,142]

Subdural Empyema

Subdural empyema, purulent infection of the subdural space, arises by direct extension through the meninges during meningitis in neonates and infants or as a complication of paranasal sinusitis or otitis in children and young adults. Rare cases of hematogenous spread from distant infection and direct contamination from trauma have also been reported.[12] The diagnosis of intracranial subdural empyema is based on clinical and radiographic findings.[53] Headache, fever, and meningismus are common complaints that can be present for 1 to 8 weeks prior to presentation.[12] Seizures and focal deficits are also common. CT and MRI readily document subdural collections; however, the mass may be isodense on CT, necessitating contrast enhancement for visualization. These imaging studies are also helpful in diagnosing concurrent sinus or mastoid infection as the etiology. The risk of lumbar puncture in a patient suspected of harboring an intracranial mass is sufficiently great to countermand the test until CT scanning has confirmed the absence of intracranial mass effect. Spinal fluid analysis is rarely diagnostic, but may show nonspecific inflammatory changes.[83]

Otorhinologic sources of subdural empyema are usually caused by streptococci, staphylococci, and anaerobic cocci.[66] Paranasal sinus disease is the most common etiologic factor in the western literature. Once the subdural space is violated, infection commonly spreads over the convexity of the brain and into the interhemispheric and Sylvian fissures. Infratentorial spread occurs in 3 to 10 percent of infections, always secondary to extension of otitis.[17] The accumulation of pus may be sufficient to produce an intracranial mass. The intense inflammatory response provokes brain swelling and edema. The clinical result is rapid neurologic deterioration, often with focal deficits, coma, and death.

Subdural empyema secondary to meningitis is commonly bilateral and less fulminant than empyema secondary to an otorhinologic infection. *H. influenzae* is the predominant organism; however, *S. pneumoniae* empyema is also commonly reported. Communicating hydrocephalus may develop when CSF resorption over the cerebral convexities is disrupted by the infection.

Prior to the advent of penicillin, subdural empyema was uniformly fatal.[12] With the use of systemic antibiotics and surgical drainage, an overall mortality rate of 25 percent was found, with poor outcomes strongly correlating with depression of consciousness prior to instituting therapy and inability to identify the pathogenic organism.[12] Bannister et al. recommended primary craniotomy with wide exposure, aggressive subdural exploration, and careful debridement of purulent material from the brain surface.[12] Two recent reports have demonstrated a significant reduction in poor outcome and mortality with a craniotomy procedure when compared to bur hole drainage.[39,88]

The source of the infection must also be treated aggressively, and a sinus or mastoid drainage procedure is often required.[66] Prophylactic use of anticonvulsants is recommended because of the high incidence of seizures.[53] Successful nonsurgical management of subdural empyema has recently been reported and a trial of antibiotic therapy alone has been advocated in patients with preserved neurologic status; normal neurologic exam; and a single, localized lesion on CT.[80,104]

Spinal subdural empyema is rare. It usually develops from local transdural extension from vertebral osteomyelitis, or through the arachnoid in the presence of meningitis. Spinal cord compression and transverse myelitis may develop. Treatment is emergent drainage by laminectomy and prolonged antibiotic administration.

Bacterial Meningitis

Bacterial meningitis is a purulent infection of the subarachnoid space. It is usually an acute, fulminating illness characterized by fever, headache, nausea, vomiting, and nuchal rigidity. Coma occurs in about 5 to 10 percent of cases and its development carries a poor prognosis. Seizures occur in approximately 20 percent of patients, and cranial nerve palsies in 5 percent. Untreated bacterial meningitis is almost always fatal. CSF classically shows polymorphonuclear leukocytosis, elevated protein, and depressed glucose; a Gram stain of the CSF demonstrates the causative organism in 75 percent of cases. CSF culture provides a diagnosis in 90 percent of cases and is indispensable in characterizing the antibiotic sensitivity profile of the microbe. Depressed level of consciousness, especially when associated with papilledema or focal neurologic deficits, should lead the investigator to CT evaluation prior to lumbar puncture to rule out a mass lesion or hydrocephalus. Diffuse intracranial hypertension, in the absence of a mass lesion, is not a contraindication to lumbar puncture. Physical evaluation should include careful examination for contiguous sites of inflammation such as otitis and sinusitus and for etiologies of bacteremia like endocarditis. Blood cultures may be positive.

Animal experiments suggest that the primary etiology of bacterial meningitis is leptomeningeal invasion by blood-borne bacteria that colonized the nasopharyngeal mucosa of the host. The common meningeal pathogens are all encapsulated bacteria. After colonizing the nasopharynx, the encapsulated bacteria traverse the epithelium and gain access to the bloodstream. Encapsulation inhibits phagocytosis by neutrophils, thus common meningeal pathogens demonstrate the ability to maintain a transient bacteremia. The subsequent mechanism by which bacteria in the bloodstream gain access to the leptomeninges and subarachnoid space is largely unknown.

Another source of bacterial meningitis is direct extension from otorhinologic infections, although its incidence has declined markedly with the advent of effective early antibiotic therapy of otitis and sinusitis. Infrequently, meningitis is caused by direct inoculation during penetrating trauma.

The treatment for acute bacterial meningitis, outlined in Table 9-2, depends on the primary source of the infection, the age of the patient, the causative organism, and its antibiotic sensitivity.[32,90,138] Treatment should be directed to both the CSF infection and the primary source. Meningitis that occurs secondary to bacteremia and direct otorhinal extension tends to be caused by organisms frequently seeding the nasopharynx. There is a significant age dependence for meningitis by these organisms. Meningitis occurring after a traumatic brain injury and skull fracture, with or without CSF otorhinorrhea, is most often caused by *S. pneumoniae*. Meningitis that develops following a penetrating wound is usually caused by staphylococcal, streptococcal, or gram-negative organisms.

Empiric therapy is subsequently modified when the causative organism is identified (Table 9-3). Penicillin G and ampicillin have been found to be equally efficacious in the majority of *S. pneumoniae* and *N. meningitidis* infection. The increasing prevalence of beta-lactamase producing *H. influenzae*, currently around 25 percent, led to the adoption of the ampicillin and chloramphenicol regimen for empiric therapy. Ceftriaxone or cefotaxime has been shown to be as efficacious and is now endorsed as the treatment of choice in neonates and children.[138,150] Although cefuroxime, a second generation cephalosporin, had been commonly used for *H. influenzae*, it is no longer recommended for CNS infections because of delayed CSF sterilization and a report of *H. influenzae* meningitis developing during systemic therapy.[7,33,76] *L. monocytogenes* is not sensitive to cephalosporins and the recommended treatment is ampicillin or penicillin G. An alternative is trimethoprim-sulfamethoxazole. Patients with *S. aureus* meningitis should be treated with nafcillin or oxacillin, with vancomycin being reserved for methicillin-resistant strains and *S. epidermidis*.

Table 9-2 Meningitis: Causative Organisms and Empiric Therapy by Source of Infection and Age

Source	Common organisms	Empiric therapy
Spontaneous age		
Neonate	*E. Coli*, group B streptococci, *L. monocytogenes*	Ampicillin + ceftriaxone or ampicillin + gentamycin
1–3 months	*E. Coli*, group B streptococci, *L. monocytogenes*, *H. influenzae*, *S. pneumoniae*	Ampicillin + ceftriaxone or ampicillin + chloramphenicol
3 months–18 years	*H. influenzae*, *N. meningitidis*, *S. pneumoniae*	Ceftriaxone or ampicillin + chloramphenicol
18–50 years	*S. pneumoniae*, *N. meningitidis*	Ampicillin or penicillin G
Over 50 yeras	*S. pneumoniae*, *N. meningitidis*, *L. monocytogenes*, gram-negative bacilli	Ampicillin + ceftriaxone
Injury		
Closed skull (±CSF Leak)	*S. pneumoniae*, other streptococcus, *H. influenzae*	Ampicillin + ceftriaxone
Penetrating	*S. aureaus*, *S. epidermidis*. Streptococcus spp, gram-negative bacilli	Vancomycin + ceftriaxone
Postoperative		
	S. aureaus, *S. epidermidis*. gram-negative bacilli	Vancomycin + ceftriaxone

Table 9-3 Specific CNS Bacterial Pathogens and Antimicrobial Therapy

Organism	Drug of choice	Alternatives
Streptococcus pneumoniae	Penicillin G (or ampicillin)	TGC, chloramphenicol
S. pyogenes	Penicillin G	TGC, chloramphenicol
S. group B	Penicillin G ± gentamycin	TGC, chloramphenicol
S. faecalis	Penicillin G + gentamycin	Vancomycin + gentamycin
Staphylococcus aureus		
Methicillin-sensitive	Nafcillin	Oxacillin, vancomycin
Methicillin-resistant	Vancomycin	Trimethoprim-sulfamethoxazole, ciprofloxicin
Staphylococcus epidermidis	Vancomycin ± rifampin	Teicoplanin
Listeria monocytogenes	Ampicillin ± aminoglycoside	Trimethoprim-sulfamethoxazole
Clostridium difficile	Vancomycin	Metronidazole
N. meningitidis	Penicillin G	Chloramphenicol, TGC
H. Influenza		
Beta-lactamase-negative	Ampicillin	TGC
Beta-lactamase-positive	Ceftriaxone	Chloramphenicol
Enterobacteriaceae (Escherichia, Klebsiella Proteus, Serratia)	Ceftriaxone	Pipercillin + aminoglycoside
P. aeruginosa	Ceftazidime ± aminogycoside	Pipercillin + aminoglycoside, imipenem
Bacteroides	Metronidizole	Clindamycin, vancomycin

TGC-third-generation cephalesporin; ceftraxone, cefotaxine, ceftazidine have been evaluated in CNS infection.

Duration of therapy for meningitis is generally empiric and based on tradition; usually 7 to 14 days for the major meningeal pathogens, and 21 days for gram-negative bacillary infections are recommended.[138]

The treatment of gram-negative bacillary meningitis has been revolutionized by the development of third generation cephalosporins. Cefotaxime, ceftazidime, and ceftriaxone penetrate into CSF to produce therapeutic concentrations allowing treatment of many episodes of gram-negative meningitis previously requiring intrathecal therapy; 78 to 94 percent cure rates in small series have been reported.[27,64,72,101] Ceftriaxone, cefotaxime, and ceftazidime have proven efficacy. Other third-generation cephalosporins, ceftizoxime and cefoperazone, have not been thoroughly evaluated. It has been recommended that ceftazidine be reserved for treatment of *P. aeruginosa* in combination with an aminoglycoside. Failure of these regimens may necessitate intrathecal or intraventricular delivery of aminoglycoside to augment therapy.

Modification of subarachnoid space inflammation by anti-inflammatory agents may lessen many of the consequences of bacterial meningitis. Recent studies of adjunctive dexamethasone therapy in infants and children with bacterial meningitis show that the incidence of long-term neurologic sequelae, particularly mental retardation and hearing loss, are lower in those treated with 0.15 mg/kg dexamethasone intravenously every 6 h for the first 4 days of therapy, and it did not adversely affect the eradication of infection.[75] A collaborative double-blind, placebo-controlled study is underway. The use of dexamethasone has been recommended in pediatric patients older than 2 months until the results of the study are known.[11,115]

Brain Abscess

Brain abscess is a circumscribed collection of purulent infection within brain parenchyma. The time course and sequential changes that occur during abscess formation have been characterized in the dog by Britt et al.[18] Acute inflammatory cells develop a center of necrotic material, surrounded by a zone of cerebritis. With maturation, a peripheral neovascularization develops and evolves into a ring of collagen-depositing fibroblasts and macrophages, terminating in a well-formed capsule. Whether cerebritis evolves into an encapsulated abscess depends upon the host-organism interaction and the effect of treatment rendered. In humans with a competent immune system the process from bacterial infiltration to encapsulated abscess takes approximately 2 weeks.[118,145] The weakest site of capsule tends to be the less vascular surface facing the ventricle; therefore, centrifugal migration of the inflammatory process with ventricular rupture and death was a common sequelae in the presurgical era.

Signs and symptoms of brain abscess are commonly related to its mass effect. Headache, focal neurologic deficits, and impaired mentation are often seen. Fever is present approximately 50 percent of the time, but there may be little or no evidence of systemic infection.[53] Seizure is present in 25 to 60 percent of patients.[53,110,151] Brain edema, mass effect, and midline shift are common; therefore, lumbar puncture is usually contraindicated and of little clinical value since CSF culture is positive in less than 10 percent of cases.

Brain abscess commonly occurs secondary to infection elsewhere, and the bacteriology is often reflective of the primary source. As with subdural empyema, direct intracranial extension from paranasal sinus or ear infections is the predominant etiology. These lesions are typically solitary and found in the frontal lobes with frontoethmoid sinusitis, temporal lobes with maxillary sinusitis, and cerebellum or temporal lobe with otologic infections.[8,29,151] Multiple brain abscesses suggest a hematogenous seeding from a distant source and common systemic infections such as bacterial endocarditis, cyanotic congenital heart disease, pneumonia, and diverticulitis should be investigated. Hematogenous spread, especially from endocarditis, may also be associated with pyogenic intracranial aneurysms.[13]

Direct contamination of the brain through a penetrating brain wound is another cause of abscess.[1,114] Indriven bone fragments and other debris are commonly found in patients with traumatic brain infection.

Abscess formation is infrequent during the course of bacterial meningitis, but is a predisposing factor in 25 percent of pediatric brain abscesses which are usually associated with neonatal *Citrobacter* or *Proteus* meningitis.[110,119] Conversely, brain abscess is frequently encountered among patients with compromised immunity secondary to chronic steroid use, lymphoproliferative disease, and organ transplantation, and these abscesses tend to be multiple.[105]

The most commonly identified organisms in brain abscesses are *Streptococcus*, *Staphylococcus*, and *Bacteroides* species, with multiple organisms present in 10 to 20 percent of cases.[86,151] Empiric antibiotic therapy based on the location of the lesion and primary source has been proposed[119]; however, the severity of the disease and the frequent occurrence of unexpected organisms has led others to recommend broad gram-positive, gram-negative, and anaerobic antibiotic coverage as empiric therapy in all cases.[53]

CT imaging is highly accurate for detecting a brain abscess. By improving early detection and allowing accurate localization, CT imaging is primarily responsible for the decrease in mortality rate from 30 to 50 percent of cases to less than 15 percent in the last two decades.[86,118]

The goals of therapy are early establishment of the responsible microbial agent and its antibiotic sensitivity, sterilization of the CNS and the primary infection, rapid correction of mass effect, and resolution of brain edema. Controversy exists as to the indication for surgery, the type of surgical intervention, and the adjuvant role of steroids. During cerebritis and the early stage of encapsulization, or in high surgical risk patients with small abscesses and a known causative organism, medical therapy with the appropriate parenteral antibiotic may be sufficient.[117] Otherwise, the preferred course of treatment is surgical drainage of the purulent material by either aspiration or excision and a minimum of 4 weeks of antibiotics.[132] Surgery reduces the mass effect and thereby reduces the most critical and dangerous aspect of this infection. Surgery also identifies the causative organism in 60 to 80 percent of cases, provided that cultures are processed carefully for both aerobic and anaerobic organisms. It is recommended that preoperative antibiotics not be given when an operation can be performed without delay because sterile cultures correlate with their use.[86] Although surgical excision has been shown to have a lower recurrence rate, most authorities currently recommend ultrasound or CT-guided stereotactic aspiration of brain abscesses, reserving excision for solitary, superficial lesions, those that contain a foreign body, or those that fail aspiration.[53,86,110,131]

Postoperative Infections

All of the pyogenic infections described in this section may develop after neurosurgical procedures. While drainage of an infected wound is a time-honored surgical principle, that method must be modified when applied to infections of the CNS. Since the dura is a critical barrier between the CSF and the external environment, drainage of an infected neurosurgical wound cannot be instituted unless the dura is sealed.

Subdural empyema can be a serious postoperative complication after bur hole exploration, craniotomy, or halo pin placement.[46] The infection is usually confined to the operative site and is commonly caused by *S. aureus* and *S. epidermidis*. It is rarely fulminant and is often detected by its subgaleal extension. Treatment includes debridement, drainage, and antibiotics. If a bone plate exists, it should be removed.

Meningitis complicates approximately 0.34 percent of cases following craniotomy, and is usually caused by *S. aureus* and *S. epidermidis* and gram-negative rods.[19] Postcraniotomy gram-negative bacillary meningitis is a serious infection usually caused by highly resistant organisms such as *Pseudomonas*, *Enterobacter*, and *Klebsiella* species. Mortality approaches 70 percent and requires prompt institution of antibiotic therapy. Vancomycin combined with a third-generation cephalosporin provides a broad spectrum of activity while awaiting specific pathogen identification. Intraventricular aminoglycosides are probably justified in critically ill patients.[94]

Eradication of infection becomes more difficult when prosthetic material or CSF shunt apparatus is involved. Shunt infection rates in recent studies range from 5 to 15 percent of the shunt procedures performed, involving 15 to 25 percent of hydrocephalic patients with shunts.[5,111,144,152,155] *S. epidermidis* and *S. aureus* are the most frequently identified organisms; however, in infants, *Enterobacteriaceae* species are also encountered.

In general, a foreign body should be removed when infection is discovered.[61,144] Sometimes, however, infections can be cleared in the presence of a shunt, provided the infection is indolent and the shunt essential.[44,49] Combined systemic and intrathecal antibiotics are usually necessary to cure the infection and salvage the shunt or prosthetic material. Pending a sensitivity profile, current therapy for shunt infections caused by *S. epidermidis* is vancomycin, for *S. aureus* is intravenous nafcillin, and for gram-negative enteric bacilli is a third-generation cephalosporin such as cefotaxime. When the patient fails to respond to antibiotic therapy promptly, removal of all hardware and external CSF drainage is required to eradicate the infection.

Operative Prophylaxis

The risk of postoperative wound infection following clean neurosurgical procedures is 2 to 5 percent in most hospitals in the absence of antibiotic prophylaxis. The use of antibiotics in clean neurosurgical cases remains controversial, despite several prospective studies showing a reduction in the wound infection rate with antibiotic prophylaxis.[16,22,37,48,122,154] Antibiotics should be administered prior to skin incision; no benefit has been documented with postoperative dosing. The commonly used agents are those that show good bacteriocidal activity against staphylococcus infection, penicillinase-resistant penicillins, second-generation cephalosporins, and vancomycin.

Antibiotics for Infections in Neurosurgical Patients

The need to provide broad spectrum activity usually leads to combination empiric therapy, which is changed to more specific therapy based on culture and sensitivity results. In the critically ill patient with CNS infection, an additional feature of therapy in some situations is the need for CNS penetration. Table 9-3 summarizes well-tested therapy options following organism identification prior to confirmation of sensitivity.[32,90,116,123,138] The parenteral dose of antibiotics is summarized in Table 9-4.

Ampicillin and penicillin G achieve good CSF levels in the face of inflammation and are most commonly used in neurosurgical settings for treating meningitis. The penicillinase-resistant penicillins such as methicillin, nafcillin, and oxacillin are central to the treatment of suspected or proven *S. aureus* infection. These compounds have no activity against gram-negative bacilli or *S. faecalis*, but do inhibit *S. pyogenes* and *S. pneumoniae* at achievable concentrations.

Methicillin-resistant *S. aureus* strains appear to have altered penicillin-binding proteins making

Table 9-4 Antibiotic Doses for CNS Infection in Adults

Antibiotic	Daily dose	Dosing inverval (h)
Penicillin G	20–40 million units	4
Ampicillin	12 g	4
Nafcillin, oxacillin	9–12	4
Vancomycin	2 g	12
Pipercillin	300 mg/kg body weight	4
Ceftriazone	50 mg/kg body weight	12
Cefotaxime	12 g	4
Ceftizoxime	6–9 g	8
Ceftazidime	6–12 g	8
Gentamycin, tobramycin	5 mg/kg body weight	8
Amikacin	14 mg/kg body weight	8
Trimethoprin/sulfamethoxazole	10 mg (Tmp)/kg body weight	12
Chloramphenicol	4–6 g	6
Metronidazole	30 mg/kg body weight	6

them resistant to all penicillins and cephalosporins. Vancomycin, a glycopeptide antibiotic, is the only antibiotic that consistently shows sensitivity to this strain and to coagulase-negative *S. epidermidis*. A newer glycopeptide, teicoplanin, is eliminated more slowly, is better tolerated, and is more potent than vancomycin.

The antipseudomonal penicillins play a role in therapy of ICU infections because of the frequency of *P. aeruginosa* in various clinical circumstances. Piperacillin is active against *P. aeruginosa* and also provides activity for other gram-negative pathogens such as *Klebsiella* and *Enterobacter*. The expanded spectrum of piperacillin has made it a popular agent in ICU settings, most commonly in combination with an aminoglycoside.

The third-generation cephalosporins have provided a major advance in therapy of complicated neurosurgical patients. Cefotaxime and cetriaxone have good CSF penetration, allowing treatment of many episodes of gram-negative meningitis previously requiring intrathecal therapy. *Klebsiella, Proteus, Serratia*, and *Enterobacter* species are usually sensitive to these extended spectrum cephalosporins. The concentrations achieved are not sufficient to be predictably active for staphylococci, however.

Metronidazole provides excellent activity for anaerobic bacteria including *B. fragilis* and penetrates the CNS well. Neurotoxicity including ataxia has been noted and can be confusing when this agent is used in a regimen for CNS infection, but fortunately these side effects are rare. In addition to excellent *B. fragilis* activity, clindamycin is a good antistaphylococcal agent.

Other unproven but promising antibiotics in the treatment of resistant gram-negative CNS infections include fluoroquinolones, imipenum, and aztreonam.

VIRAL INFECTIONS OF THE CENTRAL NERVOUS SYSTEM

Viruses are obligate intracellular parasites that carry only one type of nucleic acid. They are classified according to their nucleic acid type and subdivided by the size and shape of their protein coat. There are 10 groups of RNA viruses and 5 groups of DNA viruses. All RNA viruses replicate in the cell cytoplasm while DNA viruses, except poxviruses, replicate in the cell nucleus. Not every virus-cell contact leads to infection. Susceptible cells have appropriate receptor sites on their cytoplasmic membranes to match the polypeptide attachment molecule on the viral surface.[28] Selective vulnerability of a species or of a particular cell type to a given virus appears to be dependent upon these receptor sites.

Viruses usually enter the body through the mucous membranes of the respiratory, gastrointestinal, or urinary tracts. The epidermis is an effective barrier to viral entry, and a breach in the skin, as in animal bites or hypodermic injection, is necessary for transmission through this barrier. While some viruses remain confined to these susceptible surfaces, others are capable of wide dissemination through the lymphatic and circulatory systems. Viral entry into the CNS occurs along peripheral nerves and via the bloodstream. A peripheral neural route is very important in the migration and dissemination of rabies virus, herpes simplex, and varicella zoster. However, most viral infections of the CNS occur as the result of viremia. In the presence of a robust viremia, viruses reach brain parenchyma despite the blood-brain barrier created by endothelial cells. Viruses may be transported through the endothelial cells or may attack and infect them. Once the particles have gained entry into the CNS, they must reach susceptible cells that they can successfully infect. Not all cell types of the CNS are vulnerable to attack by a given virus and progression of the disease would be halted unless the virus contacts the appropriate cell receptor.

The production of clinical neurologic disease is dependent on the effects of the virus on the invaded susceptible cells. Herpes simplex causes such profound changes in cellular protein metabolism as to lead to early cell death. Other viruses may produce little change in the essential cellular metabolism but cause alterations in functional metabolism, such as the production of enzymes and neural transmitters, leading to major abnormalities of specialized neural physiologic functions. Yet other viruses may persist for long periods in the CNS before producing any evidence of disease. This long latency is most commonly seen with DNA viruses and is associated with chronic infections such as subacute sclerosing panencephalitis due to the measles virus and progressive multifocal leukoencephalopathy caused by papovavirus.

The wide variation of symptoms in viral diseases is due to the differing vulnerability of CNS cell populations to the various viruses. The high degree of specialization and complexity of CNS cell membranes may explain the unique vulnerability of certain groups of neurons and glia to a specific virus. For example, rabies virus involves the limbic system neurons but not neocortical neurons, papovaviruses selectively attack oligodendrocytes, and herpes virus has a predilection to the temporal lobes but can successfully infect a wide variety of cell types. Most viral infections of the CNS are caused by viruses common in the general population and are usually associated with a benign and self-limited course. Antibodies for the common viral causes of CNS infections are widely prevalent. This fact indicates that CNS infections are not due simply to an encounter with viral agents, but rather to breakdown in the usual host-defense mechanisms. The major therapeutic advance has been the development of killed and attenuated viral strains for immunization against polio, mumps, and measles.

Viral meningitis, the most common viral infection of the CNS, presents as an aseptic meningitis. Enteroviral meningitis can begin abruptly with no prodrome, a course occasionally resembling a mild SAH, and may lead to initial neurosurgical referral. As with meningitis, viral encephalitis is usually mild and self-limited; however, it may present with depressed levels of consciousness, seizures, focal weakness or paralysis, and rarely, cerebellar signs such as ataxia or nystagmus.[91] Serious consequences and even death can occur from herpes simplex encephalitis, the equine encephalitides, and polio.

Viral diseases and viral-associated diseases that may be encountered in neurosurgical practice include herpes simplex encephalitis, Jakob-Creutzfeldt disease, Reye's syndrome, and HIV infection. These will be considered in greater detail. Specific drugs for the treatment of viral diseases have generally been disappointing, but a number of newer agents have shown promise in early clinical investigation and will be discussed with respect to these diseases.

Herpes Simplex Encephalitis

Herpes simplex is a DNA virus with two antigenically distinct subtypes designated HSV type 1 and HSV type 2. HSV-1, spread by respiratory droplets and saliva, is best known as the agent of the ubiquitous and benign recurrent cold sore of the oral mucosa. Approximately 90 percent of adults have circulating antibodies to HSV-1 and about 25 percent have recurrent cold sores. For reasons that are currently unknown, this virus at times demonstrates enhanced CNS virulence and causes a localized, necrotizing encephalitis in children and adults. HSV-2, spread by sexual contact, is the cause of genital mucosal lesions and can be a devastating systemic infection in the newborn. A diffuse HSV-2 encephalitis can be a part of this process. Neonatal herpes is thought to be transferred from the mother during passage through an infected birth canal.

An important characteristic of HSV-1 is its ability to remain in a dormant, asymptomatic state for long periods of time in the cell bodies of trigeminal ganglion sensory neurons, reappearing intermittently in the form of mucocutaneous lesions around the mouth. The virus appears to reach the trigeminal ganglia by retrograde axoplasmic transport up the axons supplying the area of the oral lesion. The dormant virus can be reactivated by a variety of stimuli including fever, injury, exposure to ultraviolet light, and trauma to the trigeminal nerve; to produce a new skin lesion, presumably by centrifugal movement of virus particles down the sensory axon. No virus particles or viral antigens can be demonstrated in the trigeminal ganglia during the dormant state. The viral DNA is thus preserved without production of viral particles and without affecting the cellular integrity of metabolism of the sensory neurons. After stimulation, however, viral replication takes place rapidly.

HSV-1 encephalitis is the most common cause of fatal sporadic encephalitis in the United States. Untreated, the mortality rate is about 70 percent, much higher than most encephalitides.[148] The relationship of HSV-1 encephalitis to oral herpes infection is unclear. Although some patients have an active oral lesion at the time of onset of encephalitis, this is by no means common. A past history of herpetic lesions is present in 25 percent of encephalitis cases, a similar percentage as the general population. The mechanism of CNS infection involves HSV-1 invasion of the nasal epithelium and migration along axons of the olfactory tract to the temporal lobes.[95] The encephalitic process, generally most serious in the inferior frontal and temporal lobes, involves invasion and subsequent lysis of both glial and neuronal cells.

About 90 percent of patients show early neurologic signs indicating frontotemporal localization —hallucinations, behavioral abnormalities, and personality change. Fever and headache are almost universally present in the early stages as are seizures, either focal motor, grand mal, or partial complex. Memory impairment, implying bilateral basal temporal involvement, is seen in many patients. Focal motor deficits, usually in the face and arm, may occur and aphasia is common if a dominant frontotemporal region is involved. With progression of the disease, the frontotemporal region becomes edematous and often acts as an intracranial mass, leading to increased intracranial pressure and uncal herniation. Coma, an age greater than 30 years, and delay in antiviral therapy are indicative of a poor prognosis.[95]

Examination of the CSF has been of only modest help in confirming a diagnosis of HSV encephalitis. CSF pleocytosis is most often a mixture of neutrophils and mononuclear cells with the latter predominating. Red blood cells, very rare in other encephalitides, are frequently present and constitute a valuable diagnostic clue. Protein is moderately elevated and glucose is normal. HSV cultures have only rarely been positive from CSF and take too long to be of early diagnostic value. Tests for the detection of HSV antigens are also timely, and have not proven to be sufficiently sensitive or specific. More recently, a polymerase chain reaction technique for identification of HSV DNA in CSF has proved to be a rapid and sensitive test.[9] This test shows promise for becoming the diagnostic test of choice.

An EEG may be helpful in confirming a focal process by demonstrating periodic paroxysmal discharges or slow wave complexes in one or both temporal lobes. CT may show decreased attenuation in one or both temporal lobes as early as the third day of the disease. This decreased attenuation represents the edema and necrosis found in areas of encephalitis. The use of contrast agents can also show areas of abnormal enhancement surrounding the low-density areas. MRI is significantly more sensitive in documenting early edema changes and will hasten the recognition of nonhemorrhagic HSV encephilitic changes.[99]

Full confirmation of the diagnosis of herpes encephalitis often depends on histologic or culture results from brain biopsy. The role of biopsy in the patient suspected to have HSV encephalitis has been controversial and has prompted several authorities to perform modeling and decision analysis to define the optimal approach.[14,36,78,120,128] Most authorities would currently agree that acyclovir therapy should be instituted when the clinical constellation outlined above is found. Unfortunately, the accuracy of the diagnosis without biopsy is only about 35 to 45 percent.[128,147] In a recent review of patients who underwent biopsy for presumptive HSV encephalitis, 33 percent of results were found to be nondiagnostic, 13 percent were diagnosed but untreatable, but 9 percent identified other treatable diseases.[147] Some authorities maintain that the diagnosis of HSV encephalitis should be established for certainty by brain biopsy, arguing that biopsy has low morbidity and will identify these other conditions requiring specific therapies.[14,36,95,128] Others have found that in most cases, empiric treatment with acyclovir is slightly favored, but brain biopsy was found useful for patients who had low CSF glucose at the time of initial lumbar puncture.[120] The biopsy site is determined by MRI or CT localization. Open[121] and stereotaxic[84] methods have been described. CSF evaluation by the polymerase chain reaction may eliminate the need for biopsy in the future. Currently, the rationale of biopsy is not to confirm HSV encephalitis, but rather to detect other treatable diseases.

The treatment of choice of HSV type 1 encephalitis is acyclovir. Acyclovir is an acyclic analogue of guanosine that inhibits viral DNA synthesis by binding to the viral DNA polymerase following phosphorylation in infected cells. Therapy should begin as soon as the diagnosis is suspected since delay in the start of therapy may drastically effect patient morbidity. The dosage is 30 mg/kg per day given at 8-h intervals for at least 10 days.[146] Overall mortality has been shown to be reduced to 19 to 28 percent with acyclovir therapy, significantly less than the approximate 50 percent mortality rates reported with vidarabine treatment.[125,146] An equally important factor in the treatment of this disease is the control of increased ICP associated with frontotemporal edema. Intravenous fluids must be carefully monitored and the judicious use of hyperventilation, steroids, osmotic diuretics, and intracranial pressure monitoring are all important to the treatment program.

Jakob-Creutzfeldt Disease

The importance of Jakob-Creutzfeldt disease in neurosurgical practice is its potential for iatrogenic spread. This rapidly progressive degenerative disease is one of the subacute spongiform encephalopathies, a group that also includes kuru in humans and scrapie in sheep. These diseases are caused by prions, or "unconventional agents" that are transmissible in an unknown manner. Prions produce no immune response and are resistant to treatments that usually inactivate viruses such as heat, ultraviolet radiation, and nucleases.

Jakob-Creutzfeldt disease is worldwide in distribution, with an incidence of 1 to 2 cases per million population. About 10 to 15 percent of cases are familial. Symptoms usually begin in the fifth or sixth decade. In general, they begin with a vague prodrome of fatigue, mild gait abnormalities, and memory deficits. This is followed by a rapidly progressive dementia associated with ataxia, blindness, choreoathetosis, and, most characteristically, myoclonus. Death follows within 8 to 12 months. There are no characteristic changes in the CSF or on a CT scan. Pathologic changes include severe cerebral atrophy, neuronal loss, astrocytosis, and cytoplasmic vacuolization of neurons and astrocytes.

Nine cases of Jakob-Creutzfeldt disease have been reported following neurosurgical procedures. Extreme care should be taken during operations on patients with progressive dementia. Biopsy and ventricular shunting procedures should be carried out only after careful consideration. Surgical instruments and depth electrodes used in any procedures in patients with diseases that have no clear etiology should be handled with great respect and should be specially treated after surgery. Autoclaving at 121°C (250°F) at 15 psi for 1 h or immersion in 5% sodium hypochlorite will inactivate the agent.[45]

Reye's Syndrome

Although it is not a viral infection of the CNS, Reye's syndrome is a viral-associated illness in which neurosurgical intervention is often lifesaving. Reye's syndrome is a rare, noninflammatory encephalopathy associated with hepatic microvesicular fatty infiltration and severe hyperammonemia that occurs almost exclusively in children. First described in 1963, the syndrome is characterized by an unremarkable prodromal viral illness followed several days later by profuse vomiting and abnormal behavior, rapidly progressing to coma.[113] Hepatomegally is usually present and laboratory examination reveals elevated serum ammonia, elevated AST and ALT, lactic acidemia, and prolonged prothrombin time. CSF examination is unremarkable. Decerebrate posturing and hyperventilation become prominent as the disease progresses. EEG shows widespread neuronal dysfunction, reflecting the severity of the process, and is useful in staging the disease when combined with clinical criteria.[82]

The agent of the disease and the etiology of the biochemical abnormalities are not clearly understood but are thought to be multifactorial. In almost all cases, the encephalopathic phase is preceded by a respiratory illness or chicken pox. Epidemics of influenza B or A and varicella are associated with outbreaks of Reye's syndrome.[68] Six epidemiologic studies have documented a close relationship between aspirin usage for the prodromal viral symptoms and the subsequent development of Reye's syndrome.[43,54,55,58,130,143] The annual number of reported cases has decreased sharply since 1980; the total number of reported cases was only 25 in 1989, despite a substantial influenza B epidemic.[26] This decline is coincident with the increased public awareness of the aspirin association and a decrease in the use of aspirin-containing medication in children.[26]

The most important factor in the pathogenesis of the encephalopathy in Reye's syndrome appears to be hyperammonemia. Liver clearance of ammonia is decreased by destruction of the urea cycle enzymes. The arterial ammonia level may be as high as 1000 μg/100 mm and is directly related to the depth of coma, the severity of EEG abnormality, and the mortality rate.[31] Examination of the brain shows cytotoxic cerebral edema with swelling of astrocyte foot processes and no sign of interstitial edema, inflammation, or demyelination.[15]

Cerebral edema is almost universal in fatal cases and the high mortality in Reye's syndrome patients is closely associated with increased ICP. Reversal of coma and reduction in mortality has been documented when ICP monitoring and vigorous attempts to lower ICP are added to the protocols of supportive treatment.[69,141] Mannitol has been shown to be effective in ICP management, whereas corticosteroids appear to be ineffective.

ACQUIRED IMMUNODEFICIENCY SYNDROME (AIDS)

The infecting agent in AIDS, HIV, is a single-stranded RNA retrovirus of the lentivirus group. HIV contains a dense nucleolid of RNA, core proteins, surface glycoproteins, and a reverse transcriptase enzyme. This enzyme is a DNA polymerase that produces viral DNA capable of integrating into the host chromosome. Once integrated, it is used as the transcription message for synthesis of the virus. Integration helps the virus escape host-defense mechanisms. Lentiviruses do not have teratogenic potential like oncogenic retroviruses, but are capable of causing lysis of the cells they infect.

HIV infection appears to be restricted to cells carrying the surface receptor CD4. The helper T-lymphocyte population is especially rich in CD4 receptors, explaining the selective tropism and lysis capability of HIV to these cells. Monocytes, macrophages, and microglia also contain CD4 surface receptors, but at a much lower density. This may explain why macrophages are frequently found harboring virus, but are infrequently lysed, making them an effective viral reservoir.

In clinical series, 31 to 60 percent of patients with AIDS have neurologic abnormalities.[79,109,127] These abnormalities involve the CNS and, to a lesser extent, the peripheral nervous system. Infections involving the CNS in AIDS are of two types; opportunistic infections secondary to the immunosuppression induced by the loss of T-cell immunity, and direct HIV infection presenting as meningitis or AIDS dementia complex, a broad spectrum of clinical and biologic manifestations of HIV encephalitis.

Opportunistic Infections of the CNS in AIDS

Opportunistic infections of the nervous system in AIDS include both viral and nonviral pathogens. The most common viral syndrome is a subacute encephalitis caused by cytomegalovirus. Herpes simplex encephalitis, progressive multifocal leukoencephalopathy (PML), and vericella zoster myelitis/encephalitis occur in decreasing order of frequency.

The most common nonviral CNS infection is *Toxoplasma gondii* meningoencephalitis. Fungal infections of the meninges and/or brain occur frequently also. The most common, in decreasing order of frequency, are *Cryptococcus neoformans*, *Candida albicans*, *Coccidioides immitis*, and *Aspergillus fumigatus*. Intracranial bacterial infections are rare, but *Mycobacterium aviam-intracellulare*, *M. tuberculosis*, *E. coli*, and *Treponema pallidum* meningoencephalitides have been reported. It must also be kept in mind that CNS lesions in AIDS can be caused by neoplastic processes. Primary CNS lymphoma is found in about 3 percent of AIDS patients, and systemic lymphoma can also spread to the meninges. A few instances of Kaposi's sarcoma metastatic to the brain have been reported.

A scheme for the management of AIDS patients with neurologic symptoms was developed by Levy et al.[79] Some of these lesions respond to specific medical treatment; toxoplasmosis to pyrimethamine and sulfadiazine; cryptococcus to amphotericin B; PML to cytarabine; and lymphoma to radiation therapy. Diagnosis based on CT appearance and blood and CSF serologies is uncertain, and diagnosis can be further complicated by two or more processes being present simultaneously. Definitive diagnosis, therefore, depends on accurate biopsy of the demonstrated lesions and serial CT evaluation of the response to appropriate therapy. Early appropriate therapy is of paramount importance in the immunocompromised patient and therefore, early biopsy of an accessible lesion is critical. An MRI study may be of benefit when an inaccesible lesion is diagnosed on CT, since MRI may identify a more accessible lesion.

Protection of medical personnel during surgical procedures should include the wearing of gown and gloves when handling blood or tissue, rigorous hand washing, and the meticulous avoidance of scalpel or needle wounds.

Primary HIV Infections of the CNS

The mechanism of HIV entry into the CNS has not been determined, but is postulated to be either secondary to viremia and endothelial penetration or via transport of infected monocytes across the blood-brain barrier.[70] Approximately 30 percent of asymptomatic, HIV-seropositive patients have HIV-positive CSF cultures, suggesting that the virus penetrates the CNS early in the course of infection and often in an asymptomatic manner.[62] It is now clear that primary HIV infection causes a spectrum of clinical diseases of the CNS, meningitis, and a progressive dementia termed the AIDS dementia complex (ADC).

Two types of meningitis can occur with HIV infection; an acute febrile syndrome similar to mononucleosis within days to weeks of initial HIV exposure and an aseptic meningitis around the time of seroconversion. The symptoms of meningitis are associated with a mononuclear CSF pleocytosis and HIV-positive CSF cultures in 50 percent of patients.[89] Both of these conditions are self-limited.

ADC is a neurologic syndrome characterized by abnormalities in cognition, motor performance, and behavior.[108] Symptoms usually consist of difficulties with concentration and memory progressing to frank dementia with intact level of arousal. Slowed rapid alternating movements, hyperreflexia, and frontal releasing signs are usually illicitable on exam, with imbalance, ataxia, and axial weakness becoming prominent in more advanced stages of the disease. The end stage of ADC is nearly vegetative with vacant stare, paraparesis, and incontinence. The features of ADC are characteristic of subcortical dementias like the cognitive impairments seen in Parkinson's and Huntington's disease.[98] The presence and severity of ADC parallels the advance of systemic disease in AIDS patients. ADC is rare in healthy, seropositive patients, present in 25 to 35 percent with initial presentation of opportunistic infection, and present in nearly half of patients with advanced AIDS.[109] This parallel development of ADC, despite early exposure of the nervous system to HIV, suggests that although HIV is "neurotropic," it is relatively nonpathogenic for the brain in the absence of immunosuppression.[108]

The pathologic findings have been well characterized and recently reviewed.[20,21] The hallmark of HIV encephalitis is microglia nodules and multinucleated giant cells. The only CNS cells that have definitively shown HIV-1 antigen are macrophages, microglia, and multinucleated giant cells. Demyelination in the absence of these inflammatory changes (leukoencephalopathy), as well as vacuolar myelopathy, are also commonly seen. Absence of cytolytic infection of neurons, oligodentrocytes, and astrocytes has focused attention on the possible role of indirect mechanisms of brain dysfunction related to either virus or cell-coded toxins.

CT and MRI are relatively insensitive to HIV encephalitic changes until they are well advanced. Leukoencephalopathic changes can be demonstrated by imaging studies; MRI being significantly more sensitive than CT.[107] Brain atrophy is a common late finding.

Testing and Therapy for HIV Infection

Currently, the testing procedures in clinical use rely on the detection of HIV antibodies in patient and donor blood. The screening test, an enzyme linked immunosorbant assay (ELISA), has been shown to be 99.7 percent sensitive and 98.5 percent specific in a large national study.[25] The confirmatory test, a Western blot technique with greater specificity, is applied when a seropositive ELISA sample is encountered. Confirmation of HIV seropositivity is made when at least two HIV antibodies are isolated on Western blot, those that exhibit one antibody are "indeterminate." The FDA requires that a blood donor must test negative by ELISA and Western blot in order to qualify for donation.[42] The time between infection and the first detectable sign of antibody seropositivity is called the "window period" and is usually between 6 and 8 weeks.[126] Therefore, the risk that a seronegative blood donor is infected and infectious exists. A recent study shows that this risk is very small; only one HIV culture-positive unit was found in 61,000 units of fresh blood that tested ELISA seronegative.[126] Several newer tests are being evaluated; one that detects HIV antigen, the antigen capture test; and a second that detects HIV nucleic acids, a polymerase chain reaction method. The utility of these tests in screening has not been determined.

The current standard therapy for AIDS is 3′-azido-3′-deoxythymidine (zidovudine, AZT). AZT significantly reduces opportunistic infections and mortality in patients with HIV infection, but is not a cure.[41] AZT causes severe myelosuppression and constitutional side effects, placing limits on its dosing. Other agents, such as 2′,3′-dideoxycytidine (ddC) and 2′,3′-dideoxyinosine (ddI), are being assessed for the treatment of patients with HIV infection.[93] The most effective therapy for HIV infection may be combinations of AZT and other therapies: ddC, ddI, interferon α, and acyclovirinitial. Combination therapy trials are in progress and may allow for improved efficacy and decreased side effects.[52]

FUNGAL INFECTIONS OF THE CENTRAL NERVOUS SYSTEM

Fungi are ubiquitous organisms in the environment with low virulence that become pathogenic during special circumstances, including depression of cell-mediated immunity, neutropenia, and prolonged systemic antibiotic therapy. It is uncommon for fungi to invade the CNS.

Fungal infections are being diagnosed more frequently because of increased awareness of such infections, improved biopsy and diagnostic techniques, increasing number of patients using prolonged antibiotic therapy, and increasing travel to, and immigration from, regions of endemic infection.[153] Misdiagnosis and delays in diagnosis have been commonly described in published series of fungal infection. This problem can be generally attributed to the failure to aggressively pursue laboratory or tissue diagnosis.[153] The competency of the immune system of the host is an important factor in the preselection of the specific fungal pathogen; *Cryptococcus*, *Coccidiodes*, *Histoplasma*, and *Blastomyces* can infect otherwise healthy individuals, whereas the other fungal infections develop almost exclusively in patients with compromised cellular immunity. Involvement of the CNS may be disseminated, causing meningitis or meningoencephalitis; or focal, causing granulomatous abscesses.

In contrast to bacterial infection, fungal meningitis tends to be initially mild with gradual progression. Headache, neck stiffness, fever, lethargy, depressed mental status, and cranial nerve palsies may be present. *Cryptococcus*, *Coccidiodes*, *Candida*, and *Aspergillus* commonly present as meningitis or meningoencephalitis. The clinical signs and symptoms are indistinguishable from any other chronic meningitis. The CSF pleocytosis is lymphocytic, CSF protein is mildly elevated, and CSF glucose is usually reduced. In general, fungi are difficult to culture from blood and CSF, and serologic tests are poorly sensitive, partly because of the compromised cellular immunity common in these patients. The CT scan is not usually helpful in fungal meningitis, but it may demonstrate hydrocephalus, a complication of chronic meningitis. MRI can be effective in demonstrating basilar enhancement and inflammation.

Single and multiple brain abscesses may present with seizure, headache, depressed mental status, or focal neurologic deficits, often accompanied by pneumonia. Common pathogens are *Cryptococcus*, *Aspergillus*, *Nocardia*, *Blastomyces*, *Actinomyces*, and *Histoplasma*.

Cryptococcosis

Cryptococcus neoformans, a common soil organism, is the most common fungal meningitis encountered in the United States. Cryptococcal granulomatous abscesses have also been described, but are uncommon. Cryptococcosis occurs in both healthy and immunocompromised hosts. It is a significant cause of morbidity and mortality in AIDS, infecting approximately 10 percent of patients. The respiratory tract is the primary site of infection, and hematogenous dissemination is the most common source of CNS infection. CSF india ink smears are only positive in 50 percent of cases; however, capsular antigen is detectable by complement fixation in approximately 90 percent of cases.

Two therapeutic regimens have been adopted in recent years for the treatment of cryptococcal meningitis, based on controlled studies in populations of AIDS: intravenous amphotericin B (0.3 to 0.7 mg/kg per day) in combination with flucytosine (150 mg/kg per day) and oral fluconazole (150 to 400 mg/day). The proportion of responders with either treatment is 50 percent as is the 25 percent mortality; however, fluconazole-treated patients clear the CSF slower and had greater mortality during the first week of therapy.[74] Therefore, amphotericin B with or without flucytosine has been suggested for the initial week of therapy.[73] The less toxic, orally administered fluconazole, distinguished by its prolonged half-life, once daily oral administration, and high CSF penetrance, is preferred for the chronic course of therapy.[74]

Coccidioides

Coccidioides immitis is a natural inhabitant of the semiarid soils of the southwestern United States, Mexico, Central America, and South America. It may invade in the absence of underlying disease; almost invariably by way of the respiratory tract. Although the disease can present as an isolated CNS infection, there is usually a preceding history of respiratory complaints. In immunocompromised hosts meningitis may present as a late manifestation of lethal, systemically disseminated infection. CNS coccidiomycosis is often not recognized until the disease is well established with a thick proteinaceous basal cistern exudate; thus hydrocephalus and cranial nerve palsies may be present. Hydrocephalus can greatly complicate therapy. The complement fixation test for CSF antibody to the fungus remains an effective technique, but culture of the CSF is positive in half of the cases.

Before the introduction of amphotericin B, mortality of coccidioidal meningitis approached 100 percent. Treatment with both intravenous and intrathecal or intracisternal administration of amphotericin B lowered mortality to 30 to 50 percent. However, amphotericin B has significant adverse effects that limit its clinical application and the need for intrathecal delivery for months of therapy is difficult. Therefore, authorities have recommended placement of a subcutaneous CSF reservoir. Side effects of amphotericin B delivered in CSF include chemical meningitis, arachnoiditis, spinal cord infarction, intracisternal hemorrhage, and bacterial superinfection of reservoirs. Relapse, often years after apparently successful therapy, is common in coccidiomycosis.

Azoles have been documented to be very effective in the treatment of systemic coccidiomycosis but initial experience in the treatment of meningitis with miconazole and ketoconazole was not promising. Fluconazole has been found to be effective in the treatment of meningitis in a series of 18 patients, where it was used as either sole therapy or in combination with intrathecal amphoterecin or miconazole.[136,137] Whether a significant improvement in morbidity and mortality can be achieved will depend on further clinical experience with azole therapy.

Candidiasis

Candidiasis is rare in healthy individuals, although it is a common constituent of the oropharyngeal flora. In distinction from other fungal meningitides, the source of CNS infection is often not a respiratory primary, but from intestinal, urinary, or vascular catheter seeding.[81] Candidiasis is frequently a late complication of treatment for a variety of debilitating conditions, and a high incidence of CNS infection has been found in autopsy studies. Although meningitis is more common, there are also reports of candidal granulomatous brain abscesses.[57,59,149] *Candida albicans* and other species have been implicated in meningitis in AIDS patients and in shunt infections.[38,51,153]

Treatment with miconazole, intravenous and intravenous combined with intrathecal, has shown favorable results.[97,153] Surgical resections of granulomas following institution of antimicrobial therapy has also been reported with a favorable outcome.[60]

Aspergillosis

Aspergillus species are the most common fungi in the environment. Initially described as a rare, focal infection resulting from extension of sinus infection, aspergillosis is an increasingly prevalent disseminated infection, second only to *C. neoformans* as the most common fungal infection of the CNS in immunocompromised patients. Opportunistic CNS infections by *Aspergillus* are usually preceded by pulmonary infection and felt to arise from hematogenous spread. Meningitis, encephalitis, solitary or multiple brain abscesses, and vasculitis have been described. Vascular invasion with necrotic vasculitis and embolization is common in disseminated CNS disease, a characteristic it shares with the Phycomyces. Cerebral mycotic aneurysms may develop as a result.[13] We have recently seen two cases of community-acquired disease in immunocompetent hosts involving solitary mass lesions of the orbit apex that became disseminated following operative resection; therefore, this entity must also be considered in the noncompromised patient. An aspergillus disc space infection in a compromised host was recently reported.[96]

Amphotericin B, with or without flucytosine or rifampin, is the optimal medical therapy.[2] Objective data on dose and duration of amphotericin B is not available; however, 450 to 2300 mg cumulative doses have been described in a report of patients with successful therapy.[50] When a discrete mass is present, both craniotomy with resection and stereotactic aspiration have been described.[50] Even with aggressive therapy the prognosis for patients is poor and survival is rare.

Phycomycytes

Although hematologic spread is the primary route for most CNS infection, sometimes a fungal abscess develops after direct contamination of the brain from an adjacent infection. This is commonly seen in infections by the *Zygomyces*, particularly mucormycosis, a rather aggressive agent that often causes diffuse cerebritis.

Mucormycosis exemplifies diffuse fungal encephalitis, occurring most often in patients with diabetes mellitus and compromised immunity. This organism preferentially involves the cerebral vasculature causing ischemia, thrombosis, and infarction in addition to inflammation. Tissues of the orbit and paranasal sinuses are commonly affected. Treatment includes debridement of infected and devitalized tissue, control of the underlying disease, and systemic amphotericin B. The prognosis is poor despite treatment unless the diagnosis is made early.

Actinomycosis

Actinomyces israelii is a gram-positive anaerobic bacterium found in normal oral flora. It is discussed in this section because of its historical categorization as a fungal infection. Actinomycosis presents as either a single brain abscess, or rarely, a purulent basilar meningitis, usually by direct extension of the infection from the ear or mandible although hematogenous spread of pulmonary disease is becoming more prevalent. Treatment consists of drainage and intravenous penicillin for 3 to 4 months.

Nocardiosis

Nocardia is a gram-positive aerobe also historically categorized as a fungus-like bacteria. Nocardiosis of the CNS is usually secondary to hematogenous spread from a pulmonary infecton, and it usually presents as an abscess, though purulent meningitis also occurs. Abscesses are usually multiple and multiloculated. Capsular formation is poorly developed. In contrast to actinomycetes, nocardia tend to be penicillin-resistant. Recommended treatment is sulfamethoxazole, 4 to 8 g/day for 6 to 12 months. Drainage is indicated for accesible abscesses; however, successful nonsurgical management has been reported.

PARASITIC INFECTIONS OF THE CENTRAL NERVOUS SYSTEM

Although relatively uncommon in North America and western Europe, parasitic infection of the CNS is a major cause of disease worldwide. Many species cause CNS disease; cysticercosis, echinococcosis, toxoplasmosis, malaria, amebiasis, schistomsomiasis, paragonimiasis, gnathostomiasis, angiostrongyliasis, filariasis, ascariasis, and ancyclostomiasis.[87] In general, once CNS infestation occurs treatment options are limited and paliative at best. Three organisms of particular concern are *Taenia solium*, responsible for neurocystercicosis, *Echinococcus granulosis*, responsible for hydatid cysts, and *Toxoplasma gondii*, a common cause of meningoencephalitis in AIDS.

Neurocysticercosis

Cysticercosis is a systemic infection with the larval stage of *T. solium*, the pork tapeworm. The adult worm lives in the intestine of humans, the obligate host, and produces proglottids that are passed in the stool. The proglottids, when ingested, have the hard protective covering dissolved in the stomach and then can penetrate the gastrointestinal mucosa and are hematogenously spread through multiple organs of the intermediate host, usually the pig. The larvae survive in quiescent state for 2 to 5 years and then die. The usual intermediate host is the pig; however, when individuals intercept this chain by ingesting proglottids in feces contaminated food, or possibly when proglottids are retroperistalsed into the stomach, then they can become the intermediate host and develop cysticercosis. The muscle and CNS are especially prone to invasion with approximately 60 percent of individuals developing neurocysticercosis. The basilar cisterns are involved in the majority of patients, parenchymal and ventricular involvement being less frequent.[102] Spinal lesions have also been reported.

Neurocysticercosis manifests as a chronic meningitis, hydrocephalus, or a parenchymal mass lesion with new onset seizure disorder. Parenchymal cysts are 3 to 15 mm in diameter, whereas ventricular and subarachnoid cysts are generally smaller. On CT, parenchymal cysts appear as low-density, round, ring-enhancing lesions with or without surrounding edema. Hydrocephalus is a common finding in cases of basilar cistern involvement.

Treatment of neurocysticercosis consists of medical and surgical interventions. Albenazole, an imidazole with activity against a broad range of cestodes, is currently the drug of choice for neurocysticercosis, having replaced praziquantil. Albenazole has been shown to ameliorate parenchymal, subarachnoid, and intraventricular cysts.[34,129] The dose is 15 mg/kg per day for 8 days. CSF-diverting shunt procedures are necessary for hydrocephalus. Intraventricular cysts can cause acute obstruction and their direct excision can sometimes alleviate the need for shunting.[6] Patients who have symptoms of mass effect in the absence of hydrocephalus or after shunting for hydrocephalus may improve with surgical excision.[30]

Echinococcosis (Hydatid Cysts)

Prevalent in Central and South America, Europe, Australia, and Africa, Echinococcosis is caused by the encysted larvae of *E. granulosa*, the dog tapeworm. Intermediate hosts can include humans, sheep, cattle, and camels.[87] Children are often affected because of their close contact with dogs. CNS infestation by the larvae occurs in only 3 percent of patients with systemic echinococcus. Cysts are usually solitary lesions in white matter with a negligible inflammatory response. Patients usually present with intracranial hypertension or focal deficits secondary to very large cysts. The diagnosis is made by peripheral eosinophilia and a skin test. CT and MRI document the large cystic masses with minimal edema.

A morphologically and biologically distinct entity, alveolar hydatid disease is caused by *E. multilocularis*, a cestode infecting fox, dog, and cat. It is endemic to northern latitudes; Siberia, Alaska, Canada, and the northern United States. As in *E. granulosis* infection, CNS involvement is rare.[10]

Treatment consists of operative resection of symptomatic cysts, taking great care not to rupture the cyst as the larvae are viable and can further seed the operative field.

Toxoplasmosis

An obligate intracellular protozoan, *T. gondii*, is a frequent parasite of humans, cats, and birds. Most human infestations are asymptomatic until the host cellular immune system is compromised. The most common clinical manifestation is generalized lymphadenopathy. A chronic meningoencephalitis is the usual CNS presentation. The diagnosis is established by serologic testing. Multiple focal abscesses are typically seen on contrast CT and MRI. Treatment includes pyrimethamine and sulfadiazine.[87]

REFERENCES

1. Aarabi B: Causes of infections in penetrating head wounds in the Iran-Iraq War. *Neurosurgery* 25:923–6, 1989.
2. Abramowicz M: Drugs for treatment of deep fungal infection. *Med Lett Drugs Ther* 30:30–2, 1988.
3. Aerdts SJ, van Dalen R, Clasener HA, et al: Antibiotic prophylaxis of respiratory tract infection in mechanically ventilated patients. A prospective, blinded, randomized trial of the effect of a novel regimen. *Chest* 100:783–91, 1991.
4. Albert RK, Condie F: Handwashing patterns in medi-

cal intensive-care units. *N Engl J Med* 304:1465–6, 1981.

5. Ammirati M, Raimondi AJ: Cerebrospinal fluid shunt infections in children. A study on the relationship between the etiology of hydrocephalus, age at the time of shunt placement, and infection rate. *Childs Nerv Syst* 3:106–9, 1987.
6. Apuzzo ML, Dobkin WR, Zee CS, et al: Surgical considerations in treatment of intraventricular cysticercosis. An analysis of 45 cases. *J Neurosurg* 60:400–7, 1984.
7. Arditi M, Herold BC, Yogev R: Cefuroxime treatment failure and Haemophilus influenzae meningitis: Case report and review of literature. *Pediatrics* 84:132–135, 1989.
8. Arseni C, Ciurea AV: Cerebral abscesses secondary to otorhinolaryngological infections. A study of 386 cases. *Zentralbl Neurochir* 49:22–36, 1988.
9. Aurelius E, Johansson B, Skoldenberg B, et al: Rapid diagnosis of herpes simplex encephalitis by nested polymerase chain reaction assay of cerebrospinal fluid. *Lancet* 337:189–92, 1991.
10. Aydin Y, Barlas O, Yolas C, et al: Alveolar hydatid disease of the brain. Report of four cases. *J Neurosurg* 65:115–9, 1986.
11. Bahal N, Nahata MC: The role of corticosteroids in infants and children with bacterial meningitis. *DICP* 25:542–5, 1991.
12. Bannister G, Williams B, Smith S: Treatment of subdural empyema. *J Neurosurg* 55:82–8, 1981.
13. Barrow DL, Prats AR: Infectious intracranial aneurysms: Comparison of groups with and without endocarditis. *Neurosurgery* 27:562–72, 1990.
14. Barza M, Pauker SG: The decision to biopsy, treat, or wait in suspected herpes encephalitis. *Ann Intern Med* 92:641–9, 1980.
15. Blisard KS, Davis LE: Neuropathologic findings in Reye's syndrome. *J Child Neurol* 6:41–4, 1991.
16. Blomstedt GC, Kytta J: Results of a randomized trial of vancomycin prophylaxis in craniotomy. *J Neurosurg* 69:216–20, 1988.
17. Borovich B, Johnston E, Spagnuolo E: Infratentorial subdural empyema: Clinical and computerized tomography findings. Report of three cases. *J Neurosurg* 72:299–301, 1990.
18. Britt RH, Enzmann DR, Yeager AS: Neuropathological and computerized tomograhic findings in experimental brain abscess. *J Neurosurg* 55:590–603, 1981.
19. Buckwold FJ, Hand R, Hansebout RR: Hospital-acquired bacterial meningitis in neurosurgical patients. *J Neurosurg* 46:494–500, 1977.
20. Budka H: Human immunodeficiency virus (HIV)-induced disease of the central nervous system: Pathology and implications for pathogenesis. *Acta Neuropathol (Berl)* 77:225–36, 1989.
21. Budka H: Neuropathology of human immunodeficiency virus infection. *Brain Pathology* 1:163–175, 1991.
22. Bullock R, van Dellen JR, Ketelbey W, et al: A double-blind placebo-controlled trial of perioperative prophylactic antibiotics for elective neurosurgery. *J Neurosurg* 69:687–91, 1988.
23. Cahill DW, Love LC, Rechtine GR: Pyogenic osteomyelitis of the spine in the elderly. *J Neurosurg* 74:878–86, 1991.
24. Caplan ES, Hoyt NJ: Nosocomial sinusitis. *JAMA* 247:639–41, 1982.
25. Centers for Disease Control: MMWR update: Serologic testing for HIV-a antibody—United States, 1988 and 1989. *MMWR* 39:380–383, 1990.
26. Centers for Disease Control: Reye's syndrome surveillance—United States, 1989. *JAMA* 265:960, 1991.
27. Cherubin CE, Corrado ML, Nair SR, et al: Treatment of gram-negative bacillary meningitis: Role of the new cephalosporin antibiotics. *Rev Infect Dis* S453–64, 1982.
28. Choppin PW, Scheid A: The role of viral glycoproteins in adsorption, penetration, and pathogenicity of viruses. *Rev Infect Dis* 2:40–61, 1980.
29. Clayman GL, Adams GL, Paugh DR, et al: Intracranial complications of paranasal sinusitis: A combined institutional review. *Laryngoscope* 101:234–9, 1991.
30. Colli BO, Martelli N, Assirati JJ, et al: Results of surgical treatment of neurocysticercosis in 69 cases. *J Neurosurg* 65:309–15, 1986.
31. Corey L, Rubin RJ, Hattwick MA: Reye's syndrome: Clinical progression and evaluation of therapy. *Pediatrics* 60:708–14, 1977.
32. Dagbjartsson A, Ludvigsson P: Bacterial meningitis: Diagnosis and initial antibiotic therapy. *Pediatr Clin North Am* 34:219–30, 1987.
33. Dajani AS, Pokowski LH: Delayed cerebrospinal fluid sterilization, in vitro bactericidal activities, and side effects of selected beta-lactams. *Scand J Infect Dis Suppl* 73:31–42, 1990.
34. del Brutto OH, Sotelo J: Albendazole therapy for subarachnoid and ventricular cysticercosis. Case report. *J Neurosurg* 72:816–7, 1990.
35. Deutschman CS, Wilton PB, Sinow J, et al: Paranasal sinusitis: A common complication of nasotracheal intubation in neurosurgical patients. *Neurosurgery* 17:296–9, 1985.
36. DiSclafani A, Kohl S, Ostrow PT: The importance of brain biopsy in suspected herpes simplex encephalitis. *Surg Neurol* 17:101–6, 1982.
37. Djindjian M, Lepresle E, Homs JB: Antibiotic prophylaxis during prolonged clean neurosurgery. Results of a randomized double-blind study using oxacillin. *J Neurosurg* 73:383–6, 1990.
38. Ehni WF, Ellison RT: Spontaneous Candida albicans

meningitis in a patient with the acquired immune deficiency syndrome. *Am J Med* 83:806–7, 1987.
39. Feuerman T, Wackym PA, Gade GF, et al: Craniotomy improves outcome in subdural empyema. *Surg Neurol* 32:105–10, 1989.
40. Fink MP, Helsmoortel CM, Stein KL, et al: The efficacy of an oscillating bed in the prevention of lower respiratory tract infection in critically ill victims of blunt trauma. A prospective study. *Chest* 97:132–7, 1990.
41. Fischl MA, Richman DD, Grieco MH, et al: The efficacy of azidothymidine (AZT) in the treatment of patients with AIDS and AIDS-related complex. A double-blind, placebo- controlled trial. *N Engl J Med* 317:185–91, 1987.
42. Food and Drug Administration: *Guidelines for The Prevention of Human Immunodeficiency Virus (HIV) Transmission by Blood Products.* Rockville, 1989.
43. Forsyth BW, Horwitz RI, Acampora D, et al: New epidemiologic evidence confirming that bias does not explain the aspirin/Reye's syndrome association. *JAMA* 261:2517–24, 1989.
44. Frame PT, McLaurin RL: Treatment of CSF shunt infections with intrashunt plus oral antibiotic therapy. *J Neurosurg* 60:354–60, 1984.
45. Gajdusek DC, Gibbs CJ, Asher DM, et al: Precautions in medical care of, and in handling materials from, patients with transmissible virus dementia (Creutzfeldt-Jakob disease). *N Engl J Med* 297:1253–8, 1977.
46. Garfin SR, Botte MJ, Triggs KJ, et al: Subdural abscess associated with halo-pin traction. *J Bone Joint Surg [Am]* 70:1338–40, 1988.
47. Garner JS, Favero MS: CDC guidelines for the prevention and control of nosocomial infections. Guideline for handwashing and hospital environmental control, 1985. Supercedes guideline for hospital environmental control published in 1981. *Am J Infect Control* 14:110–29, 1986.
48. Geraghty J, Feely M: Antibiotic prophylaxis in neurosurgery. A randomized controlled trial. *J Neurosurg* 60:724–6, 1984.
49. Gombert ME, Landesman SH, Corrado ML, et al: Vancomycin and rifampin therapy for Staphylococcus epidermidis meningitis associated with CSF shunts: Report of three cases. *J Neurosurg* 55:633–6, 1981.
50. Goodman ML, Coffey RJ: Stereotactic drainage of Aspergillus brain abscess with long-term survival: Case report and review. *Neurosurgery* 24:96–9, 1989.
51. Gower DJ, Crone K, Alexander EJ, et al: Candida albicans shunt infection: Report of two cases. *Neurosurgery* 19:111–3, 1986.
52. Groopman JE: Treatment of AIDS with combinations of antiretroviral agents: A summary. *Am J Med* 90:27S–30S, 1991.
53. Haines SJ, Mampalam T, Rosenblum ML, et al: Cranial and Intracranial Bacterial Infections. In: Youmans JR (ed): *Neurological Surgery*, Philadelphia, Saunders, 1990, pp 3707–3735.
54. Hall SM: Reye's syndrome and aspirin: A review. *Br J Clin Pract Symp Suppl* 70:4–11, 1990.
55. Halpin TJ, Holtzhauer FJ, Campbell RJ, et al: Reye's syndrome and medication use. *JAMA* 248:687–91, 1982.
56. Hartenauer U, Thulig B, Diemer W, et al: Effect of selective flora suppression on colonization, infection, and mortality in critically ill patients: A one-year, prospective consecutive study. *Crit Care Med* 19:463–73, 1991.
57. Haruda F, Bergman MA, Headings D: Unrecognized Candida brain abscess in infancy: Two cases and a review of the literature. *Johns Hopkins Med J* 147:182–5, 1980.
58. Hurwitz ES, Barrett MJ, Bregman D, et al: Public Health Service study of Reye's syndrome and medications. Report of the main study. *JAMA* 257:1905–11, 1987.
59. Ikeda K, Yamashita J, Fujisawa H, et al: Cerebral granuloma and meningitis caused by Candida albicans: Useful monitoring of mannan antigen in cerebrospinal fluid. *Neurosurgery* 26:860–3, 1990.
60. Ilgren EB, Westmorland D, Adams CB, et al: Cerebellar mass caused by Candida species. Case report. *J Neurosurg* 60:428–30, 1984.
61. James HE, Walsh JW, Wilson HD, et al: Prospective randomized study of therapy in cerebrospinal fluid shunt infection. *Neurosurgery* 7:459–63, 1980.
62. Johnson RT, McArthur JC, Narayan O: The neurobiology of human immunodeficiency virus infections. *FASEB J* 2:2970–81, 1988.
63. Kaplan SL: Corticosteroids and bacterial meningitis. *Scand J Infect Dis Suppl* 73:43–54, 1990.
64. Kaplan SL, Patrick CC: Cefotaxime and aminoglycoside treatment of meningitis caused by gram-negative enteric organisms. *Pediatr Infect Dis J* 9:810–4, 1990.
65. Kaufman DM, Kaplan JG, Litman N: Infectious agents in spinal epidural abscesses. *Neurology* 30:844–50, 1980.
66. Kaufman DM, Miller MH, Steigbigel NH: Subdural empyema: Analysis of 17 recent cases and review of the literature. *Medicine (Baltimore)* 54:485–98, 1975.
67. Kerver AJ, Rommes JH, Mevissen VE, et al: Prevention of colonization and infection in critically ill patients: A prospective randomized study. *Crit Care Med* 16:1087–93, 1988.
68. Kilpatrick SL, Hale DE, Douglas SD: Progress in Reye syndrome: Epidemiology, biochemical mechanisms, and animal models. *Dig Dis* 7:135–46, 1989.
69. Kindt GW, Waldman J, Kohl S, et al: Intracranial

pressure in Reye's syndrome: Monitoring and control. *JAMA* 231:822–5,1975.
70. Koenig S, Gendelman HE, Orenstein JM, et al: Detection of AIDS virus in macrophages in brain tissue from AIDS patients with encephalopathy. *Science* 233:1089–93, 1986.
71. Kunin CM: Urinary tract infections. *Surg Clin North Am* 60:223–31, 1980.
72. Landesman SH, Corrado ML, Shah PM, et al: Past and current roles for cephalosporin antibiotics in treatment of meningitis: Emphasis on use in gram-negative bacillary meningitis. *Am J Med* 71:693–703, 1981.
73. Larsen RA: Azoles and AIDS. *J Infect Dis* 162:727–30, 1990.
74. Larsen RA, Leal MA, Chan LS: Fluconazole compared with amphotericin B plus flucytosine for cryptococcal meningitis in AIDS. A randomized trial. *Ann Intern Med* 113:183–7, 1990.
75. Lebel MH, Freij BJ, Syrogiannopoulos GA, et al: Dexamethasone therapy for bacterial meningitis. Results of two double-blind, placebo-controlled trials. *N Engl J Med* 319:964–71, 1988.
76. Lebel MH, Hoyt MJ, McCracken GJ: Comparative efficacy of ceftriaxone and cefuroxime for treatment of bacterial meningitis. *J Pediatr* 114:1049–54, 1989.
77. Ledingham IM, Alcock SR, Eastaway AT, et al: Triple regimen of selective decontamination of the digestive tract, systemic cefotaxime, and microbiological surveillance for prevention of acquired infection in intensive care. *Lancet* 1:785–90, 1988.
78. Levitz RE, Reinfrank RF, Quintiliani R: Herpes simplex encephalitis: The case against brain biopsy. *Conn Med* 47:681–4, 1983.
79. Levy RM, Bredesen DE, Rosenblum ML: Neurological manifestations of the acquired immunodeficiency syndrome (AIDS): Experience at UCSF and review of the literature. *J Neurosurg* 62:475–95, 1985.
80. Leys D, Christiaens JL, Derambure P, et al: Management of focal intracranial infections: Is medical treatment better than surgery? *J Neurol Neurosurg Psychiatry* 53:472–5, 1990.
81. Lipton SA, Hickey WF, Morris JH, et al: Candidal infection in the central nervous system. *Am J Med* 76:101–8, 1984.
82. Lovejoy FJ, Smith AL, Bresnan MJ, et al: Clinical staging in Reye's syndrome. *Am J Dis Child* 128:36–41, 1974.
83. Luken MG, Whelan MA: Recent diagnostic experience with subdural empyema. *J Neurosurg* 52:764–71, 1980.
84. Lunsford LD, Martinez AJ, Latchaw RE, et al: Rapid and accurate diagnosis of herpes simplex encephalitis with computed tomography stereotaxic biopsy. *Surg Neurol* 21:249–57, 1984.
85. Maki DG, Weise CE, Sarafin HW: A semiquantitative culture method for identifying intravenous-catheter-related infection. *N Engl J Med* 296:1305–9, 1977.
86. Mampalam TJ, Rosenblum ML: Trends in the management of bacterial brain abscesses: A review of 102 cases over 17 years. *Neurosurgery* 23:451–8, 1988.
87. Martz RD, Hoff JT: Parasitic and Fungal Disease of the Central Nervous System. In: Youmans JR (ed): *Neurological Surgery*. Philadelphia: Saunders, 1990, pp 3742–3751.
88. Mauser HW, Van HH, Tulleken CA: Factors affecting the outcome in subdural empyema. *J Neurol Neurosurg Psychiatry* 50:1136–41, 1987.
89. McArthur JC: Neurologic manifestations of AIDS. *Medicine (Baltimore)* 66:407–37, 1987.
90. McCracken GJ: Current management of bacterial meningitis. *Pediatr Infect Dis J* 8:919–21, 1989.
91. McGillicuddy JE: Infections of the Central Nervous System. In: Crockard A, Hayward R, Hoff J (eds): *Neurosurgery. The Scientific Basis of Clinical Practice*. Oxford, Blackwell, 1985, pp 676.
92. Meijer K, van Saene HK, Hill JC: Infection control in patients undergoing mechanical ventilation: Traditional approach versus a new development-selective decontamination of the digestive tract. *Heart Lung* 19:11–20, 1990.
93. Merigan TC: Treatment of AIDS with combinations of antiretroviral agents. *Am J Med* 90:8S–17S, 1991.
94. Mombelli G, Klastersky J, Coppens L, et al: Gram-negative bacillary meningitis in neurosurgical patients. *J Neurosurg* 59:634–41, 1983.
95. Morawetz RB, Whitley RJ, Murphy DM: Experience with brain biopsy for suspected herpes encephalitis: A review of forty consecutive cases. *Neurosurgery* 12:654–7, 1983.
96. Morgenlander JC, Rossitch EJ, Rawlings CE: Aspergillus disc space infection: Case report and review of the literature. *Neurosurgery* 25:126–9, 1989.
97. Morison A, Erasmus DS, Bowie MD: Treatment of Candida albicans meningitis with intravenous and intrathecal miconazole. A case report. *S Afr Med J* 74:235–6, 1988.
98. Navia BA, Jordan BD, Price RW: The AIDS dementia complex: I. Clinical features. *Ann Neurol* 19:517–24, 1986.
99. Neils EW, Lukin R, Tomsick TA, et al: Magnetic resonance imaging and computerized tomography scanning of herpes simplex encephalitis. Report of two cases. *J Neurosurg* 67:592–4, 1987.
100. Niemoller UM, Tauber MG: Brain edema and increased intracranial pressure in the pathophysiology of bacterial meningitis. *Eur J Clin Microbiol Infect Dis* 8:109–17, 1989.
101. Norrby SR: Role of cephalosporins in the treatment of

bacterial meningitis in adults. Overview with special emphasis on ceftazidime. *Am J Med* 79:56–61, 1985.
102. Obrador S: Cysticercosis cerebri. *Acta Neurochir* 10:320–364, 1962.
103. Osenbach RK, Hitchon PW, Menezes AH: Diagnosis and management of pyogenic vertebral osteomyelitis in adults. *Surg Neurol* 33:266–75, 1990.
104. Pathak A, Sharma BS, Mathuriya SN, et al: Controversies in the management of subdural empyema. A study of 41 cases with review of literature. *Acta Neurochir* 102:25–32, 1990.
105. Pendlebury WW, Perl DP, Munoz DG: Multiple microabscesses in the central nervous system: A clinicopathologic study. *J Neuropathol Exp Neurol* 48:290–300, 1989.
106. Pinilla JC, Ross DF, Martin T, et al: Study of the incidence of intravascular catheter infection and associated septicemia in critically ill patients. *Crit Care Med* 11:21–5, 1983.
107. Post MJ, Tate LG, Quencer RM, et al: CT, MR, and pathology in HIV encephalitis and meningitis. *Am J Roentgenol* 151:373–80, 1988.
108. Price RW, Brew B, Sidtis J, et al: The brain in AIDS: Central nervous system HIV-1 infection and AIDS dementia complex. *Science* 239:586–92, 1988.
109. Price RW, Sidtis JJ, Brew BJ: AIDS dementia complex and HIV-1 infection. A view from the clinic. *Brain Pathology* 1:155–162, 1991.
110. Renier D, Flandin C, Hirsch E, et al: Brain abscesses in neonates. A study of 30 cases. *J Neurosurg* 69:877–82, 1988.
111. Renier D, Lacombe J, Pierre KA, et al: Factors causing acute shunt infection. Computer analysis of 1174 operations. *J Neurosurg* 61:1072–8, 1984.
112. Reusser P, Gyr K, Scheidegger D, et al: Prospective endoscopic study of stress erosions and ulcers in critically ill neurosurgical patients: Current incidence and effect of acid-reducing prophylaxis. *Crit Care Med* 18:270–4, 1990.
113. Reye RDK, Morgan G, Baral J: Encephalopathy and fatty degeneration of the viscera, a disease entity in childhood. *Lancet* 2:749–752, 1963.
114. Rish BL, Caveness WF, Dillon JD, et al: Analysis of brain abscess after penetrating craniocerebral injuries in Vietnam. *Neurosurgery* 9:535–41, 1981.
115. Roos KL: Dexamethasone and nonsteroidal anti-inflammatory agents in the treatment of bacterial meningitis. *Clin Ther* 12:290–6, 1990.
116. Roos KL: Meningitis as it presents in the elderly: Diagnosis and care. *Geriatrics* 45:63–4, 1990.
117. Rosenblum ML, Hoff JT, Norman D, et al: Nonoperative treatment of brain abscesses in selected high-risk patients. *J Neurosurg* 52:217–25, 1980.
118. Rosenblum ML, Hoff JT, Norman D, et al: Decreased mortality from brain abscesses since advent of computerized tomography. *J Neurosurg* 49:658–68, 1978.
119. Sáez-Llorens XJ, Umana MA, Odio CM, et al: Brain abscess in infants and children. *Pediatr Infect Dis J* 8:449–58, 1989.
120. Sawyer J, Ellner J, Ransohoff DF: To biopsy or not to biopsy in suspected herpes simplex encephalitis: A quantitative analysis. *Med Decis Making* 8:95–101, 1988.
121. Schlitt MJ, Morawetz RB, Bonnin JM, et al: Brain biopsy for encephalitis. *Clin Neurosurg* 33:591–602, 1986.
122. Shapiro M, Wald U, Simchen E, et al: Randomized clinical trial of intra-operative antimicrobial prophylaxis of infection after neurosurgical procedures. *J Hosp Infect* 8:283–95, 1986.
123. Shelton MM, Marks WA: Bacterial meningitis: An update. *Neurol Clin* 8:605–17, 1990.
124. Simmons BP: CDC guidelines for the prevention and control of nosocomial infections. Guideline for prevention of intravascular infections. *Am J Infect Control* 11:183–99, 1983.
125. Skoldenberg B, Forsgren M, Alestig K, et al: Acyclovir versus vidarabine in herpes simplex encephalitis. Randomised multicentre study in consecutive Swedish patients. *Lancet* 2:707–11, 1984.
126. Sloand EM, Pitt EP, Chiarello RJ, et al: HIV testing. State of the art. *JAMA* 266:2861–2866, 1991.
127. Snider WD, Simpson DM, Nielsen S, et al: Neurologic complications of acquired immune deficiency syndrome: Analysis of 50 patients. *Ann Neurol* 14:403–18, 1983.
128. Soong SJ, Watson NE, Caddell GR, et al: Use of brain biopsy for diagnostic evaluation of patients with suspected herpes simplex encephalitis: A statistical model and its clinical implications. NIAID Collaborative Antiviral Study Group. *J Infect Dis* 163:17–22, 1991.
129. Sotelo J, del Brutto OH, Penagos P, et al: Comparison of therapeutic regimen of anticysticercal drugs for parenchymal brain cysticercosis. *J Neurol* 237:69–72, 1990.
130. Starko KM, Ray CG, Dominguez LB, et al: Reye's syndrome and salicylate use. *Pediatrics* 66:859–64, 1980.
131. Stephanov S: Surgical treatment of brain abscess. *Neurosurgery* 22:724–30, 1988.
132. Stephanov S, Joubert MJ: Large brain abscesses treated by aspiration alone. *Surg Neurol* 17:338–40, 1982.
133. Stoutenbeek CP, van SH, Miranda DR, et al: The effect of selective decontamination of the digestive tract on colonization and infection rate in multiple trauma patients. *Intensive Care Med* 10:185–92, 1984.

134. Thomas JN, Nel JR: Acute spreading osteomyelitis of the skull complicating frontal sinusitis. *J Laryngol Otol* 91:55–62, 1977.
135. Tryba M: The gastropulmonary route of infection—fact or fiction? *Am J Med* 91:135S–146S, 1991.
136. Tucker RM, Galgiani JN, Denning DW, et al: Treatment of coccidioidal meningitis with fluconazole. *Rev Infect Dis* S380–9, 1990.
137. Tucker RM, Williams PL, Arathoon EG, et al: Pharmacokinetics of fluconazole in cerebrospinal fluid and serum in human coccidioidal meningitis. *Antimicrob Agents Chemother* 32:369–73, 1988.
138. Tunkel AR, Wispelwey B, Scheld WM: Bacterial meningitis: Recent advances in pathophysiology and treatment. *Ann Intern Med* 112:610–23, 1990.
139. Ullman RF, Gurevich I, Schoch PE, et al: Colonization and bacteremia related to duration of triple-lumen intravascular catheter placement. *Am J Infect Control* 18:201–7, 1990.
140. van der Waaij D, Manson WL, Arends JP, et al: Clinical use of selective decontamination: The concept. *Intensive Care Med* S212–6, 1990.
141. Venes JL, Shaywitz BA, Spencer DD: Management of severe cerebral edema in the metabolic encephalopathy of Reye-Johnson syndrome. *J Neurosurg* 48:903–15, 1978.
142. Verner EF, Musher DM: Spinal epidural abscess. *Med Clin North Am* 69:375–84, 1985.
143. Waldman RJ, Hall WN, McGee H, et al: Aspirin as a risk factor in Reye's syndrome. *JAMA* 247:3089–94, 1982.
144. Walters BC, Hoffman HJ, Hendrick EB, et al: Cerebrospinal fluid shunt infection: Influences on initial management and subsequent outcome. *J Neurosurg* 60:1014–21, 1984.
145. Whelan MA, Hilah SK: Computed tomography as a guide in the diagnosis and follow-up of brain abscesses. *Radiology* 135:663–71, 1980.
146. Whitley RJ, Alford CA, Hirsch MS, et al: Vidarabine versus acyclovir therapy in herpes simplex encephalitis. *N Engl J Med* 314:144–9, 1986.
147. Whitley RJ, Cobbs CG, Alford CJ, et al: Diseases that mimic herpes simplex encephalitis. Diagnosis, presentation, and outcome. NIAD Collaborative Antiviral Study Group. *JAMA* 262:234–9, 1989.
148. Whitley RJ, Soong SJ, Dolin R, et al: Adenine arabinoside therapy of biopsy-proved herpes simplex encephalitis. National Institute of Allergy and Infectious Diseases collaborative antiviral study. *N Engl J Med* 297:289–94, 1977.
149. Wietholter H, Thron A, Scholz E, et al: Systemic Candida albicans infection with cerebral abscess and granulomas. *Clin Neuropathol* 3:37–41, 1984.
150. Word BM, Klein JO: Therapy of bacterial sepsis and meningitis in infants and children: 1989 poll of directors of programs in pediatric infectious diseases. *Pediatr Infect Dis J* 8:635–7, 1989.
151. Yang SY: Brain abscess: A review of 400 cases. *J Neurosurg* 55:794–9, 1981.
152. Yogev R, Davis AT: Neurosurgical shunt infections. A review. *Childs Brain* 6:74–81, 1980.
153. Young RF, Gade G, Grinnell V: Surgical treatment for fungal infections in the central nervous system. *J Neurosurg* 63:371–81, 1985.
154. Young RF, Lawner PM: Perioperative antibiotic prophylaxis for prevention of postoperative neurosurgical infections. A randomized clinical trial. *J Neurosurg* 66:701–5, 1987.
155. Younger JJ, Simmons JC, Barrett FF: Operative related infection rates for ventriculoperitoneal shunt procedures in a children's hospital. *Infect Control* 8:67–70, 1987.

CHAPTER 10

The Intensive Care Management of Patients with Head Injury

Brian T. Andrews

INTRODUCTION

Head injury is a major public health problem in the United States, accounting for 44 percent of all deaths due to trauma. Of the 500,000 significant head injuries that occur each year, 30 to 50 percent are moderately severe and 10 to 20 percent are severe.[1] Severe head injury is most common in young adults, predominantly males, 15 to 24 years of age, and most often results from motor vehicle accidents. Overall, only a small percentage of head-injured patients have surgically treatable intracranial mass lesions,[1] and therefore the vast majority are treated medically, often in an intensive care unit (ICU). For patients with severe head injury, ICU management is the hallmark of care; the goals of management are to support the patient so as to allow maximal recovery from the primary injury and to reverse or prevent secondary injury.

PRIMARY BRAIN INJURY

Cranial trauma may initiate a variety of injury mechanisms. An abrupt change in velocity and angular momentum often causes diffuse brain injury as the outer cortex rotates, shearing axons as they enter the underlying white matter. Diffuse axonal injury may also occur between the white matter and deeper sub-cortical structures, such as the basal ganglia and thalamus, and between these structures and the underlying upper brainstem. If extremely mild, a shearing injury may result in transient loss of electrical transmission and brief loss of consciousness; if more severe, it may cause more extensive cellular and axonal injury as well as more profound and long-lasting neurologic deficits.

Direct impact of certain regions of the brain, including the frontal, temporal, and occipital lobes, against the adjacent irregular inner table of the skull may result in cerebral contusions, direct cortical injury, and a variable amount of hemorrhage. Not infrequently there is contusion at opposite poles of the brain, both in the region of direct impact (coup) and at the opposite pole (contrecoup). Compound depressed skull fractures may also cause contusions or lacerations of the cortex and tearing of superficial arteries and veins.

Primary brain injury as described above cannot be treated directly. Rather, the brain must be protected from secondary injury and elevated intracranial pressure (ICP) to provide an optimal environment for spontaneous recovery.

SECONDARY BRAIN INJURY

Secondary brain injuries may be divided into developing intracranial mass lesions, such as hematomas and cerebral edema, and hypoxic-ischemic cerebral injury resulting from systemic insults, such as hypoxia, hypercarbia, hypotension, and acidosis.

Posttraumatic intracranial hematomas cause secondary brain injury by exerting a localized mass effect, altering regional cerebral blood flow, and displacing brain substance; these alterations result in further mechanical distortion and regional ischemia. Most threatening are shifts such as transtentorial herniation of the temporal lobe, which impinges upon the deep midline structures of the brain, including the brainstem, rendering them ischemic, with rapid and devastating clinical consequences.[1]

The most common traumatic intracranial hemorrhages are acute subdural and epidural hematomas. Subdural hematomas (SDHs) (Fig. 10-1) arise when bridging veins at the cortical surface tear, usually along the vertex of the skull draining toward the superior sagittal sinus and at the temporal and frontal lobes of the brain. SDH is present in about 50 percent of patients after severe head injury and is more common in older patients and those injured by low-velocity trauma, such as falls and vehicle-pedestrian injuries. Blood from the rupture of draining veins collects between the brain surface and the dura, usually over the frontal and temporal lobes, and expands to form a mass lesion affecting the underlying cortex.[2,3] Acute SDHs are often associated with significant brain tissue injury, including shearing injury and contusions, which affects the overall recovery even if the hematoma is rapidly evacuated.

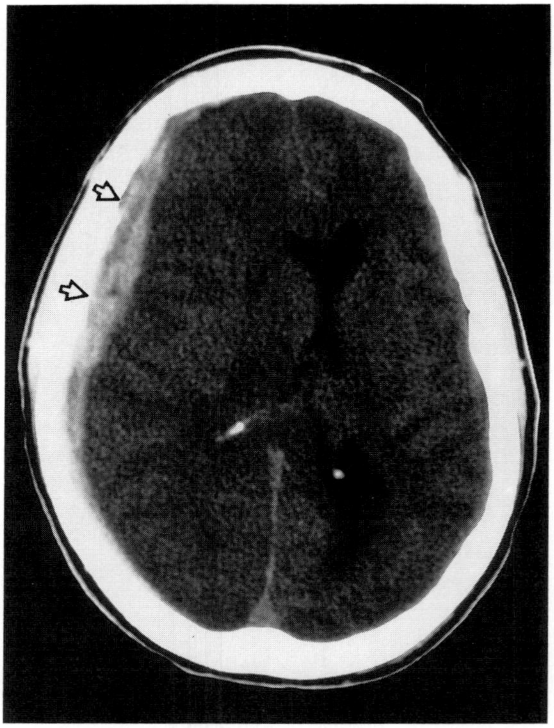

Figure 10-1 Computed tomography scan showing an acute subdural hematoma (arrows).

Acute epidural hematomas (EDHs) (Fig. 10-2) usually arise as a result of skull fractures, most commonly in the temporal region, which often lacerate the middle meningeal artery or adjacent veins. A torn artery can bleed with sufficient pressure to progressively strip the dura away from the inner table of the skull, resulting in an expanding EDH and brain compression. Acute EDHs usually occur in younger patients, often after blunt direct trauma such as blows to the head or falls. Unlike acute SDHs, EDHs are much less often associated with significant brain tissue injury; up to one-third of patients remain conscious at the time of impact,

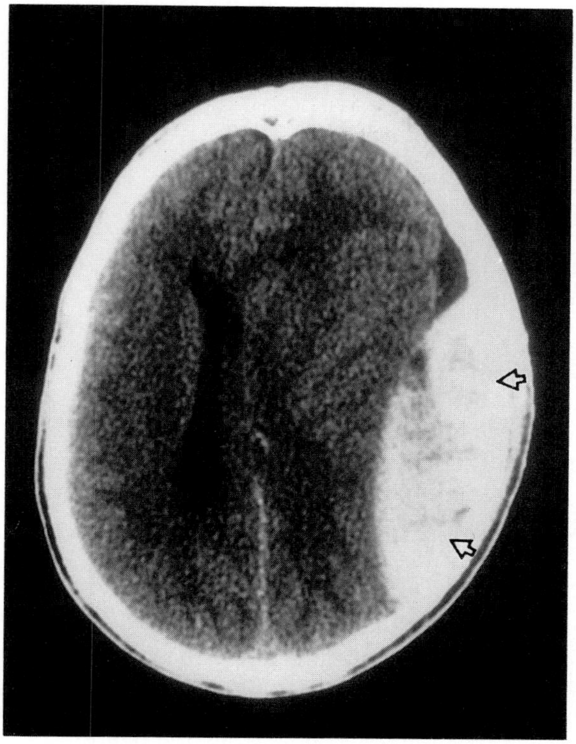

Figure 10-2 Computed tomography showing an acute epidural hematoma (arrows).

and another one-third awaken after initial unconsciousness, only to deteriorate as a result of the expanding intracranial hematoma. Because of the absence of significant brain injury in patients with acute EDHs, rapid diagnosis and surgical evacuation of the hematoma may lead to an excellent outcome.

Both SDH and EDH may be associated with the clinical triad of transtentorial herniation, including anisocoria (usually ipsilateral to the expanding mass), hemiparesis (usually contralateral to the expanding mass), and worsening level of consciousness (usually progressing to coma). Progressive development of these clinical signs often results from an expanding intracranial mass lesion. This life-threatening situation demands immediate diagnosis and management.[1]

Bleeding in a contusion or cortical laceration may cause an acute posttraumatic intracerebral hemorrhage (ICH). Posttraumatic ICH usually forms a progressively enlarging mass lesion over several hours or even days after the injury (Fig. 10-3).[4] These lesions are more common in older patients and are an important cause of delayed neurologic deterioration. ICH in the temporal lobes may cause transtentorial herniation and upper brainstem compression and usually requires urgent surgical evacuation.[5] Thus, a patient who develops delayed anisocoria, increasing hemiparesis, or worsening level of consciousness may have a posttraumatic ICH and must be promptly reevaluated. Subarachnoid hemorrhage from shearing injury, contusions, and cortical lacerations is usually of little clinical importance.

Disruption of cellular membranes and the blood-brain barrier by the primary brain injury may result in varying degrees of cerebral edema in the intracellular or interstitial space. Developing within hours to a few days after injury, cerebral edema causes localized or diffuse mass effect, which may increase ICP. Cerebral blood flow is also altered after severe head injury, often being very low initially and later becoming hyperemic.[6] This may result in secondary ischemic injury, which can be regional or diffuse. Uncontrolled elevation of ICP can decrease cerebral perfusion pressure (CPP) and increase cerebral ischemia.[7-9] Each of these secondary injury mechanisms is exacerbated by systemic hypoxemia, hypercarbia, hypotension, and acidosis.[8,10] Arterial hypercarbia, causing cerebral vasodilatation, may acutely worsen ICP elevation,[8,11,12] whereas systemic hypotension may decrease CPP; in combination, these insults may markedly enhance secondary ischemic cerebral injury.

MILD, MODERATE, AND SEVERE HEAD INJURY

Head injuries are most commonly categorized by the level of consciousness determined with the Glasgow coma scale (GCS) at the initial neurologic examination in the emergency room (see Chap. 2).[13] It is important to categorize head injuries as mild, moderate, or severe because this generally defines the form of treatment applied. Patients

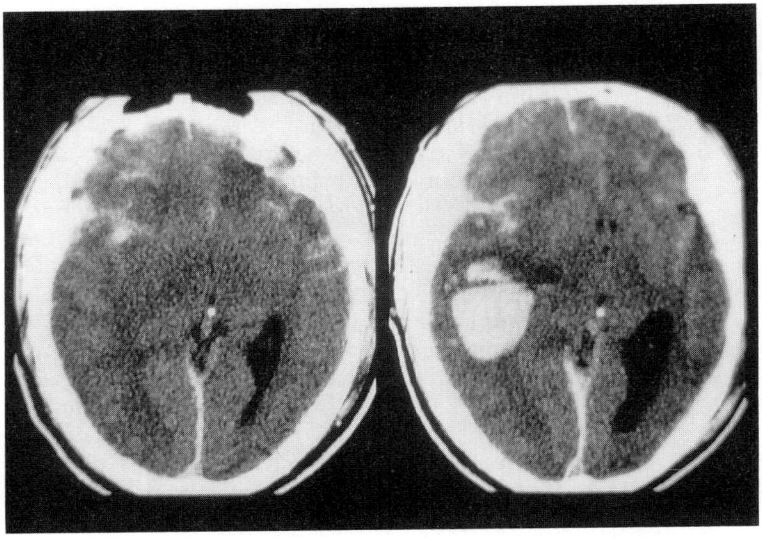

Figure 10-3 Computed tomography scan obtained at admission (left) shows small frontal contusions. Scan obtained 6 h later to evaluate clinical deterioration (right) shows a new large parenchymal hemorrhage.

with mild head injuries, who constitute the vast majority of patients admitted to the emergency room after cranial trauma, have a relatively normal level of consciousness (GCS of 13 to 15). They may be completely normal (the injury is then called a concussion) or, at worst, are slightly lethargic and confused but able to communicate and follow commands easily. Even a mild head injury may cause a distinct structural brain insult, significant and long-lasting symptoms,[14] and occasionally delayed deterioration due to complications, such as an expanding intracranial hematoma.

A moderate head injury is present when patients have a more severely altered level of consciousness but are not comatose (GCS 9 to 12). Such patients are quite lethargic or obtunded and have little understandable speech, but they can generally open their eyes and localize painful stimuli. They must be carefully evaluated not only for head injury but also for complicating clinical conditions such as drug intoxication, hypoxia, and metabolic abnormalities. These patients have a more severe degree of structural brain injury and are at even greater risk for delayed deterioration and secondary brain injury.[15]

Severe head injury is defined as having occurred in those patients rendered comatose (GCS of 8 and below) by the trauma. Such patients do not open their eyes, follow commands, or have intelligible speech, and they may range from being able to localize painful stimuli to abnormal flexor or extensor posturing or complete flaccidity. Not infrequently, a life-threatening structural brain insult has occurred and vigorous efforts may be needed to lower ICP and identify intracranial hematomas requiring evacuation. In addition, systemic hypoxia, hypercarbia, hypotension, and acidosis must be rapidly corrected to limit secondary brain injury.[16,17] Injury to other organ systems must also be quickly recognized and treated.

After initial diagnostic and therapeutic measures have been completed, including the initial assessment of neurologic function, performance of computed tomography (CT) scans or other diagnostic interventions, the evacuation of intracranial mass lesions if present, and the acute management of other systemic injuries, most patients are admitted to the ICU. The goals of intensive care include frequent assessment to allow early detection of neurologic deterioration; frequent or continuous monitoring of vital signs to prevent hypotension or excessive hypertension and to maintain an adequate CPP; respiratory monitoring; and endotracheal intubation and controlled ventilation to assure an adequate airway and tissue oxygenation, prevent hypercarbia and acidosis, and provide hyperventilation to control ICP. Continuous monitoring of ICP and treatment of ICP elevation are important aspects of the management of severe head injuries, as discussed in Chap. 4. Finally, treatment in the ICU must include attention to nutritional and infectious disease status, to allow early institution of nutritional support and prompt recognition and treatment of infections, and additional measures as necessary for the monitoring and management of other systemic and orthopedic injuries.

The decision of which head-injured patients to treat in the ICU varies from one institution to another, depending upon such factors as the frequency of head-injury admissions and what other settings are available for those with lesser injury. At our institution, a major level-one trauma center, patients are admitted to the ICU only if they have a severe head injury (GCS of 8 or less) or have had a craniotomy to evacuate an intracranial hematoma, elevate a depressed skull fracture, or treat some other complication of trauma. Those with less severe head injury (GCS of 9 to 15) may be admitted to the ICU if they have other multisystem injuries or medical complications, such as seizures, pulmonary dysfunction, or coagulopathy, that warrant intensive care management. Otherwise, patients with mild or moderate head injury are monitored in specialized neurologic observation rooms on the hospital ward by nursing staff familiar with head injury. In hospitals without such facilities or trained ward personnel, patients with head injuries of any severity should be admitted to the ICU for initial observation.

NEUROLOGIC MONITORING

During the course of ICU management, neurologic status is assessed at least hourly to identify neurologic deterioration; a uniform method of examination and record keeping is used (see Chap. 2). Delayed complications of head injury, such as intracranial hematomas, enlargement of hemorrhagic contusions with surrounding edema,[4] and increased ICP, may be reflected by a deteriorating level of consciousness or by the onset of new localizing neurologic abnormalities, such as hemiparesis or anisocoria.[1] Decreases of two or more points on the GCS and new localizing deficits are usually considered significant and should prompt an assessment of the potential causes of deterioration, such as hypoxia, hypotension, or electrolyte disturbance; CT scanning of the brain should be considered as well.

Continued neurologic monitoring may prove difficult in patients who are extremely agitated or who require sedation or pharmacologic paralysis to prevent them from injuring themselves or causing further elevation in ICP. We minimize the use of sedation but use intermittent doses of intravenous morphine (up to 0.1 mg/kg every 1 to 3 h), or lorazepam (Ativan) (0.02 to 0.05 mg/kg every 2 to 3 h). Although midazolam is a sedative favored by anesthesiologists during and after surgery, its effects on the injured brain are unknown, and we prefer not to use it.[18] For the agitated severely head-injured patients who are intubated and undergoing controlled ventilation and ICP monitoring, we administer an intravenous infusion of a short-acting paralytic such as vecuronium.[18] To allow repeated examination during paralysis, the paralytic agent is stopped temporarily to allow neurologic examination every 3 to 6 h. In conjunction with continuous monitoring of ICP, this approach is adequate to identify delayed intracranial complications.

CARDIOVASCULAR MONITORING AND MANAGEMENT

Blood pressure, pulse, and respirations must be carefully monitored. In patients with mild or moderate head injury and no other systemic insults, hourly bedside recording may suffice. In some cases, automated bedside blood pressure recording devices can provide more frequent assessment and sound an alarm if preset upper and lower limits are exceeded.[19] In patients with severe head injury, particularly those with multisystem injury or who have had a craniotomy, blood pressure should be monitored continuously with a radial artery catheter.[20,21] These catheters have little risk and allow repeated assessment of arterial blood gases and precise pharmacologic management of blood pressure. In such patients, we also frequently place a central venous catheter for added vascular access and monitoring of central blood volume.[18] In those with cardiac dysfunction, such as myocardial contusions, infarction, or congestive heart failure, a Swan-Ganz catheter is often placed to monitor pulmonary capillary wedge pressures,[20,21] Clifton[9] has recommended routine placement of a Swan-Ganz catheter to monitor pulmonary wedge pressure and cardiac output in patients with severe head injury. A more complete discussion of these and other cardiovascular monitoring methods is provided in Chaps. 1, 3, and 13.

Among patients with head injury, both hypotension and hypertension are to be avoided. Systemic hypotension [systolic blood pressure (SBP) below 90 mmHg] is of most concern because it potentially allows a decrease in CPP (calculated as the mean arterial pressure minus ICP), particularly if ICP is elevated, which may cause a devastating secondary ischemic insult to the injured brain.[7,10] An SBP of about 120 mmHg is considered optimal. We allow patients with a known history of hypertension to maintain a blood pressure at or near their normal levels, up to an SBP of approximately 180 mmHg; above this level the potential for cerebral hyperperfusion increases, which may exacerbate elevation of ICP.[16]

Hypotension after head trauma most often results from hemorrhagic shock; in the ICU, occult sources of ongoing hemorrhage must be sought, such as into the chest or abdomen, and volume resuscitation using isotonic crystalloids (0.9% normal saline), colloids, or packed red blood cells should be performed, as described in Chaps. 6 and 13. Crystalloids without additional glucose are generally used because an elevated serum glucose level appears to be harmful to the injured or ischemic brain, due to increased intracellular lactic acidosis.[18,22] During the subsequent ICU course, the serum glucose level is carefully monitored and maintained at 100 to 200 mg/dL.[18]

If fluid resuscitation proves inadequate to restore blood pressure rapidly, intravenous dopamine (Intropin) should be instituted temporarily. At lower doses (less than 5 μg/kg per min), this sympathomimetic amine acts primarily on beta-adrenergic receptors in both the heart and peripheral blood vessels, increasing cardiac rate, myocardial contractility, and cardiac output and relaxing systemic arterioles, which lowers peripheral vascular resistance and increases renal blood flow. At higher doses (5 to 10 μg/kg per min) its alpha-adrenergic effect increases, resulting in peripheral vasoconstriction, higher systemic vascular resistance, and marked increase in blood pressure.[20,23]

If an antihypertensive agent is necessary to control blood pressure in the ICU, one of the most effective classes of drugs are those that block beta-adrenergic receptors, primarily the $beta_1$ receptors in the heart, resulting in a decrease in cardiac rate, contractility, and cardiac output.[24] Beta blockers also inhibit the sympathetically mediated release of renin from the juxtaglomerular cells of the kidney, which has an additional blood pressure lowering action. Beta blockers are most indicated when hypertension is associated with a state of increased sympathetic tone, as in severe head injury,[17] resulting in tachycardia and increased cardiac output. In this setting, the drug directly counteracts the abnormal pathophysiology. Beta blockers are contraindicated in patients with congestive heart failure and pulmonary diseases, such as asthma, which may be exacerbated by beta-adrenergic blockade.

The beta blocker most often used in the intensive care setting is esmolol (Brevibloc). Its extremely short half-life allows accurate titration of its effect when administered by intravenous infusion at doses up to 300 μg/kg per min. Labetalol (Trandate, Normodyne) also has a relatively short half-life and can be given by intravenous infusion (0.3 to 1.5 mg/min or 20 to 100 mg/h). Labetalol has an additional alpha-receptor blocking action that decreases systemic vascular resistance and cardiac output. A recent clinical study of 15 patients after intracranial surgery for aneurysms or arteriovenous malformations showed that, compared with intravenous sodium nitroprusside, use of labetalol to achieve similar control of hypertension resulted in improved control of ICP in five patients and improved CPP in six.[25]

Sodium nitroprusside (Nipride) is commonly used in the general intensive care setting to control blood pressure. Although useful in severe primary hypertension, nitroprusside increases ICP both experimentally[26–28] and clinically.[29–32] The increase in ICP appears to be a direct result of cerebral vasodilation and increased cerebral blood volume.[29,31] Some have also suggested that preferential peripheral vasodilation over cerebral vasodilation by sodium nitroprusside may result in a steal effect and a relative decrease in cerebral blood flow.[23,27] For these reasons, we believe sodium nitroprusside is contraindicated in head-injured patients with potentially increased ICP.

PULMONARY MANAGEMENT

The occurrence of hypoxia, hypercarbia, and acidosis is as profound an insult to the injured brain as hypotension.[10,33] Systemic hypoxia is an extremely common initial complication of head injury and is present in 30 to 43 percent of severely head-injured patients at the time of admission.[33,34] Secondary injury mechanisms after head trauma are closely associated with ischemia and are exacerbated by hypoxia, hypercarbia, and acidosis. Hypercarbia that causes cerebral vasodilation may exacerbate elevations in ICP, resulting in decreased perfusion pressure and further ischemic injury.[8,10,11,33] Both initial management and subsequent care in the ICU should be directed to establishing and maintaining an airway, assuring adequate ventilation, and correcting these abnormalities (see Chap. 1).

Most patients with mild or moderate head injury have a normal airway, intact reflexes, and normal breathing patterns. In these patients we usually rely on nursing observation and, if needed, intermittent bedside pulse oximetry to monitor the percent of oxygen saturation. Supplemental oxygen is often used to keep the arterial P_{O_2} above 100 mmHg or the O_2 saturation above 95 percent. Patients with a moderate head injury (GCS of 9 to 12) may benefit from a nasal trumpet and supplemental O_2, or, at the lower end of the scale, endotracheal intubation and mechanical ventilation, especially if there are multiple injuries and pulmonary dysfunction; the goals of intubation in such cases are primarily to assure a patent airway, avoid aspiration of gastric contents, and maintain arterial P_{O_2} and P_{CO_2} in the physiologic range. Similarly, head-injured patients who are agitated or combative may best be managed initially by pharmacologic paralysis, intubation, and controlled ventilation to protect the airway and allow diagnostic and therapeutic interventions.[35]

At the San Francisco General Hospital, all patients with an initially severe head injury are intubated upon arrival in the emergency room. This not only protects the airway but also allows rapid correction of injury-related hypoxia and hypercarbia[33,34] and therapeutic hyperventilation.[1,8-10,36-38] In this setting it is assumed that there is an intracranial mass lesion and increased ICP. Hyperventilation to an arterial P_{CO_2} of 20 to 25 mmHg causes a respiratory alkalosis, which results in cerebral vasoconstriction, reduces cerebral blood volume,[11,18,39,40] and lowers ICP; the respiratory alkalosis also tends to reduce detrimental intracerebral acidosis.[40] Patients with a diffuse brain injury and generalized loss of cerebral autoregulation are less responsive to hyperventilation than those with more localized abnormalities or mass lesions or with injuries primarily to the brainstem.[41]

If diagnostic studies show that no mass lesion is present, and ICP monitoring fails to document elevations in ICP, hyperventilation is stopped and P_{O_2} and P_{CO_2} are maintained in the normal physiologic range. After craniotomy to evacuate a hematoma, we routinely monitor ICP in the ICU. Hyperventilation is continued until the ICP has been determined to be acceptable, and the P_{CO_2} is gradually normalized to 35 to 40 mmHg. Finally, if initially elevated ICP can be corrected with other forms of treatment, such as mannitol infusion or manipulation of the perfusion pressure, hyperventilation is gradually decreased until the P_{CO_2} is normalized. We prefer to normalize the arterial P_{CO_2} during the first several days in the ICU, both to prevent the development of regional cerebral ischemia due to vasoconstriction[42] and to allow subsequent hyperventilation if there is a delayed complication, such as intracerebral hematoma,[4] that increases ICP.

During pulmonary management in the ICU, it is not uncommon to see ICP elevations due to coughing induced by endotracheal suctioning or to Valsalva maneuvers in agitated patients "fighting" the endotracheal tube. In a randomized, prospective study at our institution, White and coworkers[43] showed that intermittent paralysis with intravenous succinylcholine was superior to lidocaine, narcotics, and barbiturates in preventing elevations in ICP during endotracheal suctioning. Restless, agitated, or thrashing patients with poor intracranial compliance may also require intermittent paralysis during the most agitated periods to prevent or correct elevations in ICP.

The criteria for weaning of ventilatory support and tracheal extubation are reviewed in Chap. 1. In head-injured patients, extubation can only be considered if the level of consciousness has improved enough that the patient can"protect" the airway from aspiration of secretions or gastric contents and if lower cranial nerve function involved with pharyngeal and tracheal reflexes is intact. Rarely, tracheostomy may be considered for patients who have a very severe neurologic deficit or a persistent vegetative state that is expected to resolve only over the course of months. The potential advantages of a tracheostomy are long-term protection of the airway and ease of pulmonary toilet; the risks include mechanical obstruction, accidental dislodgement, and tracheal strictures.

INTRACRANIAL PRESSURE MONITORING AND MANAGEMENT

The pathophysiology and general management of elevated ICP, as well as the various monitoring techniques available, have been discussed in detail in earlier chapters but will be reviewed briefly here. We monitor ICP in all patients with severe head injury (GCS of 8 or less) and in those who undergo evacuation of an acute posttraumatic intracranial hematoma or other major neurosurgical intervention, regardless of the preoperative coma score.[1,18] Continuous monitoring of ICP after head injury has several advantages. First, it identifies elevated ICP, which can result in a decrease in CPP. Treatment of ICP above 20 mmHg has been widely recommended[1,8,9,12,18,38,42,44,45] to maintain CPP above 50 mmHg. Second, ICP monitoring can provide an early warning of delayed complications of head injury; progressive elevation in ICP may indicate the development of an intracerebral hematoma or an enlarging hemorrhagic contusion and surrounding cerebral edema, which may require surgical intervention.[4,8,9,12,18,38,44] This is particularly true in deeply comatose patients, in whom the neurologic examination may not immediately reflect such complications, and in agitated patients requiring therapeutic paralysis. Narayan and coworkers,[44] after carefully reviewing a 4-year experience in 207 severely head-injured patients, suggested that ICP monitoring is particularly important if the initial CT scan is abnormal, if the patient is over 40 years of age, if the SBP is under 90 mmHg, or if there is motor posturing. The incidence of ICP elevation was 60 percent if two of these findings were present, but was only 4 percent if one or none were present.

Numerous reports have suggested a beneficial effect of ICP monitoring and treatment in patients with head injury,[9,18,44,46–50] although there are no controlled trials that show this conclusively. Among severely head-injured patients with an initial GCS of 3 to 5, the mortality rate was 39 percent when the ICP was monitored and treated and 67 percent when it was not;[48] however, patients in this study were not randomly allocated to each group. Saul and Ducker[49] reported that the mortality rate fell from 46 to 33 percent when ICP was rigorously maintained below 15 mmHg. These and other reports have generally convinced neurosurgeons who frequently treat severe head injuries that ICP monitoring is appropriate and enhances the potential for recovery.

Finally, ICP data are useful for predicting the prognosis for recovery after head injury. Patients with intractable elevation of ICP unresponsive to therapeutic measures usually die or have an extremely poor outcome.[1,8,9,12,18,38,44,45] ICP that is elevated to the level of systemic blood pressure results in total loss of cerebral perfusion and supports a declaration of brain death (see Chap. 21).

Monitoring Techniques

In comatose patients without intracranial mass lesions on initial CT scans, we usually place a percutaneous catheter into the right lateral ventricle via a frontal burr hole placed in the operating room; this may be performed in the ICU with a twist-drill technique.[18,44] Many trauma units now use the fiber-optic (Camino) catheter, which can be placed quickly and safely, using a simple twist-drill technique, in the subarachnoid space, brain parenchyma, or ventricle, for accurate ICP monitoring.[46] After a craniotomy to evacuate a hematoma or other surgical intervention such as exploratory burr-hole placement, we usually place a catheter into the subdural space; this is an extremely simple and reliable method for monitoring postoperative ICP.[1,18,51,52]

Typically, ICP catheters are left in place until the pressure remains normal for 24 h and measures such as hyperventilation and mannitol infusion are no longer necessary. If ICP monitoring is needed for longer than 7 days, it is our policy to change the catheter at that time, often placing a new contralateral ventriculostomy or a new subarachnoid fiber-optic monitor to limit the risk of infection from catheters remaining in place for longer periods. While a catheter is in place, intravenous antibiotics with anti-staphylococcal coverage, such as vancomycin, are administered daily. The ICP catheter, all tubing, and the transducer are filled with an antibiotic solution containing gentamycin, 1 mg/mL, which is stable in solution for 4 to 6 days and has wide antibacterial activity. To minimize the risk of infection, it is extremely important that the system be as closed as possible and that there be no cerebrospinal fluid (CSF) leakage at any site.[18] Additional discussion of ICP monitoring is provided in Chap. 3.

Chapter 3 provides a broad review of ICP management. In head-injured patients, we attempt to prevent or reduce ICP elevation by promptly identifying and removing intracranial mass lesions, both during initial management in the emergency department and in the ICU. We also continue to utilize hyperventilation,[1,8-10,18,36,37,39-42] hyperosmolar therapy,[1,8,9,18,42,53-55] perfusion pressure therapy,[18,50,56] and barbiturates[8,18,47,57-59] as the main components of ICP control (Table 10-1). Sedation and therapeutic paralysis are used as required in agitated or thrashing patients whose activity continually elevates ICP.

Table 10-1 Management of Elevated Intracranial Pressure

Controlled hyperventilation
Mannitol (0.25–0.5 g/kg, IV boluses)
Furosemide
Elevation of cerebral perfusion pressure
Head of bed elevation 10–20°
Sedation for restlessness
Paralysis for severe agitation
Barbiturates

Hyperventilation

In severely head-injured patients and those requiring surgical intervention, hyperventilation is usually started in the emergency room and continued through the initial period of ICP monitoring in the ICU. Arterial P_{CO_2} is generally maintained at 20 to 25 mmHg to provide cerebral vasoconstriction,[8,9,18,36,37,39,40,42] but not to a degree that reduces cerebral blood flow below the level needed to maintain normal metabolism.[18,42] Additional hyperventilation to decrease the Pa_{CO_2} below this level is generally avoided because it may not result in further vasoconstriction[11,41] and may cause metabolic complications from excessive serum alkalosis. Recently, however, in severely head-injured children, Sutton (personal communication) has used extreme hyperventilation to Pa_{CO_2} levels of 10 to 15 mmHg, with additional effect on ICP; ischemic complications due to excessive vasoconstriction are avoided by monitoring jugular venous oxygen saturation (SJ_{O_2}) and calculating the arterial-venous difference (AVD_{O_2}).[18] A widening of AVD_{O_2} from normal levels suggests increased brain oxygen extraction and the potential onset of cerebral ischemia; at this point hyperventilation is reduced slightly to allow adequate cerebral perfusion. Recently Sheinberg and coworkers[60] used this technique in 45 severely head-injured adults; venous oxygen saturation was measured with a fiber-optic catheter at the jugular bulb. The fiber-optic system provided acceptable accuracy and showed that venous desaturation occurred as a result of intracranial hypertension, excessive hypocarbia, arterial hypoxia, and systemic hypotension. This preliminary study suggests that continuous monitoring of SJ_{O_2} and AVD_{O_2} may be of clinical value in patients with head injury.

As mentioned earlier, an attempt is made to gradually normalize the P_{CO_2} while using other methods of ICP control such as osmolar therapy, to avoid inducing regional cerebral ischemia[18,42] and to avoid losing the effectiveness of hyperventilation. Muizelaar and coworkers[61] showed experimentally that continuous hyperventilation to maintain a Pa_{CO_2} of 25 mmHg results in a steady loss of pial arteriolar vasoconstriction; after 20 h, vessel diameters were essentially at baseline values, and subsequent attempts to return to normocapnia resulted in further vasodilatation and an increase in cerebral blood volume. During the same period, arterial and CSF pH had also normalized. Similar pH and blood volume findings have been described during prolonged hyperventilation in humans.[39,62] These results suggest that in the ICU management of head injury, continuous hyperventilation probably becomes ineffective after 20 to 24 h, and subsequent attempts to normalize the Pa_{CO_2} may further increase the ICP. We therefore recommend that hyperventilation be used initially, until the level of ICP can be determined, and then only to treat acute elevations in ICP[8,18] while more definitive measures, such as osmolar therapy, ventricular drainage, and the diagnosis and evacuation of progressive mass lesions, are being initiated. Hyperventilation should not be used to prevent ICP elevation, nor should it be used by itself in a prolonged fashion to maintain ICP control.[8,18]

One exception to this recommendation may be young children, in whom diffuse cerebral swelling after severe head injury may result in generalized hyperemia and increased cerebral blood flow and blood volume. This syndrome of "malignant brain edema," as described by Bruce and coworkers[45] may best be treated with more prolonged and more profound continuous hyperventilation.

Hyperosmolar Therapy

In addition to hyperventilation as a means of lowering ICP, we routinely use intravenous mannitol, and at times, other diuretics, to decrease the extracellular fluid volume within the brain. The goal is not to achieve a clinically dehydrated state, which, as expressed by Rosner in Chap. 4 and elsewhere,[50,56] may be detrimental to control of ICP due to a lack of cerebral blood flow and further vasodilatation in regions of intact autoregulation. Rather, the goal of management is to maintain a clinically euvolemic state while increasing the serum sodium, osmolality, and tonicity (see Chap. 6) to optimal levels. A serum sodium level of 145 to 155 mEq/L and serum osmolality of 300 to a maximum of 330 mOsm/L are generally desired. To avoid excessive dehydration while managing elevated ICP with diuretics, we routinely monitor central venous pressure and administer isotonic crystalloid (normal saline) or colloid (Plasmanate or salt-poor albumin) solutions to maintain a central venous pressure of 2 to 5 mmHg.[18] As previously noted, others have recommended the routine placement of a Swan-Ganz catheter in severely head-injured patients to monitor the pulmonary wedge pressure, which should be maintained at more than 5 mmHg, and to measure cardiac output.[9]

Mannitol, a 6-carbon sugar similar to glucose, is administered as an intermittent intravenous bolus (0.25 to 0.5 gm/kg body weight) as often as every 4 h.[1] Where the blood-brain barrier is intact mannitol remains within the intravascular and extracellular spaces[8,9,12,18,42,55,63,64] and has a number of effects, including an immediate increase in circulating blood volume and arterial blood pressure;[54,55] it also reduces blood viscosity by hemodilution[63,64] and by increasing red blood cell deformability.[63] Muizelaar and coworkers[64] have shown that cerebral vasoconstriction occurs in direct response to the decrease in blood viscosity after mannitol infusion. They postulate that the decrease improves red cell oxygen transport, allowing vasoconstriction in regions of the brain where autoregulation is intact. Rosner and Coley[56] showed that ICP responds better to mannitol in patients with a low initial CPP than those with a high CPP and suggested that the increases in systolic blood pressure and CPP allow direct cerebral vasoconstriction.

Mannitol infusion also results in osmotic dehydration of the brain, which reduces the volume of extracellular free water[8,9,18,55,56] and thereby decreases brain volume and ICP, and causes a urinary osmotic diuresis as well. Repeated administration of mannitol, especially in combination with furosemide,[9,55,65] usually results in a systemic hyperosmolar state and potential dehydration, which should be avoided. If it is administered repeatedly, mannitol can eventually move through the blood-brain barrier into the extracellular space, where the increased oncotic pressure can retain free water and enhance edema. Thus, mannitol use should be limited to the minimum level needed to control ICP and CPP and should not be given with furosemide unless ICP control is poor.

Furosemide (Lasix) has long been used to reduce intracerebral free water and decrease cerebral edema.[9,18,38,55,65] Furosemide acts partly through diuresis, which elevates serum sodium and osmolality, increasing intravascular oncotic pressure and withdrawing free water from the brain.[65] Furosemide also decreases CSF production.[55] Administration of furosemide in combination with mannitol may reduce ICP more effectively than either drug alone.[9,18,55,65] Roberts and coworkers[55] showed experimentally that infusion of mannitol followed 15 min later by furosemide resulted in the most profound and sustained reduction in elevated ICP; this effect did not appear to involve altered renal excretion of mannitol. We caution, however, that this combination of drugs may cause profound diuresis and rapid dehydration, which may be detrimental to the severely head-injured patient.

Barbiturate Coma

Therapeutic barbiturate coma is another way to treat otherwise intractable elevation of ICP.[4,8,18,47,57–59] Barbiturates reduce ICP by decreasing cerebral metabolism, oxygen use, and blood flow.[4,9,57-59] Barbiturate coma is usually induced with a continuous infusion of intravenous pentobarbital (10 mg/kg body weight initially, followed by 1.5 mg/kg per h). Pentobarbital levels should be checked periodically and the dosage adjusted to maintain a serum level of about 3 mg/dL. Intravenous barbiturates cause systemic hypotension[4,8,18,47,57-59] due to myocardial suppression, which can usually be managed by placement of arterial and Swan-Ganz catheters, appropriate fluid administration, and use of intravenous pressors such as dopamine to maintain an adequate cardiac output. Barbiturate coma also necessitates intubation and controlled ventilation. It also results in complete loss of responsiveness to pain or normal brainstem reflexes and should only be used during continuous ICP monitoring. After ICP control is achieved, we usually continue therapy for 2 to 3 days and then withdraw barbiturates while following ICP. If ICP cannot be controlled and rises to the level of systolic blood pressure, one can presume that there is no cerebral perfusion (CPP = 0); even if there are excessive barbiturate levels, brain death can be confirmed by bedside radionuclide testing of cerebral perfusion (see Chap. 21).

In a recent multicenter trial, Eisenberg and coworkers[59] reported that high-dose barbiturates effectively reduced ICP elevations that were uncontrollable with maximal conventional therapy. In patients whose early management had been complicated by hypotension, barbiturates were much less effective and the outcome was worse than in any other group. They concluded that barbiturates should probably be avoided in such patients. Although barbiturates can lower ICP, their effect on outcome is much less clear. In a randomized, well-controlled prospective trial of barbiturate coma for severe head injury regardless of ICP, Ward and coworkers[58] showed that there was no improvement in survival and no difference in the incidence or duration of elevated ICP. In summary, despite their apparently limited benefits, barbiturates may have a role in the treatment of severely head-injured patients with increased ICP that is unresponsive to all other treatment.

Additional Measures

The treatment of ICP elevation by increasing CPP[50,56] is discussed in detail by Rosner in Chap. 4. We generally attempt to maintain CPP at 60 mmHg or above, and control ICP elevation as described above. When ICP control is marginal or poor and continued hyperventilation or repeated doses of mannitol are required, we have in recent years begun to increase CPP to 70 to 90 mmHg, using judicious volume expansion and at times dopamine infusion. This appears to improve ICP control in some but not all patients. In a group of severely head-injured patients reported by Rosner and Daughton,[50] CPP management resulted in excellent ICP control and a mortality rate of only 21 percent; only 8 percent of the deaths were due to uncontrollable ICP.

We generally elevate the head of the bed 10 to 20 degrees to augment cerebral venous drainage and carefully avoid physical restrictions to venous drainage, such as tight endotracheal-tube ties around the neck, neck flexion, or repetitive Valsalva maneuvers due to suctioning, coughing, or agitation. The use of sedation and therapeutic paralysis has already been discussed. Rosner and Daughton[50] have suggested keeping the head of the bed flat, to augment cerebral perfusion, as one component of CPP management.

NUTRITIONAL MANAGEMENT

After major trauma, including severe head injury, a negative nitrogen balance rapidly develops as a result of hypermetabolism and hypercatabolism,[66,67] and substantial intake of both calories and protein is required to avoid significant weight loss and muscle atrophy (see Chap. 7).[66–68] Inadequate nutrition may result in impaired immune function, poor wound healing, anemia, and decreased resistance to infection. After severe head injury, enteral feeding may be poorly tolerated at first due to paralytic ileus and diarrhea.[66,68] Norton and coworkers[68] showed that the mean delay until adequate amounts of full-strength enteral nutrition could be tolerated was 11.5 days after injury; the development of increased ICP delayed tolerance even further. They recommended that total parenteral nutrition (TPN) be initiated as soon as possible after admission to begin to meet nutritional requirements and replace catabolic losses. In a prospective randomized, controlled trial comparing TPN with enteral feeding, Rapp and coworkers[69] showed improved survival among those given TPN. In a similar study, Hadley and coworkers[66] found no difference in survival among patients randomized to parenteral or enteral nutrition, although nitrogen balance was significantly better among those receiving TPN.

The expense and complications of TPN have led others to initiate enteral feeding as early as 24 to 36 h after head injury.[67,70,71] Grahm and coworkers[67] found that by placing a nasojejunal feeding tube fluoroscopically in the proximal small intestine, enteral feedings could be tolerated to a level equal to the patient's measured energy expenditure, despite the absence of bowel sounds. Compared with nasogastric feeding initiated when bowel sounds returned, jejunal feeding resulted in improved caloric intake and nitrogen balance, reduced incidence of bacterial infections, and fewer days in the ICU. We place a nasogastric tube soon after admission in all severely head-injured patients and attempt to initiate enteral feeding as soon as possible. If, after 24 to 36 h, bowel sounds remain absent or the tube has not migrated spontaneously into the jejunum as seen on plain x-ray, we advance the tube into the upper small intestine under fluoroscopic guidance to begin nasojejunal feeding. We reserve TPN for patients with multisystem injury, including abdominal trauma or burns, and those who cannot tolerate any form of enteral feeding for the first 3 or 4 days after injury.

METABOLIC MANAGEMENT

Because problems of metabolism are common after severe head injury, we monitor serum electrolytes and osmolality every 6 to 8 h for the first 36 to 48 h of ICU management. The most common metabolic abnormalities arise from electrolyte imbalance, most often hyper- and hyponatremia,[8,71] which are comprehensively reviewed in Chap. 6. Hypernatremia and a hyperosmolar state may result from the frequent use of mannitol and other diuretics combined with restriction of free-water intake to prevent or decrease cerebral edema. Excessive hypernatremia may cause neuronal dysfunction as well as cardiopulmonary and renal complications. Generally, we monitor serum sodium and osmolality carefully while mannitol and volume restriction is in use and attempt to limit hypernatremia to no more than 150 mEq/L and the hyperosmolar state to no more than 330 mOsm/L. Excessive hypernatremia is treated by replacing free-water with hypotonic crystalloid solutions, such as 0.45% normal saline.

Water intoxication and hyponatremia may occur as a result of the syndrome of inappropriate antidiuretic hormone secretion (SIADH), or cerebral salt wasting (see Chap. 6).[8,71,72] After head injury, excessive hyponatremia may increase cerebral edema and ICP elevation and, if severe, induce seizures. SIADH may appear several days after injury and account for a delayed clinical deterioration. SIADH is treated by restricting fluid intake to about 1000 mL/day and monitoring serum electrolytes.

Other complications of head injury that may affect the fluid and electrolyte status, such as diabetes insipidus, are reviewed in Chaps. 6 and 8. Diabetes insipidus may result from injury to the hypothalamus or pituitary stalk. In severe head injury, the onset of diabetes insipidus is a grave prognostic sign and may indicate impending clinical brain death. Hyperglycemia is common after head injury and may be exacerbated by enteral or parenteral feeding. Serum glucose levels should be monitored at least daily and more often if abnormally elevated; levels above 200 mg/dL should be treated with parenteral insulin, given on a sliding scale.[1]

USE OF ANTICONVULSANTS

During initial ICU management, anticonvulsants are generally administered to patients with severe head injury and those with significant localized intracranial injuries.[8,71] The drug most commonly used to control seizures in this setting is phenytoin, given in an initial loading dose of 15 to 18 mg/kg body weight intravenously, followed by 5 mg/kg per day (see Chap. 17). The duration of anticonvulsant therapy after injury has been controversial.[71,73–75] Recently Temkin and coworkers[73] showed that prophylactic treatment with phenytoin for 1 year after head injury was no more effective in preventing seizures than treatment for the first 7 days. Treatment for the first week prevents early posttraumatic epilepsy, as defined by Jennet and Teasdale,[74] which occurs in approximately 5 to 10 percent of patients after blunt trauma. Early epilepsy is most common after penetrating injury, particularly gunshot wounds, depressed skull fractures, injuries that cause focal neurologic deficits or intracranial hematomas, and in young children.[1] We therefore treat all patients with clinically severe head injuries, and those with injuries that predispose to early epilepsy, with phenytoin for at least 7 days, regardless of their clinical status.

Delayed posttraumatic epilepsy, defined as seizures which occur more than 7 days after injury, occurs in approximately 5 percent of all patients with closed head trauma,[71,74,75] 15 percent of adults with depressed skull fractures, 25 percent of those with early epilepsy, and up to 35 percent of those with intracranial hematomas. The combination of prolonged traumatic coma, depressed skull fracture, and focal brain injury (e.g., contusion or hematoma) may increase the risk of delayed epilepsy to as high as 70 percent.[1,71] Once a delayed seizure has occurred, the likelihood of further epilepsy is at least 75 percent.[71] Based upon these results, we continue anticonvulsant therapy after the first week of management in any patient with a high likelihood of later epilepsy,[75] to a minimum of 3 months of therapy. During treatment, serum anticonvulsant levels are monitored regularly, and the dosages are adjusted to maintain therapeutic levels.[75]

Carbamazepine is less likely to induce cognitive impairment than phenytoin[75] and may be a better anticonvulsant for long-term use after head injury. However, it cannot be administered parenterally and must be given daily in multiple oral doses. We routinely use phenytoin during initial ICU management but consider switching to carbamazepine therapy during the rehabilitation phase.

MANAGEMENT OF INFECTIOUS COMPLICATIONS

Pulmonary and urinary tract infections are the most common infectious complications after head injury; infections related to the injury itself, such as meningitis, brain abscess, and subdural empyemas, are much rarer.[1,71] Pulmonary infections result from the inability of the patient to clear secretions; the loss of normal mechanics, such as coughing and sighing; and prolonged endotracheal intubation. At our institution, patients who are intubated for longer than 5 days commonly develop pneumonia. Urinary tract infections are usually the result of bladder catheterization. Both sources of infection should be assessed periodically by performing appropriate stains and cultures, particularly when clinical signs warn of possible infection. A more detailed discussion of systemic infections is presented in Chap. 9.

Intracranial infections result from direct contamination of the intracranial space due to a penetrating injury, subsequent surgery, or a cranial defect, such as basilar skull fracture with leakage of CSF. Occasionally, no obvious source of contamination is found. Infections may cause delayed deterioration and must be considered if deterioration is documented. A question that sometimes arises is the safety of lumbar puncture for CSF studies and cultures in patients with possible intracranial mass lesions. In such cases, a lumbar puncture may cause a pressure gradient between the intracranial and spinal spaces and cause downward herniation of the brain through the tentorial notch or foramen magnum,[1] leading to further neurologic decline or even death. Generally, we rely on a current CT scan to identify intracranial mass lesions and avoid performing a lumbar puncture if a significant mass or obvious radiographic signs of elevated ICP are demonstrated.

We generally administer a single dose of prophylactic antibiotic (ceftriaxone, 2 g IV) before intracranial surgery. If there is an open skull fracture, especially if it is grossly contaminated, a broader-spectrum drug combination (ceftriaxone, 2 g IV every 24 h, and vancomycin, 1 g IV every 12 h) is given for a longer period. We do not advocate the use of antibiotics for a basilar skull fracture, with or without a CSF leak, as in this setting they have not proven to be efficacious, and may select for intracranial infection with more resistant bacterial strains.[1]

REFERENCES

1. Andrews BT, Pitts LH: *Traumatic Transtentorial Herniation and Its Management.* Mount Kisco, NY, Futura 1991.
2. Jamieson KG, Yelland JD: Surgically treated traumatic subdural hematomas. *J Neurosurg* 37:137, 1972
3. Stone JL, Rifai MHS, Sugar O, et al.: Subdural hematomas. I: Acute subdural hematoma: Progress in definition, clinical pathology and therapy. *Surg Neurol* 19:216, 1983.
4. Soloniuk D, Pitts LH, Lovely MP, et al.: Traumatic intracerebral hematomas: Timing of appearance and indications for operative removal. *J Trauma* 26:787, 1986
5. Andrews BT, Chiles BW, Olsen WL, et al.: The effect of intracerebral hematoma location on the risk of brainstem compression and on clinical outcome. *J Neurosurg* 69:518, 1988.
6. Marion D, Darby J, Yonas H: Acute regional cerebral blood flow changes caused by severe head injury. *J Neurosurg* 74:407, 1991.
7. Tsutsumi H, Ide K, Mizutani T, et al.: The relationship between intracranial pressure, cerebral perfusion pressure and outcome in head-injured patients: The critical level of cerebral perfusion pressure. In: Miller JD, Teasdale GM, Rowan JO, et al. (eds): *ICP VI.* Berlin, Springer Verlag, 1985, pp 661–666.
8. Pitts LH, Martin N: Head injuries. *Surg Clin North Am* 62:47, 1982.
9. Clifton GL: Management of elevated intracranial pressure. *Neurology Clinics, Baylor College of Medicine* 4:25, 1982.
10. Miller JD, Sweet RC, Narayan R, et al.: Early insults to the injured brain. JAMA 240:439, 1978.
11. Reivich M: Arterial P_{CO_2} and cerebral hemodynamics. *Am J Physiol* 206:25, 1964.
12. Marshall LF, Marshall SB: Medical management of intracranial pressure. In: Cooper PR (ed): *Head Injury*, 2d ed. Baltimore, Williams & Wilkins, 1987, pp 177–196.
13. Pitts LH: Neurological evaluation of the head-injured patient. *Clin Neurosurg* 29:203, 1981.
14. Levin HS, Mattis S, Ruff RM, et al.: Neurobehavioral outcome following minor head injury. *J Neurosurg* 66:234, 1987.
15. Rimel RW, Giordani B, Barth JT, et al.: Moderate head injury: Completing the clinical spectrum of brain trauma. *Neurosurgery* 11:344, 1982.
16. Pitts LH: Intensive care of neurologic diseases. *Curr Opin Neurol Neurosurg* 1:14, 1988.
17. Robertson CS, Clifton GL, Taylor AA, et al.: Treatment of hypertension associated with head injury. *J Neurosurg* 59:455, 1983.
18. Pitts LH, Andrews BT: Intracranial pressure monitoring and treatment of intracranial hypertension. In: Wood L (ed): *Principles of Critical Care Medicine.* New York. McGraw-Hill, 1992, pp 2985–3011.
19. Kaplan N: Hypertension in the individual patient. In: *Clinical Hypertension, 5th ed.* Baltimore, Williams & Wilkins, 1990, pp 26–53.
20. Williams FC, Spetzler RF: Hemodynamic monitoring in the neurosurgical intensive care unit. *Clin Neurosurg* 35:101, 1987.
21. Kaye W: Invasive monitoring techniques: Arterial cannulation, bedside pulmonary artery catheterization and arterial puncture. *Heart Lung* 12:395, 1983.
22. Rhencrona S, Rosen I, Seisjo B: Brain lactic acidosis and ischemic cell damage. 1: Biochemistry and neurophysiology. *J Cereb Blood Flow Metab* 1:297, 1981.
23. Thomas SJ (ed): *Manual of Cardiac Anesthesia.* New York, Churchill Livingstone, 1984.
24. Kaplan N: Treatment of hypertension: Drug therapy. In: *Clinical Hypertension*, 5th ed. Baltimore, Williams & Wilkins, 1990, pp 182–267.
25. Orlowski JP, Shiesley D, Vidt DG, et al.: Labetalol to control blood pressure after cerebrovascular surgery. *Crit Care Med* 16:765, 1988.
26. Michenfelder JD, Milde JH: The interaction of sodium nitroprusside hypotension and isoflurane in determin-

ing cerebral vasculature effects. *Anesthesiology* 69:870, 1988.
27. Davis RF, Douglas ME, Heenan TJ, et al.: Brain tissue pressure measurement during sodium nitroprusside infusion. *Crit Care Med* 9:17, 1981.
28. Ishikawa T, Funatsu N, Okamoto K, et al.: Cerebral and systemic effects of hypotension induced by trimetaphan or nitroprusside in dogs. *Acta Anaesthesiol Scand* 26:643, 1982.
29. Cottrell JE, Patel K, Turndorf H, et al.: Intracranial pressure changes induced by sodium nitroprusside in patients with intracranial mass lesions. *J Neurosurg* 48:329, 1978.
30. McDowall DG: A comparison between sodium nitroprusside and trimetaphan-induced hypotension. *Acta Anaesthesiol Belg* 31:73, 1980.
31. Anile C, Zanghi F, Bracali A, et al.: Sodium nitroprusside and intracranial pressure. *Acta Neurochir (Wein)* 58:203, 1981.
32. Griswold WR, Reznik V, Mendoza SA: Nitroprusside-induced intracranial hypertension. *JAMA* 246:2679, 1981 (Letter).
33. Miller JD: Head injury and brain ischaemia—implications for therapy. *Br J Anaesth* 547:120, 1985.
34. Katsurada K, Yamada R, Sugimoto T: Respiratory insufficiency in patients with severe head injury. *Surgery* 73:191, 1973.
35. Redan JA, Livingston DH, Tortella BJ, et al.: The value of intubating and paralyzing patients with suspected head injury in the emergency department. *J Trauma* 31:371, 1991.
36. Bruce DA, Gennarelli TA, Langfitt W: Resuscitation from coma due to head injury. *Crit Care Med* 6:254, 1978.
37. Clifton GL: Early management in the emergency room and operating room. *Neurol Clin* 4:18, 1982.
38. Saul TG: Acute head injury in adults. In: Rakel RE (ed): *Conn's Current Therapy, 38th ed.* Philadelphia, Saunders, 1987, pp 776–782.
39. Lassen NA: Brain extracellular pH: The main factor controlling cerebral blood flow. *Scand J Clin Lab Invest* 22:247, 1968.
40. Lassen NA: The luxury-perfusion syndrome and its possible relation to acute metabolic acidosis localized within the brain. *Lancet* 2:1113, 1966.
41. Paul RL, Polanco O, Turney SZ, et al.: Intracranial pressure responses to alterations in arterial carbon dioxide pressure in patients with head injuries. *J Neurosurg* 36:714, 1972.
42. Langfitt TW: Increased intracranial pressure and the cerebral circulation. In: Youmans JR (ed): *Neurological Surgery*. Philadelphia, Saunders, 1983, pp 846–930.
43. White PF, Schlobohm RM. Pitts LH, et al.: A randomized study of drugs to prevent increases in intracranial pressure during endotracheal suctioning. *Anesthesiology* 57:242, 1982.
44. Narayan RK, Kishore PR, Becker DP, et al.: Intracranial pressure: To monitor or not to monitor? A review of our experience with severe head injury. *J Neurosurg* 56:650, 1982.
45. Bruce DA, Alavi A, Bilanuik L, et al.: Diffuse cerebral swelling following head injury in children. The syndrome of "malignant brain edema." *J Neurosurg* 55:170, 1981.
46. Ostrup RC, Luerssen TG, Marshall LF, et al.: Continuous monitoring of intracranial pressure with a miniaturized fiberoptic device. *J Neurosurg* 67:206, 1987.
47. Nordstrom CH, Messeter K, Sundbarg G, et al.: Cerebral blood-flow, vasoreactivity and oxygen consumption during barbiturate therapy in severe traumatic brain lesions. *J Neurosurg* 68:424, 1988.
48. Bowers SA, Marshall LF: Outcome in 200 consecutive cases of severe head injury treated in San Diego County: A prospective analysis. *Neurosurgery* 6:237, 1980.
49. Saul TG, Ducker TB: Effect of intracranial pressure monitoring and aggressive treatment on mortality in severe head injury. *J Neurosurg* 56:498, 1982.
50. Rosner MJ, Daughton S: Cerebral perfusion pressure management in head injury. *J Trauma* 30:933, 1990.
51. Andrews BT, Lovely MP, Pitts LH, et al.: Is computerized tomography necessary after tentorial herniation? Results of immediate surgical exploration without computerized tomography in 100 patients. *Neurosurgery* 19:408, 1986.
52. North B, Reilly P: Comparison among three methods of intracranial pressure recording. *Neurosurgery* 18:730, 1986.
53. Muizelaar JP, Lutz HA, Becker DP: Effect of mannitol on ICP and CBF and correlation with pressure autoregulation in severely head-injured patients. *J Neurosurg* 61:700, 1984.
54. Wise BL, Chater N: The value of hypertonic mannitol solution in decreasing brain mass and lowering cerebrospinal fluid pressure. *J Neurosurg* 19:1038, 1962.
55. Roberts P, Pollay M, Engles C, et al.: Effect on intracranial pressure of furosemide combined with varying doses and administration of mannitol. *J Neurosurg* 66:440, 1987.
56. Rosner MJ, Coley I: Cerebral perfusion pressure: A hemodynamic mechanism of mannitol and the postmannitol hemogram. *Neurosurgery* 21:147, 1987.
57. Trauner DA: Barbiturate therapy in acute brain injury. *J Pediatr* 109:742, 1986.
58. Ward JD, Becker DP, Miller JD, et al.: Failure of prophylactic barbiturate coma in the treatment of severe head injury. *J Neurosurg* 62:203, 1985.

59. Eisenberg HM, Frankowski RF, Conant CF, et al.: High-dose barbiturate control of elevated intracranial pressure in patients with severe head injury. *J Neurosurg* 69:15, 1988.
60. Sheinberg M, Kanter MJ, Robertson CS, et al.: Continuous monitoring of jugular venous oxygen saturation in head-injured patients. *J Neurosurg* 76:212, 1992.
61. Muizelaar JP, van der Poel HG, Li Z, et al.: Pial arteriolar vessel diameter and CO_2 reactivity during prolonged hyperventilation in the rabbit. *J Neurosurg* 69:923, 1988.
62. Christensen MS: Acid-base changes in cerebrospinal fluid and blood, and blood volume changes following prolonged hyperventilation in man. *Br J Anaesth* 46:348, 1974.
63. Burke AM, Quest DO, Chein S, et al.: The effect of mannitol on blood viscosity. *J Neurosurg* 55:170, 1981.
64. Muizelaar JP, Wei EP, Kontos HA, et al.: Mannitol causes compensatory cerebral vasoconstriction and vasodilatation in response to blood viscosity changes. *J Neurosurg* 59:822, 1983.
65. Schettini A, Stahurski B, Young HF: Osmotic and osmotic-loop diuresis in brain surgery. Effects on plasma and CSF electrolytes and ion secretion. *J Neurosurg* 56:679, 1982.
66. Hadley MN, Grahm TW, Harrington T, et al.: Nutritional support and neurotrauma. A critical review of early nutritional support in forty-five acute head injury patients. *Neurosurgery* 19:367, 1986.
67. Grahm, TW, Zadrozny DB, Harrington T: The benefits of early jejunal hyperalimentation in the head-injured patient. *Neurosurgery* 25:729, 1989.
68. Norton JA, Ott LG, McClain C, et al.: Intolerance to enteral feeding in the brain-injured patient. *J Neurosurg* 68:62, 1988.
69. Rapp RP, Young B, Twyman D, et al.: The favorable effect of early parenteral feeding on survival in head-injured patients. *J Neurosurg* 58:906, 1983.
70. Hodge SH: Nutritional management. *Neurology Clinics, Baylor College of Medicine* 4:34, 1982.
71. Epstein FM, Ward JD, Becker DP: Medical complications of head injury. In: Cooper PR (ed): *Head Injury*, 2d ed. Baltimore, Williams & Wilkins, 1987, pp 390–421.
72. Lester MC, Nelson PB: Neurological aspects of vasopressin release and the syndrome of inappropriate secretion of antidiuretic hormone. *Neurosurgery* 8:735, 1981.
73. Temkin NR, Dikmen SS, Wilensky AJ, et al.: A randomized, double-blind study of phenytoin for the prevention of post-traumatic seizures. *N Engl J Med* 323:497, 1990.
74. Jennet B, Teasdale G: Neurophysical sequelae. In: Jennet B, Teasdale G (eds): *Management of Head Injuries*. Philadelphia, Davis, 1981, pp 271–288.
75. Deutschmann CS, Haines SJ: Anticonvulsant prophylaxis in neurological surgery. *Neurosurgery* 17:510, 1985.
76. O'Dougherty M, Wright FS, Walson P: Carbamazepine plasma concentration: Relationship to cognitive impairment. *Arch Neurol* 44:863, 1987.

CHAPTER 11

The Intensive Care Management of Spinal Cord Injury

Curtis A. Dickman
Volker K. H. Sonntag

The acute care of patients with a spinal cord injury (SCI) is an evolving discipline, and the neurosurgeon is an integral member of the multidisciplinary team needed to ensure optimal patient care. The therapeutic goals of treatment include preservation of existing neurologic function, maximization of neurologic recovery, treatment of associated injuries, and the prevention and treatment of complications and sequelae of neural damage.

Advances in the knowledge and technology of critical care medicine have improved patient outcome; however, the mortality from SCI remains at a peak during the initial period of hospitalization and treatment.[9,14,20,21,26] The life expectancy of survivors of SCI is reduced compared to age norms.[9,14,16,21] As our medical treatments become more sophisticated and the number of survivors increases, the emotional and financial burden associated with SCI will likewise increase.

This chapter focuses on the theoretical and practical aspects of the acute intensive care unit management of SCI.

TREATMENT OF NEURAL AND VERTEBRAL COLUMN INJURY

The early detection of spinal fractures and prevention of neurologic damage in spinal injury are essential principles that guide acute patient management. The cranium and spine should be considered interrelated, and concurrent injury is as high as 60 percent.[3,14,21] Unconscious or head-injured patients must be considered to have an SCI until proven otherwise. A full radiologic spinal survey must be obtained. Also, if a vertebral fracture occurs, an injury should be diligently sought at a distal level. Multiple noncontiguous spinal fractures occur up to 15 percent of the time.[14,21,22]

Reduction of spinal subluxations to decompress the spinal cord and spinal immobilization to protect the spinal cord are basic tenants of treatment. Cervical subluxations are reduced using spring-loaded Gardner-Wells tongs or a halo ring (Fig. 11-1). Weight is typically added in 5-lb increments to a maximum of 10 lb per level above the injured segment. The weight required for closed reduction of cervical subluxations varies with the patient's age and the type of injury.[2,3,5,13,18,21,22,24] Frequent radiographic and neurologic monitoring are essential to detect overdistraction of the vertebral column. Overdistraction is most easily detected with frequent fluoroscopic evaluation to reassess the spine during increases in traction.

Closed reductions are facilitated with muscular relaxation, which is achieved with small, intravenous doses of diazepam in 0.5 mg increments to ensure that respiratory depression does not occur. Weights are then added in 5-lb increments every 5 min until reduction is achieved or the 10 lb per level limit is reached. The amount of traction should be individualized based upon the level and type of injury.[2,3,5,13,18] Less weight is necessary to realign upper cervical injuries compared to lower cervical injuries.[3,20-22,24]

If radiographic distraction or neurologic deterioration occurs, the weights should be removed and attempts at closed reduction abandoned. If closed reduction is abandoned or if adequate realignment cannot be achieved, open reduction and internal fixation are necessary. Postural reduction or realignment of thoracic or lumbar injuries using a firm, flat surface (i.e., a Stokes bed) may be attempted cautiously. Traction has not been a popular treatment for thoracic or lumbar fractures.

Reduction of cervical dislocations in children requires consideration of skull thickness and spinal ligamentous elasticity. Traction in infants to reduce subluxation is possible with Holter traction or bilateral bur holes and wires. The total amount of traction applied to infants should be limited to 2 lb.[10] In children with thicker skulls, Gardner-Wells tongs or a halo ring permits appropriate traction. During attempted external reduction, careful evaluation of the child is necessary. If any deterioration in neurologic function occurs, external reduction of the spine should be abandoned and one should proceed to internal reduction.[5]

Early operative management may be indicated for neural decompression, internal fixation, or debridement of compound wounds.[3,5,12,21,24,26] Surgery is rarely indicated as an emergency measure for treatment of patients with spinal cord or vertebral column injuries.[24,26] All life-threatening problems must be adequately addressed before pursuing surgery in these cases. Patients with compressive pathology and incomplete neurologic deficits or progression of neurologic deficits are candidates for urgent decompression.[15,26] Elective internal fixation is pursued in patients with spinal instability, ligamentous injuries without fractures,

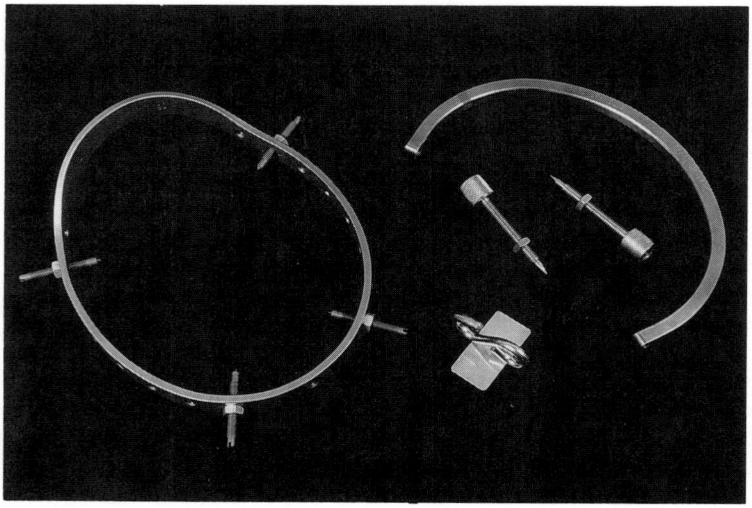

Figure 11-1 Halo ring (left) and spring-loaded Gardner-Wells tongs (right) for reduction of cervical dislocation.

progressive spinal deformity, irreducible fractures, or fractures prone to nonunion.[3-6,12,13,18,24,26]

Secondary mediators of injury are metabolic and pathophysiologic alterations that contribute to the progression of the SCI response after the primary or mechanical injury.[1,8,15,20,22,25,27] Tissue injury causes biochemical, cellular, and tissue changes that produce tissue ischemia.[15,22,25] Posttraumatic ischemia and infarction of the spinal cord are key mechanisms.[25] Posttraumatic ischemia is mediated by local and systemic effects of SCI. Systemically reduced cardiac output, hypotension, and sympathetic vasodilation occur after SCI. Locally, autoregulation can be lost and microcirculation at and adjacent to injured spinal cord segments can be reduced. Posttraumatic vascular effects should be treated to optimize recovery after SCI. Volume expansion and vasopressors are used to restore a normotensive state.[28] Spinal cord blood flow can be improved with volume expansion, steroids, nimodipine, or dopamine.[20,25]

The National Acute Spinal Cord Injury Study II (NASCIS II) performed a randomized, double-blind, placebo-controlled clinical trial that changed the history of the treatment of secondary SCI.[1] This study demonstrated that high-dose methylprednisolone (30 mg/kg bolus followed by 5.4 mg/kg per h for 23 h), if given within 8 h of SCI, improves neurologic recovery. Gangliosides are another type of agent that may enhance recovery after SCI.[8] Clinical studies with these substances are in progress.[1,8,25]

The integral role of the intensive care unit (ICU) during the acute phase of injury cannot be overemphasized. Meticulous hourly neurologic evaluations that include monitoring of sensory, motor, and reflex functions are necessary to detect progressive or ascending deficits. The maintenance of adequate tissue perfusion, ventilatory function, and detection of decompensation are vital issues.

ASSOCIATED INJURIES AND COMPLICATIONS OF SCI

The effects of an acute SCI may obscure the evaluation for other injuries and may also modify the expected responses to therapy. Sixty percent or more of the patients with SCI will have major associated injuries: head or cerebral, thoracic, abdominal, or vascular injuries.[9,20,21,24,26,27] The severity and range of potential associated injuries underscore the need for meticulous primary evaluations and for repeated, systematic reevaluation of patients after SCI. The two most common causes of death associated with SCI are aspiration and shock.[16,19,20,22,29]

Hemodynamic Management

If the patient is hypotensive, sources of hemorrhage must be sought and treated.[28] Neurogenic shock may be superimposed upon hemorrhagic shock. These conditions are not mutually exclusive.

Neurogenic shock results from the loss of adrenergic outflow from the sympathetic nervous system to the heart and peripheral vasculature after an injury above the level of T6. Hypotension, bradycardia, and hypothermia occur. Neurogenic shock impairs the distribution of intravascular volume rather than causing true hypovolemia. Atropine, dopamine, or phenylephrine should be considered for the treatment of neurogenic shock, which is unresponsive to intravascular volume replacement.[20,21,25,28]

Spinal shock differs from the physiologic syndrome of neurogenic shock. Spinal shock refers to the complete loss of sensory, motor, and segmental reflex activity with flaccidity below the level of the SCI. This condition may last as long as 6 weeks. If spinal shock persists longer than 24 h, the prognosis for ambulation is essentially nonexistent. The end of spinal shock is heralded by a return of spinal reflexes, but this phenomenon is poorly understood.

During the acute phase after injury, multiple large bore (16 gauge) peripheral intravenous lines and an arterial line blood pressure monitor are inserted and fluid resuscitation is begun. If patients with an SCI are hypotensive and unresponsive to intravenous fluids and blood products, pulmonary artery catheterization provides a diagnostic tool to guide therapeutic manipulations and to differentiate among hypovolemic, cardiogenic, and neurogenic mechanisms.[28]

The pulmonary artery catheter is the key tool for the assessment of causes of hemodynamic impairment and for judging the efficacy of intervention.[20,28] Pulmonary artery catheterization for assessment of pulmonary capillary wedge pressure and cardiac parameters is more reliable than monitoring central venous pressure.[28] Indwelling arterial catheters are inserted for monitoring blood pressure and arterial blood gases.

Pulmonary artery catheter monitoring in neurogenic shock demonstrates changes consistent with loss of sympathetic function.[20,25,27–29] Systemic vascular resistance is low (less than 800 dyne·s/cm^2). Cardiac output is variable. Renal perfusion can be compromised in these instances. Hypervolemia should be avoided. Fluid administration to maintain pulmonary capillary wedge pressure above 15 mmHg can precipitate pulmonary edema and respiratory failure if intrinsic cardiac decompensation occurs. The ideal blood pressure after SCI depends on the individual, but it should be maintained near the patient's normal preinjury level.[20,25,28]

Alpha-adrenergic agents, such as phenylephrine or norepinephrine, cause a generalized vasoconstriction and are useful for treating hypotension in neurogenic shock. Reflex bradyarrythmias sometimes occur and may require treatment. Phenylephrine HC1 is useful in conjunction with doses of dopamine (2 to 3 μg/kg per min) to augment renal perfusion.

Anticholinergic drugs are less desirable than chronotropic agents (i.e., catecholamines) and are usually reserved for emergencies. Atropine dries the mucous membranes, thickens secretions, and may exacerbate respiratory dysfunction. Ileus may also result.

Respiratory Management

Respiratory dysfunction may occur from ventilatory failure caused by the loss of neural function with paralysis of the thoracic musculature.[19–21,29] It may also be caused or exacerbated by a number of parenchymal factors (Table 11-1).[7,19,20,29] Treatment of existing pathology and prophylaxis of secondary or acquired pulmonary disease are crucial.

Frequent turning of patients with SCI (by logrolling or via oscillating beds), manual coughing, deep breathing, incentive spirometry, and continuous positive airway pressure by mask are methods to maintain lung expansion or functional residual capacity.[19,20,29] Continuous positive airway pressure by mask is an optimal method of maintaining functional residual capacity in the nonintubated patient.[20] These techniques are employed in an attempt to avoid mechanical ventilation.

Table 11-1 Parenchymal Factors Contributing to Pulmonary Dysfunction in the SCI Patient

Pneumothorax
Pulmonary contusion
Aspiration
Pulmonary embolism
Fat embolism
Bacterial pneumonia
Atelectasis
Barotrauma
Rib fractures
Adult respiratory distress syndrome
Pulmonary edema (cardiogenic)
Neurogenic pulmonary edema
Preexisting parenchymal pulmonary disease

Patients with intact phrenic nerve function (C3, C4, and C5) with a midcervical or thoracic SCI may present with initially normal blood gases and acutely deteriorate or decompensate with respiratory failure.[20,21,29] A high index of suspicion and close monitoring are indicated. The loss of innervation to the accessory muscles of respiration and to the intercostal muscles impairs the ability to expand the thorax and causes progressive atelectasis. The chest becomes functionally incompetent and less compliant in these cases. Forced vital capacity (FVC), tidal volume (*vt*), negative inspiratory force (NIF), and respiratory rate are essential parameters that must be followed serially to determine the need for intubation and mechanical ventilation.[19,20,29]

Tables 11-2 and 11-3 detail the criteria for mechanical ventilation.[20] Impaired ventilatory function, clearance of secretions, bronchopulmonary infections, and any other features that exacerbate respiratory insufficiency must be addressed to ensure effective treatment. Once mechanical ventilation is instituted, a tidal volume of 10 to 12 mL/kg is begun, with a ventilator rate to maintain the desired PA_{CO_2} level. The FI_{O_2} is adjusted to maintain Pa_{O_2} above 100 mmHg.[19,27,29]

Patients who require mechanical ventilation

Table 11-2 Criteria for Mechanical Ventilation of SCI Patients Based on Ventilatory or Mechanical Failure

Physiologic parameter	Criterion value
Tachypnea	Respiration rate > 35–40 breaths/min
Inadequate alveolar ventilation	PA_{CO_2} > 48 torr
Reduced vital capacity	Vital capacity < 10–15 mL/kg body weight
Maximal inspiratory force	Inspiratory force < −25 cmH_2O

Source: Adapted from Rosner MJ: Medical management of spinal cord injury. In: Pitts LH, Wagner FC Jr (eds): *Craniospinal Trauma*. New York, Thieme, 1990, table 17-1, p 214. Reprinted by permission of Thieme.

should receive aggressive medical therapy to minimize the length of ventilator dependency. Mobilization of secretions with frequent suctioning, use of humidified air, bronchodilator therapy, and endotracheal instillation of saline are means of reducing complications. Antibiotic prophylaxis for intubated patients is not recommended. However, specific antibiotics should be instituted immediately with active infections after obtaining sputum and blood cultures and examining for other sources of sepsis.

Table 11-3 Criteria for Mechanical Ventilation Based on Pulmonary or Parenchymal Failure

Physiologic parameter	Criterion value
Alveolar-arterial oxygen gradient	$AaDO_2$ < 300 torr ($FiO_2 = 1$)
Right-to-left shunt fraction	$Q_s/Q_t > 15$ to 20%
Wasted ventilation	$V_d/V_t > 0.6$
Compliance	<30 mL/cmH_2O

Note: $AaDO_2$ = alveolar arterial oxygen gradient (or differential)
Q_s = pulmonary shunt blood flow
Q_t = cardiac output
V_d = ventilatory dead space
V_t = tidal volume

Source: Adapted from Rosner MJ: Medical management of spinal cord injury. In: Pitts KH, Wagner FC Jr (eds): *Craniospinal Trauma*. New York, Thieme, 1990, table 17-1, p 214. Reprinted by permission of Thieme Publishers.

Tracheostomy is necessary in patients who cannot be weaned from the ventilator. At our facility, a tracheostomy is performed if more than 2 weeks of ventilation is required. Patients are weaned from the ventilator by gradually reducing intermittent mandatory ventilation while monitoring respiratory rate, end tidal CO_2, oxygen saturation, and arterial blood gases. Serial measures of pulmonary function and spirometry are helpful guides.

In weaning patients from the ventilator, the maintenance of continuous positive airway pressure at 5 to 10 cmH_2O to augment functional residual capacity can be helpful while the ventilator rate is reduced to zero.[19,20,29] Patients who demonstrate fatigue may be treated with daily cycles of 6 to 8 h of temporary ventilation, which are subsequently decreased.[19,20,29]

Nutritional and Gastrointestinal Management

Patients with acute complete SCI should be considered for either peritoneal lavage or CT of the abdomen if hemorrhage or abdominal injury is suspected. The normal signs and symptoms of intra-abdominal injury may be absent with SCI due to loss of sensation.

Acute SCI, especially in the thoracic or lumbar region, is usually associated with an ileus due to direct mechanical effects or the loss of autonomic neural function. Ileus should be treated by nasogastric suction, replacement of electrolytes, and monitoring of fluid status.

Despite paralysis, SCI patients have markedly elevated metabolic rates (50 to 100 percent above normal) and become catabolic early.[11] We advocate early nutritional therapy. Initiating nutritional support within 24 h of injury appears to reduce infections, deep vein thrombosis, and catabolic complications.[11] Indirect calorimetry is useful to measure the patient's caloric requirements.[11]

Oral feeding or enteral alimentation is preferred. A flexible duodenal tube is placed under fluoroscopy if elemental enteral hyperalimentation is anticipated. Patients with an ileus or those unable to tolerate enteral feeding should be begun on total parenteral hyperalimentation (TPN). Ulcer prophylaxis consists of administering either antihistamine agents (e.g., cimetidine, ranitidine) or antacids.

Delayed gastric emptying after injury may cause aspiration pneumonia if gastric feedings are performed. The use of duodenal feeding will avoid aspiration. Adding food coloring to the feeding formula will detect if aspiration or reflux has occurred.

Hypertonicity of feeding solutions, decreased intestinal absorption, or both can cause diarrhea with enteral feeding. This condition is managed by varying the concentration of the formula or by adding diphenoxylate hydrochloride with atropine sulfate (Lomotil) or a similar drug.

Loss of anal sphincteric function accompanying SCI can be treated once ileus and spinal shock have recovered. Administering bisacodyl (Dulcolax) suppositories with rectal manual dilatation provides a stimulus for uniform contraction of the bowel for "volitional" emptying.

Coagulation Disturbances

Disseminated intravascular coagulopathy is rarely associated with isolated SCIs compared to its frequent association with severe head injuries.[27] Instead, the paralyzed patient has a great risk of developing deep venous thrombosis and pulmonary emboli.[7,19,20,23,27,29]

Minidose heparin (5000 U administered subcutaneously 2 or 3 times a day), oscillating beds, volume expansion, elastic thigh-high stockings, pneumatic antiembolism stockings, and antiplatelet and anticoagulation therapies have all been advocated for prophylaxis;[7,19,20,23] however, no method has been proven superior. Our regimen for prophylaxis in the paraplegic or quadriplegic patient is minidose heparin and pneumatic compression stockings. Platelet counts should be monitored closely, as thrombocytopenia may complicate heparin therapy.

The diagnosis of deep vein thrombosis of the lower extremities may be confirmed by radioactive fibrinogen scan, Doppler ultrasound, or venography.[7,23] Pulmonary emboli can be detected with ventilation-perfusion scanning, but angiography may be necessary to confirm the diagnosis.[7,23] Deep venous thrombosis or pulmonary emboli are treated with systemic anticoagulation. If this therapy is contraindicated, a vena cava filter is used.

Genitourinary Management

After SCI, the bladder becomes acutely atonic.[17] an indwelling Foley catheter is initially used to monitor fluid output and to prevent bladder distention. Intermittent catheterization is begun after the patient is medically stable and is performed to maintain the volume of the bladder below 400 mL.[17,20] Intermittent, clean catheterization reduces the risk of cystitis and pyelonephritis in patients with neurogenic bladders.[17] Prophylactic antibiotics are not advocated; instead, specific infections are treated as they arise.[17]

Surgical and pharmacologic therapies are available to restore continence based upon urodynamic testing for treatment of chronic neurologic disorders. Renal failure secondary to infections was previously a major cause of mortality among chronic SCI patients, but it is now rare.[17]

Decubitus Ulcers

Decubitus ulcers readily develop in paralyzed patients due to direct dermal pressure, reduced tissue perfusion, and reduced mobility. Foam or sheepskin padding of bony prominences, frequent turning, meticulous skin care, and oscillating or air flotation beds can help prevent decubitus ulcers. Prevention of integumentary complications is of critical importance.

SUMMARY

The ICU management of patients with SCI not only focuses on the treatment of the spinal injury but also on the detection and treatment of associated injuries and complications. Specialized treatment is warranted for respiratory, hemodynamic, nutritional, genitourinary, and gastrointestinal dysfunction. This emphasis has decreased the length of stay for the SCI patient in the ICU as well as in the hospital and has decreased morbidity and mortality.

REFERENCES

1. Bracken MB, Shepard MJ, Collins WF, et al.: A randomized, controlled trial of methylprednisolone or naloxone in the treatment of acute spinal-cord injury. *N Engl J Med* 322(20):1405, 1990.

2. Dickman CA, Douglas RA, Sonntag VKH: Occipitocervical fusion: Posterior stabilization of the craniovertebral junction and upper cervical spine. *BNI Quarterly* 6(2):2, 1990.
3. Dickman CA, Hadley MN, Browner C, Sonntag VKH: Neurosurgical management of acute atlas-axis combination fractures. A review of 25 cases. *J Neurosurg* 70:45, 1989.
4. Dickman CA, Mamourian A, Sonntag VKH, Drayer BP: Magnetic resonance imaging of the transverse atlantal ligament for the evaluation of atlantoaxial instability. *J Neurosurg* 75:221, 1991.
5. Dickman CA, Rekate HL, Sonntag VKH, Zabramski JM: Pediatric spinal trauma: Vertebral column and spinal cord injuries in children. *Pediatr Neurosci* 15:237, 1989.
6. Dickman CA, Sonntag VKH, Papadopoulos SM, Hadley MN: The interspinous method of posterior atlantoaxial arthrodesis. *J Neurosurg* 74:190, 1991.
7. Frisbie JH, Sarkarati M, Sharma GVRK, Rossier AB: Venous thrombosis and pulmonary embolism occurring at close intervals in spinal cord injury patients. *Paraplegia* 21:270, 1983.
8. Geisler FH, Dorsey FC, Coleman WP: Recovery of motor function after spinal-cord injury—a randomized, placebo-controlled trial with Gm-1 ganglioside. *N Engl J Med* 324:1829, 1991.
9. Geisler WO, Jousee AT, Wynne-Jones M: Survival in traumatic transverse myelitis. *Paraplegia* 14:262, 1977.
10. Godersky JC, Menezes AH: Optimal management for children with spinal cord injury. *Contemp Neurosurg* 11:1, 1990.
11. Grahm TW, Zadrozny DB, Harrington T: The benefits of early jejunal hyperalimentation in the head-injured patient. *Neurosurgery* 25:729, 1989.
12. Hadley MN, Browner CM, Dickman CA, Sonntag VKH: Compression fractures of the thoracolumbar junction: A treatment algorithm based on 100 cases. *BNI Quarterly* 5(3):10, 1989.
13. Hadley MN, Dickman CA, Browner CM, Sonntag VKH: Acute axis fractures: A review of 229 cases. *J Neurosurg* 71:642, 1989.
14. Hardy AG: Survival periods in traumatic tetraplegia. *Paraplegia* 14:41, 1976.
15. Kliot MG, Lustgarten JH: Strategies to promote regeneration and recovery in the injured spinal cord. *Neurosurg Clin North Am* 1(3):751, 1990.
16. Kraus JF, Franti CE, Borhani NO, Riggins RS: Survival with an acute spinal-cord injury. *J Chron Dis* 32:269, 1979.
17. Maynard FM, Glass J: Management of the neuropathic bladder by clean intermittent catheterisation: 5 year outcomes. *Paraplegia* 25:106, 1987.
18. Papadopoulos SM, Dickman CA, Sonntag VKH, et al.: Traumatic atlantooccipital dislocation with survival. *Neurosurgery* 28(4):574, 1991.
19. Popp AJ, Feustel PJ, Fortune JB : ICU management of pulmonary dysfunction in neurosurgical patients. *Clin Neurosurg* 35:71, 1989.
20. Rosner MJ: Medical management of spinal cord injury. In: Pitts LH, Wagner FC Jr (eds): *Craniospinal Trauma*, New York, Thieme, 1990, pp 213–225.
21. Sonntag VKH, Douglas RA: Management of spinal cord trauma. *Neurosurg Clin North Am* 1(3):729, 1990.
22. Sonntag VKH, Hadley MN: Nonoperative management of cervical spine injuries. *Clin Neurosurg* 34:630, 1988.
23. Swann KW, Black PMcL: Deep vein thrombosis and pulmonary emboli in neurosurgical patients. A review. *J Neurosurg* 61:1055, 1984.
24. Sypert GW: Stabilization and management of cervical injuries. In: Pitts LH, Wagner FC Jr (eds): *Craniospinal Trauma*, New York, Thieme, 1990, pp 171–185.
25. Tator CH, Fehlings MG: Review of the secondary injury theory of acute spinal cord trauma with emphasis on vascular mechanisms. *J Neurosurg* 75:15, 1991.
26. Wagner FC Jr, Chehrazi B: Early decompression and neurological outcome in acute cervical spinal cord injuries. *J Neurosurg* 56:699, 1982.
27. Ward JD: Intensive care management of the head injured patient. In: Pitts LH, Wagner FC Jr (eds): *Craniospinal Trauma*, New York, Thieme Medical, 1990, pp 88–96.
28. Williams FC Jr, Spetzler RF: Hemodynamic management in the neurosurgical intensive care unit. *Clin Neurosurg* 35:101, 1989.
29. Wilson RS, Pontoppidan H, Rie MA: Acute respiratory failure. In: Ropper AH, Kennedy SK (eds): *Neurological and Neurosurgical Intensive Care*, 2d ed. Rockville, MD, Aspen, 1988, pp 85–97.

CHAPTER 12

The Intensive Care Management of Multisystem Injury

David H. Wisner

INTRODUCTION

The concept that critical illness should be cared for in a specialized, segregated area within a hospital is a relatively new one. Intensive care units (ICUs) have only been formally in existence for the last several decades, and specialized interest in critical care and management is similarly recent. That critical trauma should be cared for in specialized, designated centers with specific requirements is an even newer concept, developed within the last 10 to 15 years and taking on increasing momentum over the last several years. Expertise in critical care management and the facilities for handling critically injured patients are key factors in the delivery of optimal trauma care, and it is not by accident that facilities and expertise for caring for the critically injured are elements of the trauma center designation requirements developed by the Committee on Trauma of the American College of Surgeons. Sophisticated critical care has an impact not only on early mortality for multisystem injury but on delayed mortality from multisystem organ failure as well (Fig. 12-1).[1-3]

Several different general types of injury are encountered in patients admitted to an intensive care setting after major trauma. A simple way to subdivide these injuries is by blunt and penetrating injury mechanisms. Penetrating injury sometimes includes head injury in conjunction with serious injury to other areas of the body, but most of the time the predominant trauma is to one or the other. In situations in which the head is the sole or predominant area of injury, management can safely concentrate on the central nervous system (CNS). Likewise, when the head or spinal cord have been spared injury, management can concentrate on the other injured areas without particular attention to the neurosurgical considerations.

There are several exceptions to the general rule. One is if the patient has suffered a spinal cord injury. In this case, hemodynamics and fluid balance

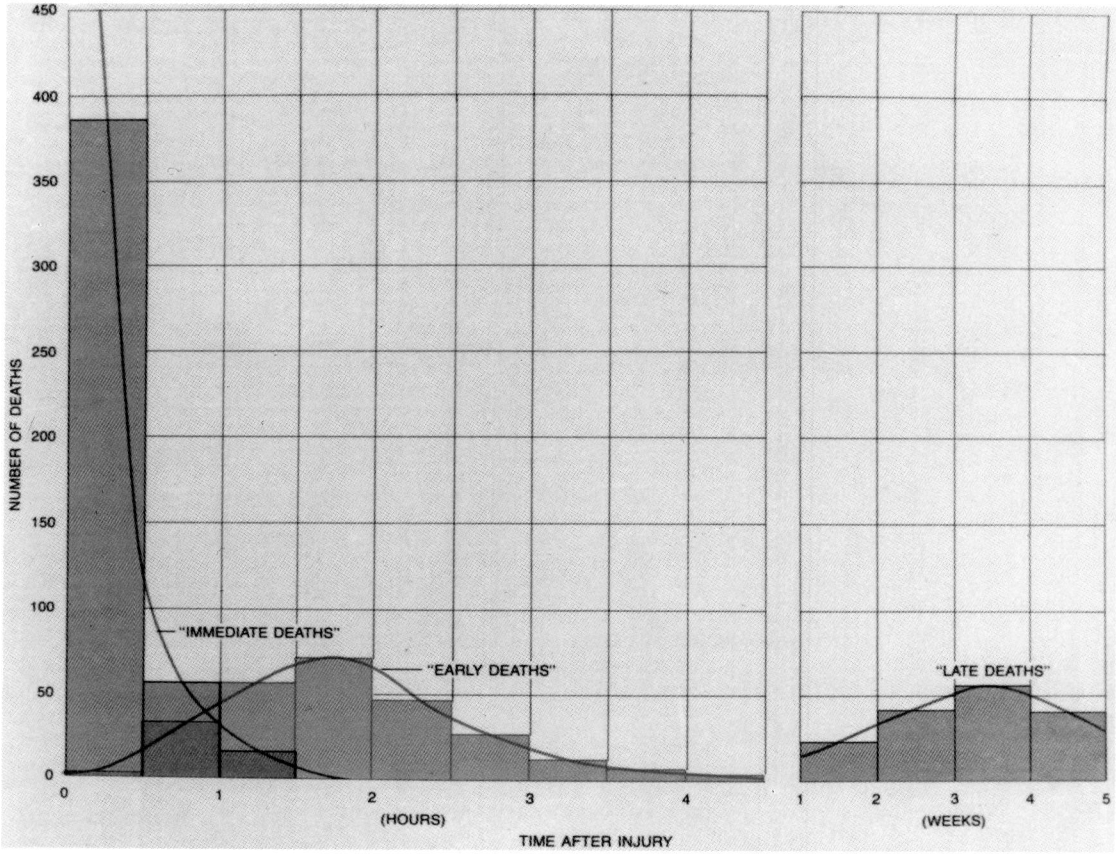

Figure 12-1 Trauma deaths occur in a trimodal distribution. The majority of deaths occur in the immediate postinjury period. Most of these are due to head injury or massive exsanguination. This is followed by a second peak within hours of injury usually due to a progressive head injury or exsanguination. The third peak occurs weeks to months later and includes deaths due to multisystem organ failure. A significant percentage of these deaths can be impacted by expert ICU management.

are profoundly affected by pooling of blood in the peripheral circulation. The patient's loss of sensation and motor function affects the examiner's ability to adequately assess the patient's physical exam even in the absence of head injury. A second situation in which neurosurgical considerations become important even in the absence of direct injury to the brain or spinal cord is in patients in profound shock states or with hypoxemia lasting for extended periods of time. In such situations, diffuse cerebral edema can occur and complicate diagnosis and management.

In contrast to penetrating injury, combinations of CNS injury and trauma to other organ systems are extremely common after blunt trauma. Estimates are that some form of head injury is present in approximately 70 percent of blunt trauma patients. There should always be the presumption that serious injury to intra-abdominal viscera or other organs is present when a patient is first seen in the emergency department setting.[4] At the same time, many patients present with the specter of a head injury of some sort. Altered mental status can be caused by a head injury but can also be due to a variety of other causes including drug or alcohol intoxication, baseline psychiatric disease or mental retardation, shock, hypercarbia secondary to hypoventilation, or hypoxemia. This scenario is particularly common in motor vehicle accident victims. Deciding whether a head injury is present can be very difficult on initial presentation.

EARLY MANAGEMENT

The initial management of patients with multiple trauma is complicated by the fact that the nature and extent of injuries may not be obvious on initial presentation. This is true both for injuries to the CNS and to the other areas of the body. Diagnostic uncertainty makes decision making about priorities of diagnosis difficult. Should the patient be sent for computed tomography (CT) scan of the head or should time first be taken to determine if there is an intra-abdominal injury? We feel that in patients with gross hemodynamic instability unresponsive to initial vigorous fluid resuscitation, the assumption should be that severe intra-abdominal or intrathoracic injury is present.[5] Many of these patients require rapid operative intervention, and this precludes the time necessary to obtain a CT study of the head. Such CT studies to rule out the presence of an operable intracranial lesion should be done as rapidly as possible after necessary operative intervention in the abdomen or chest.

Hemodynamically stable patients who are suspected of a head injury and who cannot cooperate with a physical examination are another dilemma of priorities. Absence of a large hemothorax on chest x-ray rules out immediately life threatening hemorrhage in the chest. Diagnostic peritoneal lavage should be done prior to CT scan of the head. If the diagnostic tap is grossly positive, the patient should undergo exploratory laparotomy. Such an approach delays neurosurgical intervention in a small number of patients with operable neurosurgical lesions, but this concern is balanced by the need for rapid surgical intervention in a significant number of patients with intra-abdominal hemorrhage who would otherwise deteriorate significantly in the time taken to do further workup of the CNS.[5]

While stable patients with unreliable results of a physical examination of the abdomen should undergo a diagnostic procedure to rule out the presence of catastrophic intra-abdominal injury, time should not be taken prior to the CT scan to do the full lavage procedure. If gross blood is not present on initial tap of the abdomen, the lavage fluid should be instilled and siphoned out of the abdomen while the patient is undergoing CT without interfering with the urgency of that study. Patients without gross blood are unlikely to have a catastrophic intra-abdominal hemorrhage.

Many injuries to the intrathoracic or intra-abdominal viscera require treatment and repair prior to transfer of the patient to the ICU. If the patient's general condition permits, we also feel strongly that many orthopedic injuries should be repaired during the initial operative procedure on the day of admission. This is particularly true for long bone fractures of the lower extremities and fractures that will interfere with mobilization of the patient in the postinjury period. In most cases, the earlier these fractures can be repaired the better, even for certain types of pelvic fractures such as "open book" and acetabular fractures. Femur and tibia-fibular fractures are other obvious examples. Early stabilization of these fractures is associated with improved pulmonary function and a better morbidity and mortality.[6-10] Fractures of the upper extremities, hands, and feet take a lower priority.

An occasional patient is too unstable to undergo extended operative repair of orthopedic injuries, and the fractures in these rare cases should be stabilized as well as possible and fixed on a delayed basis.[7] Patients in whom repair must be delayed include those with a coagulopathy, those in whom elaborate diagnostic procedures are necessary prior to a planned operative repair, and those with massive head injury. Orthopedic repair should still remain a priority. Initial delay can become prolonged due to the development of sepsis and multiorgan failure and concern about putting a metal foreign body into a patient at high risk for infection.

Initial management of multiple-trauma victims, particularly those with suspicion of a head injury, should include a low threshold for intubation and mechanical ventilation. High inspired concentrations of oxygen can be delivered and the airway is protected. Arterial blood gas analysis should be done frequently to ensure that an oxygen saturation of 95 to 100 percent has been achieved.

Hyperventilation of patients with suspected severe head injury is a mainstay of management of the multiple-trauma patient, and the partial pressure of carbon dioxide in the arterial blood should be maintained between 25 to 30 mmHg. Hyperventilation constricts the cerebral vasculature with a concomitant decrease in intracranial pressure.[11, 12]

Intubation and positive pressure ventilation are not without hazards. The development of a tension pneumothorax is the most common deleterious consequence. Initiation of positive pressure ventilation, because of increased intrapleural pressure, leads to decreased venous return and can compromise cardiac output in patients with decreased intravascular volume or cardiac tamponade.[13–15] Positive pressure ventilation, because of increased back pressure on the capacitance veins, can cause increased bleeding from injuries to the inferior vena cava and hepatic venous system. In rare patients, usually with penetrating trauma to the chest, initiation of positive pressure ventilation can result in the flow of air into the left-sided vasculature through a traumatic fistula between the airway and the pulmonary venous system. Air emboli thus enter the left side of the heart and can embolize to the systemic vasculature, including embolization to the cerebral vasculature with strokelike manifestations and embolization to the coronary vasculature with cardiac dysfunction.[16]

EARLY FLUID RESUSCITATION

There are also therapeutic dilemmas with respect to fluid management in the early postinjury period when a patient has the combination of a head injury and possible injuries to other areas of the body. Should fluid be restricted to minimize cerebral edema formation or should intravenous fluid be given liberally to combat shock and hypovolemia related to trauma, blood loss, and third spacing of fluid?

Hypotension is as deleterious for the outcome of a traumatic head injury as it is for the prognosis of other injuries.[17] While vigorous fluid administration should be the response to hypotension on initial evaluation, a poor response to initial fluid administration should prompt aggressive intervention. A chest x-ray should be checked early in the course of resuscitation to rule out the presence of blood in the pleural cavities, each of which can easily accommodate the entire blood volume. Persistent hypotension in spite of the administration of two or more liters of crystalloid solution suggests intra-abdominal bleeding. If hypotension is profound and unremitting, especially if the physical examination is positive for peritoneal signs, the abdomen should be emergently explored. In more questionable cases, a diagnostic peritoneal lavage should be done, as mentioned above, prior to CT scan of the head. We do not feel that patients, even those who are stable hemodynamically on presentation, should undergo routine CT scan of the abdomen because of the time that such an examination takes and the possibility that intra-abdominal bleeding will lead to shock while the diagnostic study is being done.

Even in the presence of a head injury, patients should receive adequate intravenous fluid resuscitation to ensure that hypovolemia and hypotension are avoided.[18,19] It can be difficult, however, to determine an optimal volume of fluid. The mainstays of volume status determination in the initial stages of evaluation and therapy in the emergency department are blood pressure and easily determined signs of peripheral perfusion such as skin color, skin temperature, and capillary refill. Blood pressure and capillary refill, while imperfect, are probably the most reliable of these simple measures. Abnormalities in skin color due to hypoperfusion can be difficult to evaluate, especially in dark-skinned patients, and skin temperature can be related as much to ambient temperature as it is to perfusion. Blood pressure, while simple to measure and reliable in many instances, can be misleading. With extensive endogenous catecholamine release, blood pressure can be maintained in spite of profound blood loss.[18,19] This is especially true in young people, where blood pressure can be maintained at normal or near normal levels until there is a sudden drop at critical levels of blood loss. These considerations highlight the importance of diagnostic peritoneal lavage prior to obtaining a CT study of the head in patients with altered mental status even if on initial evaluation they appear hemodynamically stable.

Other common measures of volume status are too unreliable or unwieldy for routine use in the emergency department. Urine output, helpful over prolonged periods of time, is not useful in initial evaluation because the urine drained from the bladder on initial catheterization may represent stored urine rather than the amount of urine freshly produced. Pulse rate is also unreliable in the emergency department evaluation of multiple-trauma patients.[20,21] The pulse can be elevated secondary to anxiety or pain. More important, pulse values are misleadingly low in a significant number of patients with massive injury and blood loss. Central venous pressure monitoring is sometimes of use in the early evaluation of multiple-trauma patients but is subject to interpretation errors, may not reflect the function of the left heart in patients with major pulmonary trauma or preexisting heart disease, and requires a central venous puncture in patients with a low blood volume and increased risk of pneumothorax or catheter malposition. Filling pressures and cardiac indices from pulmonary artery catheters would potentially be helpful, but filling pressures are subject to interpretation error, and placement of a pulmonary artery catheter in the immediate postinjury period is usually impractical.

While there is agreement about the need for vigorous fluid resuscitation to combat hypovolemia in the multiple-trauma patient, even in the presence of a head injury, the type of fluid that should be used is controversial.[22-24] It has been suggested that using colloid rather than crystalloid solutions minimizes secondary injury to the brain and decreased the severity of posttraumatic pulmonary dysfunction.[25,26] In animal experimentation, however, there is no difference in the degree of cerebral injury when crystalloid or colloid solutions are used to achieve identical degrees of cardiovascular resuscitation.[24] With respect to posttraumatic pulmonary dysfunction, the evidence is inconclusive that there is a benefit to the administration of colloid rather than crystalloid solutions in the early resuscitation of trauma patients. There is even some evidence that colloid resuscitation has deleterious effects on pulmonary function secondary to the leak of colloid molecules into the pulmonary extravascular space and the resultant formation of pulmonary edema.[22,27,28] Colloid molecules, most notably albumin, may also lead to deleterious effects on renal function, cardiac function, and the immune system.[29-31]

In the absence of definitive proof of the superiority of one regimen or the other, the most common practice currently employed in multiple-trauma patients is to give isotonic crystalloid solutions because of the ease of their administration and low cost.

A new approach to the resuscitation of multiple-trauma patients is the use of hypertonic crystalloid solutions, with or without the addition of colloid.[32-37] The most commonly used and widely tested solutions have an osmolarity of 2000 to 2400 mOsm/L. The effects of such solutions on the cardiovascular system of shocked animals is profound, with marked increases in blood pressure and cardiac output even when given in very small volumes. Volumes of hypertonic solution necessary to achieve restoration of blood pressure and cardiac index in the early resuscitation period after shock are approximately one-tenth those required when isotonic crystalloid solutions are used. Addition of colloid prolongs these effects for several hours. Administration of markedly hypertonic solutions leads to a sudden increase in extracellular osmolarity. This generates a powerful force across cell membranes for the flow of intracellular water into the extracellular space, with a concomitant increase in intravascular volume. The intravascular space thus receives a transient autoinfusion of fluid from the intracellular space.[38,39] When colloid, most commonly dextran 70, is added to the mixture, the colloid molecules cause preferential distribution of this infused fluid into the intravascular as opposed to the interstitial space (Fig. 12-2).

Hypertonic solutions also appear to have a direct effect on cardiac function and contractility. The exact mechanism by which this occurs is unknown but may be related to both hormonal responses and neural reflexes.[40,41]

The advantages for prehospital and emergency department resuscitation using a solution that is effective in small volumes are obvious. Minimal intravenous access is necessary, and the volumes required can be infused in very short periods of time. There are several caveats of such treatment, however. The patient can look almost too good be-

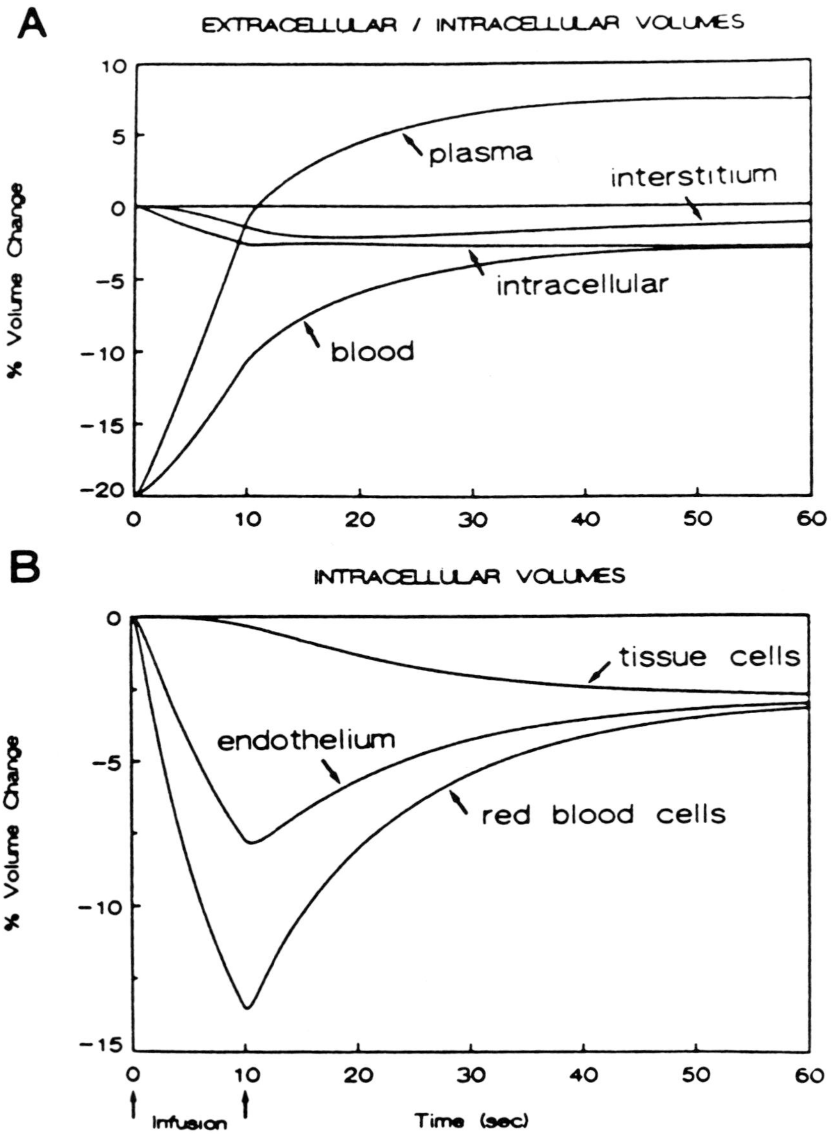

Figure 12-2 The above figures outline changes in compartmental and cell volumes during a 10-s infusion of a hypertonic saline dextran solution. Fluid initially shifts rapidly from the interstitial and intracellular spaces into the plasma space. Most of the fluid is drawn from the intracellular space.

cause of the rapidity of initial resuscitation, which can mask serious underlying injury and ongoing blood loss and lead to a false sense of security. This sense of security secondary to an elevated blood pressure is heightened by the fact that hypertonic solutions cause peripheral vasodilation and can give a misleadingly good picture of capillary refill and peripheral perfusion. Hyperchloremic acidosis can also occur because of the sudden large load of administered chloride. While the degree of acidosis commonly encountered does not appear to be harmful,[42] it can be erroneously interpreted as a lactic acidosis associated with hypoperfusion unless a chloride level is checked and the anion gap determined.

Initial research with hypertonic saline centered on resuscitation of the cardiovascular system. Recently, increasing attention has been paid to the effects of such solutions on the CNS. Hypertonic solutions such as urea and mannitol are standard components of the management of patients with head injury and suspected elevated intracranial pressure.[43,44] A theoretical advantage of hypertonic saline solutions in the resuscitation of hypovolemic shock is that at the same time that the shock state is being reversed, intracranial pressure decreases. This has been seen in animal experiments combining head injury and hemorrhagic shock (Fig. 12-3).[45–47] The effects on both intracranial pressure and blood pressure improve cerebral perfusion pressure and cerebral blood flow, a finding also found in animal experimentation. Brain water content is decreased in areas of uninjured brain, probably due to dehydration of the brain from the osmotic gradient created by administration of hypertonic solutions.[32] This is the same mechanism hypothesized to be operative after the administration of mannitol and other hypertonic fluid regimens for the treatment of intracranial hypertension.

While the effects of hypertonic saline resuscitation regimens on hemodynamics and intracranial pressure are beneficial, there is concern about the effects such sudden and profound cellular dehydration might have on cerebral function. Studies in our laboratory using both high-energy phosphate nuclear magnetic resonance and flash evoked potentials as functional measures of cerebral activity have not demonstrated any negative effects of the administration of such fluids unless the serum sodium level is driven to a value of approximately 180 mEq/L, levels not reached when hypertonic saline is used in initial resuscitation only.[48] Concerns about deleterious effects of hypertonicity may be well founded, however, if hypertonic solutions are used as repeated boluses for prolonged resuscitation.

While administration of hypertonic saline solutions has dramatic effects on both hemodynamics and the brain, these effects are not permanent and further fluid resuscitation is ultimately required.[49–51] Addition of colloid to the regimen, as mentioned above, prolongs the hemodynamic effects. The effects of the addition of colloid on the brain are still undefined. Whether there is a significant rebound phenomenon with respect to cerebral edema formation is still unknown, but early indications from animal experimentation suggest that no such phenomenon exists.[32,52]

Several clinical trials have been conducted using

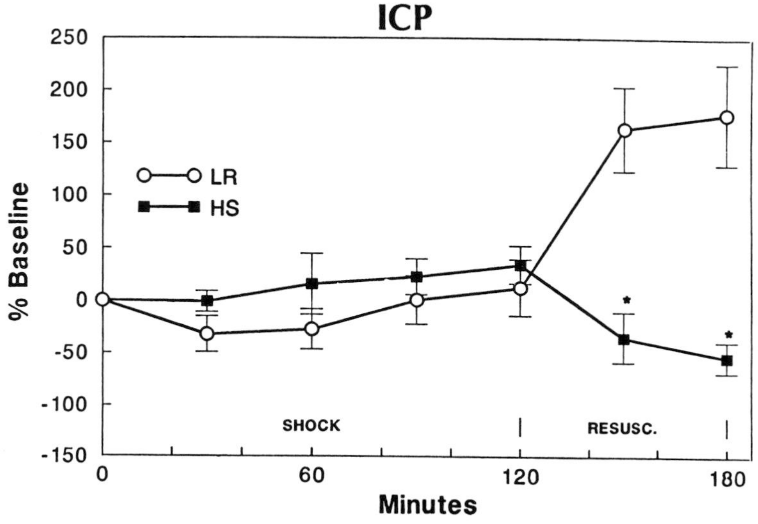

Figure 12-3 In an animal model of combined head injury and hemorrhagic shock, there was a difference in intracranial pressure between resuscitation with isotonic crystalloid (LR) and a hypertonic saline solution (HS). There was a significant increase in intracranial pressure when the isotonic solution was used, while the hypertonic solution maintained intracranial pressure at low levels.

a 7.5% hypertonic saline resuscitation regimen in the initial resuscitation of multiple-trauma patients.[35,36,42,53] Serum sodium levels with a 250-mL bolus resuscitation regimen reach approximately 150 to 155 mEq/L levels and osmolality is elevated to a range of 325 to 335 mOsm/L. Serum chloride values have been in the range of 100 to 115 mEq/L and have been associated with a slight acidemia.[42] Effects on outcome have been varied. Holcroft and coworkers showed improvement in blood pressure (Fig. 12-4) and the suggestion of improved survival, particularly in patients with head injury. Mattox and coworkers, however, could not demonstrate an improvement in survival.[53] Further clinical trials are currently under way and will be necessary to answer the question of whether hypertonic saline resuscitation regimens are helpful in reducing morbidity and mortality after major trauma and head injury.

MONITORING

Once a patient has been admitted to the ICU after multiple trauma, decisions must be made about how much monitoring is appropriate. When monitoring devices have already been placed in the emergency department or in the operating room, the decision-making process revolves around the need for additional monitoring or whether the monitoring devices already in place should be continued.

One of the simplest forms of monitoring is a central venous pressure catheter. Such catheters can be placed via a number of different routes but are most commonly inserted through the internal jugular or subclavian veins. Placement through the antecubital fossa is also possible via the cephalic vein but is more cumbersome and limits the caliber of the line, an important limitation if the line is to be used for fluid or drug infusion as well as for monitoring. Central venous lines can also be placed via a femoral venous route, but the determination of central venous pressure is more difficult because the tip of the catheter is usually in either the abdomen or the right atrium.

Advantages of a central venous catheter are that it is relatively easy to place and often gives an accurate reflection of the filling status of the heart. In patients without significant cardiac dysfunction, pulmonary dysfunction, or underlying cardiac or valvular disease, the central venous pressure is usually a reliable guide to blood volume.[54,55] No sophisticated monitoring devices are needed, and the pressure can even be measured with a handheld manometer at the bedside. When the catheter is connected to a transducer, it is important that the transducer be properly centered at the midaxillary line with the patient in the supine position so that errors in measurement related to position do not occur. Such measurement errors due to malposition of the patient or transducer, while relatively trivial when measuring high pressures such

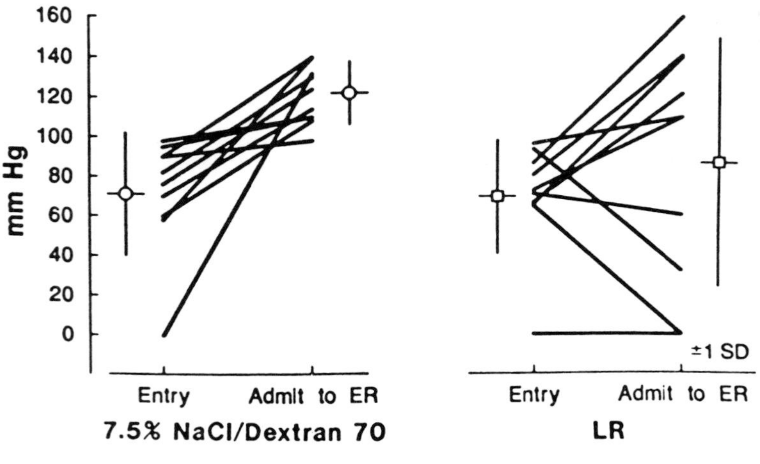

Figure 12-4 The above graphs demonstrate the individual blood pressure changes in patients given either 7.5% hypertonic saline (HS) plus dextran or lactated Ringer's (LR). Each line represents values for an individual patient. The patients given the hypertonic saline dextran solution consistently demonstrated increases in their blood pressure between the time of entry in the study and the time of their arrival in the emergency room. By contrast, patients who received isotonic solution did not demonstrate a consistent increase in blood pressure.

as the arterial pressure, are of great importance when the measured parameter is the central venous pressure.

Placement of a central venous pressure monitor usually requires puncture of a central vein. Such a puncture is safer in the operating room or intensive care setting than it is in the emergency department but is still not without risk of pneumothorax, hydrothorax, or catheter malposition. These punctures, because they put the lungs at particular risk in patients on positive pressure ventilation, can also give rise to life-threatening tension pneumothorax.

Aside from the logistic and measurement problems associated with central venous pressure monitoring, there are physiologic considerations as well. In patients with elevated pulmonary artery pressure, central venous pressures may not accurately reflect the filling of the left side of the heart.[54–56] This is particularly true if there is an element of right-sided cardiac failure. Similarly, in patients with cardiac disease and poor ventricular compliance and function, the right-sided and left-sided filling pressures may not be related and measurement of the right side only can lead to errors in management. The most critical error is to obtain a central venous pressure measurement which indicates that filling is adequate when in reality the left-sided filling pressure is low. Fluid restriction or diuresis in such situations can result in serious problems with left heart filling and function.

Another difficulty with central venous pressure is in patients who have problems with oxygenation. The goals in such patients are to provide adequate volume resuscitation without giving too much fluid and to give enough fluid to optimize blood volume and hemodynamics without overloading the patient and worsening pulmonary edema. Such patients also sometimes require inotropic support or afterload reduction.[56,57] In such instances, central venous pressure alone is inadequate as a monitoring device.

Central venous pressure monitoring is appropriate in patients in whom central venous puncture is required for administration of fluid and in whom there is minimal evidence of pulmonary or cardiac disease. The central venous pressure, along with urine output and blood pressure, can be used as a rough guide to volume status. In patients with evidence of more severe disease, particularly if there is moderate to severe pulmonary dysfunction as evidenced by difficulties with oxygenation, a pulmonary artery catheter is more appropriate.

In the trauma patient, pulmonary artery catheters are indicated for several reasons. In the early resuscitation period, pulmonary artery catheters are sometimes required in patients with massive fluid requirements when there is a question of fluid overload. A clinical diagnosis of shock is made on the basis of low blood pressure, low urine output, and poor peripheral perfusion. The differential diagnosis of this state includes hypovolemia due to hemorrhage and third spacing of fluid versus cardiac dysfunction with an element of cardiac failure. A pulmonary artery catheter is helpful in distinguishing between these two diagnoses. In the majority of cases in the early postinjury period, hypovolemia is the problem and treatment is the infusion of more fluid. Occasionally, however, particularly in elderly patients, a significant element of cardiac failure exists and the correct treatment is fluid restriction and diuresis. The pulmonary artery catheter is valuable in detecting these occasional instances.

Another instance in which pulmonary artery catheters are of value is in patients with significant cardiac or pulmonary dysfunction when sepsis with multiple organ system failure are present. It is important to optimize volume status in such patients without exacerbating the cardiac or pulmonary failure. Measuring the cardiac output and relating it to the pulmonary capillary wedge pressure, the filling pressure of the left heart, optimizes filling with respect to cardiac function. Measurement of the oxygen delivery index helps to monitor hemodynamics in patients with significant pulmonary dysfunction. The oxygen delivery index is calculated by the following formula:

$$O_2 \text{ delivery index} = 4/3 \times (\text{Hb}) \times \%\text{sat} \times \text{CI}$$

where 4/3 = constant relating amount of oxygen carried by fully saturated hemoglobin, mL/g

(Hb) = concentration of hemoglobin, dL

%sat = percent saturation of arterial hemoglobin

CI = cardiac index, liters per minute per square meter

A normal value for the oxygen delivery index in uninjured patients is 500 to 700 mL O_2/min per m^2. In the management of an acutely injured patient, however, this value is relatively unimportant because in the injured state oxygen requirements are likely to be higher than normal.

The oxygen delivery index is helpful in patients with pulmonary dysfunction and an oxygenation problem because some therapeutic maneuvers have conflicting effects on oxygen delivery.[57–60] An example is a patient given fluid in large volumes to increase the cardiac index. If administration of fluid leads to increased pulmonary edema and decreased oxygen saturation, the oxygen delivery index may decrease in spite of an increased cardiac index. In the absence of active hemorrhage, the hemoglobin concentration remains relatively constant. Similarly, in the absence of significant pulmonary dysfunction, the oxygen saturation in the arterial blood remains relatively constant because most patients remain saturated at the 90 to 99 percent level. As a result, in a majority of cases increases in cardiac index indicate increases in oxygen delivery. Occasionally in patients with severe pulmonary disease, however, the calculation of oxygen delivery index is helpful because of the reasons outlined above.

A final reason for placement of a pulmonary artery catheter is the initiation of therapeutic maneuvers designed to directly affect cardiac function. These measures can be necessary in both the early resuscitation period and later in the patient's course if pulmonary, cardiac, or multiple organ system failure occur. Inotropic support and afterload reduction are two examples of this sort of intervention. When the primary aim of the therapy is improved cardiac function, it is important to be able to measure that function directly. The pulmonary artery catheter provides the means for doing this as well as information about the filling pressures of the heart.

As outlined above, left heart filling pressures, cardiac index, oxygen delivery, and systemic vascular resistance index can be determined with a pulmonary artery catheter. The pulmonary artery catheter, by virtue of a thermistor placed at its distal end, is also able to provide on-line measurement of core body temperature which is occasionally useful in the diagnosis of systemic manifestations of infection and can be compared to the peripheral temperature to quantify the degree to which a patient is peripherally vasoconstricted. Finally, the pulmonary artery catheter is customarily placed through a large bore "straw" placed in a central vein. This large bore line allows for vigorous fluid resuscitation. The pulmonary artery catheter itself, by virtue of its multiple ports, can also be used for multiple infusions as well as for monitoring.

There are a number of disadvantages of pulmonary artery catheters. As mentioned above, placement generally involves central venous puncture with all the risks attendant to that procedure. The risks of central venous puncture are especially heightened in obese patients and in patients with clavicular fractures. The catheter can also erode through the distal pulmonary vasculature, especially if the balloon used for the measurement of pulmonary capillary wedge pressure is left inflated. The straw sheath through which the catheter is placed can also erode.

Other risks of pulmonary artery catheters are reviewed in Chap. 1 but include infectious complications,[61,62] balloon tip breakage with possible embolization, catheter position shifting, and misinterpretation of the values obtained with the catheter.

Probably the most important difficulty associated with the use of pulmonary artery catheters is the correct interpretation of the measurements obtained. There is a danger not only of erroneous measurements but also of misinterpreting or overinterpreting the values. This is particularly true for the pulmonary capillary wedge pressure measurement, one of the most important measurements obtained with the catheter.

The fact that both patient and transducer position are critical for the accurate measurement of central venous pressure has already been mentioned. The same considerations pertain to the measurement of the pulmonary capillary wedge pressure (Fig. 12–5). The patient should be supine and flat and the transducer placed at the level of the midaxillary line. Readings should always be done consistently with the patient and transducer in the same position. As with the other measured parameters obtained from the pulmonary artery catheter, pulmonary capillary wedge pressure

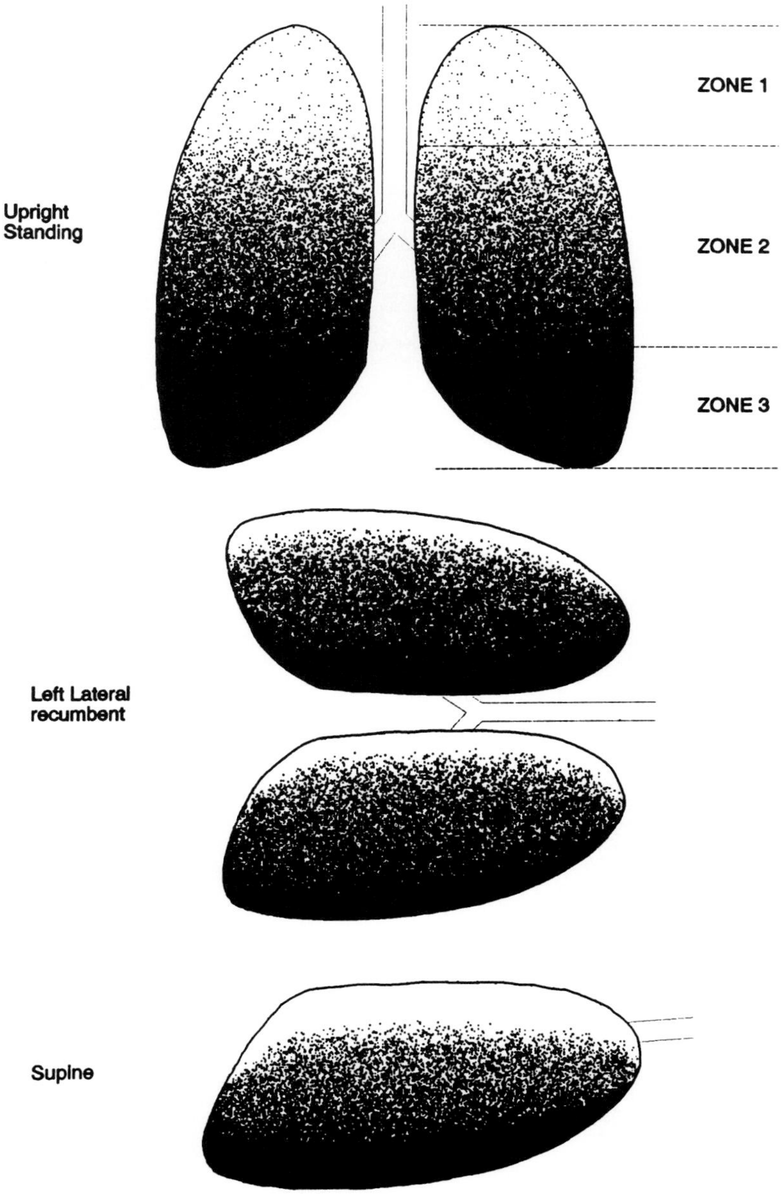

Figure 12-5 The lung in any position can be divided into three different zones based on relationships between perfusion and ventilation. See text for further details.

measurements are most important not as absolute values but as relative values obtained over time and compared to one another. This makes consistency of measurement vitally important. Insisting that all measurements by convention be done in the supine position with the transducer in the midaxillary line helps to ensure uniformity of measurement practices.

Cardiac output is another parameter measurable with placement of a pulmonary artery catheter. Cardiac output is the amount of blood flow in liters per minute. A difficulty of this approach is that the standards for a normal cardiac output vary with the size of the patient and the normal circulating blood volume, and it is difficult to define a normal value for cardiac output. A normal cardiac output of 3 L/min in a 45-kg adolescent is woefully inadequate in a 100-kg adult. The cardiac index obviates this difficulty, normalizing the cardiac output by dividing it by the body surface area. Body surface area is the morphologic measure which best correlates with physiologic measures such as blood volume and cardiac output. Dividing by the body surface area to create the cardiac index normalizes the cardiac output and results in a normal value for the cardiac index of 2.8 to 3.6 L/min per m^2, a value that is valid for all patients regardless of size.

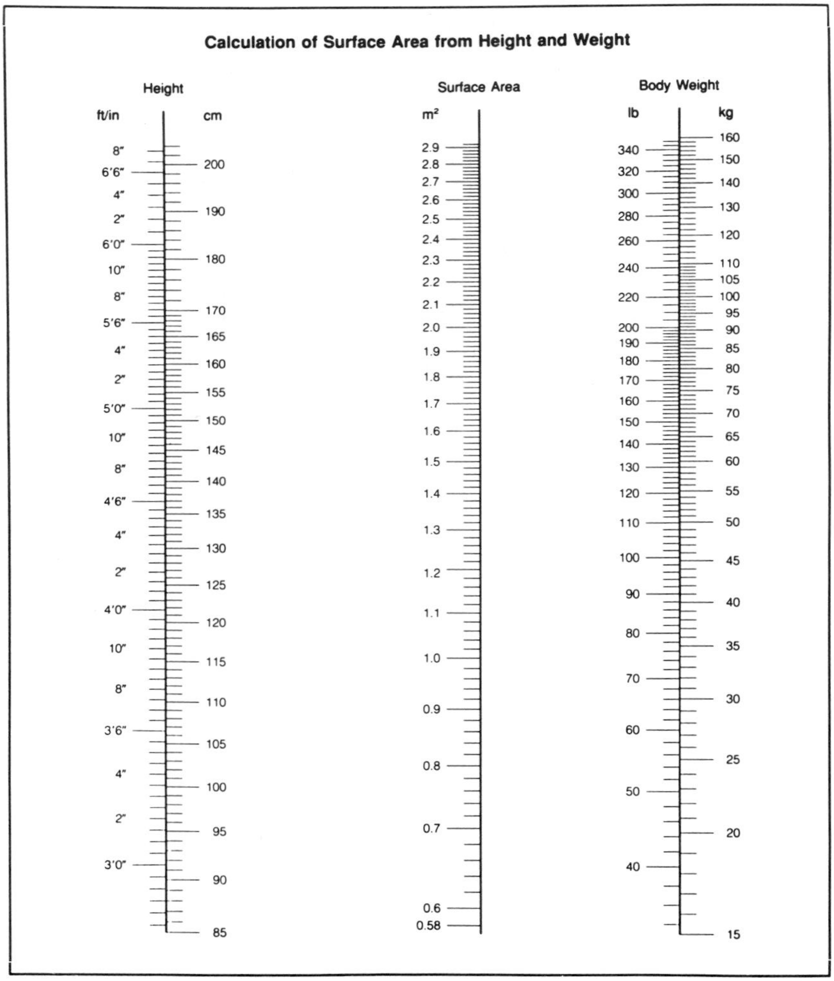

Figure 12-6 A table such as this one can calculate surface area from height and weight. The patient's height can be found on the scale on the left. The weight can be found on the scale on the right. A straight line connecting the height and weight intersects the middle scale at the patient's approximate body surface area.

Surface area is determined from nomograms or formulas relating height and weight to body surface and is easy to calculate when these two measures are known (Fig. 12-6). A difficulty with determining body surface area in critically injured patients in the ICU is that the preinjury body weight in many instances can only be estimated.

There are several technical pitfalls in the determination of cardiac index. These are largely related to technique and are easy to correct if they are noticed, but they can result in markedly misleading values if they are not recognized. Cardiac output, from which cardiac index is derived, is measured by the thermodilution method (Fig. 12-7). A fixed volume of fluid at a fixed temperature is injected through the central venous port of the pulmonary artery catheter. Either room temperature or iced saline at O°C is used. This fluid, because it is colder than body temperature, causes a temperature drop in the blood into which it is mixed. This blood is pumped through the right heart and out into the pulmonary outflow tract, causing a temperature drop at the thermistor located at the tip of the pulmonary artery catheter. Information about the change in temperature at the thermistor is fed into a bedside computer, which calculates the integral of the curve described by the change in temperature over time. The value obtained by this integration process then is multiplied by a constant relating it to the cardiac output. If the constant set on the computer does not correspond to the volume and temperature of the injectant, incorrect values for cardiac output and cardiac index are obtained.

Mixed venous oxygen tension and saturation are other parameters measurable with a pulmonary artery catheter. Measurement of the mixed venous oxygen tension and saturation allow for the calculation of oxygen consumption. The oxygen consumption index is calculated by determining the difference between the amount of oxygen delivered per unit time to the tissues and the amount of oxygen found per unit time in the mixed venous blood. The equation for calculation of the oxygen consumption index per minute per meter squared is, not surprisingly, similar to the formula for oxygen delivery:

$$O_2 \text{ consumption index} = 4/3 \times (\text{Hb}) \times (O_2\text{art} - O_2\text{mv}) \times \text{CI}$$

where 4/3 = constant relating amount of oxygen carried by hemoglobin, mL/g
(Hb) = hemoglobin concentration, g/dL
O_2art = arterial oxygen saturation (fraction)
O_2mv = mixed venous oxygen saturation (fraction)
CI = cardiac index liters per minute per square meter

A normal value for the oxygen consumption index is 120 to 160 mL/min per m^2.

Theoretically, use of the mixed venous oxygen tension and saturation is useful in diagnosing and treating shock states. In most types of shock, including hypovolemic, cardiogenic, cardiac compressive (cardiac tamponade, tension pneumothorax), and neurogenic, the mixed venous oxygen saturation decreases as the body attempts to compensate for a low flow state. The oxygen consump-

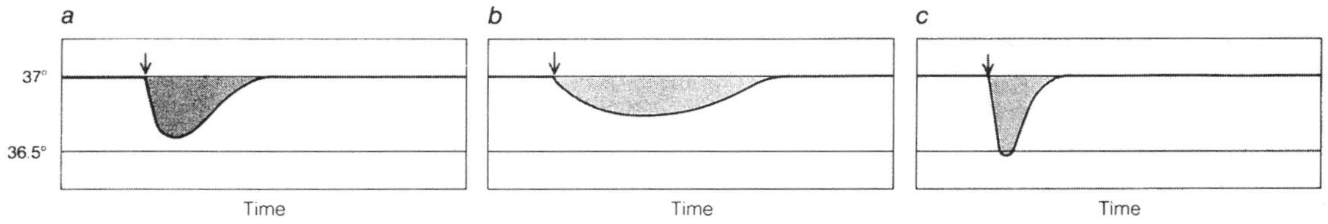

Figure 12-7 When thermodilution is used to measure cardiac output, a bolus of fluid colder than blood is injected at a specific time (arrows). This results in a temperature drop sensed at a thermistor located at the tip of the catheter. The temperature change at the thermistor and the area described by that change over time are inversely proportional to the cardiac output. The above figure outlines curves for a normal cardiac output (a), a lower than normal cardiac output (b), and a high-normal cardiac output (c). Integration of these areas and multiplication by a constant quantifies the cardiac output.

tion index thus accurately reflects whether the patient is adequately perfusing. In most of these instances, however, use of other easily measured indicators such as blood pressure and urine output leads to the same conclusions about the adequacy of peripheral perfusion, and going through the exercise of calculating the oxygen consumption index provides only confirmatory evidence.

It is in patients with sepsis and septic shock that the use of mixed venous oxygen tension and saturation is theoretically most useful.[58–60] It is thought by many that the goal of resuscitation in septic patients is to maximize oxygen consumption and that this should be the resuscitation parameter of major interest. The thought is that in under-resuscitation patients, oxygen consumption is flow-dependent and that if the delivery of oxygen can be increased, oxygen consumption will likewise increase.

Unfortunately, the meaning of oxygen consumption is more complicated in septic states than it is in nonseptic patients or other shock states.[64] When sepsis is not present, oxygen consumption is related largely to the supply of oxygen and the needs of the tissue. If oxygen delivery decreases because of a low flow state, oxygen extraction increases as the tissues try to compensate. In septic states, this ability of oxygen extraction to compensate for a decrease in oxygen delivery is impaired and the consumption of oxygen is not necessarily a reflection of the degree of peripheral perfusion.[65] There are several possible reasons why oxygen extraction is impaired and the mixed venous oxygen tensions are inappropriately high in septic states. One is that there is peripheral shunting of blood from the arterial to the venous circulation without adequate exposure to a capillary bed. Another theory to explain why mixed venous oxygen tension is inappropriately elevated in patients with sepsis is that there is dysfunction in oxygen extraction at the cellular level. Sepsis is thought to cause dysfunction of the cellular cytochromes and lead to their inability to properly use oxygen.

In addition to the theoretical inadequacies of mixed venous oxygen tension in the resuscitation of critically injured and septic patients, there are a few technical pitfalls associated with its use. The blood sample used to determine mixed venous oxygen is drawn from the distal port of the catheter in the pulmonary artery. If aspiration on the port is too strong, blood will be drawn back across the pulmonary capillary bed and will contaminate the blood sample. The sample should be pure mixed venous blood from the pulmonary artery. This ensures that none of the blood has yet been oxygenated. If the sample is aspirated too vigorously, some of the blood in the sample will have already been oxygenated and then pulled back across the pulmonary capillary bed.

An ingenious method to avoid the need for sampling of pulmonary artery blood is a pulmonary artery catheter which can do on-line measurements of oxygen saturation in the pulmonary arterial blood.[66] These continuous oximetry catheters have a sensor at their distal end which gives a continuous readout of oxygen saturation (Fig. 12-8). These catheters can be of great value in patients with significant cardiac dysfunction in whom the mixed venous saturation is an honest reflection of the state of peripheral perfusion. In the average trauma patient, however, they are of less value. In the immediate postinjury phase, placement of a pulmonary artery catheter is usually impractical. In the early stages of ICU management, determination of the state of peripheral perfusion can usually be adequately determined by using easily measured clinical parameters such as the blood pressure and urine output. If a pulmonary artery catheter is placed, mixed venous oxygen saturation values will usually decrease as cardiac index decreases, and cardiac index itself is an accurate reflection of the adequacy of resuscitation. In the later postinjury phase, if sepsis and multiorgan failure intervene, mixed venous co-oximetry values can be confusing for the reasons outlined above.

Pulmonary artery catheters allow for the direct measurement of central venous pressure, pulmonary artery pressure, pulmonary capillary wedge pressure, cardiac index, and mixed venous oxygen saturation. The catheter can also be used to derive a number of calculated variables. Probably the most commonly used variable derived in this way is the systemic vascular resistance index (SVRI). The systemic vascular resistance index is calculated by the following formula:

$$\text{SVRI} = MAP - CVP\ \text{CI}$$

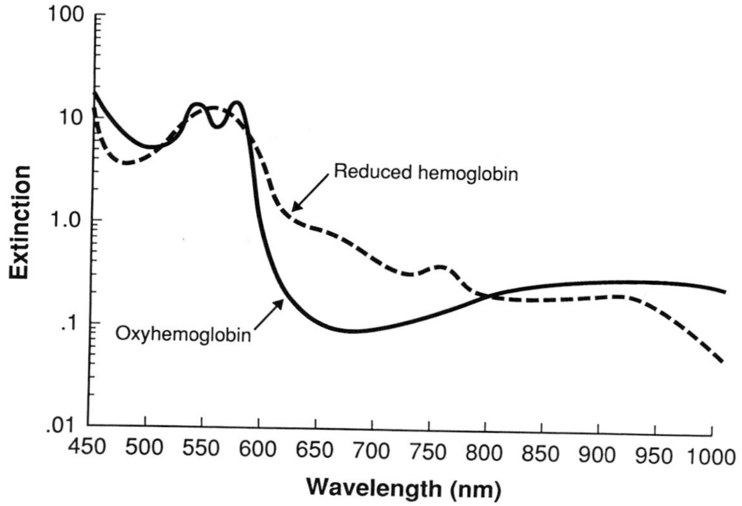

Figure 12-8 Reduced and oxygenated hemoglobin absorb light at 660 and 940 nanometers differently. This difference is used in pulse oximetry monitoring to determine the oxygen saturation of arterial blood.

where MAP = mean arterial blood pressure
CVP = central venous pressure
CI = cardiac index

The systemic vascular resistance index is useful on occasion in distinguishing between different types of shock states. Hypovolemic shock, cardiogenic shock, and cardiac compressive shock are all characterized by a high SVRI as the vasculature tries to compensate for a low flow state. Neurogenic and septic shock are different. In neurogenic shock such as seen with a spinal cord injury, the SVRI is often normal or abnormally low because of the loss of vascular tone. In septic shock, SVRI is also inappropriately low. The reasons for this are not completely understood.[67-70]

Occasional trauma patients, particularly elderly patients and those with a history of hypotension, manifest a low cardiac index in association with a high SVRI in spite of the fact that blood volume and cardiac function are adequate. Although this situation is uncommon, these patients sometimes benefit from afterload reduction with an arterial vasodilator such as sodium nitroprusside. Measurements of the SVRI in such patients helps to make the diagnosis and provides a guide to the adequacy and effectiveness of the afterload reduction.

Pulmonary vascular resistance index can also be calculated using a pulmonary artery catheter. The calculation is similar to that for the SVRI, but mean pulmonary artery pressure is substituted for the mean arterial pressure and the pulmonary artery capillary wedge pressure is substituted for the central venous pressure. This derived variable quantifies the degree of pulmonary arterial vasoconstriction or obstruction. Occasionally, the pulmonary vascular resistance index is useful if the patient is undergoing afterload reduction. Measurement of this parameter, however, is generally of minimal benefit or usefulness in trauma patients and is of more value in patients with myocardial and valvular disease.

For all calculated variables, including oxygen delivery and consumption as well as the systemic and pulmonary vascular resistance indices, the calculated variables are only as good as the directly measured variables that go into the calculation. There is some inherent error in each of the measured variables, and these errors are compounded by their combination in the formulas used to calculate derived variables. This must be borne in mind when calculating and interpreting derived parameters.

Arterial catheters are another mainstay of monitoring in the ICU. They should be placed in patients with hemodynamic instability and in patients in whom afterload or preload reduction is contemplated. An arterial catheter is also helpful in patients in whom pressors are being used to support the blood pressure and in patients being given inotropic support for cardiac dysfunction or augmentation of cardiac index.

Arterial catheters should also generally be placed in patients requiring prolonged ventilatory support. The presence of an arterial catheter provides simple and frequent determination of arterial blood gases. Arterial catheters are important in such patients, although their importance has diminished somewhat in recent years with the development of pulse oximetry and end-tidal carbon dioxide monitors.

Pulse oximetry takes advantage of the fact that oxygenated and deoxygenated blood absorb incident light differently.[71,72] Because the body contains blood with a wide spectrum of different saturations, pulse oximetry measures absorbance during both systole and diastole in order to determine what component of the absorbance is due to pulsatile arterial blood. The amount of absorbance is then compared to a standard curve of absorbance at different oxygen saturations in order to determine the patient's oxygen saturation (Fig. 12-8). Pulse oximetry does not measure oxygen tension in arterial blood as a standard arterial blood gas analysis would do. In most circumstances, this is of minimal consequence, but it should be remembered that the oxygen saturation as measured by pulse oximetry does not discriminate between patients with an arterial partial pressure of oxygen of 90 mmHg and patients with an arterial partial pressure of oxygen of 300 mmHg. In both instances the arterial oxygen saturation is close to 100 percent. The oxygen saturation as measured by pulse oximetry can therefore be falsely reassuring in patients with serious pulmonary dysfunction and oxygenation defects. Nonetheless, the advent of pulse oximetry has simplified monitoring of oxygenation in the ICU, provides a good on-line method for continuous monitoring of oxygenation, and is rapidly becoming the standard of care for critically injured and ill patients.

Patients with burns, inhalation injury, and elevated levels of carbon monoxide in their arterial blood will have falsely elevated oxygen saturation as measured by a pulse oximeter. As mentioned above, the pulse oximeter determines arterial oxygen saturation from the absorbance of the blood. Carbon monoxide turns the blood cherry red and this is interpreted by the pulse oximeter as fully saturated blood with 100 percent saturation. A standard arterial blood sample should be done in all patients with suspected inhalation injury rather than relying on the pulse oximeter.

Pulse oximetry also does not measure the arterial partial pressure of carbon dioxide. End-tidal carbon dioxide monitors are a useful new adjunct for ICU monitoring in that they provide an on-line continuous measurement of ventilation without the need for a blood gas sample. The device measures the end-expiratory carbon dioxide in exhaled gas.[73,74] This value correlates well with the partial pressure of carbon dioxide in most patients but tends to run somewhat higher in absolute value than the arterial carbon dioxide. It is useful for following trends in ventilation.

On occasion, particularly after a patient has had a long stay in the ICU during which multiple indwelling arterial catheters have been used in a number of different locations, it is difficult to place further arterial catheters because of the lack of a suitable site. If the only indication for an arterial catheter is to allow for access to the arterial blood for blood gas sampling, maintenance of mechanical ventilation and even weaning from mechanical ventilation can be done with the combination of pulse oximetry and end-tidal carbon dioxide monitoring and occasional double-checking of the noninvasive monitoring with a blood gas sample.

Arterial catheters are remarkably free from the development of complications, but they do occasionally occur, as reviewed in Chap. 1, and include distal extremity ischemia, site infection, and arterial pseudoaneurysm formation.

The correct interpretation of arterial pressures as measured by an arterial catheter is also important.[75] Pressure tracings and digital readings can be altered by movement of the catheter in the artery (artery whip). Damped tracings and digital readings can also occur, due to partial or intermittent occlusion of the catheter or an overly compliant catheter-tubing-transducer system. In the case of either catheter whip or a damped tracing, the inaccuracies produced can be minimized by concentrating on mean arterial pressure rather than on the systolic and diastolic pressure. The mean pressure is minimally altered and will be reliable.

Urinary catheters are one of the most important and simplest elements of ICU monitoring of the critically injured. They should be placed in all injured patients who require intensive care, and urinary output should be monitored on an hourly basis. Placement of a urinary bladder catheter while the patient is in the emergency department is important because quantification of urinary output can begin and discovery of gross hematuria provides clues about the possibility of a renal or bladder injury.

In the ICU, urinary output is a valuable guide to the patient's renal perfusion. This in turn is an aid in determining the adequacy of overall perfusion. Low urine output of less than approximately ½ mL/kg per h should be addressed immediately. In the majority of trauma patients, the problem is inadequate circulating blood volume, and the appropriate treatment for oliguria is administration of intravenous fluid and banked blood. In some cases, however, the cause of the oliguria is due primarily to cardiac dysfunction. When this is suspected, a pulmonary artery catheter should be placed to help define the filling status of the heart and aid in treatment of the low flow state.

In trauma patients with head injury, oliguria can also be a reflection of inappropriate antidiuretic hormone secretion, although usually the urine output appears reasonably adequate in such patients as long as renal perfusion is obtained. The diagnosis in these cases is made with electrolyte and osmolality studies of the serum and urine.

Multiple-trauma patients with a head injury can also develop diabetes insipidus. Inappropriately high urine outputs as measured in the urinary catheter are a clue that diabetes insipidus is present. The diagnosis can often be confirmed with serum and urine electrolyte studies, but occasionally the diagnosis is made largely on the basis of very large urine outputs in the setting of a patient with a head injury. The serum and urine electrolyte and osmolarity studies are sometimes unreliable because it is difficult to use them to distinguish between diabetes insipidus and compensated intravascular volume overload with an appropriate diuresis. One useful clue in making the distinction between these two diagnoses is the volume of urine. Persistent urine volumes of several hundred milliliters per hour are unusual in patients with appropriate diuresis of volume overload, and in such instances there should be a high index of suspicion for the presence of diabetes insipidus. A pulmonary artery catheter should be placed, and if the picture is inconsistent with a diagnosis of fluid overload, the patient should be treated for diabetes insipidus.

Intracranial pressure monitoring will be covered extensively in Chaps. 3 and 4 and will not be reviewed in any detail here. Monitoring of the intracranial pressure simplifies the management of multiple-trauma patients in several respects. The amount and type of fluid given in the ICU to patients with multiple trauma and head injury is extremely important. In such patients, injury and blood loss lead to diffuse capillary leak and the flux of intravascular fluid into the extravascular space and sites of injury. This leads, especially if sepsis intervenes, to the need for vigorous fluid resuscitation. Just as a pulmonary artery catheter in patients with pulmonary dysfunction can be a valuable aid to guiding fluid therapy, an intracranial pressure monitor does the same thing for monitoring the effects of fluid therapy on the CNS. The presence of an intracranial pressure monitor allows for more precise fine-tuning of ventilator and fluid therapy in patients with multiple trauma in whom there are a number of important therapeutic priorities in addition to the head injury.

MECHANICAL VENTILATION

Mechanical ventilation is a rapidly changing field, and there are several new modes of mechanical ventilation particularly useful in trauma patients. It is still true, however, that the vast majority of patients can be ventilated with standard modes of ventilatory support, which are fully reviewed in Chap. 1.

At first approximation, ventilators can be divided into volume and pressure varieties.[76] Most trauma patients can be managed with standard ventilation using a volume control mode on a volume ventilator. In volume control ventilation, the physician determines the tidal volume to be given.

This tidal volume results in a developed pressure dependent on the volume given and pulmonary compliance. Pressure ventilators are designed to administer volume until a set pressure is reached. Because supplying adequate ventilatory volume is generally more important than the generated pressure volume, ventilators are usually used in trauma patients, although two newer modes of ventilation, pressure support and pressure control, are in some respects more akin to pressure ventilators than to volume ventilators.

When a volume control mode of ventilation is used, four basic ventilatory parameters must be set. Two of these, tidal volume and ventilator rate, determine the amount of ventilation. The other two parameters, inspired oxygen concentration and the level of positive end-expiratory pressure, are the primary determinants of oxygenation.

Tidal volume is the amount of volume delivered by the ventilator with each machine breath. A tidal volume that is too low can lead to atelectasis, and the patient may be hypoventilated. Hypoventilation is of particular concern in patients with head injury because of the effects that an elevated arterial partial pressure of carbon dioxide has on cerebral blood flow and intracranial pressure. Too high a tidal volume can also be detrimental and can result in an increased incidence of barotrauma with potentially life-threatening pneumothorax. As the tidal volume increases, intrapleural pressure also increases. As intrapleural pressure increases, venous return to the heart is decreased and cardiac output goes down. High tidal volumes and increased intrapleural pressure also results in increased venous back pressure in the superior vena cava and internal jugular veins. Theoretically, this in turn can result in increases in intracranial pressure.

Normal tidal volume in a healthy, spontaneously breathing individual is approximately 5 to 6 mL/kg body weight. One approach to ventilator management is to give a machine tidal volume that is comparable to this, or approximately 500 mL for a 70-kg individual. Another feature of normal spontaneous respiration, however, is occasional deeper breaths than this at somewhat higher tidal volumes of 10 to 15 mL/kg body weight. These so-called sigh breaths help to prevent atelectasis, and when machine tidal volumes of 5 to 6 mL/kg are used, they should be added at a rate of 1 to 2 per minute.

Another approach is to give supernormal tidal volumes of 10 to 15 mL/kg body weight with each machine breath. This is the simplest and most widely used approach and is optimal for preventing gradual atelectasis. Use of high tidal volumes also compensates for dead space in the endotracheal tube and associated tubing necessary in intubated patients.

Rate is the other important determinant of ventilation. In patients without the suspicion of head injury and increased intracranial pressure, a moderate rate of 12 to 16 per minute should be set if a tidal volume of 10 to 15 mL/kg is being used. When potentially increased intracranial pressure is a consideration, initial ventilator rates of 22 to 28 are more appropriate. The partial pressure of carbon dioxide should be determined at regular intervals and adjusted by adjusting the ventilatory rate.

The inspired concentration of oxygen is an obvious determinant of oxygenation. The arterial partial pressure of oxygen should be kept between 70 and 90 mmHg. This maintains an oxygen saturation of 90 percent or greater so that the patient is maintained above the sigmoidal portion of the oxygen saturation curve (Fig. 12-9). The arterial partial pressure should not be maintained at levels higher than approximately 90 percent because to do so often requires increases in the inspired concentration of oxygen. Oxygen in high concentrations is toxic to the lungs and results in long-term damage, scarring, and restrictive lung disease. A good rule of thumb is that oxygen toxicity becomes a consideration at approximately the 50 percent level. At very high levels of inspired oxygen concentration, 80 percent or above, the additional consideration of absorption atelectasis begins to come into play. Oxygen is readily absorbed across the alveolar-capillary interface. At low inspired concentrations of oxygen, most of the lung volume is made up of nitrogen, an inert gas not absorbed across the interface. The persistent, unabsorbed nitrogen serves to keep alveoli open. At high oxygen concentrations, nitrogen volume is low and oxygen is absorbed across the alveoli. The result is gradual atelectasis.

The other primary determinant of arterial oxy-

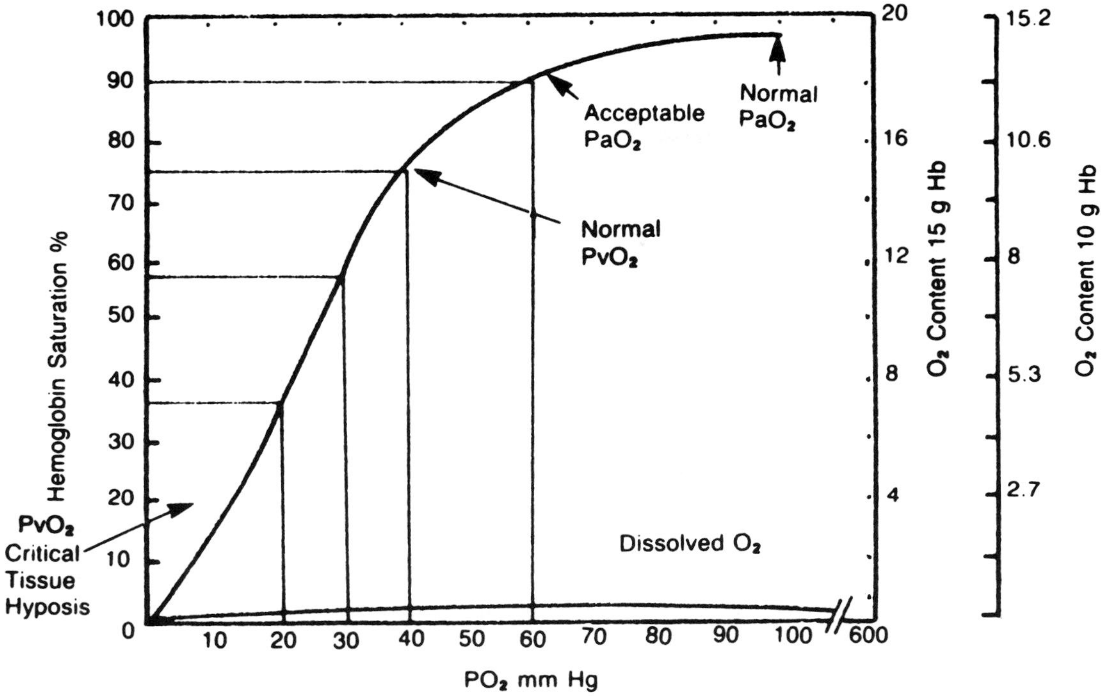

Figure 12-9 This is a graph of the partial pressure of oxygen versus the hemoglobin saturation. The shape of the curve is sigmoidal, which means that changes in P_{O_2} result in large changes in the hemoglobin saturation only on the steeply sloped part of the curve.

genation is the level of positive end-expiratory pressure. At the end of expiration, pressure in the ventilatory system falls to zero. Positive end-expiratory pressure keeps alveoli open at the end of the ventilatory cycle when they have a tendency to collapse. This tendency is particularly strong when pulmonary compliance is poor and the lungs are stiff. Collapse of alveoli leads to increased shunting of pulmonary vascular blood and a decrease in arterial oxygenation. The addition of positive end-expiratory pressure combats this tendency and improves oxygenation.

Even in patients without severe pulmonary disease and oxygenation defects, the application of low levels of positive end-expiratory pressure is a good idea.[77] In normal spontaneous ventilation the glottis closes at the end of expiration, trapping some gas in the lungs and resulting in a certain low level of physiologic positive end-expiratory pressure. Transglottic intubation with an endotracheal tube makes closure of the glottis impossible. By adding a low level of ventilator-generated positive end-expiratory pressure, the normal situation is minimized and alveolar collapse is prevented. This level of pressure is approximately 3 to 5 cmH_2O in magnitude.[78]

Positive end-expiratory pressure is not without complications. It is associated with an increased amount of barotrauma, particularly at high levels.[76,79] In addition, the same considerations outlined above for the effects of increased tidal volume on intrapleural pressure and venous return also pertain to positive end-expiratory pressure. Nonetheless, positive end-expiratory pressure is quite useful in improving oxygenation in patients with adult respiratory distress syndrome and other forms of pulmonary dysfunction that occur in multisystem injury. It is particularly helpful when high levels of inspired oxygen are required to overcome an oxygenation defect. The addition of increased levels of positive end-expiratory pressure sometimes allows for lower levels of inspired oxygen concentration with an attendant decrease in the risks of oxygen toxicity and absorption atelectasis. Our approach is to increase the inspired oxygen concentration as necessary up to a level of 50 percent. If oxygenation is still a problem, positive end-expiratory pressure is gradually increased to a level of 12 to 15 cmH_2O. If this is still insufficient to improve oxygenation saturation, other measures are necessary to improve oxygenation. Pressure control and inverse ratio ventilation, to be discussed later, are other means by which severe oxygenation defects can be treated when increased levels of positive end-expiratory pressure alone are not effective.

In addition to setting ventilatory parameters to control ventilation and oxygenation, a mode of ventilation must be determined. There are several modes of ventilation possible with a volume ventilator: controlled mandatory ventilation, assist-control ventilation, and intermittent mandatory ventilation.

Controlled mandatory ventilation is the simplest form of volume control ventilation. Mandatory ventilator-generated breaths are delivered at an interval determined by the ventilator rate. The patient's spontaneous breaths, if any, are not synchronized with the ventilator or vented through a separate circuit. Controlled mandatory ventilation is most useful in patients who are not spontaneously breathing and in whom the clinician wishes to control ventilation completely. There are alternative modes of ventilation which can be used to accomplish the same objective, and controlled mandatory ventilation is not very useful in weaning patients from the ventilator. Controlled mandatory ventilation is the least used of the three modes of volume control.

Assist control is the second mode of volume control ventilation. In this mode of ventilation, the machine is set to trigger a machine-generated breath of a present tidal volume with each inspiratory effort made by the patient. No purely spontaneous breaths are possible. If the patient makes no or only limited efforts at spontaneous ventilation, a backup rate is set on the machine so that at least a minimum number of machine-generated breaths will be given. If the patient breathes spontaneously above this backup rate, each of the additional spontaneous efforts is accompanied by a full machine breath. Advantages of assist control ventilation are patient comfort and the need for minimal patient ventilatory work. Disadvantages of this mode are the possibility of hyperventilation if the patient's respiratory rate is high because of anxiety, pain, or head injury. Assist control ventilation alone is also not useful in gradual weaning of a patient from mechanical ventilation because gradual diminution of the backup rate alone does not result in the gradual withdrawal of ventilatory support.

Intermittent mandatory ventilation is the third mode of volume control ventilation. In this mode the ventilator gives machine breaths at intervals determined by the ventilatory rate just as with controlled mandatory ventilation. As opposed to controlled mandatory ventilation, however, the patient can take spontaneous breaths between the machine breaths through a separate ventilatory circuit. Ventilation is thus a mixture of machine and spontaneous breaths. The advantage of intermittent mandatory ventilation is that the amount of ventilation provided by the ventilator can be gradually decreased by decreasing the frequency of machine breaths. This allows for slow and controlled weaning. Intermittent mandatory ventilation can be uncomfortable for patients in that the machine-generated breaths are delivered independent of the patient's spontaneous ventilatory efforts and may compete with them. Synchronized intermittent mandatory ventilation is a modification of intermittent mandatory ventilation designed to obviate this difficulty. In synchronized mandatory ventilation, the machine breaths are coordinated as much as possible with the patient's spontaneous ventilatory efforts.

New modes of ventilation have been developed within the last several years to help both with ventilation and oxygenation problems in intubated patients. There are four new modes with which a fairly broad experience has been obtained, two in the area of ventilation and weaning and two in the area of oxygenation. In the area of ventilation and weaning, the two methods are pressure support and flow-by ventilation. Pressure control and inverse ratio ventilation, usually used in combination, are the two techniques which have been applied to oxygenation problems.

Pressure support acts upon the patient's spontaneous ventilatory efforts to increase tidal volume.[80-82] This is done by the addition of positive pressure from the ventilator upon detection of a spontaneous ventilatory effort. The onset of pressure support is timed to coincide with the beginning of spontaneous inspiration and is set to stop when inspiratory flow decreases to 25 percent of its maximal value. Because of the relationship between pressure and volume, addition of pressure support acts to increase the amount of tidal volume generated with spontaneous ventilatory efforts (Fig. 12-10).

Low levels of pressure support, like low levels of positive end-expiratory pressure, can be thought of as physiologic.[83-85] Airway resistance, because it is related to the fourth power of the radius, increases markedly even with small decreases in airway size. Intubation, especially with a small endotracheal tube, substantially increases airway resistance and both inspiratory and expiratory work of breathing. Small amounts of pressure support, on the order of 3 to 5 cmH_2O, counteract this resistance increase (Fig. 12-11). Adding small amounts of pressure support is thus helpful in intubated patients, particularly those with increased work of breathing from other causes. The addition of small amounts of pressure support can also increase patient comfort. There are no known major side effects from the addition of these small amounts of pressure support.

Pressure support can also be used for weaning from mechanical ventilation. As outlined above, addition of pressure support increases the patient's spontaneous tidal volumes. Institution of pressure support is an alternative means by which minute ventilation can be given by the ventilator. Pressure support, because it adds to spontaneous breaths rather than imposing machine breaths, may be more comfortable than intermittent mandatory ventilation or even synchronized intermittent mandatory ventilation in some patients. When pressure support is used for weaning from mechanical ventilation, it can be administered either as an arbitrary amount or can be given to result in a predetermined desired spontaneous tidal volume. For example, if a patient is able to generate unaided spontaneous tidal volumes of 200 mL and the desired tidal volume is 600 mL, pressure support can be gradually added until the spontaneous tidal volume is increased by 400 mL. The number

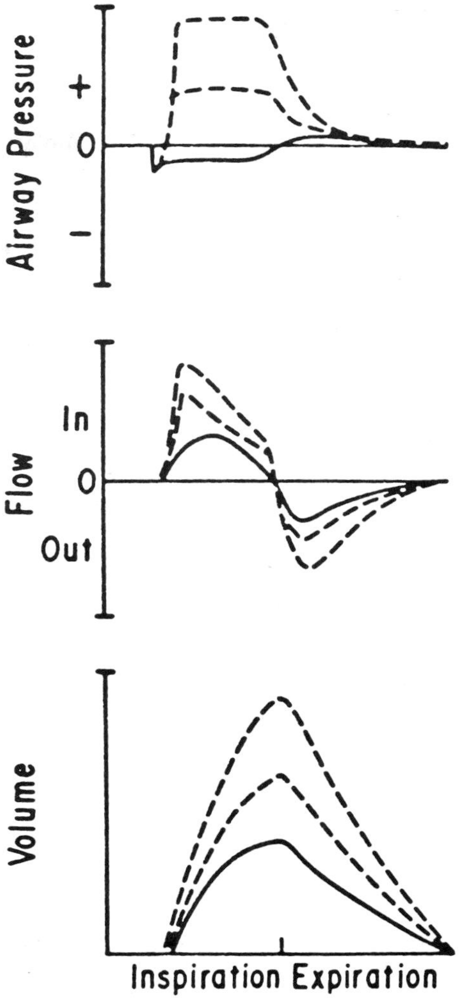

Figure 12-10 The above graphs demonstrate airway pressure, flow, and lung volume during spontaneous ventilation without pressure support (solid lines) and with two different levels of pressure support (dash lines). During pressure support the ventilator produces and maintains an inspiratory pressure that augments both flow and lung volume.

of intermittent mandatory ventilations from the ventilator can be rapidly decreased, and this is really just an exchange of minute ventilation as delivered by intermittent mandatory ventilation for minute ventilation delivered by pressure support.

When pressure is used for weaning, we generally

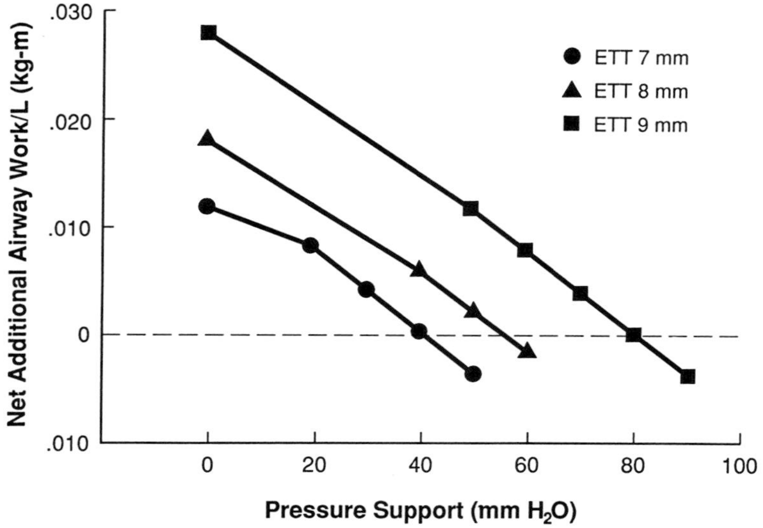

Figure 12-11 Both endotracheal tube size and the degree of pressure support have an effect on the work of breathing. As the endotracheal size increases, the work of breathing decreases markedly. Similarly, as pressure support is added, the work of breathing decreases.

add the pressure support to supplement intermittent mandatory ventilations. The intermittent mandatory ventilation breaths are then decreased in a stepwise fashion until a level of 2 to 4 per minute is reached. At this point, weaning of the pressure support in a gradual, stepwise fashion is begun and continued until it has been decreased to a physiologic level of 3 to 5 cmH_2O. In some patients, use of pressure support weaning is more effective and rapid than the use of intermittent mandatory ventilation weaning.

One caveat important in the use of pressure support for weaning is to remember that the addition of pressure support is just another way of providing minute ventilation from the ventilator. In this sense, it is no different than increasing the rate of intermittent mandatory ventilations or the tidal volumes of the machine breaths. Conversion to pressure support which results in marked decreases in the rate of intermittent mandatory ventilation should not be interpreted as an improvement in the patient's spontaneous ventilatory ability.

Flow-by ventilation is another new mode of ventilation useful in overcoming airway resistance and weaning patients from mechanical ventilation.[86–89] In flow-by ventilation, the endotracheal tube is connected to a crossbar with a high flow of gas running through it. Inspiration is aided by the entrainment of the flow-by gas, and this provides the inspiratory effort necessary to trigger ventilation. The flow-by circuit is only operative during inspiration and thus does not increase resistance to flow during expiration. Inspiratory work of breathing is decreased markedly when flow-by is instituted, and this may help in weaning the patient from the ventilator by removing the increased inspiratory work inherent in the intubated, ventilated state.

Weaning from mechanical ventilation can be done in a variety of different ways and is reviewed in Chap. 1. Multisystem-injured patients with severe pulmonary dysfunction who have required long periods of ventilatory support may be difficult to wean. We generally put such patients on a synchronized intermittent mandatory ventilation mode of ventilation and begin to gradually decrease the frequency of machine breaths so that the patient takes on more and more responsibility for ventilation. When rates of mandatory ventilation of 2 to 4 per minute are reached, the patient is tried on a trial of continuous positive airway pressure without any mandatory machine breaths. The continuous positive airway pressure (CPAP) functions in spontaneously breathing patients in much the same way as physiologic positive end-expiratory pressure functions in patients on mechanical ventilation. It ensures that the airway pressure does not drop to very low levels at the end of expiration and prevents progressive atelectasis. If the patient tolerates a prolonged trial of CPAP after gradual weaning of the intermittent mandatory ventilation rate, extubation can be safely carried out.

If a gradual decrease in the mandatory ventilation rate is unsuccessful, we try weaning from pressure control ventilation or weaning from a combination of intermittent mandatory ventilation and pressure control. The final stage of this form of weaning is also a CPAP trial. If this method of weaning is unsuccessful, we next institute "wind sprint" trials. These are intermittent periods of time on CPAP. The periods are progressively increased both in length and frequency until the patient is spending most of the time on CPAP. At this point, extubation can be considered.

The decision to extubate can be a difficult one. There are objective parameters that can be used as guidelines (Table 12-1). We rely just as heavily on more subjective criteria. The patient must be able to protect the airway and must be improving with respect to associated surgical and medical problems. A prolonged CPAP trial must be tolerated without difficulty, and the patient must be able to clear airway secretions. Objective weaning parameters can be obtained but must be put into context. Some patients with adequate pulmonary and ventilatory function may be able to tolerate extubation but may not be able to cooperate fully with the process of obtaining weaning parameters. The measurements obtained may thus be falsely discouraging. Conversely, a highly cooperative and motivated patient may be able to do quite well with respect to ventilatory function during the short period of time necessary to obtain pulmonary function tests but may not tolerate extubation and the need for prolonged spontaneous ventilation.

Table 12-1 Weaning Parameters

Spontaneous respiratory rate	< 25 per min
Tidal volume	> 5 mL/kg
Vital capacity	> 10 mL/kg
Minute ventilation	< 120 mL/kg per min
Negative inspiratory force	< -20 cmH_2O

The issue of the timing and appropriateness of tracheostomy in patients with prolonged need for mechanical ventilation is a controversial one.[90-92] Persistently altered mental status is an important reason for lowering the threshold for tracheotomy, particularly in patients with head injury. The presence of a tracheostomy may decrease the risk of aspiration, although this is somewhat unclear. Just as important, the presence of a tracheostomy simplifies pulmonary toilet in patients in whom there is a suspicion that airway protection is inadequate.

Prolonged need for mechanical ventilatory support is not always an indication for tracheostomy. It is unclear whether the incidence of airway stenosis is higher with prolonged intubation than with tracheostomy, but management is often simplified by a tracheostomy and if intubation beyond several weeks is anticipated and there is no improvement or only minimal progress with weaning, it is a good idea in most cases to perform a tracheostomy. Pulmonary toilet and discontinuation of mechanical ventilation on a trial basis are simplified greatly if there is a tracheostomy in place. Paradoxically, patients with severe adult respiratory distress syndrome (ARDS) and poor pulmonary compliance are not good candidates for tracheotomy. Leaks around the tracheostomy tube cuff due to poor pulmonary compliance and high peak inspiratory pressures are a problem in such patients, and these patients can be difficult to ventilate unless hard cuffed tubes are used. The risks of the tracheostomy outweigh the benefits in such patients, and tracheostomy should be deferred until lung compliance has improved.

Pressure control ventilation, usually used in conjunction with inverse ratio ventilation, is a relatively new mode of ventilation useful in multisystem-injured patients with severe oxygenation defects.[93-95] In pressure control ventilation, machine breaths are given to a predetermined peak inspiratory pressure and tidal volume becomes a derived rather than a determined variable. Pressure control ventilation is given in a somewhat different fashion than simple pressure ventilation, however. In simple pressure limited ventilation, volume is delivered in a steady fashion such that the pressure in the ventilatory circuit increases gradually until the present inspiratory cutoff pressure is reached. In pressure control ventilation, flow rates at the beginning of inspiration are very rapid so that the target pressure for the ventilatory system is reached quickly. Flow rates are then adjusted by a servomechanism so that the target pressure is maintained throughout the inspiratory portion of ventilation. The pressure curve of the system over time resembles a square wave rather than a parabola (Fig. 12-12). This acts to rapidly inflate the pulmonary alveoli and keep them inflated throughout inspiration. Ventilation is distributed in a more even fashion among the different alveoli with different compliances. If the lungs are filled gradually, there is a tendency for ventilation to preferentially distribute to complaint alveoli first and to fill noncompliant alveoli last. Pressure control, by using rapid initial flow rates to overcome resistance to filling, is effective in distributing volume more evenly. By maintaining a fixed pressure throughout the inspiratory phase of the ventilatory cycle, alveoli are also kept open throughout inspiration, atelectasis is minimized, and oxygenation is improved.

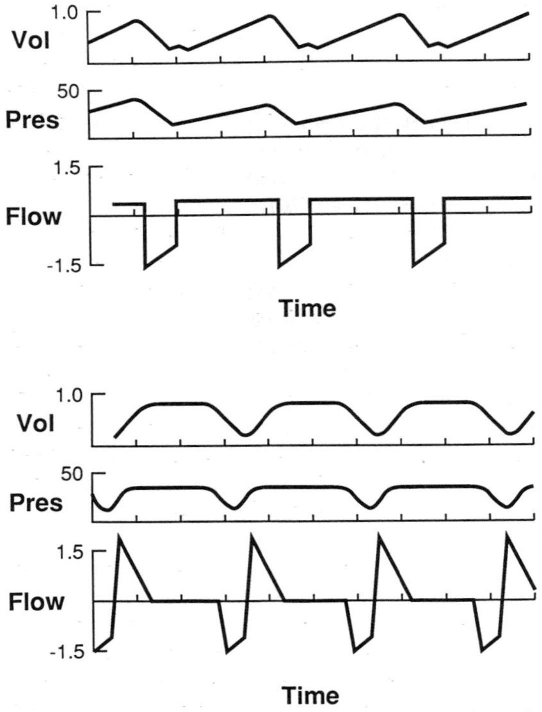

Figure 12-12 The above figures compare volume, pressure, and flow characteristics for volume control ventilation (top) and pressure control inverse ratio ventilation (bottom). With pressure control, flow is augmented at the beginning of inspiration in order to provide a square pressure waveform. When the ratio of ventilation is inverted, inspiratory time is increased at the expense of inspiratory time.

While pressure control is helpful in improving oxygenation, it is not without potential side effects. Although the peak pressure that the ventilatory system reaches is not as high with pressure control as with volume control ventilation, the rapid initial rise in airway pressure and the maintenance of this same pressure throughout inspiration unavoidably increase mean airway pressure (Fig. 12-13). This may be associated with an increase in barotrauma. The increase in mean airway pressure also means a corresponding increase in mean intrapleural pressure, which causes a decrease in venous return and a decrease in cardiac output. The inspiratory flow pattern used in pressure control ventilation is also quite different from normal ventilation and is often difficult for patients to tolerate unless they are paralyzed and sedated. The paralysis is also important in ensuring that the desired tidal volumes are delivered.

Pressure control is most useful in patients with oxygenation difficulties and usually improves the arterial partial pressure of oxygen and allows for a decrease in the inspired oxygen concentration. Pressure control can be used with positive end-expiratory pressure and the two are complementary. Pressure control ventilation is also quite useful in conjunction with inverse ratio ventilation.

Inverse ratio ventilation, like pressure control, is most useful in patients with poor compliance and disorders of oxygenation such as ARDS (Fig. 12-14). Like pressure control, inverse ratio ventilation opens alveoli that are collapsed and maintains expanded alveoli in an open state. In the normal state of spontaneous ventilation, the ratio of inspiratory to expiratory time for a normal ventilatory cycle is approximately 1:2 or 1:3; expiration lasts 2 to 3 times as long as inspiration. When standard volume control ventilation is used, the inspiratory-to-expiratory ratio is usually set at

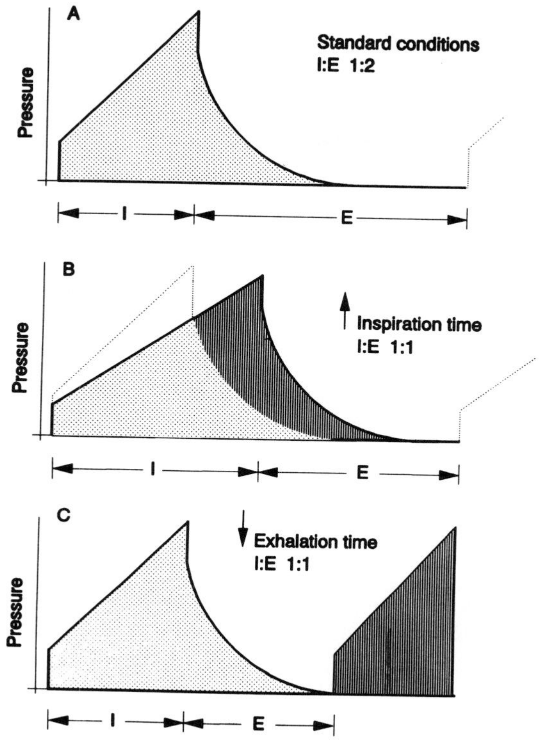

Figure 12-13 Mean airway pressure is affected profoundly by changes in the inspiratory-to-expiratory (I:E) ratio. The stippled area represents the normal area of the pressure curve. The vertical hatched region represents the increase in area of the curve and therefore the increase in mean airway pressure. *A* shows the normal area. In *B*, inspiratory time was increased by decreasing the flow rate. In *C*, exhalation time was decreased, which removes much of the expiratory pause at zero pressure.

about 1 : 2. Inverting the inspiratory-to-expiratory ratio means that the patient spends more than the normal proportion of time in inspiration. If the ratio is inverted, the lungs have less time to empty and there is some degree of air trapping. The degree of air trapping is roughly proportional to the degree to which the ratio is inverted. Air trapping maintains alveoli in an expanded state.

As the inspiratory-to-expiratory ratio is inverted and air trapping occurs there is an increased risk of barotrauma and pneumothorax if the degree of air trapping is not limited in some way.[96,97] One way to limit the degree of air trapping is to only invert the ratio as much as necessary to achieve the desired improvement in oxygenation. Another and more commonly used means of minimizing barotrauma is to use inverse ratio ventilation in conjunction with pressure control. Pressure control sets a present pressure beyond which the ventilator will not force the system. If air trapping is persistent, the airway pressure gradually rises and pressure control ensures that the pressure rise is self-limited.

Because of the complicated effects that inverse ratio ventilation has on air trapping, tidal volume, and hemodynamics, the effects on oxygenation are not entirely predictable, and when instituting inverse ratio ventilation a certain amount of trial and error is often necessary. Ratios of 1 : 1 are generally a good place to start, and arterial blood gases should be regularly followed after each ventilatory maneuver. If the desired effect on oxygenation is not achieved, the ratio should gradually be inverted further in a stepwise fashion. Ratios of up to 4 : 1 are possible and are sometimes necessary in extreme cases. Because of the effects of such extremely inverted ratios on venous return, hemodynamics should be followed closely.

SPINAL INJURIES IN THE MULTIPLY INJURED PATIENT IN THE INTENSIVE CARE UNIT

Because of the universal teaching for prehospital providers that spinal injury should be assumed in trauma victims, most patients arrive in the emergency department in spinal precautions. A challenge in the initial management of these patients is the decision about who needs radiographic clearance of the spine and who can be cleared clinically. We feel that in cooperative patients with a Glasgow coma scale of 15 and an entirely normal mental status, the spine can be cleared clinically if the patient has no vertebral pain or tenderness and no peripheral neurologic deficit.[98,99] This series of preconditions excludes patients with head injury of even moderate severity and patients with altered mental status or a difficult physical exam.

Patients who cannot be cleared clinically should be cleared radiographically whenever possible as

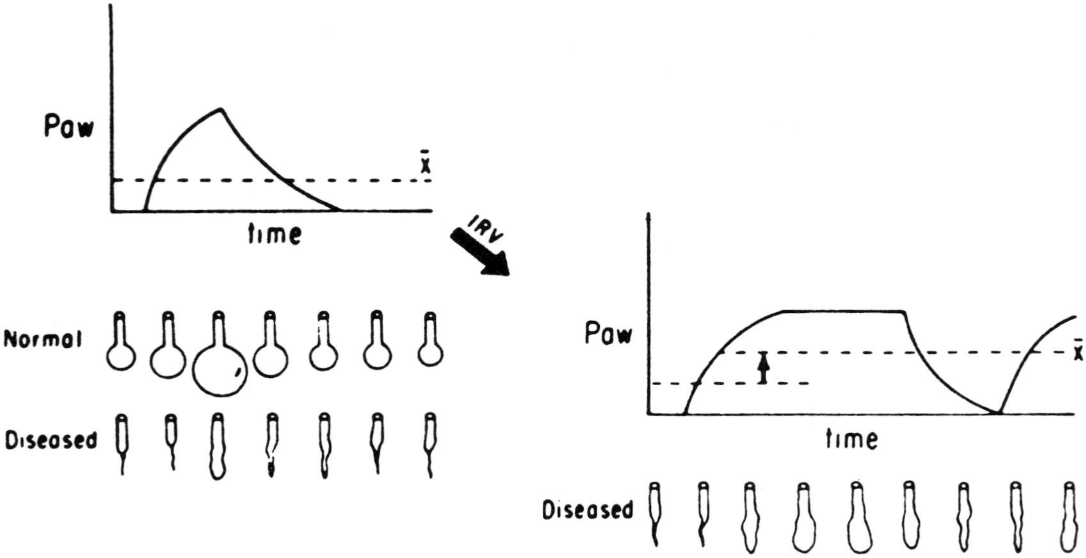

Figure 12-14 Airway pressure gradually increases during inspiration with normal ratio ventilation (left). Inspiratory volume tends to fill compliant alveoli better than diseased alveoli. Inverse ratio ventilation increases the amount of time spent in inspiration and allows for better inflation of poorly compliant alveoli and the prevention of alveoli collapse.

soon as other priorities of management allow. A dilemma in patients with severe injury is what to do when the spine cannot be cleared in the initial phases of resuscitation and the patient is transferred to the ICU without radiographic clearance of the spine having been accomplished. If the patient at this point is awake and alert and is free of pain and tenderness of the spine, clinical clearance is possible. Clinical clearance in this situation is safer than a trip to the radiology suite, particularly if the patient is unstable in any way or is intubated.[100] If the patient is stable from a hemodynamic and pulmonary standpoint and cannot be cleared clinically, he or she should be sent to the radiology suite for radiographic clearance.

In the initial stages of ICU management, the spine should be a secondary priority if the patient is at all unstable from either a hemodynamic or pulmonary point of view. Spinal precautions should be maintained. If this situation persists beyond several days, however, the risks of prolonged immobilization begin to increase and there is some urgency to discontinuing spinal precautions. If there is a high index of suspicion for spinal cord injury because of severe head or maxillofacial injuries or apparent neurologic deficit, the trip to x-ray is worth the risk unless the patient is prohibitively unstable. Another option is to perform portable cervical x-rays in the ICU to rule out spinal injury.

CHEST TRAUMA

Chest trauma is common in patients with multiple injury. Injuries of the chest wall can range from mild contusions and ecchymoses of the skin and subcutaneous tissue to grossly unstable flail segments. The lungs and great vessels can also be injured.

Pneumothorax and tension pneumothorax have been mentioned earlier with respect to initial emergency department management. They should be treated by decompression of the chest with a thoracostomy tube. In patients on positive pressure ventilation, particularly those with pulmonary dysfunction and poor pulmonary compliance, vigilance should be maintained for development of pneumothorax secondary to barotrauma. Because the patient is on positive pressure ventilation and generating high inspiratory pressures, tension pneumothorax is particularly likely. Clues to the development of a pneumothorax in this situation are the development of respiratory distress or increasing difficulty with oxygenation associated with progressive elevation of the peak inspiratory pressure (if the patient is on volume control ventilation) and hemodynamic instability. Decreased breath sounds and tracheal deviation may also occur but are not absolutely reliable. If a tension pneumothorax in this setting is suspected, the suspicious side of the chest should be immediately vented without waiting for chest x-ray confirmation.

In stable patients, x-rays of the chest may show obvious pneumothorax or the signs may be more subtle. Anterior pneumothorax is particularly difficult to diagnose from the anteroposterior chest film and is best seen on a cross-table lateral of the chest. On an anteroposterior chest film, these anterior pneumothoraces are suspected when a diffuse lucency is seen over a central portion of the lung field.

For patients with chest wall trauma, pain control is a particularly important concern. If chest wall injuries are severe, patients should be intubated and mechanically ventilated and no early attempts to wean them from mechanical ventilation should be made. The patient can be kept comfortable and relatively pain free with large doses of parenteral narcotics without fear of respiratory arrest. In less severely injured patients and in patients with massive injuries who have recovered to the point of weaning from mechanical ventilation, pain management is more complicated and is a balance between providing insufficient pain control for symptomatic relief and so much pain control that there is interference with respiratory drive. Without adequate pain control, the patient is reluctant to breathe enough to allow for weaning from mechanical ventilation. Too much pain control and respiratory drive may be reduced, complicating the weaning process. Pain management is further complicated in patients with head injury or some other cause for altered mental status. Narcotics and other analgesics cloud the neurologic exam and lead to uncertainty about how much of the altered mental status is pharmacologic and how much is due to the underlying problem. In such instances, enough analgesia should be given to alleviate subjectively obvious suffering, but the analgesia, particularly with narcotics, should otherwise be minimized. The use of nonsteroidal anti-inflammatory drugs can also be helpful in these circumstances, as they have no effects on mental status and minimal depressive effects on respiratory drive.[101,102,105] Recently, the parenteral nonsteroidal medication Ketorolac (Toradol) has been found to provide narcotic levels of analgesia while avoiding the sedative side effects of opiate-analgesics.

Epidural analgesia is quite effective in many patients with chest wall trauma.[103,104] It provides good pain control with minimal respiratory depression if given appropriately. Epidural analgesia seems to be particularly effective in elderly patients. While there are some systemic effects from this route of analgesia, they are usually not as pronounced as those seen with intravenous or intramuscular analgesia. Both immediate and delayed respiratory depression can occur. Both are rare and preventable with attention to some of the details of epidural catheter management. Immediate respiratory depression occurs due to medication errors or unrecognized placement of the catheter in the intravascular space rather than in the epidural space. Delayed respiratory depression is related to migration of the analgesic up the epidural space with central depression of the respiratory center. Careful dosing of epidural analgesic avoids this complication, as does use of highly lipid soluble narcotics as a continuous infusion into the epidural space rather than intermittent bolus injections of lipid insoluble opioids that migrate over time.

Epidural catheters are not appropriate for all patients with chest wall trauma. They should not be used in patients with severe head injury because of difficulties in determining when adequate analgesia has been administered. The presence or suspicion of vertebral column or spinal cord injury is another contraindication, as is the presence of a coagulopathy or low platelet count. Epidural catheter placement in patients with bleeding disorders can result in creation of an epidural hematoma, a potentially disastrous complication.

Patient-controlled analgesia is another form of analgesia for patients in the ICU with chest wall trauma or other sources of pain. These devices generally provide better pain control than intermittent nurse-controlled bolus administration of narcotic. Once set up, they are also less labor-intensive for the nursing staff. Patient-controlled analgesia is not appropriate in patients with altered mental status or a language barrier unless it is fully explained through an interpreter. It is also not appropriate in small children and in patients with mental retardation. Finally, it should generally be avoided in patients with head injury.

Flail chest is a severe disruption of the chest wall such that a portion of it moves independent of the rest of the chest during ventilation (Fig. 12-15). The island of chest wall is free from the support of the surrounding chest. When the rest of the chest expands, this island tends to implode. There is some debate about how important this mechanical instability is with respect to adequate ventilation. It is our feeling that the primary problem in patients with flail chest is not the mechanical instability of the chest wall but severe pain interfering with adequate chest wall excursion and ventilation and contusion of the underlying lung interfering with oxygenation.

Flail chest can occur in any part of the chest. It is most common in our experience in the anterior chest in which there is disruption of the costochondral and sternochondral margins such that the sternum is a free-floating segment of the chest

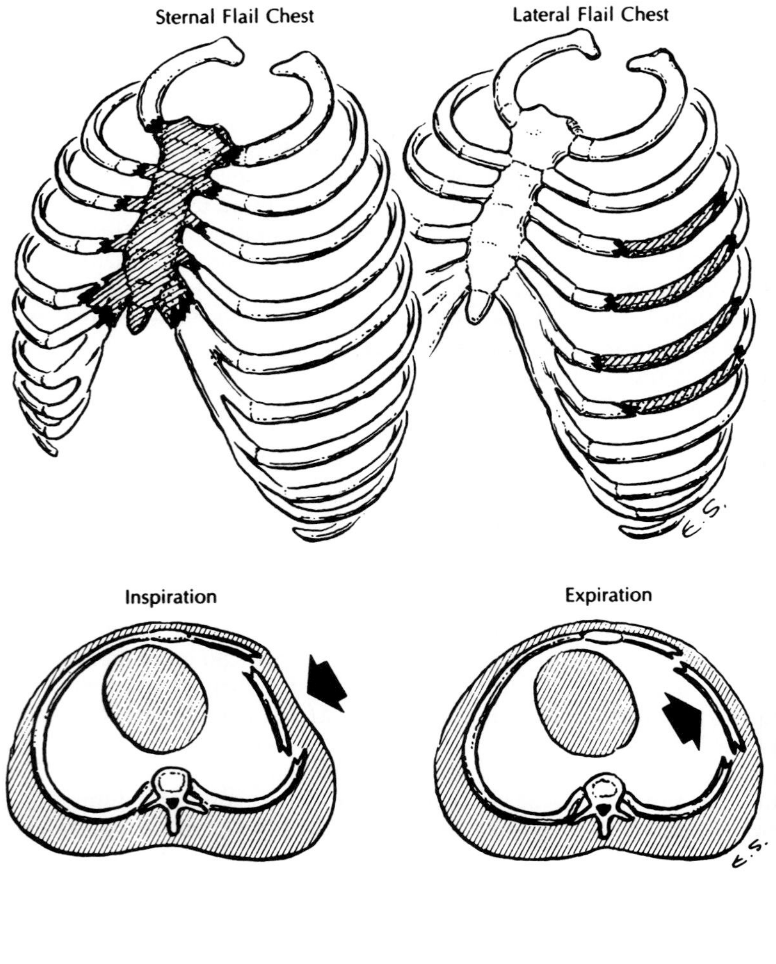

Figure 12-15 Flail chest can occur laterally or anteriorly including the sternum with separation of the costochondral junctions. The flail segment moves paradoxically compared to the rest of the chest wall with both inspiration and expiration.

wall. In addition to being the most common form of flail chest in our experience, it is also the least severe with respect to pulmonary contusion and respiratory insufficiency. Patients with anterior flail chest can often be treated effectively with good pain control. Intubation and mechanical ventilation can be avoided. This is particularly true if epidural analgesia is used, the patient is young, and there are no severe associated injuries.

Patients with lateral and posterior flail chest usually require mechanical ventilation, sometimes for prolonged periods of time. The most effective form of early ventilation is assist control ventilation in which each spontaneous ventilatory effort by the patient spurs a mechanical ventilation. With this mode of ventilation, ventilation is passive and the patient's need for ventilatory effort and excursion minimal. This minimizes pain.

Myocardial contusion is another possible injury suffered by victims of multiple trauma from blunt-force injury.[106-108] A great deal of confusion about the diagnosis of myocardial contusion exists because of the lack of a gold standard diagnostic test. A number of different diagnostic tests have been suggested, but none of them has proven a reliable predictor of the existence of the entity. Positivity in any of these tests correlates poorly with cardiac failure or cardiac arrhythmia, the two potential clinical consequences of myocardial contusion.

The important initial decision in patients with suspected myocardial contusion is about the need for a monitored bed. In massively injured patients, this is not a difficult consideration because they are admitted to a monitored bed in the ICU in any case. For stable patients who are otherwise not candidates for an ICU or telemetry bed, we feel that the mainstay of prognostic and disposition management is the admission rhythm strip electrocardiogram. If the rhythm strip does not exhibit any abnormalities other than sinus tachycardia or nonspecific ST-T wave changes, the patient can be admitted to an unmonitored bed. If the rhythm strip is positive for an abnormality, the patient should be admitted to a monitored bed for 48 h and abnormalities treated as they arise.

Blunt trauma to the chest can also result in a torn thoracic aorta.[109] The hallmark of the diagnosis is a wide mediastinum on chest x-ray.[110,111] Because the initial chest x-rays in most patients injured badly enough to have a torn aorta are anteroposterior films and this view distorts and exaggerates the width of the mediastinum, the specificity of this sign is low. It should be taken seriously, however, because failure to make the diagnosis and repair the aorta is associated with subsequent rupture of the aortic pseudoaneurysm and death in most cases. The aorta usually ruptures just distal to the takeoff of the left subclavian artery. Aortography is the definitive diagnostic test. The aorta is repaired via a left posterolateral thoracotomy, and placement of a short segment of synthetic aortic graft is usually required.

Treatment of a torn thoracic aorta in a patient with an associated head injury can be difficult. Repair requires cross-clamping of the proximal thoracic aorta, and this can have profound effects on intracranial blood flow and intracranial pressure. At the same time that intracranial and cerebrospinal fluid pressure is increased, blood pressure distal to the cross-clamp decreases markedly. This tends to compromise blood supply to the abdominal viscera, which can lead to visceral failure. These alterations in central nervous and hemodynamic pressures also put the blood supply to the thoracic spinal cord in jeopardy, and paraplegia is a well-known complication of the repair of these injuries.

We repair torn thoracic aortas with the use of left heart bypass, which helps to minimize some of the changes described above. Left heart bypass shunts oxygenated blood from the left heart or the root of the aorta to the femoral artery or the distal aorta. The shunt tubing is connected to a centrifugal pump, and the blood is thus shunted past the cross-clamped area. Left heart bypass allows for delivery of blood to the viscera and spinal cord distal to the cross-clamp. It also decompresses the proximal circulation and minimizes the increase in intracranial blood flow and pressure that occurs with placement of the cross-clamp. We also place a lumbar cerebrospinal fluid drain prior to operative repair in selected patients with either no head injury or only minor head injury in which there is minimal risk of herniation. Evoked potential monitoring is also used to follow the functional state and degree of ischemia of the thoracic and distal spinal cord after placement of the cross-clamp. This information can be used to adjust the amount of flow diverted through the bypass shunt.

The pumps used in the left heart bypass shunt require minimal or no heparinization, an important consideration in patients with head injury in which there is a risk of intracranial bleeding. Vertebral column or spinal cord injuries do not preclude operative repair of a torn thoracic aorta. A good neurologic exam should be done prior to surgery to determine the extent of neurologic impairment, if any, before the spinal cord blood supply is jeopardized with the aortic cross-clamp. Spinal precautions should also be observed during the thoracotomy. This can be difficult if the left heart bypass is placed from the left heart to the femoral artery because access to the femoral artery may be difficult, particularly in an obese individual, in the lateral decubitus position. In such situations, the distal limb of the left heart bypass should be placed in the distal descending thoracic aorta.

Occasional patients may have a head injury so severe that, even with use of left heart bypass, aortic repair should be deferred. Such patients are fortunately rare. They can be treated nonoperatively in an ICU setting with mechanical ventilation and control of blood pressure. This is done preferentially with beta blockers. Peripheral vasodilators, while they will lower the blood pressure, can increase shear forces and distention forces at the site of the aortic injury and are a second line of pharmacology in such cases. When a nonoperative approach is initially taken, the patient is followed with the above regimen, and if the head injury and general condition improve, the aorta is repaired on a delayed basis.

ABDOMINAL TRAUMA

Bleeding is the most important initial priority in the management of patients with abdominal trauma. In blunt-trauma patients, bleeding is most commonly from the liver or spleen.[112] If the patient requires laparotomy prior to arrival in the ICU, the bleeding will have been controlled in the vast majority of cases. On rare instances, the injuries and blood loss will have been so massive that the patient will develop a coagulopathy and bleeding will be ongoing upon arrival of the patient in the ICU. In such cases, treatment consists of administration of appropriate blood products to reverse the coagulopathy and maintain intravascular blood volume. It is also important to ensure that the bleeding is medical; that is, that it is diffuse bleeding which can only be corrected with transfusion and that it is not surgical bleeding amenable to operative hemostasis. In patients in whom coagulopathy is unlikely to develop in the postoperative period, hemodynamic instability and the need for large amounts of blood products should immediately raise the prospect of surgically controllable bleeding and consideration should be given to reexploration of the abdomen. If abdominal exploration has not already been performed, it should be considered in such instances.

Some hemodynamically stable patients who undergo abdominal CT scanning are candidates for nonoperative management of liver and spleen injuries.[113–116] The decision to manage such injuries conservatively is dependent on a number of factors. If the patient has serious associated injuries, hemodynamic instability, or the need for extensive transfusion, operative intervention should be carried out. If the injury appears quite severe on CT scanning, operative intervention is also indicated. If conservative management is elected, the patient should be admitted initially to the ICU. The hematocrit and abdominal exam should be checked at 4- to 6-h intervals for several days. The exact length of stay that is appropriate in the ICU is unclear but should probably be at least 48 to 72 h for both liver and spleen injuries assuming the patient remains stable and does not require extensive blood transfusion. In either of these instances, operative intervention should be undertaken.

Aside from bleeding from the liver and spleen, there are other abdominal injuries that are particularly insidious in their presentation. Penetrating trauma can result in injuries to the hollow viscera or the retroperitoneal vasculature which will manifest only over the course of a number of hours if the patient is not initially explored. We explore all gunshot wounds to the abdomen because there is an 85 to 90 percent incidence of intraperitoneal injury in such patients.[117] In patients with stab wounds to the anterior abdomen, exploration is carried out if the wound violates the abdominal fascia.[118] For stab wounds posterior to the posterior axillary line, observation is done in stable patients with minimal symptoms. If the white blood cell count does not increase and symptoms and signs remain minimal, these patients are not explored.

For blunt-trauma patients, the situation is not as simple. There are two types of serious injury which can be missed in the early postinjury course and in which delay in diagnosis can seriously increase morbidity and mortality.[119-122] These injuries are to the intestine and pancreas. Both are often missed by CT scan in the early postinjury period and should be suspected in ICU patients who are not doing well. The physical exam, in patients with a reliable exam, is helpful in making these diagnoses. In our experience, patients with blunt intestinal injury have pronounced and unmistakable peritoneal signs shortly after injury if they are awake and cooperative with an abdominal exam. In those with altered mental status from head injury or other causes, diagnostic peritoneal lavage will pick up approximately 95 percent of cases requiring operative intervention.

Pancreatic injuries are also diagnosed in awake and cooperative patients by the physical exam, although the findings are more subtle than in patients with blunt intestinal injury because of the retroperitoneal location of the pancreas.[122] Peritoneal lavage can miss these injuries, also because of the retroperitoneal location of the pancreas. Computed tomography, as mentioned above, is notoriously unreliable in making this diagnosis if done shortly after injury. If the CT scan is done on a delayed basis, sensitivity improves. Serial determination of serum amylase is also helpful in making the diagnosis of a missed pancreatic injury if the value progressively increases over time.[123] In spite of these diagnostic tools, there will be patients in whom clinical suspicion alone and a worse-than-expected initial postinjury course in the ICU should prompt abdominal exploration to rule out a missed injury before too much time passes. In these rare instances, the exploration of the abdomen can be considered an extension of the physical examination.

Development of an intra-abdominal abscess is one of the complications of multiple injury which should be borne in mind in following patients in the ICU.[124,125] A high index of suspicion should be maintained if the patient suffered intra-abdominal injuries, particularly to hollow viscera with bacterial contamination of the peritoneal cavity. Blind exploration of the abdomen in such patients based on clinical suspicion alone has a very low yield, and the preferred diagnostic study is a CT exam of the abdomen. If a suspected abscess is discovered on CT scan, a sample of abscess fluid can be obtained percutaneously under tomographic or ultrasound guidance to confirm the diagnosis and culture the organisms in the cavity.[126,127] Abscesses can sometimes be completely drained under CT guidance. If this fails or if the abscess location or contents are not amenable to such an approach, operative drainage is indicated. In patients too unstable to make the trip to the CT suite, bedside ultrasound imaging of the abdomen is an alternative, although the yield of this approach is best if the search is directed at a particular area such as the left upper quadrant or pelvis instead of being a shotgun approach to diagnosis of an abscess anywhere in the abdomen.

Patients in the ICU often appear septic, but even with the most diligent search no discrete source of sepsis or infection is discovered. Another curiosity of these patients is that in many instances when bacteria are cultured from the blood or other sites, these bacteria are flora normally found resident in the gut lumen. Bacterial translocation theory attempts to explain these phenomena.[128-130]

It is an experimental observation that a variety of traumatic and septic insults lead to atrophy and dysfunction of the gut mucosal barrier (Fig. 12-16). Since the gut lumen in the normal state contains large numbers of bacteria, the barrier function of the mucosa is an important one in protecting the patient from resident flora. Bacterial translocation theory hypothesizes that with an insult of large enough magnitude, the mucosal barrier breaks down and allows bacteria and bacterial endotoxin through the gut wall and into the lymphatic system and the portal circulation.[131] This in turn engenders an inflammatory reaction. Many of the characteristics of septic state can be replicated by injection of bacterial endotoxin,[132] and it is thought that the gut, by way of the portal venous system and the lymphatics, is a source of this endotoxin and the subsequent reaction to it. Although this is an attractive explanation for some of the events seen in severely ill and injured patients, and although it is fairly well established that bacte-

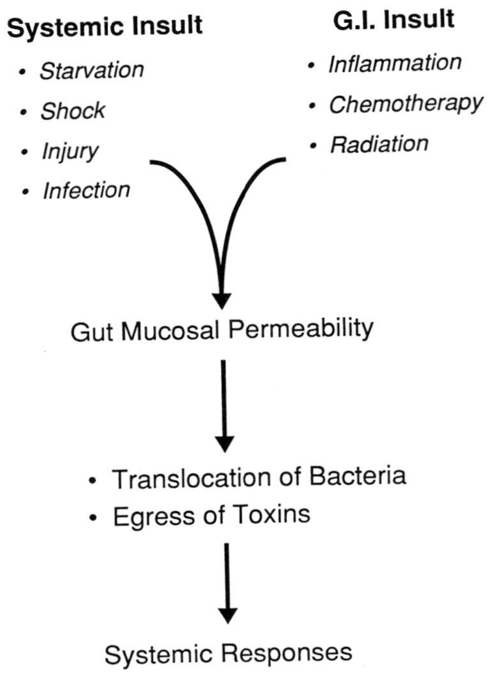

Figure 12-16 According to bacterial translocation theory, a number of different insults can lead to increased gut mucosal permeability. Increased mucosal permeability leads to the translocation of bacteria and endotoxin with a subsequent systemic inflammatory response.

rial translocation can occur under certain circumstances in both experimental animals and humans, there is debate about the degree to which translocation occurs and the clinical significance of the phenomenon in humans.

If bacterial translocation occurs and is an important clinical phenomenon, there are important therapeutic implications of the phenomenon. If the resident flora in the gut could be manipulated to decrease their number or make them less virulent, the consequences of bacterial translocation would be expected to be less severe. This line of reasoning has resulted in the development of several different regimens of gut decontamination.[133,134] These regimens have an attractive theoretical basis but remain unproven with respect to clinical efficacy, in part because of the difficulties inherent in defining sepsis and determining and therapeutic significance of culture results.

Perhaps a more important clinical implication of bacterial translocation theory pertains to enteral versus parenteral feeding. Experimental and scattered clinical experience has suggested that when the gut is unused and no enteral feedings are given, bacterial translocation is more likely to occur. There may be several explanations for this phenomenon. If the enteral route is not used, nutrients are not provided to the luminal surface of the gut mucosa. Glutamine, the predominant amino acid the gut uses for protein and energy metabolism,[129,130,135] may not be provided in sufficient amounts. Glutamine is unstable in solution and as a result is not included in standard total parenteral nutrition formulas. It is not an essential amino acid because it can be generated endogenously, but the amount thus generated may not be enough for adequate gut metabolism and maintenance of the gut mucosal barrier. Because of these considerations, it is good practice to use the enteral route of nutrition whenever possible. This is difficult in many sick ICU patients, but even if all the required nutrition cannot be delivered enterally, there is good rationale for providing as much as possible via the enteral route and supplementing with parenteral nutrition as needed.

The ease with which the gut can be used for nutritional purposes is in general inversely proportional to the severity of illness.[136,137] This can make enteral feedings difficult in the very patients in whom it would seem most important, those with major injury and critical illness. Profound ileus and gut edema accompany critical illness and make it difficult to pass a feeding tube through the pylorus into the duodenum or proximal jejunum. Placement of a feeding tube beyond the stomach is important to decrease the risk of aspiration. Unfortunately, in seriously ill patients feedings through even a distally placed tube are difficult. Feedings given even through jejunal feeding tubes placed surgically will not necessarily be tolerated by critically ill patients. We feel that the use of the enteral route is important in ICU patients whenever possible, but overly persistent attempts to force full enteral nutrition should not be allowed to interfere with the provision of adequate nutrition via the parenteral route if that is necessary. Because of concerns about bacterial translocation, giving a small amount of enteral feedings is rational in patients who will not tolerate provision of their entire nutritional requirements via the enteral route.

ORTHOPEDIC TRAUMA

Pelvic fractures are the most serious life-threatening orthopedic injuries faced in the multiple-trauma patient in the early postinjury period.[138,139] Severe pelvic fractures can easily accommodate a patient's entire blood volume and lead to death by exsanguination. We feel that the most important components of this blood loss are venous and bony bleeding and that the first priority in treatment of these fractures is stabilization. Arterial injuries amenable to treatment by angiographic embolization are rare, and the initial priorities in the management of patients with an unstable pelvic fracture should be orthopedic stabilization, volume repletion, and blood transfusion. Early and vigorous blood transfusion is particularly important in elderly patients, who, even if intravascular volume is maintained with crystalloid or colloid solutions, will not tolerate a severe drop in the hemoglobin concentration and oxygen-carrying capacity.

Stable pelvic fractures can be treated expectantly and with close follow-up of the hematocrit so that transfusion can be carried out as necessary. Unstable pelvic fractures should be stabilized as quickly and as well as possible, hopefully before massive blood loss and coagulopathy occur. Military antishock trousers (MAST) can be used in the hospital and emergency department settings to stabilize an unstable pelvis. In occasional patients MAST will also prove useful in an ICU setting. Stabilization of certain types of fractures can be obtained with external fixation or lower extremity traction, although these forms of fixation are not ideal. The best time to internally fixate an unstable pelvis is in the early postinjury period, and this should be done unless severe associated injuries and gross hemodynamic instability are present. Some of these procedures require considerable orthopedic expertise. Early stabilization of the pelvis helps considerably in minimizing subsequent blood loss and allows for early mobilization, an important factor in preventing pulmonary complications.

The same basic principles which apply to pelvic fractures also pertain to long bone fractures of the lower extremities. These should be fixed in the immediate postinjury period if at all possible. Waiting to fix these injuries in the multiply injured patient until the patient has stabilized is a failed concept unless there is gross hemodynamic or neurologic instability. After waiting for several days to repair orthopedic injuries, it is not uncommon to find that the patient's condition has actually worsened and that fixation on a delayed basis is even more dangerous than immediate fixation would have been. Early fixation obviates the profound pulmonary effects of prolonged immobilization.[7-10]

If immediate orthopedic stabilization is done, the patient with multiple long bone injuries may be in the operating room for extended periods of time in the early postinjury period. Continuous reassessment should be made of the appropriateness of continuing the orthopedic repairs, and in an occasional patient hemodynamic instability, coagulopathy, or respiratory difficulties will dictate early termination of orthopedic repair. Because of these occasional cases, in patients with multiple injuries it is important to stabilize long bone fractures of the lower extremities first and then shift attention to the upper extremities. An alternative is for multiple teams of orthopedists to work simultaneously on fracture fixation. The lower extremities are more important in this setting than the upper extremities because of their size and attendant increased amount of soft tissue injury and also because of the importance of their fixation with respect to early patient mobilization. We feel that fractures of the pelvis are the most important fractures to attempt to stabilize early, followed in order by fractures of the femur, tibia, ankle, humerus, forearm, and the foot and hand.

Another dilemma in early management of multiple trauma patients is the mangled extremity with a combination of bony, soft tissue, neurologic, and vascular injuries.[140,141] Some of these extremities are so badly injured that the decision to amputate immediately is a fairly easy one. This is particularly true in patients with severe associated life-threatening injuries. In other patients the decision-making process about whether to attempt salvage of a mangled extremity is a more difficult one. For lower extremities, we feel that salvage should be attempted unless there is clear evidence of unrepairable nerve injury. This early attempt at salvage should include debridement of nonviable soft tissue, stabilization of bony injuries, and restoration of blood supply. More strenuous attempts should be made to salvage upper extremities because of the functional importance of upper extremities as compared to lower extremities. Lower extremities are also larger, and therefore a marginally viable lower extremity is more likely to cause systemic problems for a patient than is a marginal upper extremity.

If the decision is made to salvage a severely injured extremity, the patient should be followed closely postoperatively for signs of systemic illness such as markedly positive fluid balance or deterioration of pulmonary function. If these signs develop, the extremity should be examined, and if there is evidence of marginal viability, consideration should be given to amputation. Timely and early amputation in such circumstances can be lifesaving and can improve the progress of the patient's other injuries by allowing for better perfusion and wound healing.[140]

As has already been mentioned, early mobilization of all critically ill and injured patients, particularly those with orthopedic injuries, is extremely important. Atelectasis and the development of pneumonia are decreased. Decubitus ulcers do not develop. Deep venous thrombosis and pulmonary embolus are also less likely to occur.

Mobilization is probably the most important aspect of thromboembolic prophylaxis, although other forms of thromboembolic prophylaxis are also useful both in patients who cannot be mobilized and as adjunctive measures in patients who are being mobilized.[142] Pneumatic compression devices for the lower extremities are effective in lowering the incidence of deep venous thrombosis in high-risk patients. They should be used in multiply injured patients whenever possible. Even if an injury limits use of the device to one lower extremity only, a compression device should be placed on the other lower extremity. Compression devices work not only mechanically by squeezing blood through the venous system and thereby avoiding stasis but also by activating systemic fibrinolysis.

Heparin can also be used both for prophylaxis and therapy of thromboembolic complications. Subcutaneous heparin in a dose of 5000 U twice a day is probably effective in some patients, but we feel more vigorous prophylaxis is necessary in high-risk situations. We use intravenous heparin in a dose high enough to increase the partial thromboplastin time to approximately 20 percent above the control value. The heparin is titrated to this level in an attempt to document an effect on antithrombin III, an important mediator in the development of thromboembolic disorders.[142] If a patient develops deep venous thrombosis or pulmonary embolus, the dose of heparin is increased. We often use a dose high enough to increase the partial thromboplastin time to 2 to 2.5 times the control value, but in some patients with clinical evidence of continued deep venous thrombosis or pulmonary embolus, the heparin is further increased as necessary to achieve the desired clinical effect.

When heparin is either contraindicated, such as in severe head injury, or is ineffective, more invasive forms of therapy are necessary. In drastic cases, the vena cava can be ligated by a transabdominal approach. Caval clips can also be placed surgically. Increasingly, caval filters are being placed in such patients. This can usually be done percutaneously under fluoroscopic guidance, has a low rate of complications, and is effective. In instances where patients are at very high risk for the development of thromboembolic complications, caval filters can be placed prophylactically. The long-term morbidity of this prophylactic approach is still under investigation, but initial experience is promising.[143]

NUTRITION

Provision of adequate nutrition after injury is a high priority.[144,145] While it may be desirable in some respects to begin nutrition as early as possible, there are difficulties with this approach. As outlined above, the gut is difficult to use in critically injured patients, and this situation is especially pronounced in the immediate postinjury period. This effectively rules out use of the enteral route in the early phases after injury except in selected patients, those with isolated head injury or burns for example. Parenteral nutrition is also not appropriate in the immediate postinjury period in critically injured multiple-trauma patients because it interjects an unnecessary complicating variable at a time when fluid management is already complex and difficult. Because the response to injury includes an endogenous hyperglycemia, premature institution of parenteral nutrition can complicate fluid balance by further raising the blood glucose and inducing an osmotic diuresis. The early postinjury period is also not the ideal time to ensure that central catheters placed for the administration of parenteral nutrition are put in under sterile conditions. For these reasons, after multiple trauma we wait to begin nutrition until the second or third day after injury when patients are stable hemodynamically and with respect to fluid management.

While precocious attempts at the administration of nutrition are ill-advised, so to is waiting too long to give a patient nutritional support. Aggressive nutritional support should be given to multiple-trauma patients in the ICU if there is any doubt about the rapidity with which they will recover and be able to feed themselves adequately. This includes patients with head injury in which the outlook for improvement in mental status is at all questionable. It also includes patients with serious multiple injuries in whom the development of organ failure is a possibility. In such patients, early provision of adequate nutrition is prophylactic as well as therapeutic. Major injury induces a catabolic state. Nutritional support in such situations will not usually convert the patient to an anabolic state but does minimize the degree of catabolism. If a severe catabolic state is allowed to persist, the effects on the immune system, pulmonary function, and wound healing are disastrous.

A variety of formulas can be used initially to calculate a patient's nutritional requirements after multiple trauma.[146–148] While formulas are reasonable guidelines for the initial administration of nutrition, the patient's nutritional state should be followed on a regular basis to determine if the nutritional repletion being given is adequate. This should take the form of a nitrogen balance study to determine if the patient is in positive or negative nitrogen balance. More sophisticated measures such as calorimetry sometimes provide valuable further information about a patient's nutritional state, particularly with respect to carbohydrate and fat metabolism. The respiratory quotient can be calculated and the mix of protein, fat, and carbohydrate nutrients appropriately adjusted. This is sometimes useful in patients who are difficult to wean from the ventilator because of carbon dioxide retention. The respiratory quotient determination can help to determine if the amount of carbohydrate being provided should be reduced.

MENTAL STATUS CHANGES

There are a large number of reasons for mental status changes in ICU patients with multiple injury, and more than one of them is operative in many patients. Some of the most obvious sources for mental status changes are the sequelae of head injury, both primary and secondary. Withdrawal from alcohol and drugs is another common cause of mental status changes. Electrolyte disturbances are also a possibility. Although electrolyte disturbances are uncommon, they are relatively easy to correct and should always be included in the differential diagnosis of such patients. Another potentially correctable source of mental status changes is the overly enthusiastic administration of narcotic and sedative drugs. These should be given in amounts necessary to alleviate pain and anxiety, but care should be taken not to overadminister them and cloud a patient's sensorium unnecessarily.

Another source of mental status changes in patients in the ICU for long periods of time has been termed *ICU psychosis* and seems to be related to a sense of disorientation caused by unfamiliar surroundings, pain, anxiety, and the administration of narcotic and sedative drugs. Particularly common in the elderly, treatment is to minimize drug administration, try to bring in friends and relatives or familiar objects to reorient the patient, and wait.

A final cause of mental status changes in the critically ill and injured is related to sepsis. Why the clinical syndrome of sepsis should include mental status changes is unclear, but it is a remarkably common observation that mental status changes occur in septic patients and that one of the hallmarks of improvement is an improvement in mental status. Early investigations in animals suggest that the cause of these changes is not related to cerebral edema or metabolic changes in the brain; the exact causative factors are still unknown. Treatment for the mental status changes related to sepsis is supportive, and efforts are directed toward treating the source of the sepsis.

REFERENCES

1. Smith JS, Martin LF, Young WW, et al.: Do trauma centers improve outcome over non-trauma centers: The evaluation of regional trauma care using discharge abstract data and patient management categories. *J Trauma* 30:1533, 1990.
2. Trunkey DD: Trauma. *Sci Am* 249:20, 1983.
3. West JG, Williams MJ, Trunkey DD, et al.: Trauma systems: Current status—Future challenges. *JAMA* 259:3597, 1988.
4. Gurdjian ES, Gurdjian ES: Acute head injuries. *Surg Gynecol Obstet* 146:805, 1978.
5. Gutman MB, Moulton RJ, Sullivan I, et al.: Relative incidence of intracranial mass lesions and severe torso injury after accidental injury: Implications for triage and management. *J Trauma* 31:974, 1991.
6. Latenser BA, Gentilello LM, Tarver AA, et al.: Improved outcome with early fixation of skeletally unstable pelvic fractures. *J Trauma* 31:28, 1991.
7. Seibel R, LaDuca J, Hassett JM, et al.: Blunt multiple trauma (ISS 36), femur traction, and the pulmonary failure-septic state. *Ann Surg* 202:283, 1985.
8. Bone LB, Johnson KD, Weigelt J, et al.: Early versus delayed stabilization of femoral fractures. *J Bone Joint Surg* 71-A:336, 1989.
9. Johnson KD, Cadambi A, Seibert GB.: Incidence of adult respiratory distress syndrome in patients with multiple musculoskeletal injuries: Effect of early operative stabilization of fractures. *J Trauma* 25:375, 1985.
10. Goris RJA, Gimbrere JSF, VanNiekerk JLM, et al.: Early osteosynthesis and prophylactic mechanical ventilation in the multitrauma patient. *J Trauma* 22:895, 1982.
11. Heffner AE, Sahn SA: Controlled hyperventilation in patients with intracranial hypertension. *Arch Intern Med* 143:765, 1983.
12. Cold GE, Jensen FT, Malmros R: The effects of PA_{CO_2} reduction on regional cerebral bloodflow in the acute phase of brain injury. *Acta Anaesthesiol Scand* 21:359, 1977.
13. Luce JM: The cardiovascular effects of mechanical ventilation and positive end-expiratory pressure. *JAMA* 252:807, 1984.
14. Shelhamer JH, Natanson C, Parrillo JE: Positive end expiratory pressure in adults. *JAMA* 251:2692, 1984.
15. Pick RA, Handler JB, Murata GH, et al.: The cardiovascular effects of positive end-expiratory pressure. *Chest* 82:345, 1982.
16. Holcroft JW, Blaisdell FW: Trauma to the torso. In: Wilmore DW, Brennan MF, Harken AH, et al. (eds): American College of Surgeons *Care of the Surgical Patient, vol 1*. New York, Scientific American, 1988, pp IV;1:1.
17. Price DJE, Murray A: The influence of hypoxia and hypotension on recovery from head injury. *Injury* 3:218, 1972.
18. Buchman TG, Menker J, Lipsett PA: Strategies for trauma resuscitation. *Surg Gynecol Obstet* 172:8, 1991.
19. Levison M, Trunkey DD: Initial assessment and resuscitation. *Surg Clin North Am* 62:9, 1982.
20. Shenkin HA, Cheney RH, Govons SR, et al.: The diagnosis of hemorrhage in man. *Am J Med Sci* 208:421, 1944.
21. Little RA, Jones RO, Eltraifi AE: Cardiovascular reflex function after injury. *Prog Clin Biol Res* 264:191, 1988.
22. Sturm JA, Wisner DH: Fluid resuscitation of hypovolemia. *Intensive Care Med* 11:227, 1985.
23. Demling RH: The pathogenesis of respiratory failure after trauma and sepsis. *Surg Clin North Am* 60:1373, 1980.
24. Wisner DH, Busche F, Sturm J, et al.: Traumatic shock and head injury: Effects of fluid resuscitation on the brain. *J Surg Res* 46:49, 1989.
25. Jupa-Marcinkowski V: Osmotic and oncotic therapy in neurosurgical practice. In: deVlieger M, deLange SA, Beks JW (eds): *Brain Edema Vliegar*. New York, Wiley, 1981, pp 155–164.
26. Albright AL, Latchaw RE, Robinson AG: Intracranial and systemic effects of osmotic and oncotic therapy in experimental cerebral edema. *J Neurosurg* 60:481, 1984.
27. Sturm JA, Carpenter MA, Lewis FR, et al.: Water and protein movement in the sheep lung after septic shock: Effect of colloid versus crystalloid resuscitation. *J Surg Res* 26:233, 1979.
28. Holcroft JW, Trunkey DD: Extravascular lung water following hemorrhagic shock in the baboon: Comparison between resuscitation with Ringer's lactate and plasmanate. *Ann Surg* 180:408, 1974.
29. Dahn MS, Lucas CE, Ledgerwood AM, et al.: Negative inotropic effect of albumin resuscitation for shock. *Surgery* 86:235, 1979.
30. Lucas CE, Weaver D, Higgins RF, et al.: Effects of albumin versus non-albumin resuscitation on plasma volume and renal excretory function. *J Trauma* 18:564, 1978.

31. Lucas CE, Bouwman DL, Ledgerwood AM, et al.: Differential serum protein changes following supplemental albumin resuscitation for hypovolemic shock. *J Trauma* 20:47, 1980.
32. Wisner DH, Schuster L, Quinn C: Hypertonic saline resuscitation of head injury: Effects on cerebral water content. *J Trauma* 30:75, 1990.
33. DeFelippe J, Timoner J, Velasco IT, et al.: Treatment of refractory hypovolemic shock by 7.5% sodium chloride injections. *Lancet* 2:1002, 1980.
34. Traverso LW, Bellamy RF, Hollenbach SJ, et al.: Hypertonic sodium chloride solutions: Effect on hemodynamics and survival after hemorrhage in swine. *J Trauma* 27:32, 1987.
35. Maningas PA, Mattox KL, Pepe PE, et al.: Hypertonic saline-dextran solutions for the prehospital management of traumatic hypotension. *Am J Surg* 157:528, 1989.
36. Shackford ST, Fortlage DA, Peters RM, et al.: Serum osmolar and electrolyte changes associated with large infusions of hypertonic sodium lactate for intravascular volume expansion of patients undergoing aortic reconstruction. *Surg Gynecol Obstet* 164:127, 1987.
37. Lopes OU, Pontieri V, Rocha e Silva M, et al.: Hyperosmotic NaCl and severe hemorrhagic shock: Role of the innervated lung. *Am J Physiol* 241:H883, 1981.
38. Halvorsen L, Blaisdell FW, Holcroft JW: Recent advances in prehospital fluid resuscitation: Hypertonic saline. In Cleveland H (ed): *Advances in Trauma, vol. 5*. Chicago, Mosby 1991, pp 1–18.
39. Mazzoni MC, Borgstrom P, Arfors KE, et al.: Dynamic fluid redistribution in hypertonic resuscitation of hypovolemic hemorrhage. *Am J Physiol* 255:H629, 1988.
40. Templeton GH, Mitchell JH, Wildenthal K: Influence of hyperosmolarity on left ventricular stiffness. *Am J Physiol* 222:1406, 1972.
41. Wildenthal K, Mierzwlak DS, Mitchell JH: Acute effects of increased serum osmolarity on left ventricular performance. *Am J Physiol* 216:898, 1969.
42. Vassar MJ, Perry CA, Holcroft JW: Analysis of potential risks associated with 7.5% sodium chloride resuscitation of traumatic shock. *Arch Surg* 125:1309, 1990.
43. Takagi H, Saitoh T, Kitahara T, et al.: The mechanism of ICP reducing effect of mannitol. In: Ishii S, Nagai H, Brock M (eds): *Intracranial Pressure V*. Berlin-Heidelberg, Springer-Verlag, 1983, pp 729.
44. Mahoney BD, Ruiz E: Acute resuscitation of the patient with head and spinal cord injuries. *Emerg Med Clin North Am* 1:583, 1983.
45. Battistella FD, Wisner DH: Combined hemorrhagic shock and head injury: Effects of hypertonic saline (7.5%) resuscitation. *J Trauma* 31:182, 1991.
46. Walsh JC, Zhuang J, Shackford SR: A comparison of hypertonic to isotonic fluid in the resuscitation of brain injury and hemorrhagic shock. *J Surg Res* 50:284, 1991.
47. Gunnar W, Jonasson O, Merlotti G, et al.: Head injury and hemorrhagic shock: Studies of the blood brain barrier and intracranial pressure after resuscitation with normal saline solution, 3% saline solution, and dextran-40. *Surgery* 103:398, 1988.
48. Wisner DH, Battistella FD, Freshman SP, et al.: Nuclear magnetic resonance as a measure of cerebral metabolism: Effects of hypertonic saline resuscitation. *J Trauma* 32(3):351, 1992.
49. Kramer GC, Perron PR, Lindsey DC, et al.: Small-volume resuscitation with hypertonic saline dextran solution. *Surgery* 100:239, 1986.
50. Smith GJ, Kramer GC, Perron P, et al.: A comparison of several hypertonic solutions for resuscitation of bled sheep. *J Surg Res* 39:517, 1985.
51. Hands R, Holcroft JW, Perron PR, et al.: Comparison of peripheral and central infusions of 7.5% NaCl/6% dextran 70. *Surgery* 103:684, 1988.
52. Zornow MH, Scheller MS, Shackford SR: Effect of a hypertonic lactated Ringer's solution on intracranial pressure and cerebral water content in a model of traumatic brain injury. *J Trauma* 29:484, 1989.
53. Mattox KL, Maningas PA, Moore EE, et al.: Prehospital hypertonic saline/dextran infusion for post-traumatic hypotension. *Ann Surg* 213:482, 1991.
54. Risk C, Rudo N, Falltrick R, et al.: Comparison of right atrial and pulmonary capillary wedge pressures. *Crit Care Med* 6:172, 1978.
55. Rice CL, Hobelman CF, John DA, et al.: Central venous pressure or pulmonary capillary wedge pressure as the determinant of fluid replacement in aortic surgery. *Surgery* 84:437, 1978.
56. O'Quin R, Marin JJ: Pulmonary artery occlusion pressure: Clinical physiology, measurement, and interpretation. *Am Rev Respir Dis* 128:319, 1983.
57. Wisner DH, Holcroft JW: Surgical critical care. In: Wells SA, Austen WG, Fonkalsrud EW, et al. (eds): *Current Problems in Surgery*. St. Louis, Mosby, 1990, pp 471–569.
58. Wilson RF, Christensen C, LeBlanc LP: Oxygen consumption in critically-ill surgical patients. *Ann Surg* 176:801, 1972.
59. Cain SM: Peripheral oxygen uptake and delivery in health and disease. *Clin Chest Med* 4:139, 1983.
60. Gutierrez G, Pohil RJ: Oxygen consumption is linearly related to O_2 supply in critically ill patients. *J Crit Care* 1:45, 1986.
61. Michel L, Marsh M, McMichan JC, et al.: Infection of pulmonary artery catheters in critically ill patients. *JAMA* 245:1032, 1981.
62. Applefeld JJ, Caruthers TE, Reno DJ, et al.: Assessment of the sterility of long-term cardiac catheteriza-

tion using the thermodilution Swan-Ganz catheter. *Chest* 74:377, 1978.
63. West JB (ed.): Blood flow. In: *Respiratory Physiology—the Essentials.* Baltimore, Williams & Wilkins, chap 4, 1974, pp 42–45.
64. Dahn MS: Visceral organ resuscitation. In: Cerra FB, Chernow B, Fuhrman BP, et al. (eds): *Perspectives in Critical Care, vol 4.* St. Louis, Quality Publishing, 1991, pp 1–41.
65. Rackow EC, Astiz ME, Weil MH: Cellular oxygen metabolism during sepsis and shock. *JAMA* 259:1989, 1988.
66. Rasanen J, Cane RD: Continuous oximetry: Is it beneficial? In: Cerra FB, Chernow B, Fuhrman BP, et al. (eds): *Perspectives in Critical Care, vol 4.* St. Louis, Quality Publishing, 1991, pp 133–151.
67. Harkema JM, Dean RE, Stephan RN, et al.: Cellular dysfunction in sepsis. *J Crit Care* 5:62, 1990.
68. Winslow EJ, Loeb HS, Rahimtoola SH, et al.: Hemodynamic studies and results in therapy in 50 patients with bacteremic shock. *Am J Med* 54:421, 1973.
69. Parker MM, Parrillo JE: Myocardial function in septic shock. *J Crit Care* 5:47, 1990.
70. Parker MM, Parillo JE: Septic shock: Hemodynamics and pathogenesis. *JAMA* 250:3324, 1983.
71. Kelleher JE: Pulse oximetry. *J Clin Monit* 5:37, 1989.
72. Alexander CM, Teller LE, Gross JB: Principles of pulse oximetry: Theoretical and practical considerations. *Anesth Analg* 68:368, 1989.
73. Carlon GC, Ray C, Miodownik S, et al.: Capnography in mechanically ventilated patients. *Crit Care Med* 16:550, 1988.
74. Wiedemann HP, McCarthy K: Noninvasive monitoring of oxygen and carbon dioxide. *Clin Chest Med* 10:239, 1989.
75. Abrams JH, Cerra F, Holcroft JW: Cardiopulmonary monitoring. In: Wilmore DW, Brennan MF, Harken AH, et al. (eds): American College of Surgeons *Care of the Surgical Patient, vol 1.* New York, Scientific American, 1988, pp II;1:1.
76. Dupuis YG: *Ventilators: Theory and Clinical Application,* 2d ed. St. Louis, Mosby 1986.
77. Bergmen NA, Tien YK: Contribution to the closure of pulmonary units to impaired oxygenation during anesthesia. *Anesthesiology* 59:395, 1983.
78. Bartlett RH: Use of the mechanical ventilator. In: Wilmore DW, Brennan MF, Harken AH, et al. (eds): American College of Surgeons *Care of the Surgical Patient, vol. 1.* New York, Scientific American, 1988, pp II;5:1.
79. Peterson GW, Baier H: Incidence of pulmonary barotrauma in a medical ICU. *Crit Care Med* 11:67, 1983.
80. Murphy DF, Dobb GD: Effect of pressure support of spontaneous breathing during intermittent mandatory ventilation. *Crit Care Med* 15:612, 1987.
81. Prarkash O, Meij S: Cardiopulmonary response to inspiratory pressure support during spontaneous ventilation vs conventional ventilation. *Chest* 88:403, 1985.
82. MacIntyre NR: New forms of mechanical ventilation in the adult. *Clin Chest Med* 9:47, 1988.
83. Fiastro JF, Habib MP, Quan SF: Pressure support compensation for inspiratory work due to endotracheal tubes and demand continuous positive airway pressure. *Chest* 93:499, 1988.
84. Viale JP, Annat GJ, Bouffard YM, et al.: Oxygen cost of breathing in postoperative patients. *Chest* 93:507, 1988.
85. Brochard L, Harf A, Lorino H, et al.: Inspiratory pressure support prevents diaphragmatic fatigue during weaning from mechanical ventilation. *Am Rev Respir Dis* 139:513, 1989.
86. Gibney RTN, Wilson RS, Pontoppidan H: Comparison of work breathing on high gas flow and demand valve continuous positive airway pressure systems. *Chest* 82:692, 1982.
87. Cox D, Tinloi SF, Farrimond JG: Investigation of the spontaneous modes of breathing of different ventilators. *Intensive Care Med* 14:532, 1988.
88. Saito S, Tokioka H, Kosaka F: Efficacy of flow-by during continuous positive airway pressure ventilation. *Crit Care Med* 18:654, 1990.
89. Sassoon CSH, Giron AE, Ely EA, et al.: Inspiratory work of breathing on flow-by and demand-flow continuous positive airway pressure. *Crit Care Med* 17:1108, 1989.
90. Pemberton LB: Tracheostomy and two alternative airways. *Contemp Surg* 23:27, 1983.
91. Colice GL: Prolonged intubation versus tracheostomy in the adult. *J Intensive Care Med* 2:85, 1987.
92. Berlauk JF: Prolonged endotracheal intubation vs. tracheostomy. *Crit Care Med* 14:742, 1986.
93. Tharratt RS, Allen RP, Albertson TE: Pressure controlled inverse ratio ventilation in severe adult respiratory failure. *Chest* 94:755, 1988.
94. Lain DC, DiBenedetto R, Morris SL, et al.: Pressure control inverse ratio ventilation as a method to reduce peak inspiratory pressure and provide adequate ventilation and oxygenation. *Chest* 95:1081, 1989.
95. Gurevitch MJ, Van Dyke J, Young ES, et al.: Improved oxygenation and lower peak airway pressure in severe adult respiratory distress syndrome. *Chest* 89:211, 1986.
96. Berman LS, Downs JB, Van Eeden A, et al.: Inspiration:expiration ratio. *Crit Care Med* 9:775, 1981.
97. Papadakos PJ, Halloran W, Hessney JI, et al.: The use of pressure-controlled inverse ratio ventilation in the surgical intensive care unit. *J Trauma* 31:1211, 1991.
98. Roberge RJ: Facilitating cervical spine radiography in blunt trauma. *Emerg Med Clin North Am* 9:733, 1991.

99. Kreipke DL, Gillespie KR, McCarthy Mc, et al.: Reliability of indications for cervical spine films in trauma patients. *J Trauma* 29:1438, 1989.
100. Indeck M, Peterson S, Smith J, et al.: Risk, cost, and benefit of transporting ICU patients for special studies. *J Trauma* 28:1020, 1988.
101. Rockwell WB, Ehrlich HP: Ibuprofen in acute-care therapy. *Ann Surg* 211:78, 1990.
102. *The Medical Letter*, Vol 32, in Abramowicz M, Rizack MA (eds). New Rochelle, The Medical Letter, Inc, 1990.
103. Staren ED, Cullen ML: Epidural catheter analgesia for the management of postoperative pain. *Surg Gynecol Obstet* 162:389, 1986.
104. Wisner DH: A stepwise logistic regression analysis of factors affecting morbidity and mortality after thoracic trauma: Effect of epidural analgesia. *J Trauma* 30:799, 1990.
105. Kehlet H: Postoperative pain. In: Wilmore DW, Brennan MF, Harken AH, et al. (eds): American College of Surgeons *Care of the Surgical Patient, vol 1.* New York, Scientific American, 1988, pp II;12:1.
106. Wisner DH, Reed WH, Riddick RS: Suspected myocardial contusion. *Ann Surg* 212:82, 1990.
107. Fabian TC, Cicala RS, Croce MA, et al.: A prospective evaluation of myocardial contusion: Correlation of significant arrhythmias and cardiac output with CPK-MB measurements. *J Trauma* 21:653, 1991.
108. Beresky R, Klingler R, Peake J: Myocardial contusion: When does it have clinical significance? *J Trauma* 28:64, 1988.
109. Merrill WH, Lee RB, Hammon JW, et al.: Surgical treatment of acute traumatic tear of the thoracic aorta. *Ann Surg* 207:699, 1988.
110. Gundry SR, Burney RE, Mackenzie JR, et al.: Assessment of mediastinal widening associated with traumatic rupture of the aorta. *J Trauma* 23:293, 1983.
111. Richardson JD, Wilson ME, Miller FB: The widened mediastinum. *Ann Surg* 211:731, 1990.
112. Cox EF: Blunt abdominal trauma. *Ann Surg* 199:467, 1984.
113. Wisner DH, Blaisdell FW: When to save the ruptured spleen. *Surgery*. In press.
114. Pachter HL, Spencer FC, Hofstetter SR, et al.: Experience with selective operative and nonoperative treatment of splenic injuries in 193 patients. *Ann Surg* 211:583, 1990.
115. Luna GK, Dellinger EP: Nonoperative observation therapy for splenic injuries: A safe therapeutic option. *Am J Surg* 153:462, 1987.
116. Cogbill TH, Moore EE, Jurkovich GJ, et al.: Nonoperative management of blunt splenic trauma: A multicenter experience. *J Trauma* 29:1312, 1989.
117. Feliciano DV, Burch JM, Spjut-Patrinely V, et al.: Abdominal gunshot wounds. *Ann Surg* 208:362, 1988.
118. Blaisdell FW: General assessment, resuscitation and exploration of penetrating and blunt abdominal trauma. In: Blaisdell FW, Trunkey DD (eds): *Trauma Management, vol. 1.* New York, Thieme-Stratton, 1982, chap 1, pp 1–18.
119. Wisner DH, Wold RL, Frey CF: Diagnosis and treatment of pancreatic injuries. *Arch Surg* 125:1109, 1990.
120. Wisner DH, Chun Y, Blaisdell FW: Blunt intestinal injury. *Arch Surg* 125:1319, 1990.
121. Dauterive AH, Flancbaum L, Cox EF: Blunt intestinal trauma. *Ann Surg* 201:198, 1985.
122. Stone HH, Fabian TC, Satiani B, et al.: Experiences in the management of pancreatic trauma. *J Trauma* 21:257, 1981.
123. Moretz JA, Campbell DP, Parker DE, et al.: Significance of serum amylase level in evaluating pancreatic trauma. *Am J Surg* 130:739, 1975.
124. Pine RW, Wertz MJ, Lennard S, et al.: Determinants of organ malfunction or death in patients with intra-abdominal sepsis. *Arch Surg* 118:242, 1983.
125. Saini S, Kellum JM, O'Leary MP, et al.: Improved localization and survival in patients with intraabdominal abscesses. *Am J Surg* 145:136, 1983.
126. Gerzof SG, Johnson WC, Robbins AH, et al.: Expanded criteria for percutaneous abscess drainage. *Arch Surg* 120:227, 1985.
127. Haaga JR, Weinstein AJ: CT-guided percutaneous aspiration and drainage of abscesses. *AJR* 135:1187, 1980.
128. Peitzman AB, Udekwu AO, Ochoa J, et al.: Bacterial translocation in trauma patients. *J Trauma* 31:1083, 1991.
129. Edmiston CE, Condon RE: Bacterial translocation. *Surg Gynecol Obstet* 173:73, 1991.
130. Wilmore DW, Smith RJ, O'Dwyer ST, et al.: The gut: A central organ after surgical stress. *Surgery* 104:917, 1988.
131. Deitch EA, Winterton J, Berg R: The gut as a portal of entry for bacteremia. *Ann Surg* 205:681, 1987.
132. Michie HR, Manogue KR, Spriggs DR, et al.: Detection of circulating tumor necrosis factor after endotoxin administration. *N Engl J Med* 318:1481, 1988.
133. Stoutenbeek CP, van Saene HKF, Zandstra DF: The effect of selective decontamination of the digestive tract on colonization and infection rate in multiple trauma patients. *Intensive Care Med* 10:185, 1984.
134. Ledingham IM, Eastaway AT, McKay IC, et al.: *Lancet* 1:785, 1988.
135. Alverdy JC, Aoys E, Moss GS: Total parenteral nutrition promotes bacterial translocation from the gut. *Surgery* 104:185, 1988.
136. Hayashi JT, Wolfe BM, Calvert CC: Limited efficacy of early postoperative jejunal feeding. *Am J Surg* 150:52, 1985.

137. McDonald WS, Sharp CW, Deitch EA: Immediate enteral feeding in burn patients is safe and effective. *Ann Surg* 213:177:1991.
138. Cryer HM, Miller FB, Evers BM, et al.: Pelvic fracture classification: Correlation with hemorrhage. *J Trauma* 28:973, 1988.
139. Flint L, Babikian G, Anders M, et al.: Definitive control of mortality from severe pelvic fracture. *Ann Surg* 211:703, 1990.
140. Roessler MS, Wisner DH, Holcroft JW: The mangled extremity: When to amputate? *Arch Surg* 126:1243, 1991.
141. Johansen K, Daines M, Howey T, et al.: Objective criteria accurately predict amputation following lower extremity trauma. *J Trauma* 30:568, 1990.
142. Blaisdell FW: Acquired and congenital clotting syndromes. *World J Surg* 14:664, 1990.
143. Addonizio VP: Thrombotic problems. In: Wilmore DW, Brennan MF, Harken AH, et al. (eds): American College of Surgeons *Care of the Surgical Patient, vol 2.* New York, Scientific American, 1988, p VII;8:1.
144. Fink JA, Jones BT: The Greenfield filter as the primary means of therapy in venous thromboembolic disease. *Surg Gynecol Obstet* 172:253, 1991.
145. Cerra FB: Hypermetabolism, organ failure, and metabolic support. *Surgery* 101:1, 1987.
146. Rombeau JL, Rolandelli RH, Wilmore DW: Nutritional support. In: Wilmore DW, Brennan MF, Harken AH, et al. (eds): American College of Surgeons *Care of the Surgical Patient, vol 1.* New York, Scientific American, 1988, pp II;10:1.
147. Shizgal HM: Body composition and nutritional support. *Surg Clin North Am* 61:729, 1981.
148. Apelgran K, Wilmore D: Nutritional care of the critically ill patient. *Surg Clin North Am* 63:497, 1983.

CHAPTER 13

The Intensive Care Management of Patients with Subarachnoid Hemorrhage

Neil Martin
Rohit Khanna
Gerald Rodts

INTRODUCTION

Intensive care plays a more important role in the management of subarachnoid hemorrhage (SAH) than in any other neurosurgical disorder. In no other disease is a patient, admitted to the hospital in good condition, who undergoes a technically adequate (or even perfect) surgical procedure, more likely to experience a poor outcome from potentially preventable or treatable delayed complications. In this disorder, excellence in neurologic diagnosis and in operative neurosurgery must be accompanied by excellence in intensive care.

It is not surprising that patients who are stuporous or comatose after SAH generally have a bad outcome, as it can be presumed that in such cases the initial hemorrhage has caused permanent brain damage. However, a surprisingly high number of patients who are admitted to the hospital alert or only slightly drowsy, who apparently have not been profoundly damaged by the initial hemorrhage, die or are left with severe neurologic damage. A review of the overall management results of the International Cooperative Study on the Timing of Aneurysm Surgery underlines the frequency with which delayed complications cause poor outcome (Table 13-1).[26] Even patients admitted in good condition (alert) are able to return to a normal way of life in only 75 percent of cases. When all patients are considered, less than 60 percent have a good recovery. It is clear that even in very recent neurosurgical experience the delayed complications of SAH continue to exact a high toll in terms of morbidity and mortality.

In recent years we have seen the addition of a number of techniques that promise to improve outcome in SAH, including the use of transcranial Doppler ultrasonography for the early detection of vasospasm, the treatment of vasospasm with balloon dilatation angioplasty and intraarterial infusions of vasodilator drugs, and endovascular oc-

Table 13-1 Aneurysmal Subarachnoid Hemorrhage: Causes of Death and Disability

Cause	Death, %	Disability, %	Total, %
Direct effect of bleed	7.0	3.6	10.6
Vasospasm	7.2	6.3	13.5
Rebleeding	6.7	0.8	7.5
Hydrocephalus	0.3	1.4	1.7
Other medical complications	1.3	1.0	2.3
Complications of surgery	1.7	2.3	4.0
Complications of medical therapy	0.7	0.1	0.8

Source: Adapted from Kassell N, et al.[26]

clusion of aneurysms in patients not amenable to surgery. While some of these techniques have yet to be proven efficacious, they are destined to be incorporated in the contemporary management of aneurysmal SAH patients. The primary focus of this chapter will be on the important neurologic complications that are often the cause of a poor outcome after SAH: vasospasm, rebleeding, hydrocephalus, and seizures. The medical complications of SAH will be covered as well. Standard techniques, including the newest developments, for diagnosis, monitoring, and management of each of these disorders will be discussed.

SUBARACHNOID HEMORRHAGE MANAGEMENT PROTOCOL

The management of SAH requires the integration of clinical diagnosis and management in the emergency room, urgent neuroimaging evaluation, special operative and anesthetic considerations, as well as conventional intensive care unit (ICU)–based critical care. The intelligent approach to intensive care, therefore, requires an appreciation of the overall management protocol. Table 13-2 provides an overview of the management of SAH patients at the University of California, Los Angeles (UCLA) Medical Center.

The key initial steps in the emergency room are to consider, and then establish, the diagnosis of SAH while stabilizing the vital signs. The hallmark of SAH is headache, and characteristically the headache is sudden, unusual, and often unilateral and associated with neck pain or stiffness. Alternatively, the SAH patient may present with obtundation or coma, with or without focal neurologic deficit. SAH must be suspected in such cases, and computed tomography (CT) is the necessary next step (Fig. 13-1). CT is diagnostic of SAH in approximately 90 percent of cases and can detect important immediate complications such as intracerebral hemorrhage (ICH), intraventricular hemorrhage, and hydrocephalus. Lumbar punc-

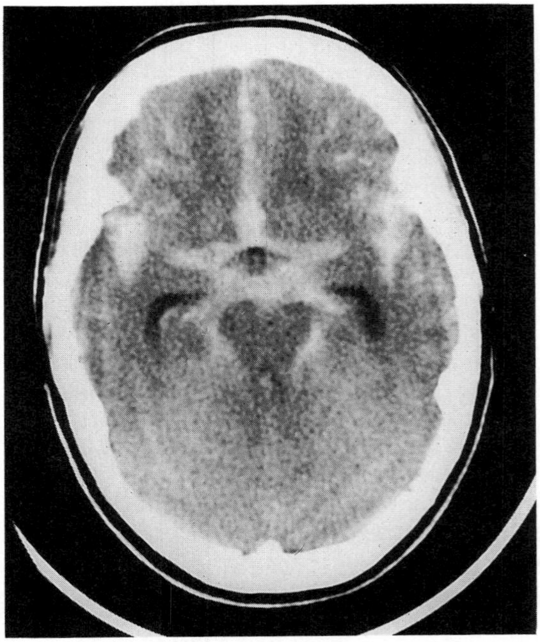

Figure 13-1 This cranial CT scan (done without contrast infusion) demonstrates the typical appearance of a severe SAH. Notice the thick layer of clot found in the suprasellar cisterns, the sylvian cisterns bilaterally, and the anterior interhemispheric fissure.

Table 13-2 Comprehensive Management of Subarachnoid Hemorrhage

A. Emergency room
   1. Control of hypertension
   2. Intubation (if comatose)
   3. Emergency CT scan
   4. Lumbar puncture (if CT negative)
   5. Ventriculostomy (for symptomatic acute hydrocephalus)

B. Angiography
   1. Done as soon as possible after admission
   2. Careful clinical monitoring
   3. Four-vessel study

C. Surgery
   1. Performed within 24 h of admission in most cases
   2. Surgery delayed (for 10–12 days) if more than 3 days since hemorrhage and significant vasospasm is present

D. ICU
   1. Nimodipine
   2. Anticonvulsants
   3. Volume expansion (with colloid)
   4. Clinical monitoring
   5. Physiologic monitoring
      a. Blood pressure
      b. Pulmonary artery pressure or central venous pressure
      c. ICP (if ventriculostomy in place)
      d. Transcranial Doppler
      e. Cerebral blood flow
   6. Hypervolemia, hemodilution, hypertension for vasospasm
   7. Transluminal angioplasty for medically refractory vasospasm

ture is a necessary diagnostic step only when the index of suspicion is high but the CT scan is negative.

Management in the emergency room also includes stabilization of vital signs and the initiation of treatment for systemic arterial hypertension, which often is present after SAH. The blood pressure should be controlled in order to minimize the risk of early rebleeding. We prefer to use a rapidly reversible intravenous agent such as sodium nitroprusside. The goal is to avoid severe systolic hypertension and to stabilize systolic blood pressure below 150 mmHg. Hypotension is avoided in order not to reduce cerebral blood flow (CBF) to a dangerous level. Because of the risk of seizure-induced arterial hypertension, all patients are given anticonvulsants.

The comatose patient is treated with intubation and mild hyperventilation in order to ensure airway protection and adequate oxygenation during the initial diagnostic and therapeutic maneuvers, as well as to mitigate the effects of elevated intracranial pressure (ICP). Only patients demonstrating signs of brainstem compression (pupillary abnormalities) are given mannitol. A ventricular catheter is inserted in comatose patients in order to monitor ICP and to drain cerebrospinal fluid if necessary.[17]

After the patient has been stabilized in the emergency room and a diagnosis of SAH has been established, a cerebral angiogram is performed in most cases with no delay. Carotid and vertebral angiography is performed to identify the site of hemorrhage and to evaluate for multiple aneurysms. It is important that the patient be carefully monitored during angiography, with particular attention paid to arterial blood pressure, ICP (if a ventriculostomy is in place), and neurologic condition.

After completion of the angiogram, surgery is carried out within 24 h. The anesthetic management during surgery emphasizes maintenance of normal arterial blood pressure with avoidance of pronounced hypotension or hypertension, mild hyperventilation in conjunction with mannitol infusion, and ventricular drainage to provide brain relaxation. A pulmonary artery (PA) catheter is routinely inserted for hemodynamic monitoring. Barbiturate cerebral protection may be employed during aneurysm dissection, being used to protect the brain should temporary arterial occlusion be required. Deep hypotension, once used to reduce the risk of aneurysm rupture during dissection, has been abandoned in favor of temporary arterial occlusion in order to avoid exposing the already compromised brain to global ischemia. After clipping the aneurysm, the surgical results are generally confirmed using intraoperative angiography. During recovery from anesthesia, the patient's blood pressure is maintained at a normal or slightly hypertensive level to ensure adequate cerebral perfusion.

In patients showing signs of brainstem compression whose initial cranial CT scan demonstrates an ICH with mass effect in addition to SAH, angiography should be deferred and the patient taken to the operating room for immediate decompressive surgery.[6] In many of these cases the topography of the ICH suggests the location of an underlying aneurysm, and exploration of the appropriate vessels may be carried out after decompression of the hematoma. Alternatively, intraoperative angiography can be performed immediately after removing the hematoma in order to localize the aneurysm.

Postoperative management in the ICU includes the administration of nimodipine (60 mg by mouth or nasogastric tube every 4 h) and colloid infusion (5% albumin, 250 mL every 6 to 12 h) as prophylaxis for delayed cerebral ishcemia. The administration of fluid is titrated to maintain optimal central venous or pulmonary artery pressure. Ventricular drainage is continued as needed to maintain ICP at less than 15 mmHg and to promote clearance of blood breakdown products.

Monitoring in the ICU is centered on frequent clinical neurologic examinations, ICP monitoring, and evaluation for vasospasm using transcranial Doppler and CBF studies. At the first sign of neurologic deficit or of impairment of CBF due to vasospasm, hypervolemic-hemodilution-hypertensive (triple-H) therapy is initiated; a PA catheter should be placed if not already present. If this fails to reverse the neurologic deficit or the decline in CBF, follow-up angiography is performed. If severe arterial vasospasm is present, balloon dilatation angioplasty is considered. Monitoring in the ICU is continued until ventricular drainage is no longer necessary and until the neurologic condition, transcranial Doppler results, and CBF values have stabilized.

The patient remains in the hospital until posthemorrhage day 8 to 10. The patient can be discharged at this point if medically and neurologically stable and if transcranial Doppler studies have not demonstrated evidence of vasospasm. If spasm is detected, the patient remains in the hospital until its resolution.

NEUROLOGIC COMPLICATIONS OF SUBARACHNOID HEMORRHAGE

The neurologic complications that follow aneurysmal SAH are, in order of their relative frequency and importance, vasospasm, rebleeding, hydrocephalus and elevated ICP, and seizures. Vasospasm is the most important cause of a poor outcome in patients admitted to the hospital in good condition and will be covered in greatest detail.

VASOSPASM

Vasospasm (cerebral arterial spasm) is the most frequent cause of morbidity and mortality in patients admitted to the hospital after an SAH.[26] Numerous experimental and clinical studies have demonstrated that vasospasm is related to the dense periarterial clot that is present after aneurysm rupture.[51] Vasospasm does not occur acutely after aneurysm rupture but rather makes its appearance 4 to 10 days after the hemorrhage.[7,30] The severity of vasospasm peaks during the second week after SAH and resolves during the third week (Fig. 13-2). It is important to differentiate between the angiographic finding of arterial narrowing (angiographic vasospasm) and "symptomatic vasospasm," which is characterized by neurologic deterioration due to cerebral ischemia. Angiographic arterial narrowing may be seen in 60 to 70 percent of patients when it is performed 10 to 12 days fol-

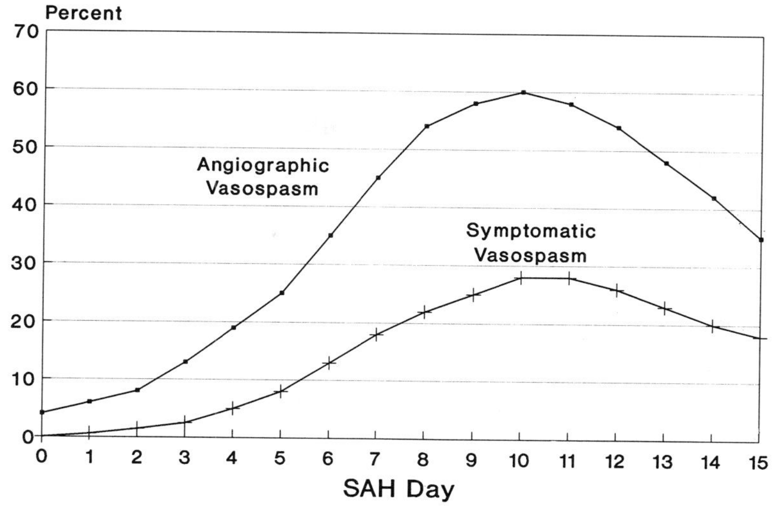

Figure 13-2 Prevalence of angiographic or symptomatic vasospasm by post-SAH day. (Adapted from Torner J, et al.[48a]).

lowing SAH. However, ischemic neurologic deficit due to arterial narrowing occurs only in approximately 30 percent of patients.

Vasospasm generally involves the major cerebral vessels at the base of the brain: the supraclinoid internal carotid artery, the middle cerebral artery (MCA), the anterior cerebral artery, the intracranial vertebral arteries, the basilar artery, and the posterior cerebral arteries (PCAs). When the SAH extends into the sylvian fissure and insular cistern, or when it involves the interhemispheric fissure, peripheral arterial narrowing may occur.

Prediction of Vasospasm

As vasospasm is caused by periarterial blood clot, it is not surprising that the amount of subarachnoid blood seen on the initial CT scan is the strongest predictor of vasospasm. Takemae and colleagues, in 1978, first demonstrated the association of subarachnoid clot with vasospasm.[49] In 1980 Fisher and colleagues developed a system for grading the amount of subarachnoid clot that can be used for defining the highest-risk group for vasospasm.[12] They found that the CT demonstration of a localized subarachnoid clot correlated strongly with the subsequent development of significant arterial narrowing in the adjacent artery. Currently, the amount and pattern of subarachnoid blood seen on the initial CT scan is the most widely used feature for estimating the risk for vasospasm in individual patients (Fig. 13-1). A number of other clinical and radiographic features have been associated with the occurrence of vasospasm (poor clinical grade, hydrocephalus, intraventricular hemorrhage), but it is likely that these features also simply reflect the magnitude of the initial hemorrhage.

Diagnosis and Monitoring of Vasospasm

Clinical Observation Headache has been cited as an early symptom of vasospasm, but the clinical hallmark is the progressive development of impaired consciousness or focal neurologic deficit over the course of minutes to hours. Other signs, such as fever, tachycardia, and hypertension, may develop, but the relative nonspecificity of these signs limits their value in the diagnosis of vasospasm.

Because the neurologic deficit associated with arterial narrowing often consists of a subtle, mild change in level of consciousness, or a slight pronator drift or aphasia, careful sequential neurologic examination of these patients is essential. When the ischemic deficit of vasospasm is detected at this stage, prompt institution of treatment can often result in complete resolution of the deficit. When treatment is delayed until a dense neurologic deficit has developed, irreversible infarction may occur. Rapid laboratory evaluation and CT scanning is necessary to rule out other systemic causes (hyponatremia, hypotension, hypoxia) or neurologic causes (hydrocephalus, rebleeding) of deterioration.

Transcranial Doppler Ultrasonography In the past a determination of the degree of arterial narrowing could only be made with angiography. However, the invasiveness of this technique limits its usefulness for diagnosis and makes it unsuitable as a monitoring technique. The development of transcranial Doppler ultrasonography has made it possible to assess noninvasively the degree of arterial narrowing in the major arteries at the base of the brain.[1,2] Transcranial Doppler employs a very low frequency ultrasonic signal that has the capacity to penetrate thin areas of the cranium in order to study the intracranial arteries. The ultrasonic energy is reflected from flowing blood cells, and the resulting Doppler frequency shift is used to determine flow direction and velocity. While the systolic and diastolic velocities can be determined, the mean velocity is generally reported. Three cranial "windows" are used to assess the major intracranial arteries. The transorbital window is used to assess the carotid syphon and supraclinoid internal carotid artery. The transtemporal window provides ultrasonic access to the proximal segments of the anterior and middle cerebral arteries. The suboccipital window is used for evaluating vertebral and basilar arteries.

Arterial stenosis of any cause results in an increase in blood flow velocity through the stenotic segment. Flow velocity increases rapidly when the degree of stenosis exceeds 50 percent. A close correlation between flow velocity and degree of arterial narrowing has been demonstrated when transcranial Doppler recordings have been compared with angiograms of patients with vasospasm. The normal mean blood flow velocity in the MCA is approximately 60 cm/s, with a range of 30 to 80 cm/s.[2] A blood flow velocity in the MCA of greater than 120 cm/s is found when the angiogram demonstrates mild to moderate arterial spasm, and a velocity of greater than 200 cm/s indicates severe arterial narrowing (Fig. 13-3).

The proximal, horizontal segment of the MCA is most suited for monitoring vasospasm. When vasospasm occurs in patients with ruptured anterior circulation aneurysms, the proximal MCA is

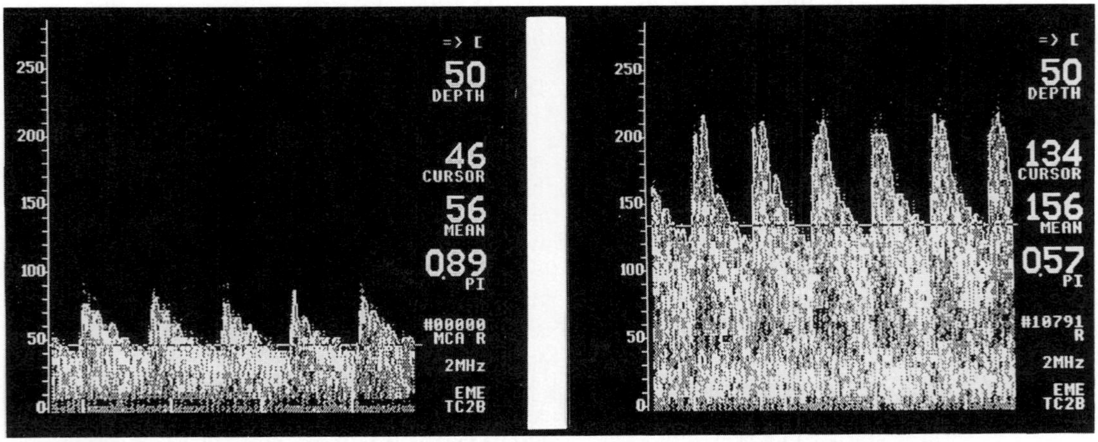

Figure 13-3 Transcranial Doppler in vasospasm. The waveform on the left was obtained from the right middle cerebral artery, at a depth of 50 mm, on the second posthemorrhage day after rupture of a right internal carotid artery aneurysm. This tracing demonstrates a normal waveform with a normal mean velocity of 56 cm/s. The waveform on the right was obtained on the ninth posthemorrhage day, again from the right middle cerebral artery. This transcranial Doppler evaluation demonstrated evidence of right middle cerebral artery spasm, with significant elevation of the mean velocity to 156 cm/s.

almost always narrowed. Newell and associates found that less than 8 percent of patients with anterior circulation aneurysms had spasm only of distal MCA branches (a situation in which transcranial Doppler would miss the spasm).[40] Other investigators have confirmed that Transcranial Doppler has a sensitivity of 85 percent and a specificity of 90 percent or more for detecting MCA spasm.[32,46,47]

There have been few studies of flow velocity in the posterior circulation in SAH. The blood flow velocity values that correspond to significant spasm of the vertebral and basilar arteries have not yet been defined, but the demonstration of rapidly increasing velocities in these vessels, particularly in patients with ruptured posterior circulation aneurysms, can be presumed to denote vasospasm.

Because this noninvasive technique can be performed at the bedside in the ICU, transcranial Doppler can be used serially to monitor SAH patients for the development of vasospasm. The experience of a number of clinical investigators has demonstrated that there is a characteristic pattern of velocity changes associated with neurologic deterioration from vasospasm. Patients who develop rapidly rising MCA velocities during the first posthemorrhage week, and patients who develop mean MCA velocities higher than 200 cm/s, are at significant risk for the development of symptomatic cerebral ischemia.[46,47]

It is important to remember that the demonstration of high flow velocities does not necessarily indicate dangerous cerebral ischemia. Just as some patients with angiographically demonstrated vasospasm remain asymptomatic, a proportion of patients with transcranial Doppler evidence of vasospasm never develop cerebral ischemia. Furthermore, normal velocity measurements do not provide a guarantee that injurious cerebral ishcemia will not occur because spasm may involve arterial segments not accessible to transcranial Doppler study. For these reasons the direct measurement of CBF is a valuable adjunct to transcranial Doppler for monitoring SAH patients.

Cerebral Blood Flow Measurement A number of techniques are available for the measurement of regional CBF, including radioactive xenon clearance (using the intravenous or inhalational technique), stable xenon CT, single photon emission computed tomography (SPECT), and positron emission tomography (PET).[11,28,36,41,44,45,54] All these techniques permit intermittent measurement of CBF in both cerebral hemispheres and each has advantages and disadvantages, but only xenon-133 clearance technique can be applied using portable equipment in the ICU. At UCLA, we have employed the intravenous xenon-133 technique. This technique allows measurement of average hemispheric blood flow and is weighted toward the MCA territory. This portable technique avoids the need to transport unstable patients from the ICU to a scanner. Other investigators, however, have used the tomographic CBF techniques or other methods successfully for the management of SAH patients.[8,54]

The xenon-133 technique has been used for clinical research and clinical studies for more than 20 years, has been repeatedly validated, and provides CBF measurements that are stable and reliable. The dose of xenon-133 employed for the test is small enough so that patient radiation exposure is low (equivalent to or less than that of one chest x-ray). The xenon-133, which is cleared from the body through the lungs, is exhaled into a closed system and collected in a lead-shielded charcoal trap. Careful monitoring of technologist exposure and of ambient air radioactivity in the ICU at UCLA has demonstrated a high level of safety.

The intermittent measurement of CBF in patients at risk for vasospasm complements the information derived from transcranial Doppler ultrasonography. The transcranial Doppler can be thought of as a detector for arterial narrowing. The CBF techniques measure the net effect of vasospasm on cerebral perfusion. CBF is dependent not only on the severity of spasm, but also on blood pressure, ICP, blood viscosity, $PaCO_2$, the competency of collateral pathways, and the integrity of the autoregulatory responses. The normal mean hemispheric CBF is approximately 50 mL/100 g per min, but neurologic deficit does not occur until CBF falls below 20 to 25 mL/100 g per min. Clearly, there can be a significant impairment in hemispheric blood flow without any clinically detectable sign of cerebral hypoperfusion. Once an ischemic neurologic deficit appears, a relatively small additional decrease in CBF (below 15 to 18 mL/100 g per min) may result in irreversible neuronal injury and cerebral infarction.[20,21,27,44,54] Therefore, CBF measurement allows for the detection of a fall in CBF long before the development of an ischemic neurologic deficit. The clinical examination only detects cerebral hypoperfusion when the patient has developed signs of ischemia (when CBF has fallen dangerously close to the threshold for irreversible brain damage).

Management of Vasospasm

Prophylactic Treatment

Calcium Antagonists Allen and associates reported the first prospective clinical trial which compared the use of the calcium antagonist nimodipine to placebo in aneurysm patients.[3] This study demonstrated a substantial reduction in the incidence of severe deficit or death in patients treated with nimodipine. In the largest study, by Pickard and coworkers, aneurysm patients of all grades were given either nimodipine or placebo.[43] Nimodipine reduced the incidence of cerebral infarction (nimodipine—22 percent; placebo—33 percent), and reduced the incidence of poor outcome (nimodipine—20 percent; placebo—33 percent). Several subsequent noncontrolled clinical studies using intravenous or cisternal administration of nimodipine confirmed the benefits of this calcium antagonist in the treatment of patients with aneurysmal SAH.[4,33] It is interesting to note that the studies of calcium antagonists show that angiographic arterial narrowing is not reduced by the use of calcium antagonists.[3,43] Rather more probable, the mechanism of action involves an effect on leptomeningeal pathways to improve collateral flow, or a direct protective effect on neuronal cells.[37]

The weight of clinical evidence supports the prophylactic use of calcium antagonists in patients with ruptured intracranial aneurysms. Nimodipine is the most thoroughly studied calcium antagonist and is the only one approved by the Food and Drug Administration (FDA) for use in aneurysmal SAH. Currently, it is recommended that nimodipine be administered to all patients with a ruptured intracranial aneurysm beginning upon admission. Nimodipine is currently available only as an oral preparation, and the recommended dosage is 60 mg every 4 h (to be continued for 21 days). In some cases nimodipine administration results in decreased systemic arterial blood pressure, and in such cases the dosage should be reduced or divided into 30 mg every 2 h. In patients unable to swallow medications, nimodipine may be administered via nasogastric tube.

Volume Expansion CBF gradually declines during the first week after SAH and reaches its low point during the second week before gradually increasing toward normal.[20] While vasospasm is a primary cause of the progressive blood flow reduction, a reduction in circulating blood volume also appears to contribute to this effect. Maroon and Nelson demonstrated reductions in both blood volume and red blood cell mass in a study of SAH patients.[35] Others have confirmed these findings.[18] The cause for this reduction in circulating blood volume may include cerebral salt-wasting, bed rest with supine diuresis, decreased erythropoiesis, iatrogenic blood loss, or sympathetic hyperactivity.[31]

In order to counteract the hypervolemia that follows subarachnoid hemorrhage, fluid therapy is a key component of preventive management. Colloid, generally in the form of 5 percent albumin, is administered empirically in a dose of 250 mL two to three times daily (in patients without cardiac dysfunction or pulmonary edema), or titrated to maintain a CVP of 5–10 torr, or a pulmonary capillary wedge pressure of 12–15 torr.

Hypervolemic Hemodilution and Arterial Hypertension (Triple-H Therapy) The reduction in CBF that results from cerebral vasospasm is accompanied by a disturbance in cerebral autoregulation. Under these physiologic circumstances, induced arterial hypertension results in an increase in CBF. A number of investigators have demonstrated improvement in ischemic neurologic deficit with arterial hypertension. Muizelaar and Becker[38] and Rosenstein and coworkers[45] have demonstrated that hypertensive treatment improves CBF. Kosnik and Hunt in 1976 reported the resolution of delayed ischemic deficit in vasospasm patients using induced arterial hypertension in combination with hypervolemia.[29] This strategy was brought into broad clinical use by the report of Kassell and associates, who successfully used this therapy in a large series of patients with symptomatic vasospasm.[24] They advocated aggressive volume expansion and very aggressive induction of hypertension (often to a systolic pressure of more than 200 mmHg) and achieved neurologic improvement in 74 percent of their patients.

Hemodilution alone has been demonstrated to decrease blood viscosity and improve blood flow in regions of hypoperfusion.[52] Hemodilution almost invariably results from aggressive volume expansion using colloid infusion, and only a few clinical investigators have advocated adding phlebotomy in order to lower hematocrit.[42] It is generally agreed that the optimal hematocrit to provide a lowered blood viscosity without unduly reducing the oxygen carrying capacity of the blood is approximately 35 percent.

As the first step of the triple-H therapy, a central venous pressure or a PA catheter is inserted for hemodynamic monitoring. Volume expansion is carried out with a goal of achieving a central venous pressure of approximately 10 mmHg, or a pulmonary artery wedge pressure of approximately 15 mmHg. Albumin (5%) is the agent of choice. Colloid infusion generally results in a lowering of the hematocrit, and it is rare to require phlebotomy in order to achieve a hematocrit of approximately 35 percent. In anemic patients it may be necessary to infuse packed red blood cells as a component of volume expansion to achieve the desired hematocrit. The systemic arterial pressure often rises with volume expansion, and this can be promoted by withdrawal of antihypertensive agents. However, in many cases pressor therapy is required. Dopamine is the agent used initially, but even at high doses this ocassionally cannot achieve the desired blood pressure. In such cases phenylephrine is employed. When used in conjunction with hypervolemia, phenylephrine is very effective at inducing marked arterial hypertension. The systolic blood pressure is raised to the range of 160 to 200 mmHg in patients with clipped aneurysms. In some refractory cases, systolic blood pressures of 220 mmHg or more have been used. Severe hypertension is dangerous in patients with unclipped aneurysms, and in such cases the upper limit is approximately 170 mmHg. With this degree of hypervolemia and systemic arterial hypertension, many younger patients will develop a very high urine output. In these cases the volume of colloid infused is adjusted to maintain the desired central venous or pulmonary artery pressure. When the urine output is extremely high (greater than 200 to 300 mL/h) the diuresis may be suppressed with florinef (generic) or vasopressin (Pitressin).[24] When these agents are added, it is particularly important to monitor the serum electrolytes and observe carefully for the development of hyponatremia.

As one might expect, medical complications may result from this triple-H therapy. The most common medical complication is that of pulmonary edema, and patients must be auscultated frequently and daily chest x-rays should be obtained. Oxygen saturation should be continuously monitored as well with pulse oximetry. Cardiac arrhythmia and myocardial ischemia occur in rare cases, and continuous electrocardiogram (ECG) monitoring is necessary. Somewhat surprisingly, cerebral edema and cerebral hemorrhage are rare complications, almost certainly because the arterial spasm prevents the transmission of the high systemic arterial pressure to the distal cerebral vasculature. However, recurrent SAH may occur in patients treated before their aneurysms have been clipped. In order to avoid this complication, the degree of arterial hypertension is limited in patients with unclipped aneurysms. This is one of the reasons that acute or early aneurysm surgery is advantageous.

Angioplasty Even with the aggressive application of hypervolemic hemodilution and arterial hypertension, a significant number of patients with symptomatic vasospasm develop permanent neurologic deficit. In the report by Awad and associates, 40 percent of patients with ischemic neurologic deficit due to vasospasm failed to improve with aggressive hemodynamic therapy.[5] Sixteen percent of the patients in fact continued to progress despite maximal therapy, and 19 percent of the patients were left with a major neurologic deficit or died.

The limitations of triple-H therapy have resulted in a search for new therapeutic modalities for severe, medically refractory vasospasm. Angioplasty is an endovascular technique that employs a balloon catheter for the mechanical dilatation of regions of vessel stenosis. Balloon dilatation angioplasty has been widely used for atherosclerotic lesions involving the coronary arteries, but more recently has been applied to cerebral vasospasm following SAH (Fig. 13-4).[9,10,19] The microballoon catheters available for angioplasty of vasospasm vary in diameter from 2.5 to 3 mm and in length from 12 to 15 mm. The balloon microcatheters are long enough that they can be introduced transfemorally and supple enough that they can be directed into the major intracranial arteries at the base of the brain.

Angioplasty is indicated for patients with delayed ischemic deficit due to vasospasm who have failed to improve with aggressive hypervolemic hemodilution and arterial hypertension, and in whom a CT scan does not demonstrate an established infarction. Transluminal angioplasty has been reported to result in neurologic improvement in patients with medically refractory vasospasm in 60 to 70 percent of cases.[10,19,55] Angioplasty appears to result in a long-lasting dilation of the narrowed arterial segment. Serial transcranial Doppler studies and follow-up angiography have generally not demonstrated recurrent spasm.

Early intervention is a critical factor in the use of angioplasty for vasospasm. Most of the clinical failures can be attributed to the occurrence of irreversible ischemic injury prior to treatment. Furthermore, it appears that narrowed arteries are easier to dilate in the early stages of vasospasm. In the later stages of spasm the vessel appears to be more rigid, and higher dilatation pressures are required to reverse arterial narrowing.[10]

Several problems attend the use of transluminal angioplasty for vasospasm. Mechanical dilatation for spastic arteries may be injurious to the vessel wall. There have been cases reported of fatal arterial rupture due to angioplasty, as well as reports of distal embolization related to endothelial dam-

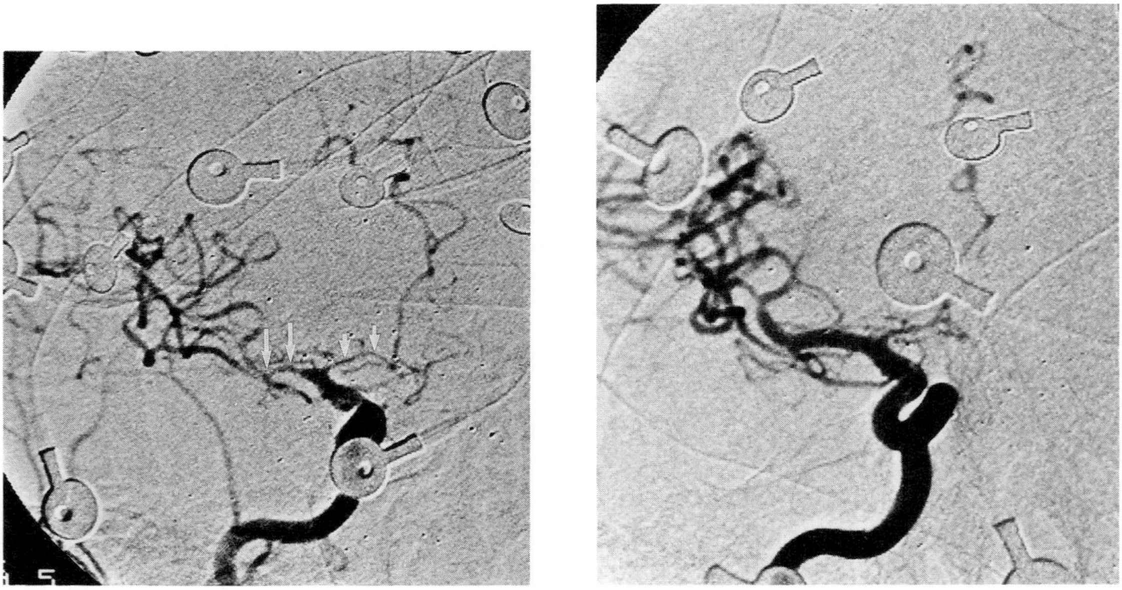

A B

Figure 13-4 Internal carotid angiography, anteroposterior view. *A*. The angiogram demonstrates severe spasm of the middle cerebral artery (arrows) and the anterior cerebral artery (small arrows). *B*. The angiogram performed after balloon dilatation angioplasty of the middle cerebral artery demonstrates return of the vessel diameter to normal. The anterior cerebral artery, which originated at a right angle from the internal carotid artery, could not be entered to allow angioplasty.

age.[10] Delayed intracerebral hemorrhage involving the territory of the dilated artery has also been reported, presumably due to reperfusion of previously infarcted region areas.

Technical constraints limit the application of transluminal angioplasty to the larger basal cerebral arteries. The proximal anterior cerebral artery, because it often takes off at a right angle from the internal carotid artery, may be difficult to catheterize and dilate. The secondary MCA branches generally are often too small for angioplasty, and distal branches of both the MCA and PCA are currently inaccessible.

A new development in endovascular treatment of arterial vasospasm may provide treatment for medically refractory ischemia due to narrowing in small peripheral vessels. Intraarterial high-dose papaverine infusion has been demonstrated to dilate areas of severe arterial spasm in a small number of cases.[16] If further experience with this technique confirms its efficacy, intraarterial infusion of vasodilators may provide a therapeutic technique for spasm of the arterial branches inaccessible to balloon angioplasty.

Integrated Management of Vasospasm Several therapeutic protocols have been employed for the management of vasospasm following aneurysm rupture. The "classic" strategy, which is the standard at most medical centers, involves prophylactic management with nimodipine and maintenance of normovolemia or moderate hypervolemia, augmented by aggressive hypervolemic hemodilution and systemic arterial hypertension only when patients develop the clinical signs of ischemic neurologic deficit. (Angioplasty is employed, when it is available, in patients refractory to medical management) (Table 13-3). This strategy requires extremely close clinical neurologic monitoring and has the shortcoming that aggressive therapy is instituted only when arterial spasm is severe enough to decrease CBF to the point at which it is dangerously close to the threshold for permanent, irreversible infarction. Using this strategy, permanent neurologic damage can only be avoided if aggressive treatment is begun very shortly after the onset of deficit. Clinical experience with this strategy indicates that symptomatic vasospasm can be treated effectively in many cases, but that neurologic improvement fails to occur in as many as 25 to 40 percent of patients.[5,22,26] In patients with deficits due to cerebral vasospasm, it may be difficult to be sure that the deficits are due to reversible ischemia rather than to irreversible infarction, and aggressive treatment may result in the complication of bleeding into infarcted tissue.

A second therapeutic strategy combines the use of nimodipine with moderate hypervolemia, hemodilution, and induced arterial hypertension for all patients, symptomatic or not.[42] Results using this protocol have suggested that it is effective in *preventing* the gradual decline in CBF that generally occurs after SAH. This regimen is also useful in reducing (but not eliminating) ischemic neurologic deficit from vasospasm. While controlled

Table 13-3 Vasospasm Management Protocol (without TCD/CBF monitoring)

Ischemic deficit	Treatment
All SAH patients	Nimodipine 60 mg by mouth or nasogastric tube every 4 h
	5% albumin 250 mL intravenously every 6 h
Deficit present	ICU admission
	Volume expansion (to PCWP 15 mmHg)
	HCT 33–37% hypertension (to BP 170–220 mmHg systolic)
Deficit refractory to medical treatment	Transluminal angioplasty
Deficit resolved	Gradual withdrawal of hypervolemia, hypertension

PCWP = pulmonary capillary wedge pressure; HCT = hematocrit; BP = blood pressure.

clinical trials of this technique have not been carried out, the results have been encouraging. This protocol, however, has the significant drawback that many patients not destined to develop ischemic deficit from vasospasm are exposed to costly and in some cases risky medical therapy.

We have employed a third strategy at UCLA. This includes prophylactic treatment of all patients following SAH with nimodipine and colloid infusion to induce moderate hypervolemia. All patients are monitored serially with transcranial Doppler and bedside CBF studies in order to detect the development of vasospasm and low CBF before clinically apparent ischemic neurologic dysfunction occurs. Aggressive hypervolemic therapy and induced arterial hypertension are introduced only when the TCD and/or the CBF testing demonstrates progressive and significant disturbance of cerebral hemodynamics. These measures are employed before the development of symptomatic ischemia. The most aggressive therapeutic measures (marked arterial hypertension, angioplasty) are reserved for the patients who develop clinically apparent neurologic deterioration. This protocol has several important advantages. First, patients who never develop significant vasospasm are not exposed to the risks and costs of intensive hemodynamically directed therapy. Second, therapy is initiated before the development of ischemia in patients with significant vasospasm, thereby preventing these high-risk patients from developing neurologic deterioration. Third, patients at high risk for severe cerebral ischemia are identified and are therefore monitored extremely closely. When these patients develop ischemic deficit, it is detected immediately, and intensive treatment can be started before irreversible damage occurs.

Table 13-4 demonstrates the management protocol, based on physiologic data obtained with transcranial Dopper and CBF measurements, currently employed at UCLA. Using this protocol over the last 2 years we have reduced the incidence of ischemic neurologic deficit due to vasospasm to less than 5 percent in our aneurysmal SAH patients. Future improvements in pharmacologic therapy for the prevention of vasospasm and developments in the therapy of established vasospasm should bring the incidence of permanent ischemic damage due to this problem even lower.

Figures 13-5 and 13-6 demonstrate the typical TCD and CBF findings with application of this protocol in a patient with moderate vasospasm (treated with triple-H therapy) and in a patient with severe, medically refractory vasospasm (treated with angioplasty).

REBLEEDING

Aneurysm rebleeding remains an important cause of death and disability in patients surviving the initial hemorrhage. Rebleeding occurs in approximately 20 percent of cases during the first 2 weeks after initial aneurysm bleeding if the aneurysm remains untreated. The period of highest risk for rebleeding appears to be the first 24 h after initial hemorrhage, when the risk is approximately 4 percent. Thereafter the risk falls to 1 to 2 percent daily (Fig. 13-7).[25,26] The mortality of rebleeding episodes approaches 70 percent. Several therapeutic steps can be taken to reduce the risk of rebleeding.

Table 13-4 Vasospasm Management Protocol (with TCD/CBF monitoring)

TCD velocity	CBF	Ischemic deficit	Treatment
All SAH patients	All patients	Absent	Nimodipine 60 mg by mouth or nasogastric tube every 4 h 5% Albumin 250 mL intravenous every 6 h
>150 cm/s	Normal	Absent	Careful clinical and physical monitoring
>150 cm/s	Low	Absent	ICU, hypertension to 150–170 mmHg systolic
>150 cm/s	Low	Present	ICU, volume expansion, hypertension to 170–220 mmHg systolic
>150 cm/s	Low	Present, refractory	Transluminal angioplasty
<150 cm/s	Normal	Resolved	Withdrawal of hypertension

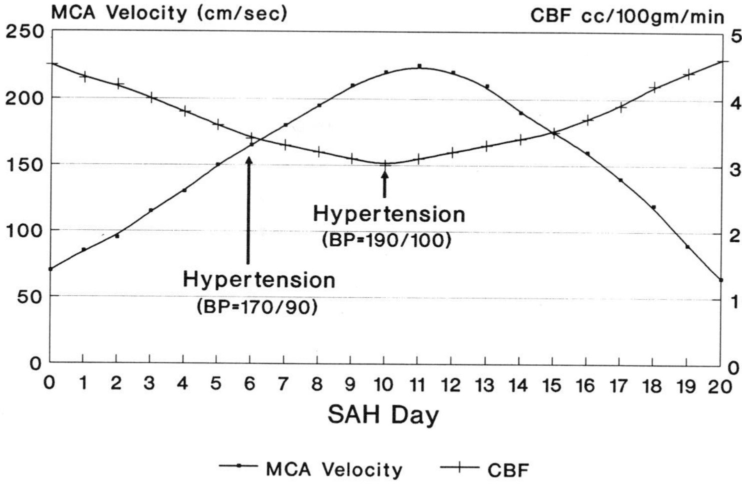

Figure 13-5 The time course of evolution of middle cerebral artery velocity and cerebral blood flow are demonstrated in a patient treated with induced arterial hypertension. At the first arrow (day 6) the patient was treated with moderate hypertension because of the rising middle cerebral artery velocity, associated with the falling cerebral blood flow. At the second arrow (day 10) the blood pressure was raised further, resulting in gradual improvement in cerebral blood flow. This hypothetical case demonstrates treatment of arterial spasm based on transcranial Doppler and cerebral blood flow studies rather than on the patient's clinical condition.

Immediately after admission, it is important to ensure that marked arterial hypertension is avoided. In many cases this requires the careful use of antihypertensive agents; we generally use nifedipine for moderate hypertension, and sodium nitroprusside for more severe or refractory hypertension. It is important not to overtreat; the brain already injured from SAH may be particularly vulnerable to hypotension because of autoregulatory impairment. Our goal is generally to reduce the systolic arterial pressure to less than 150 mmHg, although a slightly higher level may be advisable in patients with chronic arterial hypertension.

Early Surgery

The most effective strategy to prevent aneurysm rebleeding is to perform surgery as soon as possible after admission. However, the timing of aneurysm surgery has been a controversial topic for the past 30 years.[48a] Early aneurysm surgery has the advantage that it prevents rebleeding, it may reduce the

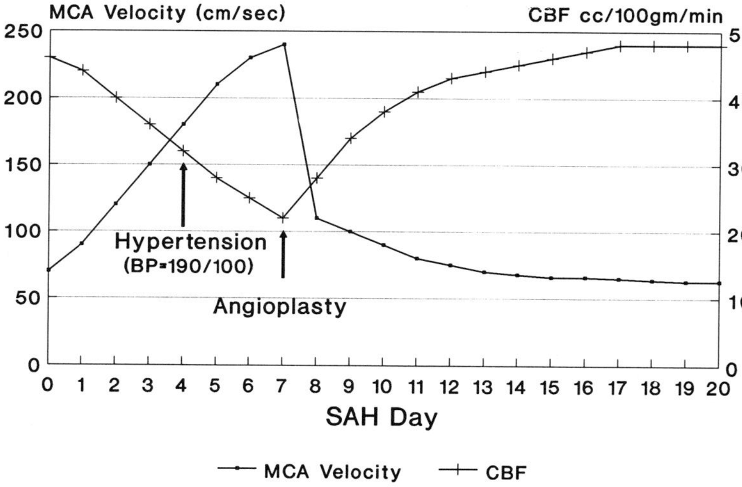

Figure 13-6 Typical pattern of middle cerebral artery velocity and cerebral blood flow in severe vasospasm treated with angioplasty. At the first arrow (day 4) hypertensive therapy is initiated because of rising middle cerebral artery velocity associated with falling cerebral blood flow. At the second arrow (day 7) angioplasty is performed because of the development of ischemic neurologic deficit refractory to hypertensive therapy. Note that the middle cerebral artery velocity rapidly returns to normal after angioplasty, at the same time that cerebral blood flow gradually increases and returns toward normal.

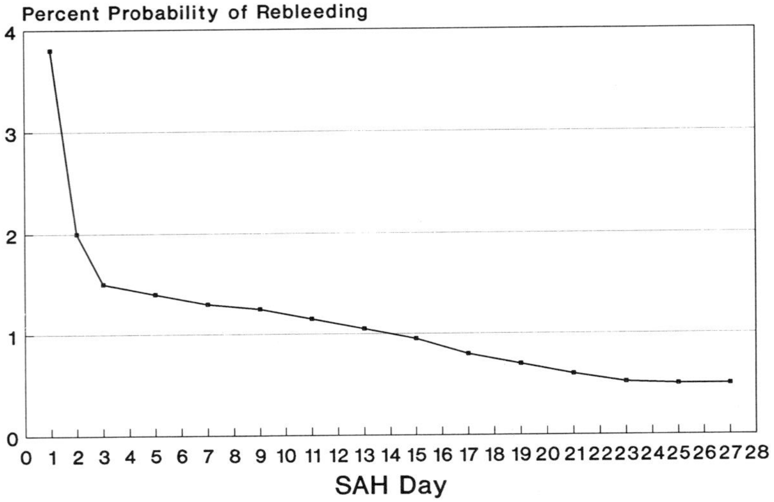

Figure 13-7 The risk of recurrent bleeding following the initial SAH is highest during the first 24 h after onset. The risk of rebleeding is between 1 and 2 percent per day after the first 24-h period. (Adapted from Kassell N and Torner J.[25])

severity of vasospasm by removing the periarterial clot that appears to be the underlying cause of spasm, and it permits more aggressive medical treatment of vasospasm (with induced arterial hypertension). However, clinical investigators in the past have suggested that early surgery was associated with a higher morbidity and mortality because of the technical problems in dealing with the swollen brain and with the fragile recently ruptured aneurysm. Delayed surgery (10 to 14 days after hemorrhage) has the advantage that the brain is less swollen and may be more tolerant to surgical manipulation, resulting in lower operative morbidity. However, many patients die or become disabled because of the effects of rebleeding or cerebral vasospasm which occur during the delay before surgery. The International Cooperative Study on the Timing of Aneurysm Surgery evaluated the relationship of surgical interval to outcome.[26] When the planned interval to surgery was studied, they found that the outcome with early surgery was the same (days 0 to 3 after hemorrhage) as with delayed surgery (11 or more days after hemorrhage). The outcome, however, appeared to be significantly worse when surgery was planned for the interval of 4 to 10 days after the hemorrhage, presumably because of the fact that this is the period of highest risk for cerebral ischemia due to vasospasm. The fact that early surgery did not demonstrate a clear-cut advantage to delayed surgery was somewhat disappointing. It appears that although rebleeding (as a major cause of poor outcome) was reduced in the early surgery group, morbidity and mortality due to vasospasm compensated for this factor. It seems that many patients, particularly patients in grades III and IV, are at high risk from both rebleeding and vasospasm. While early surgery may protect these patients from rebleeding, they later succumb to the effects of vasospasm. This study was carried out in the early 1980s, before widespread use of nimodipine, before the refinement of triple-H therapy, and before the introduction of angioplasty. It can be expected that the application of these treatments for vasospasm will, in combination with early surgery to prevent rebleeding, result in improved overall management outcome in SAH.

Antifibrinolytic Therapy

Antifibrinolytic drugs have been used in the management of patients with ruptured intracranial aneurysms for more than 20 years. Epsilon-aminocaproic acid (EACA, AMICAR) has been most commonly employed in North America. Antifibrinolytic therapy has been used to retard dissolution of the fibrin clot sealing the rent in the aneurysm, thereby reducing the risk of rebleeding in patients for whom delayed surgery is planned. A number of clinical trials of antifibrinolytic therapy have confirmed that these drugs reduce the incidence of rebleeding, but this effect appears to be balanced by an increased risk for the development of focal cerebral ischemia. A number of recent trials have indicated that the use of antifibrinolytic therapy does not result in an improvement in overall clinical outcome.[14] Because of these findings, the use of antifibrinolytic therapy has declined dramatically over the last decade, at the same time that the practice of early surgery has increased. Given the present state of knowledge, antifibrinolytic drugs should be used cautiously, if at all, and only in patients who are believed not to be candidates for early surgery.[14] Patients receiving this therapy must be monitored closely for the development of cerebral ischemia, and the antifibrinolytic drug should be discontinued if signs of symptomatic vasospasm appear.

When EACA is to be administered, an initial loading dose of 48 g by intravenous infusion is given daily for the first 2 days, followed by an infusion of 36 g daily until the aneurysm has been treated surgically. The medication is discontinued 6 h before any planned operation, or before angiography.

Endovascular Aneurysm Occlusion

The development of endovascular techniques has provided a new alternative for the treatment of acutely ruptured intracranial aneurysms in patients who, because of poor neurologic or medical condition, are not candidates for early surgery. The most promising technique, currently undergoing evaluation, involves the positioning and electrolytic detachment of fine platinum coils within the aneurysm sack.[13] This method (developed at UCLA) has been used successfully in a number of cases since 1990. The technique has proved especially valuable for the treatment of patients with severe medical disorders (e.g., neurogenic pulmonary edema, myocardial ischemia) or with severe vasospasm. Such patients, who fall into a very high risk group for acute surgery, have been treated with the endovascular detachable platinum coil technique successfully in a number of cases. In these circumstances the endovascular technique appears to expose the patient to less physiologic stress than does open surgical treatment. In one of the patients treated at UCLA, regrowth of the aneurysm after acute endovascular treatment was seen on a follow-up angiogram. As the patient had recovered by that point, elective surgical clipping of the residual aneurysm was well tolerated and successful. The use of endovascular techniques for the treatment of acutely ruptured aneurysms in patients who are not good candidates for early surgery may become an important technique for the prevention of rebleeding.

HYDROCEPHALUS

Hydrocephalus occurs in approximately 20 percent of SAH patients.[15] Heros has described three patterns of hydrocephalus following SAH (acute, subacute, and late).[17,18] Acute hydrocephalus is seen on the admission cranial CT scan generally in poor-grade patients and is often associated with intraventricular hemorrhage. When this condition is accompanied by a significant depression in the level of consciousness or with progressive neurologic deterioration, immediate ventricular drainage is indicated. When there is filling of the ventricular system with blood, bilateral ventriculostomies are often necessary. Rapid cerebrospinal fluid drainage should be avoided, as the abrupt change in ICP may precipitate aneurysm rupture. Generally the ventricular pressure is not lowered below 15 cmH_2O. Tunneling of the ventriculostomy catheter beneath the scalp and the use of prophylactic antibiotics reduces the risk of infection. If ventricular drainage is required for more than 5 to 7 days, the ventriculostomy catheter is removed and replaced at another site in order to reduce the risk of bacterial colonization and ventricular infection. A ventricular peritoneal shunt is inserted if cerebrospinal fluid drainage is required in order to chronically control ICP. The insertion of a permanent shunt is generally delayed until there is clearing of gross blood from the cerebrospinal fluid, which can cause occlusion of the shunt.

Subacute hydrocephalus is a common finding after SAH and generally develops during the first week. The type is usually communicating hydrocephalus, and in many cases it is not associated with significant neurologic deterioration. Treatment of this type of ventriculomegaly is reserved for those patients demonstrating progressive neurologic impairment. This type of hydrocephalus often resolves without the need for permanent shunting. Serial cranial CT scanning is performed in these patients to ensure that progressive ventricular enlargement does not occur.

Late hydrocephalus appears weeks or months after the initial hemorrhage and often conforms to the clinical syndrome of normal pressure hydrocephalus. Gait ataxia, followed by dementia and in some cases incontinence, are the classic symptoms. This condition responds well to ventricular shunting.

SEIZURES

Seizures occur in association with SAH in 10 to 25 percent of cases.[17] Anticonvulsant therapy, therefore, is particularly important during the acute phase in order to avoid seizures and the arterial hypertension that often accompanies them. We have generally employed phenytoin (Dilantin) in a loading dose of approximately 1000 mg (18 mg/kg for adults) followed by a maintenance dose of approximately 300 to 400 mg daily (with dosage guided by phenytoin levels and seizure activity). Phenobarbital may be substituted for Dilantin in patients in whom a sedative effect is desired. In the absence of seizures, it is not clear how long anticonvulsant therapy should be continued after recovery from SAH. Our practice is to continue anticonvulsants for 3 to 6 months and then taper them in patients who have never had seizures.

MEDICAL COMPLICATIONS OF SUBARACHNOID HEMORRHAGE

In addition to the well-recognized neurologic complications of SAH, numerous medical problems can result and may lead to serious morbidity and even death (Table 13-5). Among the more common medical complications of SAH are cardiac arrhythmias and ischemia, pulmonary edema, pneumonia and adult respiratory distress syndrome (ARDS), anemia, gastrointestinal bleeding, and syndrome of inappropriate antidiuretic hormone secretion (SIADH). These and other medical problems can be very disabling and need to be recognized early and treated aggressively.

Table 13-5 Aneurysmal Subarachnoid Hemorrhage Medical Complications

Complication	Percent of patients
Cardiovascular	
Hypertension	18.3
Arrhythmia	3.6
Hypotension	3.0
Cardiac failure	2.0
Thrombophlebitis	1.4
Myocardial infarction	0.7
Angina	0.6
Pulmonary	
Pneumonia	7.0
Atelectasis	2.3
ARDS	2.0
Pulmonary edema	1.7
Asthma	1.2
Pulmonary embolism	0.8
Other	
Anemia	4.9
Gastrointestinal bleeding	3.7
SIADH	3.6
Diabetes mellitus	2.2
Hepatic failure	1.9
Renal failure	1.4
Hepatitis	1.1

Source: Adapted from Kassell N, et al.[26]

Cardiac Complications

Electrocardiographic abnormalities occur in 60 to 100 percent of the patients with SAH.[34,50] The ECG abnormalities are more common during the first 48 h following SAH and include prolonged QT interval, T-wave inversion, prominent U waves, ST segment elevation or depression, and rhythm abnormalities. The most common arrhythmias are supraventricular tachycardia, atrial flutter or fibrillation, premature atrial and ventricular contractions, and ventricular flutter and fibrillation. Myocardial ischemia, especially subendocardial hemorrhage and necrosis, has been observed in 1 percent of these patients. Most arrhythmias in these patients, however, are not related to myocardial ischemia. The high incidence of cardiac abnormalities is thought to be related to excessive neurogenic and humoral sympathetic stimulation following SAH. Myocardial ischemia is also possible secondary to triple-H therapy and occurs in 2 percent of the patients.[24]

Beta-adrenergic blockers (propranolol) have been used effectively in the treatment of these arrhythmias and have also been found to prevent subendocardial lesions.[34] Ventricular flutter or fibrillation is treated with defibrillation and antiarrhythmic medication.[34,50]

Pulmonary Complications

Neurogenic pulmonary edema is seen occasionally in patients with SAH and is more common in fatal cases.[34] This syndrome is related to excessive sympathetic stimulation secondary to an elevated ICP. The high pressure and flow in the pulmonary vasculature secondary to the sympathetic discharge leads to an injured endothelium resulting in altered permeability. Cardiac decompensation is a rare cause of pulmonary edema following SAH. The edema fluid of neurogenic pulmonary edema has a high protein content compared to cardiogenic pulmonary edema. Treatment is geared toward improvement of systemic oxygenation by intubation and mechanical ventilation using positive end-expiratory pressure. Control of ICP with diuretics, mannitol, and cerebrospinal fluid drainage is also necessary.

Pulmonary edema can also be seen secondary to triple-H therapy and occurs in about 17 percent of the cases.[24,42] This iatrogenic complication is secondary to volume overload and can be avoided with meticulous control and monitoring of the degree of volume expansion.

Deep venous thrombosis occurs in about 2 percent of the patients following aneurysmal rupture, and 1 percent of the patients will have a pulmonary embolus.[26] For patients developing this complication during the preoperative or early postoperative period, treatment consists of vena caval filter insertion. Prophylaxis for deep venous thrombosis is generally recommended and includes passive exercises, elastic and intermittent pressure stockings, early mobilization, and (in high-risk patients) low-dose heparin.

Gastrointestinal Complications

Gastrointestinal bleeding secondary to stress ulceration occurs in about 4 percent of the patients following SAH.[26] An increased incidence has been observed in comatose and fatal cases. The hypersecretion of acid and gastrin commonly seen in patients with ICP is accompanied by breakdown of gastric mucosal defenses, predisposes these patients to develop ulcers in the esophagus, stomach, or duodenum with an increased risk of perforation (Cushing's ulcer). Treatment consists of nasogastric intubation with suctioning, saline lavage, fluid replacement, and transfusion. Aggressive antacid and H_2-antagonist therapy should be instituted. If uncontrollable bleeding continues, partial gastrectomy with vagotomy may be indicated. Prophylaxis with antacids and H_2-antagonists is generally used in all SAH patients.

Hyponatremia

Hyponatremia occurs in approximately 4 percent of cases following aneurysmal rupture.[26,39] The presence of elevated ADH (SIADH) accompanied by continued water intake can lead to expansion of the extracellular fluid volume and hyponatremia. Hyponatremia can also result from natriuresis rather than SIADH, a syndrome known as cerebral salt wasting. Both SIADH and cerebral salt wasting present with hyponatremia and decreased serum osmolality, but the hyponatremia in cerebral salt wasting is accompanied by a decrease in blood volume, whereas the hyponatremia in SIADH is a dilutional effect secondary to free-water retention. Recently, it has been documented that a majority of patients with hyponatremia following SAH are volume-depleted, suggesting that cerebral salt wasting is the primary cause of hyponatremia in these patients.[39] Symptoms in both syndromes are related to the degree of hyponatremia and include anorexia, nausea, vomiting, irritability, lethargy, neurologic abnormalities, seizures, and coma.

Patients with SIADH are treated with fluid restriction and, if severe hyponatremia (<115 mmol/L) is present, 3 percent saline infusion accompanied by fluid restriction is used. Patients with cerebral salt wasting require both sodium and volume replacement.

SUMMARY

Intensive care of a patient with SAH should focus on the prevention or immediate treatment of the common sequelae of this disorder: vasospasm, rebleeding, hydrocephalus, seizures, and associated medical problems.

The extent of SAH on the CT scan can identify those patients at highest risk for the development of vasospasm, and all patients must be closely monitored in the ICU with serial neurologic testing, transcranial Doppler, and CBF examinations. Calcium-channel blocking agents and volume (colloid) expansion is recommended prophylactically for all patients. Aggressive hypertensive, hemodilutional, hypervolemic therapy (including PA catheter placement) is indicated for symptomatic vasospasm. Transluminal angioplasty can be used in selected cases of vasospasm refractory to these aforementioned measures.

The frequency of rebleeding can be lessened by early surgery, antifibrinolytic therapy (for the first week after SAH), and endovascular aneurysmal occlusion. Hydrocephalus can occur acutely, subacutely, or several weeks or months following SAH and is treated effectively with external (acute hydrocephalus) or internal cerebrospinal fluid diversion. Seizures, which can cause increased arterial hypertension, high cerebral metabolic demand, and delayed neurologic injury, should be prevented with prophylactic use of anticonvulsants.

Timely integration of these techniques, in addition to early recognition and treatment of associated cardiac and pulmonary complications, will lead to a continually improving outcome in patients with aneurysmal SAH.

REFERENCES

1. Aaslid R, Huber P, Nornes H: Evaluation of cerebrovascular spasm with transcranial Doppler ultrasound. *J Neurosurg* 60:37, 1984.
2. Aaslid R, Markwalder TM, Nornes H: Noninvasive transcranial Doppler ultrasound recording of flow velocity in basal cerebral arteries. *J Neurosurg* 57:769, 1982.
3. Allen GS, Ahn HS, Preziosi TJ, et al.: Cerebral arterial spasm—a controlled trial of nimodipine in patients with subarachnoid hemorrhage. *N Engl J Med* 308:619, 1983.
4. Auer LM: Acute operation and preventive nimodipine outcome in patients with subarachnoid hemorrhage. *Neurosurgery* 15:57, 1984.
5. Awad IA, Carter LP, Spetzler RF, et al.: Clinical vasospasm after subarachnoid hemorrhage: Response to hypervolemic hemodilution and arterial hypertension. *Stroke* 18:365, 1987.
6. Bailes JE, Spetzler RF, Hadley MN, et al.: Management morbidity and mortality of poor-grade aneurysm patients. *J Neurosurg* 72:559, 1990.
7. Barker FG II, Heros RC: Clinical aspects of vasospasm. *Neurosurg Clin North Am* 1:277, 1990.
8. Carter LP, Grahm T, Bailes JE, et al.: Continuous post-operative monitoring of cortical blood flow and intracranial pressure. *Surg Neurol* 35:36, 1991.
9. Dion J, Duckwiler G, Vinuela F, et al.: Preoperative micro-angioplasty of refractory vasospasm secondary to subarachnoid hemorrhage. *Neuroradiology* 32:232, 1990.
10. Eskridge JM, Newell DW, Pendleton GA: Transluminal angioplasty for treatment of vasospasm. *Neurosurg Clin North Am* 1:387, 1990.
11. Ferguson G, Farrar J, Meguro K, et al.: Serial measurements of CBF as a guide to surgery in patients with ruptured aneurysms. *J Cereb Blood Flow Metab* 1(suppl 1):S518, 1981.
12. Fisher CM, Kistler JP, Davis JM: Relation of cerebral vasospasm to subarachnoid hemorrhage visualized by computed tomography scanning. *Neurosurgery* 6:1, 1980.
13. Guglielmi G, Vinuela F, Sepetka I, et al.: Electrothrombosis of saccular aneurysms via endovascular approach. Part 1: Electrochemical basis, technique and experimental results. *J Neurosurg* 75:1, 1991.
14. Haley EC, Torner JC, Kassell NF: Antifibrinolytic therapy and cerebral vasospasm. *Neurosurg Clin North Am* 1:349, 1990.
15. Hasan D, Vermeulen M, Wijdick EFM, et al.: Acute hydrocephalus after subarachnoid hemorrhage. *Stroke* 20:747, 1989.
16. Helm G, Meekin G, Phillips D, et al.: Intra-arterial papaverine for the treatment of cerebral vasospasm. *41st Annual Meeting of the Congress of Neurological Surgeons* Orlando, Florida, 1991.
17. Heros RC: Preoperative management of the patient with a ruptured intracranial aneurysm. *Semin Neurol* 4:430, 1984.
18. Heros RC: Acute hydrocephalus after subarachnoid hemorrhage. *Stroke* 20(6):715, 1989. Editorial.
19. Higashida RT, Halbach VV, Cahan LD, et al.: Transluminal angioplasty for treatment of intracranial arterial vasospasm. *J Neurosurg* 7:648, 1989.
20. Ishii R: Regional cerebral blood flow in patients with a ruptured intracranial aneurysm. *J Neurosurg* 50:587, 1979.
21. Jones TH, Morawitz RB, Crowell RM, et al.: Thresholds of focal cerebral ischemia in awake monkeys. *J Neurosurg* 54:773, 1981.

22. Kassell NF, Boarini DJ: Patients with a ruptured aneurysm: Pre- and postoperative management. In: Wilkins RH, Rengachary SS (eds): *Neurosurgery*. New York, McGraw-Hill, 1985, pp 1367–1371.
23. Kassell NF, Haley EC, Torner JC, et al.: Nicardipine and angiographic vasospasm. *J Neurosurg* 74:341A, 1991.
24. Kassell NF, Peerless SJ, Durward QJ, et al.: Treatment of ischemic deficits from vasospasm with intravascular expansion and induced arterial hypertension. *Neurosurgery* 11:337, 1982.
25. Kassell NF, Torner JC: Aneurysmal rebleeding: A preliminary report from the cooperative aneurysm study. *Neurosurgery* 13:479, 1983.
26. Kassell NF, Torner JC, Haley EC Jr, et al.: The international cooperative aneurysm study on the timing of surgery. Part 1: Overall management results. *J Neurosurg* 73:18, 1990.
27. Kelly PJ, Gorten RJ, Rose JE, et al.: Cerebral infarction and ruptured intracranial aneurysms. In: Wilkins RH (ed): *Cerebral Arterial Spasm: Proceedings of the Second International Workshop.* Baltimore: Williams & Wilkins, 1980, pp 366–371.
28. Kety SS, Schmidt CF: The deterioration of cerebral blood flow in man by the use of nitrous oxide in low concentrations. *Am J Physiol* 143:53, 1945.
29. Kosnik EJ, Hunt WE: Postoperative hypertension in the management of patients with intracranial arterial aneurysms. *J Neurosurg* 45:148, 1976.
30. Kwak R, Niizuma H, et al.: Angiographic study of cerebral vasospasm following rupture of intracranial aneurysms: Part I. Time of the appearance. *Surg Neurol* 11:257, 1979.
31. Levy ML, Giannotta SL: Induced hypertension and hypervolemia for treatment of cerebral vasospasm. *Neurosurg Clin North Am* 1:357, 1990.
32. Lindegaard KF, Nornes H, Bakke SJ, et al.: Cerebral vasospasm after subarachnoid hemorrhage investigated by means of transcranial Doppler ultrasound. *Acta Neurochir* 42(suppl):81, 1988.
33. Ljunggren B, Brandt L, Saveland H, et al.: Outcome in 60 consecutive patients treated with early aneurysm operation and intravenous nimodipine. *J Neurosurg* 61:864, 1984.
34. Marion DW, Segal R, Thompson ME: Subarachnoid hemorrhage and the heart. *Neurosurgery* 18:101, 1986.
35. Maroon JC, Nelson PB: Hypovolemia in patients with subarachnoid hemorrhage: Therapeutic implications. *Neurosurgery* 4:223, 1979.
36. Merory J, Thomas D, Humphrey P, et al.: Cerebral blood flow after surgery for recent subarachnoid hemorrhage. *J Neurol Neurosurg Psychiatry* 43:214, 1980.
37. Meyer FB: Calcium antagonists and vasospasm. *Neurosurg Clin North Am* 1:367, 1990.
38. Muizelaar JP, Becker DP: Induced hypertension for the treatment of cerebral ischemia after subarachnoid hemorrhage. Direct effect on cerebral blood flow. *Surg Neurol* 25:317, 1986.
39. Nelson PB, Seif SM, Maroon JC, et al.: Hyponatremia in intracranial disease: Perhaps not the syndrome of inappropriate secretion of antidiuretic hormone (SIADH). *J Neurosurg* 55:938, 1981.
40. Newell DW, Grady MS, Eskridge JM, et al.: Distribution of angiographic vasospasm after subarachnoid hemorrhage: Implications for diagnosis by transcranial Doppler ultrasonography. *Neurosurgery* 27:574, 1990.
41. Nilsson BW: Cerebral blood flow in patients with subarachnoid hemorrhage studied with an intravenous isotope technique: Its clinical significance in the timing of surgery of cerebral arterial aneurysm. *Acta Neurochir (Wien)* 37:33, 1977.
42. Origitano TC, Wascher TM, Reichman OH, et al.: Sustained increased cerebral blood flow with prophylactic hypertensive hypervolemia hemodilution ("triple-H") therapy after subarachnoid hemorrhage. *Neurosurgery* 27:729, 1990.
43. Pickard JG, Murray GD, Illingworth R, et al.: Effect of oral nimodipine on cerebral infarction and outcome after subarachnoid hemorrhage: British aneurysm nimodipine trial. *Br Med J* 298:636, 1989.
44. Powers WJ, Grubb RL, Baker RP, et al.: Regional cerebral blood flow and metabolism in reversible ischemia due to vasospasm. *J Neurosurg* 62:539, 1985.
45. Rosenstein J, Suzuki M, Symon L, et al.: Clinical use of a portable bedside cerebral blood flow machine in the management of aneurysmal subarachnoid hemorrhage. *Neurosurgery* 15:519, 1984.
46. Seiler RW, Grolimund P, Aaslid R, et al.: Relation of cerebral vasospasm evaluated by transcranial Doppler ultrasound to clinical grade and CT-visualized subarachnoid hemorrhage. *J Neurosurg* 64:594, 1986.
47. Sekhar LN, Weschler LR, Yonas H, et al.: Value of transcranial Doppler examination in the diagnosis of cerebral vasospasm after subarachnoid hemorrhage. *Neurosurgery* 22:812, 1988.
48. Solomon RA, Post KD, McMurty JG III: Depression of circulating blood volume in patients after subarachnoid hemorrhage: Implications for the management of symptomatic vasospasm. *Neurosurgery* 15:354, 1984.
48a. Torner J, Kassell N, Haley EC: The timing of surgery and vasospasm. *Neurosurg Clin North Am* 1:335, 1990.
49. Takamae T, Mizukami M, Kim H, et al.: Computed tomography of ruptured intracranial aneurysms in acute stage – relationship between vasospasm and high density on CT scan. *No To Shinkei* 30:861, 1978.
50. Vidal BE, Dergal EB, Cesarman E, et al.: Cardiac ar-

rhythmias associated with subarachnoid hemorrhage: Prospective study. *Neurosurgery* 5:657, 1979.

51. Weir B: The effect of clot removal in cerebral vasospasm. *Neurosurg Clin North Am* 1:377, 1990.
52. Wood JH, Snyder LL, Simeone FA: Failure of intravascular volume expansion without hemodilution to elevate cortical blood flow in region of experimental focal ischemia. *J Neurosurg* 56:80, 1982.
53. Yamamoto M, Meyer J, Naritomi H, et al.: Non-invasive measurement of cerebral vasospasm in patients with subarachnoid hemorrhage. *J Neurol Sci* 43:301, 1979.
54. Yonas H, Johnson D: Irreversible ischemia determined by xenon-enhanced computed tomographic cerebral blood flow studies. In: Yonas H (ed): *Cerebral Blood Flow Measurement with Stable Xenon-Enhanced Computed Tomography*. New York, Raven Press, 1992, pp 170–174.
55. Zubkov YN, Nikiforov BM, Shustin VA: Balloon catheter technique for dilatation of constricted cerebral arteries after aneurysmal SAH. *Acta Neurochir (Wien)* 70:65, 1984.

CHAPTER 14

The Intensive Care Management of Nontraumatic Intracerebral Hemorrhage

William G. Obana
Brian T. Andrews

INTRODUCTION

Spontaneous intracerebral hemorrhage (ICH) accounts for 6.3 to 12 percent of all new strokes in the United States each year, two-thirds of which are fatal.[1] The average annual incidence of spontaneous ICH in the United States is 9 per 100,000 population. Men are more commonly affected than women, and about two-thirds are between 45 and 75 years old.

Computed tomography (CT) has improved localization and facilitated earlier and more accurate diagnosis of spontaneous ICH.[2–5] Although several recent series have evaluated nonoperative versus operative treatment, timing of surgery, and usefulness of intracranial pressure (ICP) monitoring in determining management, the optimal treatment of nontraumatic ICH remains unsettled. Regardless of the treatment employed, the majority of these patients require monitoring and management in the intensive care unit (ICU).

ETIOLOGY AND PATHOPHYSIOLOGY

Arterial Hypertension

Hypertensive cerebrovascular disease accounts for 70 to 90 percent of spontaneous ICH.[6,7] However, this percentage appears to be decreasing because of improved methods of blood pressure control in hypertensive patients.[8] The most common sources of hemorrhage are small penetrating arteries (80 to 300 μm), including the thalamoperforating and lenticulostriate arteries and paramedian branches of the basilar artery.[9] There appears to be hypertension-induced degeneration of the media of the arterial wall, or fibrinoid necrosis, resulting in progressive weakening and/or development of microaneurysms.[9–11] What precipitates the actual hemorrhage is unclear, although sudden elevations in blood pressure coincident with exertion or activity are common.[12,13]

The predilection of hypertension-induced pathologic changes for small subcortical and perforating arteries helps explain the typical anatomic location of these hemorrhages. The most commonly affected region is the caudate and putamen (35 to 45 percent) (Fig. 14-1), followed by the subcortical white matter (25 percent), thalamus (20 percent), cerebellum (10 to 20 percent), and pons (5 percent).[8,14-16] Notably, 90 percent of pontine hemorrhages are due to hypertension, while about 60 to 75 percent of putaminal, thalamic, and cerebellar hemorrhages have a hypertensive etiology.[8] Hypertension does not appear to be a significant etiologic factor in lobar hemorrhages.[17,18] Rebleeding is considered rare,[4] although a recent review of 518 hypertensive hemorrhages found a recurrent bleeding rate of 2.7 percent.[19] The main cause of delayed deterioration is secondary to cerebral edema and ischemic necrosis of surrounding brain tissue or hydrocephalus (Fig. 14-1).[13]

Intracranial Aneurysms

Hemorrhage from ruptured intracranial aneurysms is usually into the subarachnoid space and less frequently into the lateral ventricles or brain parenchyma. However, reviews of spontaneous ICH have shown ruptured aneurysms to be the cause in 18 to 23 percent of cases.[15,20] Hemorrhage is usually into the frontal or temporal lobes and is due to internal carotid or middle cerebral artery aneurysms. The probability of aneurysmal rebleeding is about 4 percent within the first 24 h following the initial hemorrhage, and then 1.5 percent daily. The incidence of rebleeding averages about 19 percent during the first 2 weeks, 64 percent at 1 month, and up to 78 percent at 2 months.[21]

The pathogenesis of aneurysm formation and bleeding is controversial. These lesions are thought by some to be due to a congenital weakness in the muscular layer which allows the intima to bulge through, eventually rupturing the elastic membrane. Others think that these lesions are acquired and that degenerative changes in the internal elastic membrane allow the intima to herniate through a weakened area. Some think it is a combination of both processes which leads to the de-

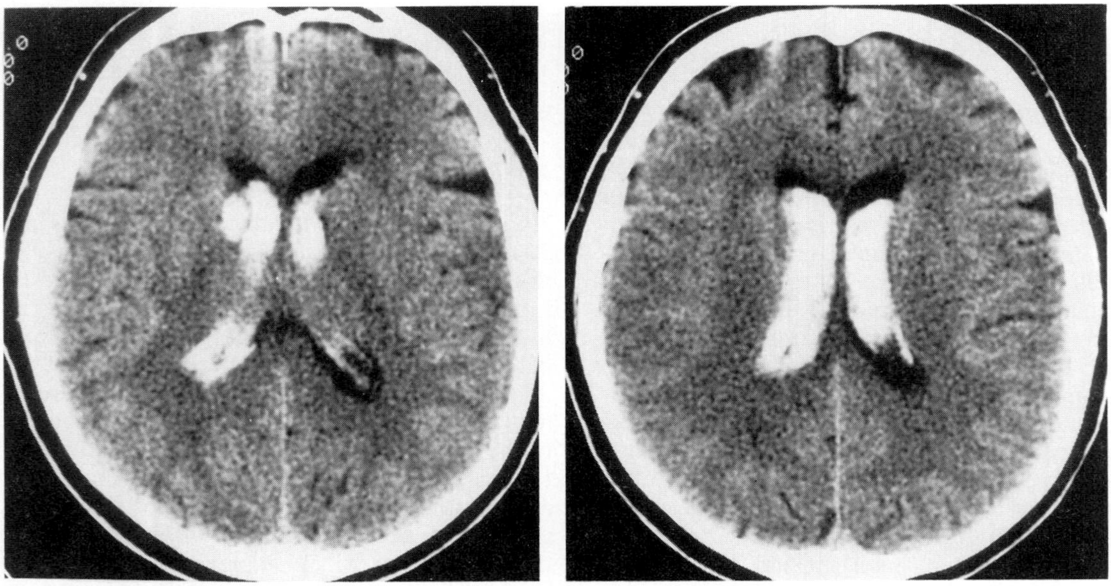

Figure 14-1 Axial CT scans of the head showing a right caudate hemorrhage with ventricular rupture in a 52-year-old hypertensive woman with headache and confusion. Shortly thereafter, the patient showed signs and symptoms of obstructive hydrocephalus and was treated with a ventriculostomy. She recovered with only a mild deficit in mentation.

velopment of these lesions. The management of aneurysmal subarachnoid hemorrhage is more fully discussed in Chap. 13.

Mycotic aneurysms, which account for 1 to 2 percent of all cerebral aneurysms, result most often from septic emboli to the brain from bacterial endocarditis.[22,23] They bleed most commonly into brain parenchyma due to their location distal to the circle of Willis and usually into the parietal lobe[5] (Fig. 14-2).

Intracranial aneurysms may rarely occur following head trauma, usually along the pericallosal artery adjacent to the falx or on distal branches of the middle cerebral artery on the cortical surface adjacent to skull fractures. Traumatic aneurysms usually result in parenchymal hemorrhage weeks, months, or years following major head injury.[24]

Cerebral Amyloid Angiopathy

Cerebral amyloid angiopathy is probably the third most common cause of ICH behind arterial hypertension and intracranial aneurysms, accounting for up to 10 percent of spontaneous ICH.[25] Forty to seventy percent of patients with autopsy-proven cerebral amyloid angiopathy die from the effects of hemorrhage.[26,27] Cerebral amyloid angiopathy is a condition characterized by deposits of amyloid fibrils in the media and intima of small and medium-sized arteries in the brain and leptomeninges of the elderly patient.[8,25–29] Bleeding may be due to either rupture of a weakened vessel wall or a microaneurysm.[8,26,29] The incidence of amyloid angiopathy on postmortem examination has been reported to be 8 percent in the seventh decade and

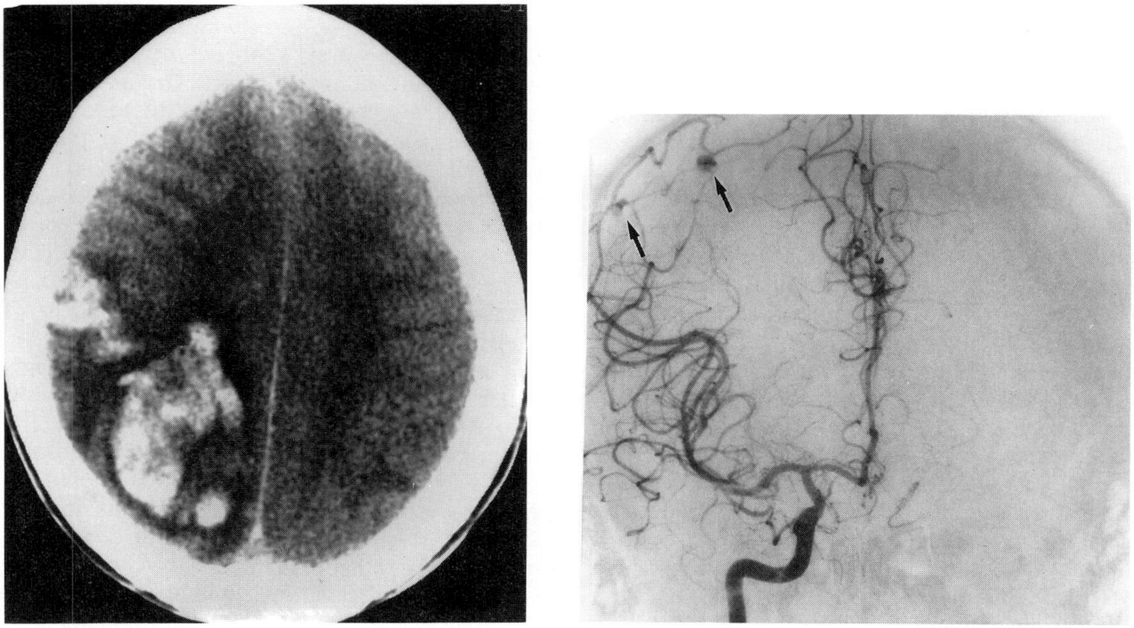

Figure 14-2 Axial CT scans of the head (left) showing a right parietal hemorrhage in a 24-year-old intravenous drug abuser with bacteremia. Cerebral angiography (right) demonstrates multiple bacterial aneurysms on distal branches of the middle cerebral artery (arrows). A craniotomy was performed for evacuation of the hematoma, and the bilateral bacterial aneurysms were subsequently treated using stereotactic guidance. The patient remains neurologically intact.

almost 60 percent in the tenth decade.[8] In one series, amyloid angiopathy was demonstrated at autopsy in 7 of 41 (17.1 percent) patients who died of spontaneous ICH and in 3 of 39 (7.7 percent) surgically treated patients with nonfatal lesions.[29]

Cerebral amyloid angiopathy is not associated with systemic amyloid angiopathy and occurs sporadically, although familial occurrences have been reported.[25,30,31] An association with Alzheimer's has been postulated since senile plaques have been seen in over 50 percent of cases and 10 to 30 percent of patients exhibit progressive dementia.[8,25,26,29] In contrast to hypertensive hemorrhages, it has a predilection for the superficial layers of the cerebral cortex, especially the parietal and occipital lobes, and is rarely seen in the deep white or gray matter.[25,28] Multiple spontaneous hemorrhages in a normotensive elderly patient are most likely to be due to amyloid angiopathy.[25] Recurrent hemorrhage is not uncommon in both operative and nonoperative cases.[8,25,29,32]

Vascular Malformations

Intracranial vascular malformations are generally divided into four pathologic types: (1) arteriovenous malformations (AVMs), (2) capillary telangiectasias, (3) cavernous malformations ("angiomas"), and (4) venous malformations ("angiomas").[33,34]

Arteriovenous malformations account for 6 to 13 percent of spontaneous ICHs.[15,20] They are congenital abnormalities which develop between the fourth and eighth weeks of embryonic life.[33–35] There is persistence of a direct communication between the arterial and venous system without an intervening capillary bed. A nidus of tortuous vessels is fed by arteries, which progressively enlarge over time because of the high flow volume resulting from the low peripheral resistance of the arteriovenous shunt. Sustained elevations in venous pressure and high flow volumes cause progressive enlargement of the draining veins.[35] The development of venous outflow restriction or varicies may increase the risk of hemorrhage.

Arteriovenous malformations are located predominantly in the cerebral hemispheres (70 to 93 percent) and most commonly involve branches of the middle cerebral artery. In general, the risk of subarachnoid or intraparenchymal hemorrhage from an intraparenchymal AVM following diagnosis is about 3 to 4 percent per year.[35–39] Although the risk of hemorrhage in patients who present with seizures and have no history of bleeding has been reported to be lower (1 to 2.3 percent),[36,40] a recent series of 166 patients with an average of 24 years' follow-up reported a similar hemorrhage rate (3.9 and 4.3 percent) regardless of the manner of presentation.[39] The rate of hemorrhage may be higher during the first year following diagnosis even in patients without a history of hemorrhage.[37,41] There is no conclusive data to show that smaller AVMs are more likely to bleed than larger ones.[37]

Capillary telangiectasias are small, solitary, abnormally dilated capillaries with intervening brain parenchyma. They are found predominantly in the pons and the roof of the fourth ventricle. They are only occasionally associated with spontaneous hemorrhage.[33–35,42]

Cavernous malformations are dilated sinusoidal vascular anomalies without intervening neural tissue except at the margins. They vary in size, occasionally are multiple, and are found mainly in the cerebral hemispheres. With the advent of magnetic resonance imaging (MRI), diagnosis of angiographically occult lesions has led to a clearer understanding of the natural history of the disease.[43,44] These lesions most commonly present with headache, seizures, or focal neurologic deficits.[43,44] Although MRI usually shows evidence of occult bleeding, overt hemorrhage is infrequent. The estimated risk of clinically significant hemorrhage is 0.25 to 0.7 percent per person-year of exposure.[43,44]

Venous malformations are collections of veins which are arranged in a radial fashion and drain into a central vein.[33,34,42] There is intervening neural parenchyma within the vascular malformation. They are located usually in the frontal or parietal lobes or in deep cerebellar white matter. Diagnosis is incidental. Although previous reports have found a rather high incidence of hemorrhage (17 to 22 percent) associated with these lesions,[45,46] these studies included only those patients who were diagnosed after the development of significant complications. If all patients with radiographically identifiable venous angiomas are included, the estimated risk of hemorrhage has been reported to be 0.22 percent per year[47] (Garner, 1991). These findings justify a conservative approach.

A venous varix, once considered a separate pathologic type of vascular malformation,[33] is now thought to be a variant of a venous malformation.[34] It consists of a single dilated vein not associated with an arteriovenous shunt.[34] Spontaneous hemorrhage of a varix is extremely rare.

Brain Tumors

Spontaneous hemorrhage into a brain tumor has been reported to be less than 1 percent in most series of brain tumors, whereas underlying tumors are found in 2 to 10 percent of patients with ICH.[11,48,49] The most common types of tumors to hemorrhage are malignant gliomas and metastases, most often melanoma, renal cell carcinoma, choriocarcinoma, and bronchogenic carcinoma.[48-50] The propensity of malignant tumors to bleed is thought to be related to their tendency to undergo spontaneous necrosis due to rapid growth and their rich but friable vasculature.[8] Benign tumors rarely demonstrate spontaneous hemorrhage.

Anticoagulants

Warfarin sodium, an oral anticoagulant, is often used to prevent venous or arterial embolism. Approximately 8 percent of patients taking warfarin sodium have bleeding complications.[51] Although intracranial hemorrhages account for only 0.5 to 1.5 percent of all these complications, the consequences are usually devastating. Patients who are orally anticoagulated have an 11 times higher risk of ICH than nonanticoagulated patients with similar risk factors.[52] About 80 percent of anticoagulated patients suffering an ICH have excessively prolonged prothrombin time (greater than 16 to 18 s), although the therapeutic range varies among studies.[8] Although some have found that increasing age, a preceding cerebral infarction, hypertension, and increased duration of anticoagulant therapy increase the risk of ICH, others have found no such relationship.[52-55] Head trauma does not appear to be a significant etiology of ICH in these patients.[55] The most common location of hemorrhage is the subdural space followed by brain parenchyma and then subarachnoid hemorrhage.[55]

Hereditary Bleeding Disorders

Hemophilia and von Willebrand's disease account for over 90 percent of severe hereditary bleeding defects.[56] Hemophilia is an X-linked recessive deficiency of factor VIII (hemophilia A) or less frequently factor IX (hemophilia B).[4,56,57] There is prolongation of partial thromboplastin time. Clinical presentations of this disorder vary, based on the degree of factor deficiency as determined by in vitro clotting assays. Intracranial hemorrhages can occur spontaneously or arise from apparently trivial head trauma.

Von Willebrand's disease is an autosomal dominant disorder characterized by a deficiency in factor VIII activity, a prolonged bleeding time, and abnormal ristocetin platelet aggregation.[56] Major events such as surgery do not present as severe a risk to patients with von Willebrand's disease as it does to patients with hemophilia. Spontaneous ICH is uncommon.

Thrombocytopenia

Thrombocytopenia (platelet counts below 80,000/mm^3) is the most common cause of abnormal bleeding resulting from either decreased platelet production or increased peripheral sequestration or destruction.[4,56] Causes of decreased platelet production include aplastic anemia, leukemia, other bone marrow failure states, and following cytotoxic chemotherapy. Causes of increased platelet destruction include idiopathic (autoimmune) thrombocytopenic purpura, secondary and drug-induced immune thrombocytopenias, thrombotic thrombocytopenia purpura, hemolytic uremic syndrome, disseminated intravascular coagulation, and vasculitis. In general, platelet counts greater than 50,000/mm^3 are not associated with significant hemorrhagic complications, and severe spontaneous bleeding is rare with platelet counts greater than 20,000/mm^3.[56] Although uncommon, spontaneous ICH does occur and is characterized by insidious onset of headache followed by a deterioration in the level of consciousness.[4] Subdural hematomas are less frequent.

Sympathomimetic Drugs

Amphetamines,[58] phenylpropanolamine,[59] and cocaine[60] are sympathomimetic drugs which have been most commonly associated with hemorrhagic stroke. Specifically, cocaine use in the United States has risen dramatically over the past decade, and this has been paralleled by an increase in cocaine-related strokes.[60] In a recent review of 47 patients with cocaine-related strokes, the average age of occurrence was 32 years, with patients in their twenties being most commonly affected.[60] ICH occurred in 49 percent of patients, subarachnoid hemorrhage in 29 percent, and cerebral infarction in 22 percent. Twenty-three of 32 (72 percent) patients undergoing cerebral angiography were found to have abnormalities, including aneurysms,[12] AVMs,[5] vasculitis,[2] and arterial vasospasm, occlusions, or stenosis.[6] Two patients had two anomalies.

It has been postulated that transient elevations in blood pressure following administration of these drugs may be responsible for rupture of cerebral blood vessels, including intracranial aneurysms and AVMs.[8,60] In addition, hemorrhage due to angiographically proven vasculitis has been seen, raising the possibility of a drug-induced angiopathy.[8,60,61] In this case, pathologically, there is a necrotizing angiitis characterized by fibrinoid degeneration and necrosis of the media and intima of medium-sized and small arteries and arterioles.[8,61] Whether these changes are due to a direct toxic effect of the drug or a hypersensitivity reaction to the drug or its vehicle is unclear.[8]

CLINICAL PRESENTATION

Spontaneous ICH is characterized by abrupt onset and relatively rapid evolution of symptoms over minutes, hours, or occasionally days.[62] Hemorrhages secondary to anticoagulant therapy usually have a slower progression of symptoms. There are typically no warning signs; patients commonly feel entirely normal immediately preceding the ictus.

At the time of presentation, 72 percent of all patients with ICH are comatose and 8 percent are stuporous,[1] although lobar hemorrhages appear to have a lower incidence of coma.[17] Among noncomatose patients, 60 percent are hemiplegic, 43 percent have speech difficulties, 13 percent have pupillary abnormalities, and 16 percent have seizures.[7]

Headaches are present in only 33 percent of patients at the onset of symptoms and in 60 percent before, during, or after the development of neurologic deficits.[1] Severe headaches or progressively worsening headaches in conjunction with a neurologic deficit should alert one to the possibility of an ICH. Although headaches are usually nonspecific, Ropper and Davis found that their location may be helpful in predicting the site of lobar hemorrhages.[17]

Vomiting occurs in about 51 percent of patients.[1] It occurs much more commonly at the onset of ICH than with infarction.[62]

Neurologic symptoms and signs depend on the location and size of the hemorrhage. Clinical syndromes based on hemorrhages in certain anatomical locations have been delineated and will briefly be reviewed. These are most commonly related to hypertension.

Putamen

Putaminal hemorrhage is characterized by a progressive onset in almost two-thirds of patients, while less than one-third develop symptoms which are abrupt and nearly maximal at onset.[4,13] In one series of 27 consecutive patients, headaches were present at the onset of symptoms in only 14 percent and at any time in only 28 percent; all these patients displayed some form of motor deficit and about 65 percent had an alteration in response to pinprick.[13]

Small putaminal hemorrhages cause moderate contralateral motor and sensory deficits. Moderate-sized hemorrhages may present initially with a flaccid hemiplegia, hemisensory deficit, conjugate deviation of the eyes to the side of the hemorrhage, homonymous hemianopia, and dysphasia if the dominant hemisphere is involved. Progression to a massive hemorrhage results in stupor and then coma, respiratory variations, fixed and dilated pupils, loss of extraocular movements, abnormal motor posturing, and bilateral Babinski responses.[4,13,62,63]

Thalamus

The clinical syndrome of thalamic hemorrhage has been well characterized.[2,10,62,64] In general, small thalamic hemorrhages result in more pronounced neurologic deficits compared to putaminal hemorrhages. As with putaminal hemorrhages, a contralateral hemiparesis is seen when the internal capsule is compressed. However, there is a characteristic dense contralateral hemisensory loss encompassing the head, face, arm, and trunk. Extension of the hemorrhage into the subthalamus and brainstem produces classic ocular features including limitation of vertical gaze, downward eye deviation, and small but reactive or sluggish pupils.[2,64] Anisocoria, absence of convergence, unreactive pupils, skew deviation, visual field deficits, ptosis, and retraction nystagmus are also seen. Anosognosia associated with right-sided hemorrhages and speech disorders associated with left-sided lesions are not uncommon. Headache is present in 20 to 40 percent of patients.[2] Hydrocephalus can also develop due to compression of cerebrospinal fluid pathways.[4]

Pons

Pontine hemorrhages are the most uniformly devastating of all brain hemorrhages. Even small hemorrhages usually lead to immediate coma, pinpoint (1 mm) but reactive pupils, disturbances of lateral ocular movements, cranial nerve abnormalities, quadriplegia, and extensor posturing.[4,7,62] Headache, nausea, and vomiting are rare.

Cerebellum

The clinical syndrome of cerebellar hemorrhage was first clearly delineated by Fisher and coworkers.[65] Characteristically, there is a sudden onset of nausea, vomiting, and inability to walk or stand.[65] Depending on the evolution of the hemorrhage, different severities of neurologic dysfunction occur. Hypertension is an etiologic factor in the majority of cases.[66]

In a retrospective study of 56 patients with spontaneous cerebellar hemorrhage, over two-thirds had an altered level of consciousness and were still responsive at the time of admission; only 14 percent were comatose on admission.[66] Fifty percent of patients became comatose by 24 h and 75 percent by 1 week after onset.[66] Nausea and vomiting were present in 95 percent, headaches (commonly bioccipital) in 73 percent, and dizziness in 55 percent.[66] Of the 32 patients questioned, inability to walk or stand was present in 94 percent.[66] Among the noncomatose patients, cerebellar signs were common and included gait ataxia (78 percent), truncal ataxia (65 percent), and ipsilateral appendicular ataxia (65 percent).[66] Other findings including peripheral facial nerve palsy (61 percent), ipsilateral gaze palsy (54 percent), horizontal nystagmus (51 percent), and miosis (30 percent).[66] Hemiplegia or hemiparesis have been found to be rare, and when present are usually attributable to previous or concomitant occlusive strokes,[65,66] The clinical triad of appendicular ataxia, ipsilateral gaze palsy, and peripheral facial palsy was thought to be suggestive of a cerebellar hemorrhage.[66]

Midline cerebellar hemorrhages pose more of a diagnostic dilemma on clinical examination. In general, these patients have a more fulminant course and present with total ophthalmoplegia, areflexia, and flaccid quadriplegia.[66]

In comatose patients, the clinical diagnosis of cerebellar hemorrhage is more difficult due to severe brainstem dysfunction. Among the comatose patients in the aforementioned series, 83 percent had complete external ophthalmoplegia, 53 percent had respiratory irregularities, and 54 percent had ipsilateral facial weakness.[66] Pupils were uniformly small; there was no pupillary reaction to light in 40 percent of the cases.[66]

Lobar

The acute clinical syndromes of lobar hemorrhage in 26 patients have been outlined by Ropper and Davis.[17] Chronic hypertension was present in only 31 percent of the patients, and only one patient was comatose at the time of admission. Occipital hemorrhage typically caused severe pain around the ipsilateral eye and dense hemianopsia. Left temporal hemorrhage was characterized by mild pain in or just anterior to the ear, fluent dysphasia with poor auditory comprehension but relatively good repetition. Frontal hemorrhage caused severe contralateral arm weakness, minimal face and leg weakness, and frontal headache. Parietal hemorrhage began with anterior temporal ("temple") headache and hemisensory deficit, sometimes involving the trunk to the midline. A more rapid but not instantaneous evolution of symptoms over several minutes combined with one of these syndromes helped distinguish lobar hemorrhages from other types of stroke.[17] Most AVMs and tumors have a lobar location.

Cortical

The clinical manifestations of spontaneous cortical hemorrhage are dependent on the size and location of the hemorrhage. When these lesions occur in normotensive, demented, elderly patients, the most likely cause is cerebral amyloid angiopathy.[25] Multiple or repeated hemorrhage further solidifies the diagnosis. Although they can be lobar in location, they differ from lobar hemorrhages in that they arise from the cortex. They occasionally extend into deep white matter and rupture into the lateral ventricle or superficially into the subarachnoid or subdural space.

Intraventricular

Spontaneous intraventricular hemorrhage is not associated with any distinct acute clinical syndrome. However, the sudden onset of a severe headache and nuchal rigidity should alert one to the possibility of a ruptured cerebral aneurysm, which occasionally ruptures into the ventricular system. In addition, progressive neurologic deterioration following onset of nonfocal symptoms could be suggestive of acute obstructive hydrocephalus from intraventricular blood.

In general, symptoms and signs of intraventricular hemorrhage are related to the etiology of the hemorrhage and associated ICH. About 78 percent of ventricular hemorrhages are associated with a subarachnoid or parenchymal hemorrhage.[67] In a series of 32 patients with hypertensive hemorrhages, 62 percent had ruptured into the ventricular system.[68] A ruptured aneurysm or intraventricular AVM should be highly suspected if there is no associated parenchymal hemorrhage.

DIAGNOSIS AND IMAGING STUDIES

Careful review of the present illness and past medical history of the patient may provide important clues to the cause of the hemorrhage. In addition, a detailed general physical examination and neurologic examination are essential. Based on these findings and a knowledge of the previously mentioned clinical presentations of ICH, one should not only be alert for an intracranial mass lesion but also have an idea of its likely etiology and location. Computed tomographic scanning allows for rapid and accurate diagnosis of spontaneous ICH, including its size and location. The CT appearance of the hemorrhage is often suggestive of specific lesions (Fig. 14-1). Computed tomography scans with intravenous contrast may reveal an adjacent mass suggestive of a tumor of AVM, identifying the probable cause of the hemorrhage.

Further radiographic evaluation using MRI with intravenous gadolinium is indicated in a clinically stable patient if spontaneous hemorrhage occurs in a nonhypertensive patient with normal coagulation studies, the hemorrhage is in an unusual location in a hypertensive patient, the clinical presentation is suggestive of a nonhypertensive cause, or the initial CT scan is suggestive of an underlying lesion such as a tumor. Cerebral angiography should be performed in all patients suspected of having ICH due to an aneurysm, arteriovenous fistula, vascular malformation, or vasculitis (Fig. 14-2). Occasionally, the initial angiogram may be negative due to compression of the vascular abnormality by the hematoma. When an underlying vascular lesion is highly suspected, repeat angiography should be performed 2 to 3 weeks after the hematoma has resolved and edema decreased.

MEDICAL MANAGEMENT

Initial Evaluation and Management

The management of spontaneous ICH depends predominantly on the clinical state of the patient and the etiology, size, and location of the hemorrhage. However, irrespective of whether conservative or surgical therapy is employed, the initial evaluation and medical management of the patient is the same.

At the time of admission or consultation, evaluation and initial management should occur simultaneously without unnecessary delays. The initial neurologic examination, which can be performed in 10 min, should be comprehensive. This information is critical not only for determining prognosis but also for making subsequent treatment decisions. Serial neurologic examinations are performed thereafter as outlined in Chap. 2.

Standard measures for maintaining airway, breathing, and circulation are employed as described in Chap. 1. Hypoxia must be treated promptly in order to avoid secondary cerebral injury due to ischemia. Meticulous monitoring and control of blood pressure is essential in both hypertensive and nonhypertensive patients. An arterial line should be placed for continuous monitoring of blood pressure. Following ICH, most patients are hypertensive. It is important not to precipitously decrease blood pressure in a patient with an intracranial mass lesion and increased ICP, since there will be a concomitant drop in cerebral perfusion pressure. Initially, efforts should be made to maintain blood pressure at about 160 mmHg systolic in the awake patient and at about 180 mmHg in the comatose patient, although these values are somewhat arbitrary and will vary according to the individual patient. Those with a history of severe and poorly controlled hypertension may be allowed to maintain blood pressure at above 180 mmHg systolic, but usually below 210 mmHg, to avoid enlarging the hemorrhage by further rebleeding. For initial management of hypertension, we prefer to use labetalol, a competitive alpha-1, beta-1, and beta-2 antagonist. A nitroglycerin drip may be necessary in selected cases.

Arterial blood gases are obtained to assess oxygenation and the acid-base status of the patient. If the patient cannot safely protect his or her airway or an intracranial mass lesion with high ICP is suspected in an obtunded or comatose patient, endotracheal intubation is performed. Care must be taken to avoid anesthetic agents which will increase ICP such as nitrous oxide. Short-acting anesthetic agents are preferred. If increased ICP is suspected, hyperventilation is instituted to maintain a P_{CO_2} of 25 to 30 mmHg, and after a Foley catheter is placed, mannitol (1.5 g/kg) is given intravenously. These measures are also instituted in patients with progressive neurologic deterioration such as worsening hemiparesis, progressive anisocoria, or decreasing level of consciousness. An electrocardiogram is obtained, and heart rate is monitored.

Blood is obtained at the time an intravenous line is started. Complete blood count, platelet count, electrolytes, blood urea nitrogen, serum creatinine, prothrombin time, partial thromboplastin time, and liver function tests are evaluated. Plain radiographs are obtained as necessary.

Following this rapid evaluation and initial stabilization of the patient, a head CT scan without contrast is obtained. Once the diagnosis of ICH is made, the patient is taken for further radiographic studies as necessary, or to the ICU, operating room, or ward depending on clinical status, extent and location of hemorrhage, and etiology of the bleed. The initial goals of management are to prevent rebleeding and reduce mass effect, while subsequent treatment focuses on general medical care and prevention of complications.

Prevention of Rebleeding

Rebleeding is rare in hypertensive hemorrhages. By the time the patient presents to a physician, the active bleeding has usually ceased. Similarly, the risk of rebleeding from AVMs and tumors is also low. The main measure taken to prevent rebleeding in these patients is controlling increased blood pressure as previously outlined. In cases of hemorrhage from ruptured cerebral aneurysms, the risk of rebleeding is considerably higher. Efforts are made to maintain blood pressure at 10 to 20 percent above normotensive levels to prevent vasospasm but low enough to minimize the risk of hemorrhage. Some advocate the use of aminocaproic acid, an antifibrinolytic agent. However, its efficacy and indications for use remain unsettled.[69,70]

In cases of abnormal coagulation, the risk of rebleeding or continued bleeding is significant unless the coagulopathy is corrected. Patients with ICH due to anticoagulant therapy require prompt correction of their coagulation factors. Intravenous heparin (half-life of 1 to 2 h) should be discontinued, and protamine sulfate administered to immediately reverse the effects of heparin. Patients with ICH who are receiving warfarin should be given fresh frozen plasma to immediately reverse anticoagulation. Vitamin K (phytonadione), which takes less than 6 h to restore normal coagulation parameters, should also be given to aid in maintaining hemostasis. Coagulation studies should be monitored and additional fresh frozen plasma and vitamin K given as necessary.

Patients with ICH due to von Willebrand's disease or hemophilia A or B should have a prompt hematologic consultation. Patients with von Willebrand's disease should receive cryoprecipitate. Patients with hemophilia A should be given cryoprecipitate or lyophilized concentrates of factor VIII. Patients with hemophilia B may be given intravenous fresh frozen plasma or concentrates rich in factors II, VII, IX, and X. Blood levels of the clotting factors should be kept at least at 20 to 30 percent of normal if surgery to evacuate the hematoma is not performed and at 50 to 100 percent of normal if surgery is necessary. If ICH occurs in a patient with a yet to be identified congenital bleeding defect, fresh frozen plasma should be given. This will provide all clotting factors except platelets.

Patients with ICH due to thrombocytopenia should receive platelet transfusions regardless of the etiology of the thrombocytopenia to maintain platelet counts of at least $100{,}000/mm^3$. In patients with decreased platelet production, platelet survival time is usually normal, so the platelet count can be maintained by repeated transfusions. In cases of increased platelet destruction, platelet survival is markedly shortened and transfused platelets may circulate for as brief a period as 1 h. Thus, platelet transfusions are of much more limited value. In these cases, after the initial transfusion of platelets, corticosteroids are often helpful in raising platelet counts. Oftentimes, splenectomy is necessary to remove the area of massive platelet sequestration.

Reduction of Mass Effect

Reduction of mass effect can be accomplished both medically and surgically. In patients with increased ICP and/or more focal areas of mass effect, nonoperative efforts to decrease mass effect are important in preventing secondary cerebral ischemia and life-threatening brainstem compression. Management of increased ICP is discussed in detail in Chap. 3. Measures which we use to reduce increased ICP include (1) head-of-bed elevation to 30° in order to decrease intracranial venous volume and improve venous drainage; (2) intravenous mannitol (1.5 g/kg bolus initially, then 0.5 g/kg every 4 to 6 h to keep serum osmolarity at 295 to 310 mOsm/L; (3) mild fluid restriction (at 67 to 75 percent of maintenance) with supplement fluid boluses using colloid solutions as necessary; (4) ventriculostomy with ICP monitoring and drainage of cerebrospinal fluid to maintain an ICP less than 20 mmHg; and (5) endotracheal intubation and hyperventilation, maintaining the P_{CO_2} at 25 to 30 mmHg.

In awake patients with regional mass effect from ICH, head-of-bed elevation, fluid restriction, and mannitol are usually sufficient. These measures are designed to improve cerebral perfusion pressure and minimize secondary ischemic injury. It must be emphasized that cerebral perfusion pressure is equal to mean arterial blood pressure minus intracranial pressure, so systemic blood pressure must be maintained at normal or, preferably, at slightly higher than normal levels. We aim for a cerebral perfusion pressure of at least 70 mmHg, using vasopressors such as intravenous dopamine or phenylephrine if necessary.

Awake patients are monitored with serial neurologic examinations, and ICP monitoring is rarely required. In comatose patients who are not moribund, we routinely monitor ICP. We prefer a ventriculostomy, since this allows us to drain cerebrospinal fluid and thus more easily control ICP. In the case of intraventricular hemorrhage, this is essential because hydrocephalus often develops due to loss of cerebrospinal fluid outflow. In addition, we prefer drainage of cerebrospinal fluid via a ventriculostomy over hyperventilation for more long-term control of ICP. Monitoring ICP facilitates assessment of the efficacy of medical management and helps one decide whether surgical intervention is necessary. Although many have shown ICP monitoring to be useful in guiding treatment of ICH, it has not conclusively been shown to improve outcome.[16,17,71-73]

The use of corticosteroids to reduce focal cerebral edema associated with ICH has been reported to be beneficial in many anecdotal cases and is often advocated. However, its efficacy in ICH has yet to be clearly demonstrated in a controlled trial of spontaneous ICH. There have been only two studies evaluating the effect of corticosteroids on intracerebral hemorrhage.[74,75]

One randomized study on the effect of dexamethasone on ICH found no beneficial effect,[74] but there were several shortcomings of the study including lack of stratification according to level of consciousness, outcome measures, small study population, and lack of uniformity among cases of the disease under treatment.[75] The other study was a double-blind randomized trial evaluating the effect of dexamethasone in primary supratentorial hemorrhage.[75] In this study, dexamethasone (10 mg IV initially, followed by 5 mg IV every 6 h for 6 days, 5 mg IV every 12 h for 2 days, and 5 mg IV for 1 day) was found to have no beneficial effect on outcome. Furthermore, those patients treated with dexamethasone had significantly more complications (infection and diabetes) compared to the placebo group, leading to early termination of the study. Nevertheless, we commonly use high-dose dexamethasone (4 mg every 6 h IV) in patients with parenchymal hemorrhage who show CT evidence of marked cerebral edema.

General Care

The benefits of nimodipine in the management of subarachnoid hemorrhage from ruptured cerebral aneurysms is well known.[76,77] In patients with intraventricular hemorrhage or combined subarachnoid and parenchymal hemorrhage due to aneurysmal rupture, nimodipine (60 mg by mouth or nasogastric tube every 4 h) should be administered. However, its use in nonaneurysmal ICH has not been established. At present, we do not use nimodipine in patients with spontaneous nonaneurysmal ICH.

Anticonvulsants are given once the diagnosis of a supratentorial ICH is made unless the hemorrhage is limited to the thalamus or basal ganglia. We initially prefer phenytoin since therapeutic blood levels can be attained in 1 h with intravenous administration, it is easy to administer, and it is effective in preventing generalized seizures. In adults, a 1-g IV load (50 mg/min) is given followed by 300 to 400 mg IV or orally daily. Blood pressure must be monitored during intravenous loading since too-rapid infusion can result in abrupt decreases in blood pressure. In addition, the electrocardiogram should be monitored since phenytoin has been associated with cardiac arrhythmias including widening of the PR interval and Q waves with subsequent vascular collapse. Phenytoin levels should be monitored frequently and doses adjusted until the serum phenytoin level is within the therapeutic range (10 to 20 μg/mL) and the patient is seizure-free.

Other anticonvulsants used include phenobarbital (60 mg IV or orally twice daily; therapeutic blood levels 20 to 40 μg/mL) and carbamazepine (200 mg orally 3 to 4 times daily, therapeutic levels 4 to 12 μg/mL). Seizures can be associated with dramatic increases in ICP and systemic blood pressure, which may lead to rehemorrhage and thus must be avoided. Furthermore, hypoxia and acidosis are frequently seen during seizure activity, potentially adding to secondary cerebral injury.

Careful metabolic management of patients with ICH is necessary. Fluid status, serum electrolytes, and renal function should be assessed frequently, especially in those patients who are fluid-restricted, receiving mannitol or other diuretics, or not eating. Adequate nutrition is essential. These areas are reviewed in greater detail in other chapters.

Aggressive pulmonary care is used to prevent mucous plugs, aspiration, and pneumonia. Pneumatic compression stockings and antiembolic hose are placed to prevent deep venous thrombosis. Physical therapy is started early, emphasizing range of motion. Wrist and ankle splints are placed in comatose patients to prevent flexion contractures.

Additional Studies

Further imaging studies should be performed if the etiology of the hemorrhage is initially unclear. This might include repeated MRI scans with and without intravenous gadolinium and/or cerebral angiograms. Follow-up head CT scans should be obtained at least once per week for several weeks following the hemorrhage in order to assess resolution of the hematoma and also to check for the development of communicating hydrocephalus, particularly in cases of intraventricular hemorrhage. Delayed hydrocephalus could be responsible for lack of clinical improvement or deterioration in some patients. Computed tomography scans thus should be obtained more frequently if the patient exhibits any evidence of rehemorrhage or neurologic deterioration.

SURGICAL MANAGEMENT

Indications for Surgery

The indications for surgical treatment of ICH remain controversial but depend predominantly on the etiology, location, and size of the hemorrhage and the clinical state of the patient. It remains to be seen whether stereotactic evacuation of intraparenchymal hematomas will have a significant impact on general management, especially in cases of deep-seated lesions. This area has been reviewed extensively and will be discussed only briefly.

Etiology of Hemorrhage The role of surgery in hypertensive ICH remains unsettled, but it appears that in the majority of cases conservative therapy is as efficacious as surgical therapy. Only in selected circumstances such as cerebellar hemorrhage or occasionally in lobar or putaminal hemorrhages with progressive neurologic deterioration can surgery be strongly advocated. This is discussed further in the next section. On the other hand, the benefit of surgery in nonhypertensive ICH is more clear.

Surgical treatment of spontaneous ICH due to cerebral amyloid angiopathy should be avoided. Surgery can be associated with uncontrollable intraoperative bleeding and postoperative hemorrhage. In a recent review of 35 cases of surgically treated cerebral amyloid angiopathy, postoperative mortality was 37 percent.[25] Of those who survived, 43 percent had subsequent fatal hemorrhages within 3 months to 4 years after the initial event.[25] Most patients who are in good neurologic condition do not have increased ICP and do not require surgical decompression. Those who are in poor neurologic condition and undergo immediate operative treatment uniformly die or are severely disabled. It has been recommended that treatment of patients with massive cerebral hemorrhage due to amyloid angiopathy diagnosed by its characteristic CT appearance should be restricted to supportive measures.

Arteriovenous malformations, which have bled, rarely require emergent operative intervention. Only when there is life-threatening increased ICP or impending brainstem compression from the hematoma should immediate surgery for hematoma removal be considered. Even in these instances, all efforts should be made to manage the patient medically, since such procedures not infrequently result in catastrophic and uncontrollable bleeding. Since the risk of rebleeding is low, we prefer to wait at least a week before surgical intervention. This allows time for cerebral edema to resolve and for the patient to improve, and enables us to obtain an angiogram with less distortion from mass effect for precise surgical planning. Endovascular and open surgical approaches are used alone or in combination.[78]

The timing of surgery for ruptured cerebral aneurysms should not be influenced by an associated ICH unless the patient is deteriorating due to mass effect. If evacuation of the hematoma is necessary, all efforts should be made to repair the aneurysm at the same operation.[4] The treatment of ruptured cerebral aneurysms is discussed in more detail in Chap. 13.

Spontaneous ICH from a suspected brain tumor warrants surgical exploration and biopsy of the hematoma cavity. This need not be performed emergently unless there is life-threatening increased ICP or a progression of a neurologic deficit. A preoperative MRI scan and, if necessary, cerebral angiogram should be obtained.

Surgical removal of spontaneous ICH in patients with a coagulopathy is dependent on the clinical state of the patient and on the ability to correct the bleeding disorder. A patient with a progressive neurologic deficit, correctable coagulation abnormalities, and an accessible lesion is a candidate for surgical evacuation of the hematoma. Those with uncorrectable bleeding diathesis should not be considered for operative treatment. If ICH was due to anticoagulant therapy, anticoagulants should not be restarted for at least 1 week postoperatively. In cases of ICH due to thrombocytopenia, the platelet count should be kept above $100{,}000/mm^3$ for 1 week postoperatively. In patients with hemophilia or von Willebrand's disease, blood levels of clotting factors should be maintained at 50 to 100 percent of normal for 7 to 10 days postoperatively.

The role of surgery for ICH associated with the

use of sympathomimetic agents in patients without vascular abnormalities is the same as hypertensive hemorrhages. Those patients with drug-induced rupture of cerebral aneurysms or AVMs are considered for surgery as previously outlined.

Location and Size of Hypertensive Hemorrhage The surgical indications for removal of hypertensive putaminal hemorrhages remain unsettled. It is generally agreed that patients with hemorrhages less than 3 cm in diameter or with larger hemorrhages which extend into the midbrain or are associated with evidence of brainstem compression do not benefit from surgical evacuation.[4,63,79–84] In the latter group, surgical evacuation can be lifesaving, but improvement to better than a vegetative or severely disabled state is rare.

The management of patients with "moderate" hemorrhages is less clear. Some series have shown no benefit of surgery over nonsurgical management in these patients,[80] while others have reported improved outcome with surgical evacuation within 6 h of the hemorrhage[79,81] or when patients show rapid neurologic deterioration.[84] Fujitsu and coworkers[84] reported on a series of 180 patients with hypertensive putaminal hemorrhages, 69 of which were treated surgically. They divided patients based on their neurologic examination 6 h following the hemorrhage. They evaluated functional outcome at 6 months. They concluded that only those patients with rapidly progressive neurologic deterioration showed a functional benefit from surgery. Those who had slow or nonprogression of symptoms during the first 6 h or who had a fulminant course showed no functional benefit from surgical evacuation. Thus, it appears that surgery should be considered only in those patients who have moderate-sized hematomas (3 to 6 cm) and who are deteriorating neurologically but have no evidence of brainstem compression.

Hypertensive thalamic hemorrhages are best managed nonoperatively.[4,81,83] A ventriculostomy may be necessary if there is ventricular extension of hemorrhage or evidence of obstructive hydrocephalus (Fig. 14-1). Patients with hemorrhages less than 1 cm in diameter rarely have associated ventricular rupture and recover well. Those with hemorrhages from 1 to 3 cm in diameter also recover well but often with some disability. However, recovery from hemorrhages greater than 3 cm in diameter is rare.[2,64,85] In two series of 41 hypertensive thalamic hemorrhages, all patients with lesions greater than 3.3 cm in diameter died.[2,64] Similarly, Kwak and coworkers found hemorrhages larger than 3 cm in diameter to be associated with nonfunctional outcomes.[85] At present, there is no evidence to suggest that patients with larger hematomas benefit from surgical removal.

Spontaneous cerebellar hemorrhage is a surgically treatable disease.[4,16,65,66,81,83,86–88] Ojemann and Heros have emphasized the importance of treating the patient before mass effect causes an alteration in the level of consciousness and an unstable clinical situation, since neurologic deterioration from brainstem compression is often unpredictable and irreversible once set in motion.[4] Ott and coworkers reported a mortality rate of 17 percent in patients who were alert or lethargic preoperatively compared to a mortality rate of 75 percent in those who were stuporous or comatose before surgery.[66] Nevertheless, it is important to note that surgical evacuation of cerebellar hematomas is indicated even in the comatose patient with evidence of brainstem compression.

Little and coworkers found that 60 percent of their patients with cerebellar hemorrhages greater than 3 cm in diameter on CT were comatose or rapidly progressed to coma, while those patients with hematomas less than 3 cm in diameter were awake and alert and had a benign course.[87]

We recommend surgical evacuation of large cerebellar hematomas (>3 cm in diameter) diagnosed within 1 week of onset even in awake patients, since surgical morbidity is minimal. These lesions tend to displace the fourth ventricle and often cause obstructive hydrocephalus or brainstem compression. If the patient is seen more than 1 week following the hemorrhage, then the risk of further deterioration is small and conservative management is justified.[88] Lesions less than 3 cm in diameter are less likely to displace the fourth ventricle or cause brainstem compression and usually can be successfully managed medically in the ICU.[4,16,66,81,83,89] However, surgical evacuation of even small hematomas (<3 cm) should not be delayed if there is evidence of neurologic deterioration.

We routinely place a ventriculostomy at the time of surgery and use this for postoperative-ICP monitoring. However, ventriculostomy as the sole treatment of spontaneous cerebellar hemorrhage may be associated with upward herniation and a fatal outcome.[86]

Lobar hemorrhages are predominantly nonhypertensive in etiology. However, those attributed to hypertension are initially treated medically unless there is evidence of progressive neurologic deterioration.[4,8,16,17]

There is little role for surgery in the management of hypertensive pontine hemorrhages.[4,16,81,83] Lesions greater than 1 cm on CT are almost uniformly fatal, while those less than 1 cm cause severe disability in those who survive regardless of treatment.[90] Although O'Laorie and coworkers reported improvement in all six of their patients undergoing evacuation of pontine hemorrhages, the etiology of these hemorrhages was unknown.[91] Furthermore, none of the six patients had a history of hypertension, and five out of six were less than 29 years of age.[91]

Intraventricular hemorrhage associated with a hypertensive ICH is managed by ventriculostomy, if necessary. This can be lifesaving in cases of acute obstructive hydrocephalus.

Clinical State The level of consciousness at the time of presentation is an important prognostic indicator in spontaneous ICH. With the exception of hypertensive cerebellar hemorrhages, those who present in a coma with evidence of brainstem compression are unlikely to benefit from surgical decompression. Likewise, patients who are awake and alert should not be considered surgical candidates, unless they have a cerebellar hemorrhage greater than 3 cm in diameter. Those patients with progressive neurologic deterioration may benefit from surgical evacuation of their hematoma in cases of hypertensive putaminal and lobar hemorrhages. In nonhypertensive hemorrhages, surgical management will be dependent largely on the etiology of the hemorrhage as previously discussed.

Timing of Surgery

The timing of surgical intervention has been reported to influence outcome in a number of studies.[79,82,83,92,93] While some advocate early (<24 h) or ultra-early (<6 h) surgery following the ictus, others prefer delayed surgery. Since the indications for surgery and study designs vary considerably, no conclusions can be confidently reached regarding the ideal time to operate. It is generally agreed, however, that surgery should be strongly considered in any patient demonstrating neurologic deterioration.

OUTCOME

Outcome from spontaneous ICH may be influenced by several factors including etiology, size, location, ventricular rupture, age of the patient, and medical and/or surgical decision-making. This has been discussed in detail in several reports[3,4,7,9,10,14,16,18,20,25,48-50,57,60,63-67,71,72,79-97]

Overall, mortality from spontaneous ICH in the CT era has been estimated to be 38 percent with a range of 15 to 57 percent.[20] In the largest clinical series of hypertensive ICH reported to date, Kanaya and coworkers found a surgical mortality rate of 22 percent in 5255 cases.[95] It is important to remember that any mortality figures will underestimate the actual death rate, since about 35 percent of patients with spontaneous ICH die before medical treatment can be instituted.[14] In addition, mortality figures do not take into account those who are vegetative or severely disabled. Eighty-five to ninety percent of all deaths from spontaneous ICH occur within 1 month from the time of hemorrhage, and most of these are within the first few days.[4,6]

REFERENCES

1. Weinfeld FD (ed): The national survey of stroke. *Stroke* 12(suppl 1):1, 1981.
2. Walshe TM, Davis KD, Fisher CM: Thalamic hemorrhage: A computed tomographic-clinical correlation. *Neurology* 27:217, 1977.
3. Kaneko M, Koba T, Yokoyama T: Early surgical treatment for hypertensive intracerebral hemorrhage. *J Neurosurg* 46:579, 1977
4. Ojemann RG, Heros RC: Spontaneous brain hemorrhage. *Stroke* 14:468, 1983.
5. Drury I, Whisnant JP, Garraway WM: Primary intracerebral hemorrhage: Impact of CT on incidence. *Neurology* 34:653, 1984.

6. Mohr JP, Caplan LR, Melski JW, et al.: The Harvard Cooperative Stroke Registry: A prospective registry. *Neurology* 28:754, 1978.
7. Ducker TB: Spontaneous intracerebral hemorrhage. In: Wilkins RH, Rengachary SS (eds): *Neurosurgery*, New York, McGraw-Hill, 1985, pp 1510–1517.
8. Kase CS: Intracerebral hemorrhage: Non-hypertensive causes. *Stroke* 17:590, 1986.
9. Fisher CM: Pathological observations in hypertensive cerebral hemorrhage. *J Neuropath Exp Neurol* 30:356, 1971.
10. Fisher CM: The pathologic and clinical aspects of thalamic hemorrhage. *Trans Am Neurol Assoc* 84:56, 1959.
11. Russell DS: The pathology of spontaneous intracranial haemorrhages. *Proc R Soc Med* 47:689, 1954.
12. Zulch KJ: Pathological aspects of cerebral accidents in arterial hypertension. *Acta Neurol Belg* 71:196, 1971.
13. Ojemann RG, Mohr JP: Hypertensive brain hemorrhage. *Clin Neurosurg* 23:220, 1975.
14. Freytag E: Fatal hypertensive intracerebral hematomas: A survey of the pathological anatomy in 393 cases. *J Neurol Neurosurg Psychiatry* 31:616, 1968.
15. Jellinger K: Pathology and aetiology of ICH. In: Pia HA (ed): *Spontaneous Intracerebral Haematomas*. Berlin, Springer-Verlag, 1980, pp 13–29.
16. Borges LF: Management of nontraumatic brain hemorrhage. In: Ropper AH, Kennedy SF (eds): *Neurological and Neurosurgical Intensive Care*. Rockville, MD, Aspen, 1988, pp 209–217.
17. Ropper AH, Davis KR: Lobar cerebral hemorrhages: Acute clinical syndromes in 26 cases. *Ann Neurol* 8:141, 1980.
18. Kase CS, Williams JP, Wyatt DA, Mohr JP: Lobar intracerebral hematomas: Clinical and CT analysis of 22 cases. *Neurology* 32:1146, 1982.
19. Lee KS, Bae HG, Yun IG: Recurrent intracerebral hemorrhage due to hypertension. *Neurosurgery* 26:586, 1990.
20. Tsementzis SA: Surgical management of intracerebral hematomas. *Neurosurgery* 16:562, 1985.
21. Espinosa F, Weir B, Noseworthy T: Nonoperative treatment of subarachnoid hemorrhage. In: Youmans JR (ed): *Neurological Surgery*. Philadelphia, Saunders, 1990, pp 1661–1668.
22. Bingham WF: Treatment of mycotic intracranial aneurysms. *J Neurosurg* 46:428, 1977.
23. Frazee JG, Cahan LD, Winter J: Bacterial intracranial aneurysms. *J Neurosurg* 53:633, 1980.
24. Fleisher AS, Patton JM, Tindall GT: Cerebral aneurysms of traumatic origin. *Surg Neurol* 4:223, 1975.
25. Leblanc R, Preul M, Robitaille Y, et al.: Surgical considerations in cerebral amyloid angiopathy. *Neurosurgery* 29:712, 1991.
26. Okazaki H, Reagan TJ, Campbell RJ: Clinicopathologic studies of primary cerebral amyloid angiopathy. *Mayo Clin Proc* 54:22, 1979.
27. Cosgrove GR, Leblanc R, Meagher-Villemure K, et al.: Cerebral amyloid angiopathy. *Neurology* 35:625, 1985.
28. Vinters HV, Gilbert JJ: Cerebral amyloid angiopathy: Incidence and complications in the aging brain. II. The distribution of amyloid vascular changes. *Stroke* 14:924, 1983.
29. Kalyan-Raman UP, Kalyan-Raman K: Cerebral amyloid angiopathy causing intracranial hemorrhage. *Ann Neurol* 16:321, 1984.
30. Gudmundsson G, Hallgrimsson J, Jonasson TA, Bjarnason O: Hereditary cerebral hemorrhage with amyloidosis. *Brain* 95:387, 1972.
31. Wattendorff AR, Bots GTAM, Went LN, Endtz LJ: Familial cerebral amyloid angiopathy presenting as recurrent cerebral haemorrhage. *J Neurol Sci* 55:212, 1982.
32. Finelli PF, Kessimian N, Bernstein PW: Cerebral amyloid angiopathy manifesting as recurrent intracerebral hemorrhage. *Arch Neurol* 41:330, 1984.
33. McCormick WF: The pathology of vascular ("arteriovenous") malformations. *J Neurosurg* 24:807, 1966.
34. McCormick WF: Pathology of vascular malformations of the brain. In: Wilson CB, Stein BM (eds): *Intracranial Arteriovenous Malformations*. Baltimore, Williams & Wilkins, 1984, pp 44–63.
35. Garretson HD: Intracranial arteriovenous malformations. In: Wilkins RH, Rengachary SS (eds): *Neurosurgery*. New York, McGraw-Hill, 1985, pp 1448–1458.
36. Perret G, Nishioka H: Arteriovenous malformations. An analysis of 545 cases of cranio-cerebral arteriovenous malformations and fistulae reported to the cooperative study. *J Neurosurg* 25:467, 1966.
37. Samson DS, Batjer HH: Preoperative evaluation of the risk-benefit ratio for arteriovenous malformations of the brain. In: Wilkins RH, Rengachary SS (eds): *Neurosurgery Update II*. New York, McGraw-Hill, 1991, pp 129–133.
38. Crawford PM, West CR, Chadwick DW, et al.: Arteriovenous malformations of the brain: Natural history in unoperative patients. *J Neurol Neurosurg Psychiatry* 49:1, 1986.
39. Ondra SL, Troupp H, George E, Schwab K: The natural history of symptomatic arteriovenous malformations of the brain: A 24-year follow-up assessment. *J Neurosurg* 73:387, 1990.
40. Forster DMC, Steiner L, Hakanson S: Arteriovenous malformations of the brain. A long-term clinical study. *J Neurosurg* 37:562, 1972.
41. Itoyama Y, Uemura S, Ushio Y, et al.: Natural course of unoperative intracranial arteriovenous malformations: Study of 50 cases. *J Neurosurg* 71:805, 1989.
42. Rengachary SS, Kalyan-Raman UP: Other cranial intradural angiomas. In: Wilkins RH, Rengachary SS

(eds): *Neurosurgery*. New York, McGraw-Hill, 1985, pp 1465–1473.
43. Curling OD Jr, Kelly DL Jr, Elster AD, Craven TE: An analysis of the natural history of cavernous angiomas. *J Neurosurg* 75:702, 1991.
44. Robinson JR, Award IA, Little JR: Natural history of the cavernous angioma. *J Neurosurg* 75:709, 1991.
45. Handa H, Moritake Y: Venous angiomas of the brain: In: Fein JM, Flamm ES (eds): *Cerebrovascular Surgery*. New York, Springer-Verlag, 1985, vol IV, pp 1139–1149.
46. Malik GM, Morgan JK, Boulous RS, et al.: Venous angiomas: An underestimated cause of intracranial hemorrhage. *Surg Neurol* 30:350, 1988.
47. Garner TB, Curling OD, Kelly DL Jr, Laster DW: The natural history of intracranial venous angiomas. *J Neurosurg* 75:715, 1991.
48. Scott M: Spontaneous intracerebral hematoma caused by cerebral neoplasms. Report of eight verified cases. *J Neurosurg* 42:338, 1975.
49. Little JR, Dial B, Bellanger G, Carpenter S: Brain hemorrhage from intracranial tumor. *Stroke* 10:283, 1979.
50. Mandybur TI: Intracranial hemorrhage caused by metastatic tumors. *Neurology* 27:650, 1977.
51. Coon WW, Willis PW: Hemorrhagic complications of anticoagulant therapy. *Arch Int Med* 133:386, 1974.
52. Wintzen AR, de Jonge H, Loeliger EA, Bots GTAM: The risk of intracerebral hemorrhage during oral anticoagulant treatment: A population study. *Ann Neurol* 16:553, 1984.
53. Lieberman A, Hass WK, Pinto R, et al.: Intracranial hemorrhage and infarction in anticoagulated patients with prosthetic heart valves. *Stroke* 9:18, 1978.
54. Furlan AJ, Whisnant JP, Elveback LR: The decreasing incidence of primary intracerebral hemorrhage: A population study. *Ann Neurol* 5:367, 1979.
55. Kase CS, Robinson RK, Stein RW, et al.: Anticoagulant-related intracerebral hemorrhage. *Neurology* 35:943, 1985.
56. Abbey EE: Bleeding disorders. In: Campbell JW, Frisse M (eds): *Manual of Medical Therapeutics*. Boston, Little, Brown, 1983, pp 285–296.
57. Seeler RA, Imana RB: Intracranial hemorrhage in patients with hemophilia. *J Neurosurg* 39:181, 1973.
58. Delaney P, Estes M: Intracranial hemorrhage with amphetamine use. *Neurology* 30:1125, 1980.
59. Fallis RJ, Fisher M: Cerebral vasculitis and hemorrhage associated with phenylpropanolamine. *Neurology* 35:405, 1985.
60. Klonoff DC, Andrews BT, Obana WG: Stroke associated with cocaine use. *Arch Neurol* 46:989, 1989.
61. Citron BP, Halpern M, McCarron M, et al.: Necrotizing angiitis associated with drug abuse. *N Engl J Med* 283:1003, 1070.
62. Adams RD, Victor M: *Principles of Neurology*. New York, McGraw-Hill, 1989, pp 663–667.
63. Heir DB, Davis KR, Richardson EP, Mohr JP: Hypertensive putaminal hemorrhage. *Ann Neurol* 1:152, 1977.
64. Barraquer-Bordas L, Illa I, Escartin A, et al.: Thalamic hemorrhage. A study of 23 patients with diagnosis by computed tomography. *Stroke* 12:524, 1981.
65. Fisher CM, Picard EH, Polak A, et al.: Acute hypertensive cerebellar hemorrhage: Diagnosis and surgical treatment. *J Nerv Ment Dis* 140:38, 1965.
66. Ott KH, Kase CS, Ojemann RG, Mohr JP: Cerebellar hemorrhage: Diagnosis and treatment. *Arch Neurol* 31:160, 1974.
67. Little JR, Blomquist GA Jr, Ethier R: Intraventricular hemorrhage in adults. *Surg Neurol* 8:143, 1977.
68. Wiggins WS, Moody DM, Toole JF, et al.: Clinical and computerized tomographic study of hypertensive intracerebral hemorrhage. *Arch Neurol* 35:832, 1978.
69. Kassell NF, Torner JC, Adams HP Jr: Antifibrinolytic therapy in the acute period following aneurysmal subarachnoid hemorrhage: Preliminary observations from the cooperative aneurysm study. *J Neurosurg* 61:225, 1984.
70. Adams HP: Antifibrinolytics in aneurysmal subarachnoid hemorrhage. *Arch Neurol* 44:114, 1987.
71. Janny P, Colnet G, Georget A, Chazal J: Intracranial pressure with intracerebral hemorrhages. *Surg Neurol* 10:371, 1978.
72. Papo I, Janny P, Caruselli G, et al.: Intracranial pressure time course in primary intracerebral hemorrhage. *Neurosurgery* 4:504, 1979.
73. Ropper AH, King RB: Intracranial pressure monitoring in comatose patients with cerebral hemorrhage. *Arch Neurol* 41:725, 1984.
74. Tellez H, Bauer RB: Dexamethasone as treatment in cerebrovascular disease. A controlled study in intracerebral hemorrhage. *Stroke* 4:541, 1973.
75. Poungvarin N, Bhoopat W, Viriyavejakul A, et al.: Effects of dexamethasone in primary supratentorial intracerebral hemorrhage. *N Engl J Med* 316:1229, 1987.
76. Allen GS, Ahn HS, Preziosi TJ, et al.: Cerebral arterial spasm—a controlled trial of nimodipine in patients with subarachnoid hemorrhage. *N Engl J Med* 308:619, 1983.
77. Auer LM: Acute operation and preventive nimodipine improve outcome in patients with ruptured cerebral aneurysms. *Neurosurgery* 15:57, 1984.
78. Andrews BT, Wilson CB: Staged treatment of arteriovenous malformations of the brain. *Neurosurgery* 21:314, 1987.
79. Kaneko M, Tanaka K, Shimada T, et al.: Long-term evaluation of ultra-early operation for hypertensive intracerebral hemorrhage in 100 cases. *J Neurosurg* 58:838, 1983.

80. Waga S, Yamamoto Y: Hypertensive putaminal hemorrhage: Treatment and results. Is surgical treatment superior to conservative one? *Stroke* 14:480, 1983.
81. Kanno T, Sano H, Shinomiya Y, et al.: Role of surgery in hypertensive intracerebral hematoma. A comparative study of 305 nonsurgical and 154 surgical cases. *J Neurosurg* 61:1091, 1984.
82. Waga S, Miyazaki M, Okada M, et al.: Hypertensive putaminal hemorrhage: Analysis of 182 patients. *Surg Neurol* 26:159, 1986.
83. Castel JP, Kissel P: Spontaneous intracerebral and infratentorial hemorrhage. In: Youmans JR (ed): *Neurological Surgery.* Philadelphia, Saunders, 1990, pp 1890–1917.
84. Fujitsu K, Muramoto M, Ikeda Y, et al.: Indications for surgical treatment of putaminal hemorrhage. *J Neurosurg* 73:518, 1990.
85. Kwak R, Kadoya S, Suzuki T: Factors affecting the prognosis in thalamic hemorrhage. *Stroke* 14:493, 1983.
86. McKissock W, Richardson A, Walsh R: Spontaneous cerebellar haemorrhage. A study of 34 consecutive cases treated surgically. *Brain* 83:1, 1960.
87. Little JR, Tubman DE, Ethier R: Cerebellar hemorrhage in adults. *J Neurosurg* 48:575, 1978.
88. Yoshida S, Sasaki M, Oka H, et al.: Acute intracerebellar hemorrhage with signs of lower brain stem compression. *Surg Neurol* 10:79, 1978.
89. Heiman TD, Satya-Murti S: Benign cerebellar hemorrhages. *Ann Neurol* 3:366, 1978.
90. Sano K, Ochai C: Brain stem hematomas: Clinical aspects with reference to indications for treatment. In: Pia HW, Langmaid C, Zierski J (eds): *Spontaneous Intracerebral Hematomas.* New York, Springer-Verlag, 1980, pp 366–371.
91. O'Laoire SA, Crockard HA, Thomas DGT, Gordon DS: Brain stem hematoma. A report of six surgically treated cases. *J Neurosurg* 56:222, 1982.
92. Paillas JE, Alliez B: Surgical treatment of spontaneous intracerebral hemorrhage. Immediate and long-term results in 250 cases. *J Neurosurg* 39:145, 1973.
93. Juvela S, Heiskanen O, Poanen A, et al.: The treatment of spontaneous intracerebral hemorrhage. A prospective randomized trial of surgical and conservative treatment.. *J Neurosurg* 70:755, 1989.
94. Duff TA, Ayeni S, Levin AB, Javid M: Nonsurgical management of spontaneous intracerebral hematoma. *Neurosurgery* 9:387, 1981.
95. Kanaya H, Saiki I, Ohuchi T, et al.: Hypertensive intracerebral hemorrhage in Japan: Update on surgical treatment. In: Mizukami M (ed): *Hypertensive Intracerebral Hemorrhage.* New York, Raven, 1983, pp 147–163.
96. McKissock W, Richardson A, Taylor J: Primary intracerebral haemorrhage. A controlled trial of surgical and conservative treatment in 180 unselected cases. *Lancet* 2:221, 1961.
97. Nakajima K: Clinicopathological study of pontine hemorrhage. *Stroke* 14:485, 1983.

CHAPTER 15

The Intensive Care Management of Cerebral Ischemia*

Fredric B. Meyer

INTRODUCTION

Although the human brain is only 2 percent of total body weight, it requires 20 percent of the inspired oxygen at rest, 15 percent of the cardiac output (approximately 750 mL/min), and the liver's entire output of glucose in the fasting state. Since it has no appreciable stores of glycogen, it is dependent on oxidative phosphorylation for the production of high-energy phosphates. Resting cerebral blood flow (CBF) is approximately 50 mL/100 g of brain tissue per minute. Although total CBF is relatively stable throughout variations in body activity, cardiac output, and blood pressure, focal CBF is closely coupled to metabolism and increases significantly with activation of a cortical region.

In neurosurgical practice, the etiologies of acute cerebral ischemia can be divided into three general categories. First, the most common cause of acute cerebral ischemia is embolic or thrombotic stroke usually due to atherosclerosis or cardiac disease. Although this clinical situation is usually managed by the neurologist, the principles of intensive care unit (ICU) management can be extended to those more typically encountered by the neurosurgeon. The second category involves perioperative vascular insults during neurosurgical procedures such as arterial dissection or thrombosis, or prolonged temporary vessel occlusion. The third major category of acute cerebral ischemia is subarachnoid hemorrhage-induced delayed ischemic deficits secondary to vasospasm. In all three general categories of acute ischemia, ICU management consists of interventions designed to increase CBF or provide direct neuronal protection. In order to construct a framework for analyzing treatment modalities, this chapter will first deal with the pathophysiology of ischemic brain injury. Subsequently, current and potential future treatment regimens will be discussed.[1]

**Acknowledgment:* Work performed in the author's laboratory was supported by NIH R01 25374.

PATHOPHYSIOLOGY OF ISCHEMIC BRAIN INJURY

It is important to recognize that there are significant differences between focal and global cerebral ischemia. A typical clinical situation of focal ischemia is that which occurs with embolic occlusion of the middle cerebral artery (MCA). Alternatively, global ischemia occurs in patients suffering from cardiac arrest. Patients with global ischemia have no CBF during the ischemic insult as opposed to those with focal ischemia in which the potential for low-level residual blood flow from collateral circulation exists. This residual perfusion in focal ischemia may provide sufficient substrate delivery to maintain a low level of metabolic activity which may preserve membrane integrity thereby retarding the evolution of irreversible neuronal injury. However, this low-level residual blood flow results in a more complex biochemical situation including the delivery of glucose under anaerobic conditions which may worsen brain acidosis. This review will concentrate on the pathophysiology of focal cerebral ischemia since it is by far the more common clinical situation treated by the neurosurgeon.

Thresholds of Ischemia

In 1948, Dr. Kety and Dr. Schmidt first demonstrated that CBF in humans was approximately 50 mL/100 g brain tissue per min. Subsequently, it was demonstrated in patients undergoing carotid endarterectomy that reductions in CBF to approximately 18 mL/100 g brain tissue per min caused attenuation or suppression in the electroencephalogram (EEG). Subsequent laboratory studies revealed that when CBF was reduced to approximately 15 mL/100 g brain tissue per min, there was suppression of somatosensory evoked potentials.[2] Accordingly, a threshold of electrical failure was quantitated at a range of critical CBF of 18 to 15 mL/100 g brain tissue per minute. More recent investigations in a large number of experimental models have shown that this threshold of electrical failure is reproducible but may vary depending on the type and degree of anesthesia. In 1977, Astrup and colleagues[3] demonstrated that a reduced CBF of approximately 12 to 10 mL/100 g brain tissue per min resulted in significant alterations in the extracellular ionic concentrations of cations such as K^+ and Ca^{2+}. This second reduced level of blood flow was termed the threshold of ionic failure. Since neuronal tissue is critically dependent on a continuous delivery of oxygen and glucose for aerobic metabolism, declines in CBF to this approximate level of 12 to 10 mL/100 g brain tissue per min will result in a rapid depletion in adenosine triphosphate (ATP) (Fig. 15-1). With depletion of

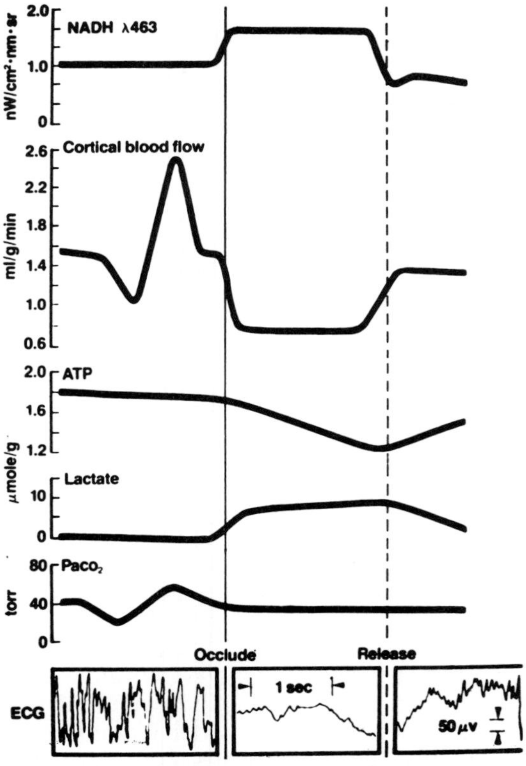

Figure 15-1 Correlation of cortical NADH fluorescence, CBF, and parenchymal ATP with lactic acid levels at various PA_{CO_2} and during ischemia. Note that NADH remains at a constant level throughout a wide range of PA_{CO_2} and CBF but increases significantly during MCA occlusion. Parallel to the increase in NADH is an increase in lactic acid and decline in ATP also due to the ischemic injury. This failure of energy production is associated with EEG attenuation. (From Sundt TM Jr, Anderson RE, Sharbrough FW: Effects of hypocapnia, hypercapnia, and blood pressure on NADH fluorescence, electrical activity, and blood flow in normal and partially ischemic monkey cortex. *J Neurochem* 27:1125, 1976.)

ATP, there is failure of the Na^+/K^+ ATPase pump, which is essential for maintaining ionic gradients. Because of the difference in the extracellular and intracellular concentration of these two cations, there is an efflux of K^+ along with an influx of Na^+ into neurons leading to membrane depolarization. In addition to these initial ionic fluxes, there is a rapid rise in intracellular lactic acid concentrations due to anaerobic metabolism. During severe reductions in CBF, lactic acid concentrations increase fourfold during the first 30 min. With prolonged ischemia, lactic acid concentrations continue to climb to approximately 14 μmol/g brain tissue.[4] Although the tolerance of neuronal tissue for these reduced flows of approximately 10 mL/100 g brain tissue per min is unknown, experimental evidence indicates that after 3 to 4 h, irreversible neuronal injury may occur. In fact, specific brain regions are extremely vulnerable to these low CBF levels. For example, hippocampal CA 4, CA 3, and CA 1 neurons demonstrate ischemic neuronal injury after 3 to 5 min of significant flow reduction.

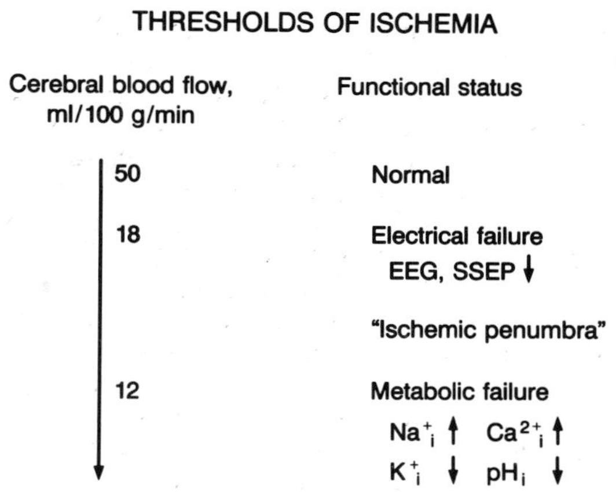

Figure 15-2 Schematic diagram of the thresholds of cerebral ischemia. Normal CBF in humans is approximately 50 mL/100 g per min. When CBF declines to about 18 mL/100 g per min, there is loss of functional activity as evidenced by EEG attenuation. When CBF declines to approximately 12 to 10 mL/100 g per min, there is rapid alteration in extracellular ionic concentrations, representing depletion of ATP. This is ionic or membrane failure. Between these two thresholds of electrical failure and ionic failure, there is a circumscribed range of reduced CBF in which membrane activity is preserved, despite functional loss, implying reversible ischemic neuronal damage.

Between these two thresholds of electrical failure and ionic failure, there exists a small circumscribed range of CBF at which, despite functional loss, membrane homeostasis and structural integrity are maintained (Fig. 15-2). This circumscribed range of CBF has been termed the *ischemic penumbra*.[5] This concept may explain why patients suffering from an acute stroke may have the potential for recovery if there is sufficient collateral flow to satisfy basic energy requirements necessary for maintenance of membrane integrity. Perhaps the best clinical example of the ischemic penumbra is the patient suffering from a reversible ischemic neurologic deficit (RIND). Presumably during the RIND, CBF is reduced below the threshold of electrical failure and the patient therefore has a neurologic deficit. However, since the patient recovers, it is reasonable to postulate that there is sufficient collateral CBF to retard cerebral infarction. The original intent of the term *ischemic penumbra* was to describe a zone of electrically silent but structurally intact parenchyma surrounding the core region of infarction during an acute focal cerebral ischemic insult (Fig. 15-3). However, the question of ischemic penumbra stability remains unresolved. More recently, the ischemic penumbra has been characterized by two states.[6] Type 1 is

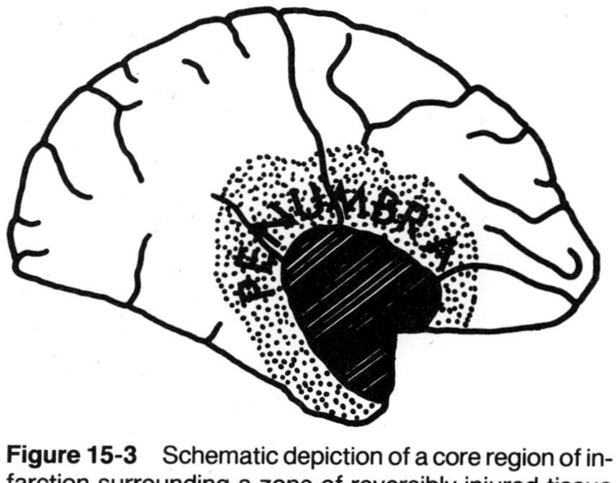

Figure 15-3 Schematic depiction of a core region of infarction surrounding a zone of reversibly injured tissue termed the *ischemic penumbra*. [From Symon L: The relationship between CBF, evoked potentials, and the clinical features in cerebral ischemia. *Acta Neuronal Scand* 62(suppl 78):175, 1980.]

manifested by EEG suppression, CBF reduction, and neuronal structural preservation. Type 2 is defined by EEG attenuation, critical CBF reduction, and repetitive transient increases in K^{+}_{e}. The type 2 ischemic penumbra is associated with varying degrees of neuronal loss. When considering the stability of the ischemic penumbra, the element of time must be considered. For example, CBF reductions to 18 mL/100 g brain tissue per min in permanent MCA occlusion in the *Macaca* monkey lead to infarction suggesting either deterioration in CBF or poor tolerance of neuronal tissue for prolonged reductions in blood flow.

It is therefore reasonable to assume that the ischemic penumbra is actually in a dynamic state that has the potential to deteriorate over time. This deterioration may reflect a progressive decline in residual collateral blood flow due either to fatigue of collaterals, ischemic vasoconstriction, or progressive edema. Therefore, the clinical outcome following vascular occlusion reflects both the severity and duration of reduced CBF (Fig. 15-4).[7] A variety of experimental studies have been performed to try to determine the maximum time of MCA occlusion that can be tolerated without infarction. Early research suggested that MCA occlusion could be tolerated for 1 h in the squirrel monkey or 6 h in the cat without severe infarction. Subsequent detailed experiments in the *Macaca* monkey demonstrated that 15 to 18 min of MCA occlusion was tolerated without any evidence of infarction. When MCA occlusion was extended to 30 min, there were rare subcortical gray matter infarcts. If MCA occlusion was further extended to 60 min, there was a heterogeneous pattern of neuronal injury spanning from no infarction to gross macroscopic lesions. Following 4 h of MCA occlusion, there were multiple nonconfluent infarctions involving both the basal ganglia and subcortical gray matter. If the time of MCA occlusion was extended beyond 4 h, single large confluent infarctions involving both deep and superficial brain structures were observed. Collation of focal ischemia experiments in the primate suggests that 30 min of MCA occlusion is well tolerated, whereas occlusion periods of 60 min frequently result in multiple small infarcts with a perivascular localization. As the time of MCA occlusion extends to approximately 4 h, these microinfarcts coalesce into large infarcts involving both superficial and deep structures in the distribution of the MCA. These animal studies also suggest that reperfusion or restoration of blood flow within 4 to 8 h can ameliorate the extent of infarction. It is important to note, however, that reperfusion may exacerbate the degree of brain injury. For example, in early primate studies of MCA occlusion, reperfusion after 3 or 6 h of ischemia tended to increase the degree of vasogenic edema. It has been hypothesized that reperfusion injury may be due to reoxygenation with the production of free radicals.[8]

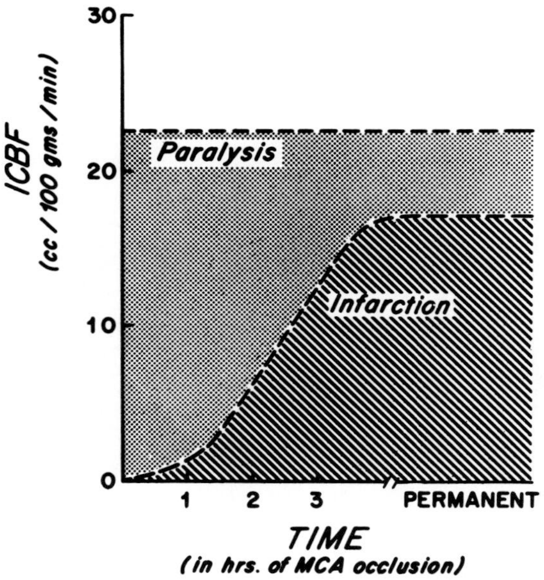

Figure 15-4 An analysis of ischemic thresholds relating time and severity of ischemia with morphologic injury. (From Jones TH, Morawetz RB, Crowell RM, et al.: Threshold of focal cerebral ischemia in awake monkey. *J Neurosurg* 54:773, 1981.)

Metabolic Events

The deleterious metabolic cascades which occur at profound CBF reductions are multifactorial and complex. Some of these initial major metabolic insults include brain acidosis, altered membrane permeability to Ca^{2+} and Na^{+}, and release of sequestered Ca^{2+}_{i}. In fact, these events can all be related to energy failure (Fig. 15-5). For example, the release of excitatory amino acids, opening of

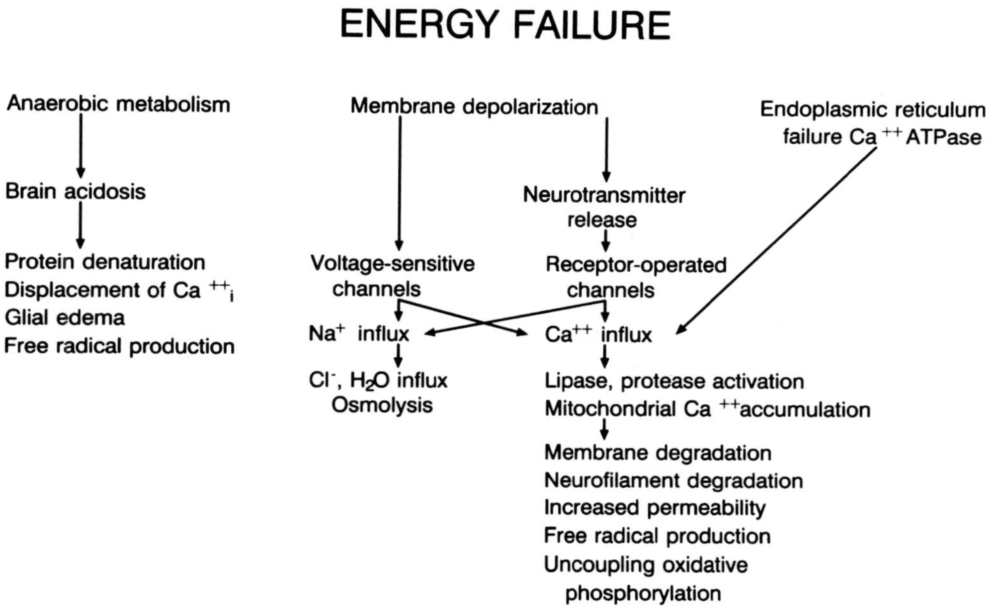

Figure 15-5 Schematic depiction of the relationship between energy failure and the major degradative metabolic pathways causing ischemic neuronal damage.

membrane voltage-dependent calcium channels, and intracellular acidosis can all be linked to the failure of aerobic metabolism resulting from the depletion of ATP secondary to decreased glucose and oxygen delivery. Each of these critical events will be reviewed in detail.

It is now well established that Ca^{2+} plays a critical role in normal cellular events including secondary messenger, metabolic regulator, and effecting neurotransmitter release. It is also recognized that abnormal Ca^{2+} accumulation can mediate anoxic death. In 1977, it was demonstrated that extracellular Ca^{2+} concentrations decreased in hypoxic cerebellar cortex. Subsequent studies demonstrated that Ca^{2+} also declined in hippocampal anoxia, status epilepticus, and hypoglycemia. These observations resulted in an integrative hypothesis implicating calcium-related cell damage as the final common pathway for neuronal injury.[9] This theory hypothesized that Ca^{2+} entered neurons through voltage-dependent calcium channels which opened following membrane depolarization. Under anaerobic conditions, the rapid depletion of ATP would lead to failure of the Na^+/K^+ ATPase pump. This would ultimately lead to membrane depolarization with an influx of calcium. Since Ca^{2+}_i is largely sequestered in the endoplasmic reticulum by a Ca^{2+} ATPase, it was also postulated that with energy failure there would be a release of intracellular calcium which could contribute to neuronal injury independent from transmembrane calcium fluxes. The differences in vulnerability to ischemic injury between different neuronal populations were postulated to be due to differences in the density of membrane calcium channels.

This original calcium hypothesis of neuronal injury was challenged by several experiments. First in vitro studies demonstrated that neurons could die from a hypoxic insult in culture mediums devoid of Ca^{2+}. Second, there was a poor correlation between location of certain voltage-dependent calcium channels and ischemic vulnerability. Third, the role of neurotransmitters such as glutamate and aspartate in hypoxic injury was demonstrated.

Rothman and Olney first hypothesized that certain excitatory amino acids such as glutamate or aspartate were cytotoxic and if permitted to overexcite postsynaptic receptors, could result in dendrosomatic injuries.[10] This *excitotoxic hypothesis* has been subsequently implicated in both anoxic and hypoglycemic injury which is concordant with the concept that overexcitation could involve either increased release or decreased reuptake of cytotoxic neurotransmitters. The mechanism of excitotoxic injury was subsequently elucidated by a series of eloquent experiments in which both an early and delayed form of irreversible injury were observed. The early injury was ascribed to Na^+ influx and the delayed injury to Ca^{2+} entry.

As depicted in Fig. 15-6, there are at least three receptors for these excitotoxic amino acids which have been defined pharmacologically by analog binding: The N-methyl-D-aspartate (NMDA), kainic acid/quisquolate, and the AMPA receptors. In the excitotoxic hypothesis of ischemic neuronal injury, early cell damage has been attributed to Na^+ influx followed by obligatory Cl^- and H_2O entry with resultant cellular edema and osmolysis. This Na^+ influx is hypothesized to occur primarily through channels gated by the kainic acid/quisquolate receptor or the AMPA receptor. It is also possible that Na^+ could enter cells by following its concentration gradient through membrane voltage channels independent from these receptor-operated channels. During ischemia with decreased ATP production, there is a failure of the Na^+/K^+ ATPase pump. The delayed neuronal injury is thought to be secondary to Ca^{2+} influx primarily through the NMDA receptor which gates a receptor-operated calcium channel. Similar to Na^+ influx, it is reasonable to suggest that with energy failure and membrane depolarization, Ca^{2+} could also enter the cell through voltage-depen-

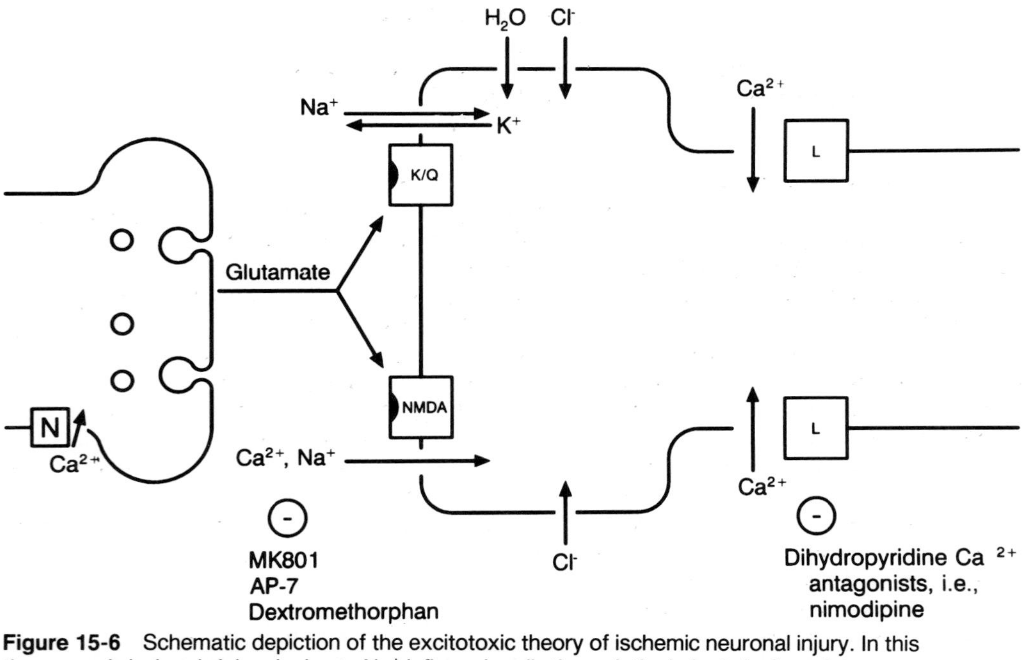

Figure 15-6 Schematic depiction of the excitotoxic theory of ischemic neuronal injury. In this theory, early ischemic injury is due to Na^+ influx primarily through the kainate/quisquolate-operated channels. With this Na^+ influx, there is passive Cl^- and H_2O influx which leads to dendritic edema and subsequent osmolysis. The delayed ischemic injury is due to Ca^{2+} influx through the NMDA receptor. Note that presynaptically, Ca^{2+} influx through the N-type voltage-dependent calcium channel would lead to additional neurotransmitter release. In addition to NMDA receptor-operated channels, calcium could enter neurons through L-type voltage-dependent calcium channels. These L channels tend to be located closer to the cell soma. (Modified from Siesjo BK: Calcium, ischemia, and death of brain cells. *Ann NY Acad Sci* 522:638, 1988.)

dent calcium channels independent of these receptor-operated channels. Therefore, the concept of calcium-related cell death in the more recent excitotoxic hypothesis is to a large degree similar to the original calcium hypothesis.[11]

Evidence to support the importance of these excitotoxic mechanisms in ischemic injury consists of several experimental observations. First, the extracellular levels of glutamate and aspartate increase considerably during experimental hypoxia. Second, deafferentation of CA1 neurons by Schafferotomy (elimination of glutamatergic input) and local injection of a glutamate antagonist prevent decreases in extracellular calcium during ischemia. Third, competitive and noncompetitive glutamate receptor antagonists appear to ameliorate both in vitro and in vivo ischemic injury.[12-14] Fourth, antagonists to the NMDA receptor and more recently the AMPA receptor decrease both in vitro and in vivo ischemic neuronal injury. Fifth, the excitotoxic theory may explain the phenomenon of selective vulnerability. Brief periods of forebrain ischemia in the Wistar rat or gerbil result in injury limited to the subiculum and CA1 and CA4 regions of the hippocampus. With more prolonged ischemic results, there is injury to hippocampal CA3, cortical pyramidal neurons, the caudate nucleus, and the putamen. Radiographic agonist binding studies have demonstrated that the NMDA receptor is concentrated in the Schaeffer collateral terminations of CA1 and CA4, while the kainic acid/quisquolate receptors are localized at the mossy fiber terminations of CA3, pyramidal neurons, caudate, and putamen. Therefore, the distribution of the receptor sites for these excitatory amino acids corresponds well to brain regions with low ischemic tolerance.

Since increases in intracellular Ca^{2+} are currently thought to be the major catalyst for ischemic neuronal injury, it is worthwhile to consider both neuronal calcium regulation and the mechanisms by which calcium could lead to neuronal injury. Given the fact that extracellular Ca^{2+} concentrations are approximately 10^{-3} versus an intracellular concentration of 10^{-7}, small alterations in calcium metabolism can have profound effects on intracellular Ca^{2+}-mediated events including contraction, excitation, and secretion. These processes transpire at micromolar concentrations of ionized calcium. Inward calcium fluxes are driven by a high concentration gradient between extracellular and intracellular calcium through both voltage-dependent and receptor-operated calcium channels. Currently, there are three recognized voltage-dependent membrane calcium channels: T, N, and L channels. Receptor-operated calcium channels refer to channels such as those regulated by the NMDA receptor for the excitatory amino acids. In addition to these membrane channels, other major regulators of Ca^{2+} include the Na^+/Ca^{2+} antiport pump which is electrogenic with a ratio of approximately 3 : 1 in which the direction of calcium exchange may be either inward or outward depending on Na^+ gradients, a Ca^{2+}-ATPase pump located both in the cytoplasmic and endoplasmic reticulum membranes, mitochondria which electrophoretically accumulate Ca^{2+} when intracellular free calcium rises, and intracellular calcium-binding proteins such as calmodulin.

The major mechanisms by which increases in $Ca^{2+}{}_i$ may contribute to ischemic neuronal injury include the following:

1. Activation of degradative enzymes including proteases, endonucleases, and lipases which catabolize cellular membranes and neurofilaments. A loss of membrane phospholipids increases the permeability of mitochondrial membranes causing interference with residual oxidative phosphorylation, while injury to neurofilament structures retards neuronal transport mechanisms. In addition, the accumulated free fatty acids from membrane phospholipid degradation are thought to be oxidized through a lipooxygenase or cyclooxygenase pathway during reperfusion. The net result of these pathways is the production and release of prostaglandins, leukotrienes, and possibly free radicals. The prostaglandin thromboxane A_2 is a potent vasoconstrictor, leukotrienes alter membrane permeability and lead to vasoconstriction, and free radicals if present attack cellular membranes.

2. In an attempt to buffer rising $Ca^{2+}{}_i$ concentrations, mitochondria electrophoretically accumulate calcium. This uncouples residual oxidative phosphorylation at a time when energy production is already limited to anaerobic metabolism.

3. An increase in $Ca^{2+}{}_i$ leads to neurotransmitter release including the punitive neurotransmitters such as glutamate or aspartate propagating this degradative cycle.

It is important to consider the effects of brain acidosis when considering ischemic neuronal injury. Intracellular brain pH is approximately 7.01 to 7.03. Within 10 min of severe reductions in CBF, brain pH_i can deteriorate to approximately 6.60. This reflects the rapid increase in intracellular lactic acid concentrations. This profound brain acidosis has been found to have the following detrimental effects: (1) the denaturating of proteins with loss of enzymatic function, (2) increasing glial edema with the potential to compromise collateral flow by extravascular compression thereby reducing residual CBF, (3) contributing to increase in $Ca^{2+}{}_i$ by H^+ competing for intracellular Ca^{2+} binding sites, (4) creating an internal mileau that is favorable for free-radical production, and (5) suppressing the cerebral metabolic rate for glucose and the regeneration of NADH. It has been demonstrated experimentally that hyperglycemia worsens intracellular acidosis in core regions of ischemia and has a detrimental effect on survival in experimental studies. In addition, hyperglycemia may impair postischemic cerebral perfusion along with ATP and phosphocreatine recovery, which results in tissue accumulation of lactic acid. Although hyperglycemia has been shown to have the above detrimental effects in core regions of ischemia, there is also contrary data which suggest that hyperglycemia may be neuroprotective in the ischemic penumbra.

Microcirculatory Alterations

In addition to the metabolic alterations which occur during ischemia, there are also blood flow changes referable to the microcirculation which can contribute to ischemic neuronal injury. First, following vessel occlusion there is sludging of the blood which has been termed *particulate flow.* It has been postulated that this particulate flow is due to a reduction in the shearing forces which tend to keep cellular blood components dispersed. Because of the sludging, blood viscosity increases with increased resistance to flow.

Second, experiments which have observed the cortical surface conducting vessels during focal ischemia have demonstrated the following progression. Initially, there is an immediate slight increase in vessel diameter due to local extracellular acidosis. During this vasodilatation, vasomotor paralysis occurs such that blood flow through these dilated vessels correlates directly with cerebral perfusion pressure. In fact, there is a loss of blood pressure autoregulation wherein drops in arterial blood pressure can lead to significant reductions in CBF. Within a variable time period following this local vasodilatation, vasoconstriction of these same surface conducting vessels occurs. This vasoconstriction has been termed *ischemic vasoconstriction* or *secondary vasospasm* to distinguish it from subarachnoid hemorrhage–induced vasospasm.[15] This ischemia-induced vasoconstriction can be partially blocked by the use of certain calcium antagonists which block voltage-dependent L channels suggesting that it may, in part, be due to Ca^{2+} influx into smooth muscle cells. Presumably, the decline in ATP leads to smooth muscle cell depolarization with Ca^{2+} influx and subsequent actin and myosin cross-linking. An alternative theory involves an increase in extracellular K^+ or the release of endogenous vasoconstrictors such as norepinephrine or serotonin. If norepinephrine does play a critical role in ischemic vasoconstriction, it is important to note that the deactivation of norepinephrine is energy-dependent since it must undergo reuptake at the presynaptic terminal. Irrespective of the etiology of ischemic vasoconstriction, the end result is a reduction in microcirculatory blood flow.

A third microcirculatory change which can be observed following focal ischemia is postischemic hypoperfusion.[16] Postischemic or delayed hypoperfusion following an ischemic brain insult was originally described as the *no reflow phenomenon.* In fact, the use of the term *no reflow* is a misnomer in that the degree of postischemic hypoperfusion depends on the severity of the ischemic injury. If the ischemic insult is mild, typically there will be no postischemic hypoperfusion. Following a severe ischemic event, however, postischemic hypoperfusion following flow restoration can be profound. During postischemic hypoperfusion, there is an increase in both oxygen extraction and metabolism suggesting that a mismatch between metabolic demand and substrate delivery exists which may injure surviving neurons after an ischemic insult. The pathophysiology of postischemic hypoperfusion has been attributed to the following: (1) intravascular rheologic factors including increased platelet aggregation or blood viscosity, or polymorphonuclear leukocyte injury to endothelium; (2) vascular wall alterations including smooth muscle contraction, microvilli formation, or endothelial edema; and (3) extravascular edema including glial tissue causing mechanical capillary bed compression.

TREATMENT OF ACUTE FOCAL CEREBRAL ISCHEMIA

Before discussing specific treatment modalities for acute brain ischemia, it is important to establish that different putative mechanisms require different approaches and treatments. For example, a patient suffering from an MCA embolus from a cardiac mural thrombus might be treated with intravascular thrombolytic therapy. Alternatively, intravascular thrombolytic therapy in the context of a surgical patient suffering from ischemia due to prolonged intraoperative vascular occlusion would be contraindicated due to the risk of hemorrhage and absence of intraluminal clot. Similarly, intravascular thrombolytic therapy would be ill-advised in the subarachnoid hemorrhage patient suffering from ischemic deficits due to vasospasm. Accordingly, prior to instituting any treatment, it is critical to attempt to ascertain by history, physical examination, and appropriate diagnostic studies the presumptive etiology of the ischemic insult.

Once the cause of the ischemic insult is identified, a rational treatment plan can be devised based on the pathophysiology of ischemic brain injury which was discussed in the preceding sections. In essence, there are two general principles for the treatment of acute stroke—increasing collateral CBF and providing direct neuronal protection.

Thromboembolic Stroke

The etiology of thromboembolic stroke is heterogeneous and complex. This type of acute cerebral ischemia is the most common cause of stroke and would include diffuse pathophysiologies such as embolus from a cardiac mural thrombus, embolus from a carotid stenosis, or thrombosis of an intracranial or extracranial vessel. Because of the diffuse possible mechanisms, the treatment of thromboembolic stroke must be tailored to each individual patient. For example, occlusion of a lenticulostriate artery results in a lacunar infarct. Since these lenticulostriates are end arteries without any collateral flow, it is likely that treatments to increase collateral blood flow will be ineffective. Likewise, agents that might be neuroprotective would also be ineffective due to the inability to deliver the agent to the ischemic brain tissue.

The first step in diagnosis is to perform a good history and physical examination. A history of diabetes or hypertension may support the diagnosis of a lacunar infarct, while a history of prior transient ischemic attacks (TIAs) including amaurosis fugax would favor cardiac or carotid disease. A critical part of the neurologic examination includes auscultation for cervical bruits and cardiac murmurs, palpation of the superficial temporal artery pulse, and ophthalmoscopic examination of the retina for evidence of emboli or venous-stasis retinopathy. Following the examination, an emergency CT scan should be performed to rule out nonischemic causes of acute neurologic deficit such as intracerebral hemorrhage or neoplasm. The CT scan may also yield secondary signs of infarction such as embolus in the MCA or cerebral edema in a vascular distribution. Finally, the CT scan may demonstrate old ischemic insults such as prior lacunar or watershed infarctions.

The choice of further diagnostic studies depends in large part on clinical suspicion and the degree of aggressiveness of the treating physician. For example, if no significant intervention is planned, then an argument can be made to not obtain any further imaging studies. Diagnostic tests to be considered which could provide important information include carotid ultrasound, transcranial Doppler, oculoplethysmography, transfemoral cerebral angiogram, MR angiography, and transesophageal or transthoracic echocardiography. In the ideal setting in a patient without evidence of small vessel disease, an argument can be made to proceed directly from CT scan in the emergency room to angiography to define the anatomic pathology if an aggressive treatment such as surgical or medical thrombolytic therapy is contemplated.

Treatment

Treatment of thromboembolic stroke depends in large part on the etiology. At present there is no effective treatment for an acute lacunar infarct. Fortunately, many of these patients have significant neurologic recovery. Although there are currently no clear-cut pharmacologic agents for the treatment of acute thromboembolic stroke, a variety of potential neuroprotective agents such as Ca^{2+} antagonists, excitatory amino acid antagonists, and free-radical scavengers are undergoing clinical trials. Therefore, at the present time the following treatment steps can be advocated:

1. It is our general practice to keep the patient euvolemic. It should be noted that it is the practice of some experienced clinicians to utilize hemodilution techniques including phlebotomy to decrease blood viscosity thereby theoretically increasing microcirculatory flow.[17] Our reluctance to practice hemodilution is based on the experimental evidence which suggests that this might increase cerebral edema combined with the negative results of two prospective European trials.[18]

2. The patient is hydrated with either 0.45 or 0.9% NaCl devoid of glucose. This is based on the evidence that hyperglycemia aggravates brain acidosis.[19]

3. Consider thrombolytic therapy. This controversial area can be divided into medical and surgical thrombolytic therapy. Currently, medical thrombolytic therapy includes the use of heparin or tissue plasminogen activating factor (tPA). The goal of intravenous heparin is prophylactic, to prevent repeat embolism such as that from a cardiac mural thrombus or to prevent propagation of a thrombus up the circle of Willis arteries. Although it was initially hypothesized that heparin might increase microcirculatory flow, there is little experimental evidence to support this postulate. Alternatively, most clinicians would agree with the use of heparin in a patient with a cardiac embolus due to atrial fibrillation or from a paradoxical embolus. The use of heparin to prevent extension of a thrombosis has rare clinical applications in spontaneous stroke. More typically, heparin might be used for this specific indication in a patient undergoing a carotid occlusion for treatment of an intracranial aneurysm. Prior to starting heparin, a CT scan should be obtained to rule out a hemorrhagic stroke.

The use of tPA for emergent clot lysis is currently being investigated with several prospective clinical trials. Clearly, the most effective technique to significantly increase blood flow would be to restore flow through the occluded vessel.[20] The greatest potential risk of intravascular thrombolytic therapy is the risk of hemorrhagic infarction.[21] In support of this concern is the evidence that the use of streptokinase for the treatment of peripheral deep vein thrombosis is associated with a 3 percent incidence of intracerebral hemorrhage. Current issues of concern in medical trials for the treatment of acute stroke with tPA and other neuroprotective agents include defining the etiology and time of entry of patients into the clinical trial.

Surgical thrombolytic therapy refers to the surgical extirpation of the embolus or thrombosis by emergency MCA embolectomy or carotid endarterectomy. Although there are published clinical reports demonstrating the potential benefits of this aggressive treatment, this practice is not well established. Surprisingly, the risk of intracerebral hemorrhage following surgical revascularization has been found to be quite low. Although it is reasonable to presume that medical thrombolytic therapy would be preferable to surgical revascularization, no firm conclusions can be drawn until the results of the tPA trials are analyzed. Until these data are published, it remains worthwhile noting that occasionally an emergency MCA embolectomy or carotid endarterectomy can be extremely beneficial in salvaging neurologic function in select patients.[22]

Irrespective of surgical versus medical thrombolytic therapy, the issue of time of ischemia and time of flow restoration remains central. As noted in the background discussion, the experimental data would indicate that after 4 h of focal ischemia, major cerebral infarction occurs. These experimental data also indicate that flow restoration even after 4 to 5 h of ischemia can be beneficial in reducing the size of infarction. Review of the time of ischemia and flow restoration in the surgical reports of MCA embolectomy and carotid endarterectomy did not demonstrate a definitive cutoff time in which flow restoration after that time period was ineffective. Clearly, the sooner emergent treatment is started, the better the chance of clinical improvement. Most clinicians and researchers would accept the 4- to 6-h cutoff time for attempting to restore flow through aggressive medical or surgical interventions.

4. Consider cerebral protective agents. Currently, there are no clear-cut neuroprotective agents which can be strongly advocated for the treatment of acute stroke. The dihydropyridine calcium antagonist nimodipine has been demonstrated to be neuroprotective in several European acute stroke trials.[23] Alternatively, this result has not been reproduced by several clinical trials in the United States.[24] Part of the discrepancy may be due to the time of entry of patients, which was up to 48 h after the onset of the acute stroke. Other potential neuroprotective agents which are currently undergoing clinical testing include free-radical scavengers and excitatory amino acid antagonists. It is reasonable to postulate that in the near future, a cocktail approach might emerge in which the use of tPA is combined with neuroprotective agents, each dedicated to antagonizing a specific mechanism of ischemic injury.

Perioperative Ischemia

Fortunately, perioperative cerebral ischemia is infrequently seen due to the advances in microsurgical technique. Occasionally, the neurosurgeon may need to treat a patient who is suffering from perioperative ischemia due to prolonged intraoperative vessel occlusion or intraoperative vessel injury including dissection or thrombosis. In this situation, there is usually a high index of suspicion regarding the etiology based on the operative scenario. An emergency CT scan should be performed to eliminate the possibility of a postoperative hemorrhage mimicking a vascular insult. The clinician must also be wary of postoperative seizures such as periodic lateralized epileptiform discharges (PLEDs) that can occasionally mimic an acute ischemic insult. If blood vessel injury is suspected, an emergency angiogram should be performed to define the anatomic pathology. It has been our preference to perform early angiography as opposed to limited noninvasive studies such as transcranial Doppler. In this way, if a postoperative dissection or thrombosis is visualized, early aggressive management can be initiated. In most situations, perioperative ischemia is due to prolonged vessel occlusion occurring during treatment of difficult lesions such as giant aneurysms.

Treatment

The treatment of acute perioperative ischemia depends in large part on the etiology and includes the following:

1. The patient should be kept euvolemic with 0.45 or 0.9% NaCl devoid of glucose. We do not practice hemodilution for fear of increasing postoperative cerebral edema. In addition to intravenous (IV) hydration, a colloid such as albumin 250 mL is administered IV 2 to 4 times daily. The role of therapy is to maximize the volume expansion, thereby increasing collateral flow without increasing cerebral edema or intracranial pressure.

2. From a neuroprotective perspective, it is reasonable to consider giving a calcium antagonist such as nimodipine 60 mg by mouth every 4 to 6 h. This is based on the experimental data which demonstrate that calcium antagonists like nimodipine can increase CBF and the clinical experience with subarachnoid hemorrhage which demonstrates that nimodipine decreases the severity of ischemic deficits following subarachnoid hemorrhage.

3. If the patient's neurologic deficit is severe, we will occasionally administer thiopental 3 to 5 mg/kg continuous IV drip or alternatively phenobarbital 15 mg/kg intramuscular or IV loading dose followed by maintenance of therapeutic serum levels. The advantage of thiopental is that its half-life is shorter than that of phenobarbital. The rationale for administering a barbiturate is based on the experimental observation of a direct neuronal protective effect in progressive ischemia.[25–27] In addition, barbiturates may be beneficial by decreasing cerebral edema, which would decrease intracranial pressure, thereby increasing cerebral perfusion pressure. The disadvantages of using barbiturates include obscuration of the neurologic examination and the need for intubation and controlled ventilation.

4. Occasionally, surgical intervention may be warranted. For example, if a postoperative angiogram demonstrated thrombosis or dissection, an emergency embolectomy or bypass procedure could be considered. The risk of perioperative hemorrhage would contraindicate intravascular thrombolytic therapy with agents like tPA. Rarely, an emergency temporal lobectomy can be beneficial both by reversing transtentorial herniation and by increasing cerebral perfusion pressure through the reduction of intracranial pressure.

Subarachnoid Hemorrhage-Induced Ischemic Deficits

Treatment of subarachnoid hemorrhage is authoritatively discussed in Chapter 13 in this textbook. The initial diagnosis of vasopasm should be a clinical one by a physician with a high index of suspicion. Transcranial Doppler or angiography are imaging studies which may support this diagnosis in the demonstrated absence of hydrocephalus on CT scan.

Treatment

Our techniques to treat subarachnoid hemorrhage-induced ischemia are the following:

1. It is our practice to institute hypertensive hypervolemia as the initial treatment for vasospasm once the aneurysm has been repaired.[28] This is contrary to the practice of many neurosurgeons who utilize hemodilution techniques. Hypertensive hypervolemia therapy is initiated by IV hydration with saline solutions at approximately 125 to 150 mL/h. This is supplemented with albumin 250 mg IV every 6 h. If there is no significant cardiac history, the cardiac output is increased by infusing either isoproterenol or dopamine to elevate the blood pressure to approximately 160 mmHg. With infusion of isoproterenol, it will occasionally be necessary to use lidocaine 1 to 2 mg IV to suppress cardiac irritability.

2. Based on results of multiple prospective randomized trials demonstrating that nimodipine decreases the incidence and severity of ischemic deficits, it is our routine to place patients on nimodipine upon admission to the hospital. However, we appreciate that nimodipine is not a magic bullet; if a patient does develop an ischemic deficit, early angiography is performed to determine if angioplasty may be of benefit. Our early experience with angioplasty has provided some promising results.

3. Consider placing a ventricular catheter for drainage of cerebrospinal fluid. In the setting of vasospasm with mild hydrocephalus, removal of cerebrospinal fluid may significantly improve CBF.

FUTURE PHARMACOLOGIC OPTIONS

A critical analysis of the above regimens for the treatment of acute stroke and perioperative ischemia quickly reveals that there are limited pharmacologic interventions which are currently available. Given the rapid advancements in understanding the pathophysiology of ischemic brain injury, it is likely that additional drugs will be developed which will provide neuroprotection by blocking specific mechanisms involved with ischemic cell damage or by increasing collateral blood flow.

Potential Neuroprotective Agents

Excitatory Amino Acid Antagonists Recent advancement and understanding of the role of excitatory amino acids has fostered a tremendous interest in developing both competitive and noncompetitive antagonists to the NMDA receptor and more recently the AMPA receptor. Noncompetitive NMDA antagonists include ketamine, dizocilpine (MK-801), and phenylcyclidine (PCP). These agents block NMDA-gated ion channels. These agents readily penetrate the blood-brain barrier since they are lipid-soluble. Their ability to block the ion channel is voltage-dependent and raises the concern that they may be less effective during massive depolarization or severe ischemia. Competitive NMDA receptor antagonists include the phosphonates such as 2-amino-5-phosphonovalerate (APV), 2-amino-7-phosphonoheptanoate (APH), and more recent compounds with improved blood-brain barrier penetration (CPP, CGS19755). More recently, AMPA receptor antagonists have been developed (CNQX, NBQX). NMDA antagonists have been found to be beneficial in experimental focal ischemia induced by MCA occlusion. A reduction in infarct size by both noncompetitive and competitive antagonists has been demonstrated in multiple experimental models. Some of these agents such as MK-801 have been found to be beneficial when administered up to 1 to 2 h after the onset of focal ischemia. These experimental studies suggest that NMDA antagonists decrease injury in penumbra tissue. Although it is reasonable to presume that these agents decrease Ca^{2+} influx through NMDA receptor-operated calcium channels, there is also some evidence to suggest that they may have a beneficial effect on CBF. Recently, the AMPA receptor antagonist MBQX has also been demonstrated to reduce infarct size when given up to 90 min after MCA occlusion.

There are multiple ongoing clinical trials assessing the effects of NMDA antagonists as a treatment for acute stroke. It is probable that some of these excitatory amino acid antagonists will prove to be beneficial and assume a primary role in the treatment of focal ischemia.

Calcium Antagonists Calcium antagonists could be beneficial either by decreasing the influx of calcium through voltage-dependent calcium channels or by increasing CBF. There is minimal evidence to indicate that calcium antagonists prevent calcium entry into ischemic neurons. A rise in intracellular free calcium during ischemia could occur through multiple avenues including voltage-dependent calcium channels, receptor-operated calcium channels, and release from the endoplasmic reticulum. Within the subgroup of voltage-dependent calcium channels, there are actually three channels, with only one (L channel) being modulated by calcium antagonists such as nimodipine. Other calcium antagonists like flunarizine and nicardipine may also have effects on voltage-dependent T channels. In any event, the effects of calcium antagonists on focal ischemia are equivocal. Although there is general agreement that calcium antagonists, specifically those of the dihydropyridine class such as nimodipine, nicardipine, or PN-200-110 increase CBF in both ischemic and nonischemic conditions, results regarding their effects on size of infarction are inconsistent.[29] Postulated mechanisms of improvement in CBF by calcium antagonists include the reversal of ischemic vasoconstriction, dilation of pial collateral blood vessels, or reduction of platelet aggregation with reduced blood viscosity. More recently, a calcium antagonist with serotonin effects called S-emopamil has been demonstrated to ameliorate damage following MCA occlusion.[30]

Despite the inconsistent experimental data, nimodipine has been demonstrated to decrease the incidence and severity of ischemic deficits following subarachnoid hemorrhage. In addition, several European studies have observed that the administration of nimodipine in patients with acute stroke significantly reduced deaths in males and led to improved long-term functional outcome. Therefore, it is likely that some voltage-dependent calcium antagonists like nimodipine or nicardipine will secure a role in the treatment of acute stroke perhaps as part of a therapeutic cocktail.

Free-Radical Scavengers There is accumulating evidence that oxygen-free radical-mediated lipid perioxidation plays a detrimental role in focal ischemia.[31] It has been demonstrated that endogenous antioxidants such as α-tocopherol, ascorbate, and glutathione decrease during focal ischemia. Free-radical scavengers such as polyethylene glycol–conjugated superoxide dismutase and catalase have been demonstrated to decrease infarct size in focal ischemia experiments. More recently, a group of 21-amino steroids (lazaroids) have been developed.[32] These amino steroids have no glucocorticoid activity but act as free-radical scavengers and iron chelators. These compounds have been demonstrated to be beneficial in experimental head trauma, subarachnoid hemorrhage, focal ischemia, and global ischemia. If these results are verified, the 21-amino steroids may prove beneficial in the treatment of acute stroke. As with all free-radical scavengers, administration prior to the period of reperfusion during peak free-radical production must be accomplished. Mannitol has also been reported to be a free-radical scavenger and therefore beneficial in focal ischemia, leading some experienced neurosurgeons to routinely administer mannitol intraoperatively prior to vessel occlusion during aneurysm surgery.

CONCLUSION

A rational approach to the neurosurgical ICU management of acute cerebral ischemia depends on an understanding of the mechanisms of ischemic neuronal injury. In focal cerebral ischemia, there is a heterogeneous pattern of blood flow reduction. In the core region of dense ischemia, it is unlikely that interventions will be beneficial in reversing neuronal damage. Alternatively, surrounding the core region of ischemia is a moderate ischemic zone termed the *ischemic penumbra*, which is potentially salvageable tissue. Techniques to salvage this reversibly injured tissue can be divided into methods to increase collateral blood flow and those designed to offer direct neuronal protection. In the nonoperative acute stroke, intravascular thrombolysis may ultimately prove to be the technique of choice to provide early flow restoration. Alternatively, in postoperative ischemia, methods of volume expansion or possibly hemodilution are the techniques of choice. Currently available drugs which might offer direct neuronal protection include the dihydropyridine calcium antagonist nimodipine and barbiturates. In the future, agents which attenuate specific degradative pathways including NMDA and AMPA receptor antagonists and free-radical scavengers may prove effective.

REFERENCES

1. Weinstein PR, Faden AL: *Protection of the Brain from Ischemia*, Baltimore, Williams & Wilkins, 1990.
2. Bransten NM, Simon L, Crockard HA, et al.: Relationship between the cortical electrical potential and local cortical blood flow following acute middle cerebral artery occlusion in the baboon. *Exp Neurol* 45:195, 1974.
3. Astrup J, Simon L, Branston NM, et al.: Cortical evoked potential in extracellular K^+/H^+ at critical levels of brain ischemia. *Stroke* 8:51, 1977.
4. Michenfelder JD, Sundt TM Jr: Cerebral ATP and lactate levels in the squirrel monkey following occlusion of the middle cerebral artery. *Stroke* 2:319, 1971.
5. Simon L, Bransten NM, Strong AJ, et al.: The concept of thresholds of ischemia in relation to brain structure and function. *J Clin Pathol* 30(suppl 11):149, 1977.
6. Strong AJ, Venables GS, Gibson G: The cortical ischemic penumbra associated with occlusion of the middle cerebral artery in the cat. 1. Topography of changes in blood flow, potassium activity, and EEG. *J Cereb Blood Flow Metab* 3:86, 1983.
7. Morawetz RB, Crowell RH, DeGiorlami U, et al.: Regional CBF thresholds during cerebral ischemia. *Fed Proc* 48:49, 1979.
8. Ianotti F, Hoff J: Ischemic brain edema with and without reperfusion: An experimental study in gerbils. *Stroke* 14:562, 1983.
9. Siesjö BK: Cell damage in the brain: A speculative synthesis. *J Cereb Blood Flow Metab* 1:155, 1981.
10. Rothman SM, Olney JW: Glutamate in the pathophysiology of hypoxic-ischemic brain damage. *Ann Neurol* 19:105, 1986.
11. Siesjö BK, Bengtsson F: Calcium fluxes, calcium antagonists, and calcium related pathology in brain ischemia, hypoglycemia, and spreading depression: A unifying hypothesis. *J Cereb Blood Flow Metab* 9:127, 1989.
12. Simon RP, Swan JH, Griffith T, et al.: Blockade of N-methyl-D-aspartate receptors may protect against ischemic damage in the brain. *Science* 226:850, 1984.
13. Oyzuart E, Graham DI, Woodruff GN, et al.: Protective effect of glutamate antagonist MK801 in focal cerebral ischemia in the cat. *J Cereb Blood Flow Metab* 8:138, 1988.
14. Park CK, Nehls DG, Graham DI, et al.: Focal cerebral ischemia in the cat: Treatment with the glutamate antagonist MK801 after induction of ischemia. *J Cereb Blood Flow Metab* 8:757, 1988.
15. Meyer FB, Sundt TM Jr, Anderson RE, et al.: Ischemic vasoconstriction and parenchymal brain pH. *Ann NY Acad Sci* 522:502, 1988.
16. Crowell RM, Olsson Y: Impaired microvascular filling after focal cerebral ischemia in monkeys. *J Neurosurg* 36:303, 1972.
17. Wood J, Simeone F, Fink E, et al.: Correlative aspects of hypervolemic hemodilution with low molecular weight dextran after experimental cerebral artery occlusion. *Neurology* 34:24, 1984.
18. Scandinavian Stroke Study Group: Multicenter trial of hemodilution in acute ischemic stroke. *Stroke* 18:691, 1987.
19. Myers RE: Lactate acid accumulation as cause of brain edema in cerebral necrosis resulting from oxygen deprivation. In: Korobkin R, Guilleminault C (eds): *Advances in Perinatal Neurology*, vol. 1. New York, Spectrum Publications, 1979, pp 85–114.
20. Zivin JA, Fisher M, DeGirolami U, et al.: Tissue plasminogen activator reduces neurological damage after cerebral embolism. *Science* 230:1289, 1985.
21. Del Zoppo GJ, Zeumer H, Harker LA: Thrombolytic therapy in stroke: Possibilities and hazards. *Stroke* 17:595, 1986.
22. Meyer FB, Sundt TM Jr, Yanagihara T, Anderson RE: Focal cerebral ischemia: Pathophysiologic mechanisms and rationale for future avenues of treatment. *Mayo Clin Proc* 62:35, 1987.
23. Gelmers HJ, Gorter K, de Weerdt CJ, et al.: A controlled trial of nimodipine in acute stroke. *N Engl J Med* 318:203, 1988.

24. Sherman DG, Easton JD, Hart RG, et al.: Nimodipine in acute cerebral infarction. A double blind study of safety and efficacy. In: Battistini N, Fiorani P, Courbier R, et al. (eds): *Acute Brain Ischemia. Medical and Surgical Therapy.* New York, Raven, 1986, pp 257–262.
25. Smith AL, Hoff JT, Nielsen SL, et al.: Barbiturate protection in focal cerebral ischemia. *Stroke* 5:1, 1974.
26. Steen PA, Michenfelder JD: Mechanisms of barbiturate protection. *Anesthesiology* 53:183, 1980.
27. Selman WR, Spetzler RF, Roessmann UR, et al.: Barbiturate induced coma therapy for focal cerebral ischemia: Effect after temporary and permanent MCA occlusion. *J Neurosurg* 55:220, 1981.
28. Sundt TM Jr, Onofrio BM, Merideth J: Treatment of cerebral vasospasm from subarachnoid hemorrhage with isoproterenol and lidocaine hydrochloride. *J Neurosurg* 38:557, 1973.
29. Mohammed AA, Mendelow AD, Teasdale GM, et al.: Effect of the calcium antagonist nimodipine on local CBF and metabolic coupling. *J Cereb Blood Flow Metab* 5:26, 1985.
30. Nakayama H, Ginsberg MD, Dietrich WD: S-emopamil, a novel calcium channel blocker and S_2 antagonist, markedly reduces infant size following middle cerebral artery occlusion in the rat. *Neurology* 38:1667, 1988.
31. Demopoulos HB, Flamm ES, Pietronigro DD, et al.: The free radical pathology in the microcirculation in the major central nervous system disorders. *Acta Physiol Scand* 42:91, 1980.
32. Hall ED, Yonkers PA: Attenuation of postischemic cerebral hypoperfusion by the 21-aminosteroid U74006F. *Stroke* 19:340, 1988.

CHAPTER 16

The Intensive Care Management of the Neurointerventional Patient

Stanley L. Barnwell

HISTORY OF INTERVENTIONAL NEURORADIOLOGY

Occlusion of blood vessels by an endovascular approach was first described by Brooks in 1930 for treatment of a traumatic arteriovenous fistula.[1] This approach to lesions in the central nervous system was not developed until more recently because of limitations in catheter technology and imaging. Luessenhop and Spence described the first endovascular approach to treating a cerebral arteriovenous malformation in 1960.[2] As advances occurred in radiologic imaging, the field of interventional neuroradiology developed.[3] Djindjian led the way in this area by developing catheters which could be used to superselectively catheterize branches of the external carotid artery, and ultimately the intracranial circulation.[4] Serbinenko invented a detachable balloon catheter which has led to the development of a wide variety of embolic devices.[5] These developments of balloon technology have largely been made by Debrun.[6] Luessenhop has pointed out that many developments in this field were being made in the Soviet Union by Serbinenko, Scheglov, and others, but because of restricted access, these advances have only recently been noted.[3,6,7]

Endovascular therapy became a more routine part of radiology in the 1970s, with the development of better imaging and catheters.[3] The treatment of cerebral arteriovenous malformations became a prime motive for developing interventional neuroradiology because of difficulty with the surgical treatment of this disease.

Because neurointerventional techniques are used for patients with complex intracranial lesions, often with a risk of ischemia or hemorrhage during or after treatment, it is common to place such patients in the ICU afterwards for neurologic observation, blood pressure control, and at times, hemodynamic management. This chapter will review the methodology and techniques of neurointerventional therapy, and highlight the place of ICU care for these patients.

METHODOLOGY

Advances in neurointerventional radiology have in large part been dependent on imaging technology. Subtraction angiography allows visualization of small vessels without interference of overlapping bony structures.[8] This technique is performed by having the first image acquired at a time when no contrast is present. This produces a transparent positive image. This mask image is placed over an image with contrast, and a final print subtracts the bone from the angiogram. The result is a detailed view of the vessels.

The majority of work presently performed uses digital angiography rather than direct imaging of x-rays on photographic film.[9] Image intensifier tubes allow a noiseless amplification of a light signal from cesium iodide crystals used as detectors. Television cameras can detect small differences in radiation exposure more reliably than conventional photographic plates. The digital memory and electronic subtraction produce real-time images that can be subtracted instantly. Real-time subtraction angiography involves automatically subtracting a mask image from an averaged real-time fluoroscopy image. This technique allows continuous imaging of blood vessels, from the early arterial phase through a late venous phase without interference of overlying bones. Real-time subtraction allows one to reliably confirm results of therapy instantly.

The technique of road-mapping adds greatly to the ease and efficacy of endovascular surgery. Road-mapping involves projecting a subtracted vascular pathway, such that the blood vessel is continuously displayed, much as a road map, under live fluoroscopy without imaging the bones. This technique allows the interventionalist to follow the course of a moving catheter through a blood vessel. The interventionalist may direct a catheter into a selected pedicle supplying an arteriovenous malformation, or a balloon into an aneurysm, for example, without the image being obstructed by overlying bones.

SUPERSELECTIVE CATHETERIZATION FOR ANALYSIS OF THE ANGIOARCHITECTURE AND FLOW

Prior to embolization it is critical to obtain highly selective angiograms of every feeder to a lesion before it is occluded.[10] This information is not necessarily apparent on global proximal artery injections where there is rapid obscuring of the angioarchitecture of the nidus and feeding vessels. Superselective catheterization allows one to evaluate the anatomy of the lesion, with particular attention directed at finding aneurysms and evaluating normal vessels in the area. When combined with high-speed acquisition of images, up to 30 images per second, information on flow and aneurysms can be obtained that may otherwise not be forthcoming. Information regarding flow through the lesion is critical in determining which embolic agents to use and for proper preparation of the agents in terms of size of particles or polymerization times of liquid adhesives.[11] Data obtained from this superselective catheterization add greatly to the safety of the procedure.[10]

USE OF PROVOCATIVE TESTING PRIOR TO EMBOLIZATION

Prior to occluding a vessel that supplies a lesion, testing is performed that may predict any functional loss that may occur from blocking that vessel. The use of superselective injection of amobarbital into intracranial arteries before embolization has been performed for over 10 years.[12–14] This test is a variation of the Wada and Rasmussen test, wherein amobarbital is injected into the internal carotid artery to test for language function.[15] The test is generally considered to be reliable, although there may be false positives or false negatives. Pressure and speed of the injection of the drug should replicate what will be used with the embolic agents. Overinjection may cause reflux into normal vessels, giving false-positive results.[14,16] Underinjection, or sumping of the drug into the malformation and bypassing normal branches, may lead to false-negative tests. As the embolization of a pedicle proceeds and flow is altered, it is necessary to retest the vessel since normal vessels that previously did not fill may subsequently fill. A negative test does not necessarily indicate that it will be safe to embolize that pedicle.

Amobarbital is typically used for intracranial circulation but will not affect cranial nerve function. The use of lidocaine is more effective for testing of cranial nerve function and sight.[14] Lidocaine is toxic to the central nervous system, and caution should be taken to ensure it does not enter the cerebral circulation through reflux or via collateral between the external carotid artery and intracranial circulation.[14]

NEUROLOGIC TESTING DURING EMBOLIZATION

The neurologic exam on an awake patient is probably the most sensitive indicator of the effect of an embolization. When the embolization is preceded by a full understanding of the vascular anatomy, provocative testing with amobarbital, and under constant neurologic monitoring, it is generally a safe procedure. The majority of reports with large numbers of patients note the importance of doing the procedures in awake patients while closely monitoring the clinical exam, especially for cerebral arteriovenous malformations.[10,12,17–27] The use of neuroleptic analgesia is generally advocated for these procedures to make them more tolerable for the patient.[28]

At times it becomes necessary to perform these procedures under a general anesthetic, for example, with patients who are moribund or uncooperative or for children. In these cases, the use of electroencephalography, continuous recording of brainstem acoustic responses, and somatosensory-evoked cortical potentials may be used for monitoring both hemispheric and brainstem functions.[29]

EMBOLIC AGENTS

A wide variety of agents have been used to produce vascular occlusion for the treatment of vascular lesions. These agents can be grouped into agents that result in proximal occlusion of vessels supplying the lesion and agents which penetrate into the nidus of the lesion.

Proximal occlusion of vessels is useful in treating lesions prior to surgery. This blockage can reduce the size and pressure within the nidus and diminish the number of feeding pedicles allowing for easier surgery. The disadvantage to proximal occlusion is that it generally cannot be used as the sole form of therapy because there will be enlargement of collateral feeders. The hypertrophy of these feeders results ultimately in reconstitution of the nidus and return of high flow. Proximal occlusion also prevents later use of the pedicle if more selective catheterization and embolization is planned for the future.

Proximal occlusion of vessels can be obtained with detachable balloons (Interventional Therapeutic Corp., South San Francisco) and platinum coils.[22,24] The use of balloons has the advantage of allowing neurologic testing before permanent occlusion. In the largest series of balloon occlusions in preparation for cerebral arteriovenous malformation surgery, 36 feeders were occluded in 31 patients.[22] There were only two strokes as a result of these occlusions, and surgery was judged to be significantly less difficult. Occlusion can also be performed with platinum coils. These coils do not interfere with magnetic resonance imaging and are small enough to be delivered to pedicles very close to the malformation. Small straight or curved coils may also be particularly useful in obliterating small vessels with associated aneurysms.

Agents that penetrate into the small vessels composing the nidus of lesion include cyanoacrylates, polyvinyl alcohol particles, ethanol, and microfibrillar collagen. The most commonly used agents are cyanoacrylates and polyvinyl alcohol. All these agents have the potential for causing proximal vessel occlusion if they are delivered proximally.

The majority of large series of patients with cerebral arteriovenous malformations treated by embolization show the results using isobutyl 2-cyanoacrylate (IBCA). The use of this agent for embolization was first described by Cromwell and Kerber in 1979.[30] Because of concerns over the carcinogenicity of this agent, n-butyl 2-cyanoacrylate (NBCA) has been substituted for its use.[31] There are no data that show the risk with this agent is less than IBCA, and they perform very similarly in vivo. The polymerization time may be adjusted for these agents by adding glacial acetic acid.[11] The polymerization time is adjusted based on the flow through the malformation and distance between the catheter tip and the nidus. The glue is not inherently radiopaque and an oil-based contrast agent with tantalum powder is added to make it visible on fluoroscopy. The long-term effects of IBCA, and presumably NBCA, show pathologic changes in the vessel's wall, including angionecrosis.[32] Although generally thought to be a permanent occlusive agent, there can be dissolution and resorption of the glue over a period of months.[32,33] Liquid glues have the advantage of being able to be delivered through flow-directed catheters, which are very soft and less likely to cause vascular perforations than the stiffer catheters through which particles are delivered.

Polyvinyl alcohol (Contour, Interventional Therapeutics Corp., South San Francisco) is the particulate agent most frequently used in the treatment of many lesions.[34-36] The advantage of particles over glue is the reduced risk of causing proximal vessel occlusion and gluing the delivery catheter into the brain or blood vessel.[36] The particles are sized from 150 to 1000 μm in diameter or may be hand cut from larger pieces. Particle size is chosen based on an estimation of the size of shunts within the malformation. Occlusion is best obtained if the particles lodge in the nidus rather than proximally. There is a well-demonstrated need for the appropriate choice of particle size. Particles which are too small will pass through the malformation and can lodge in the lung, causing fatal pulmonary insufficiency.[37] Small particles may also pass into vessels which cannot be seen on angiography due to limitations of the equipment. Occluding these small vessels which may be end arteries can result in infarction.[35] While the particles are radiolucent, their effect on closing vessels is evaluated by the flow patterns of contrast in which the particles are suspended. The occlusive mechanism of polyvinyl alcohol appears to be adherence to the walls of vessels, such that small particles may not pass through a malformation even if the vessel diameter is larger than the particle.[38] Vessels that have been occluded by polyvinyl alcohol show an angionecrosis similar to IBCA.[39] The combination of polyvinyl alcohol with Gelfoam (Upjohn, Kalamazoo) as an embolic agent has been recommended as a way to reduce the friction which occurs as the particle flows through a catheter.[34]

Fistulous connections within the nidus of a lesion may complicate the endovascular treatment. These large connections allow most emoblic agents to pass through and into the venous side of the lesion. These agents which pass through the lesion may occlude the venous outflow or go to the lung. The use of silk suture has been shown to be effective in closing large fistulous connections within arteriovenous malformations.[40] Larger, handcut pieces of polyvinyl alcohol may also be useful in closing fistulous connections. Both have the disadvantage of being radiolucent, although if used in selected instances with contrast it is safe. As the fistulous connections are closed, smaller agents may be used.

There are a variety of agents under investigation as embolic agents.[41-43] Ethylene vinyl alcohol copolymer and metrizamide dissolved in dimethylsulfoxide forms an ethylene vinyl alcohol copolymer sponge that obstructs both the feeding artery and nidus.[43] This agent may be advantageous over glues in that it stays liquid and will not hold the catheter in the blood vessel, despite its ability to occlude the nidus of a lesion. Ethyl alcohol results in occlusion of blood vessels when administered in sufficient concentration.[41] It may be useful in obliterating the nidus of a lesion and is relatively easy to deliver.

INTRACRANIAL ANEURYSMS

The treatment of choice for most aneurysms is surgical clipping. There are, however, aneurysms that by virtue of size or location cannot be safely treated by surgery. Some patients are judged too ill to undergo a surgical procedure requiring a general anesthetic, or they may refuse to undergo a surgical procedure. The natural history of these previously untreatable aneurysms is dismal. Interventional neuroradiologic techniques have emerged as an alternative to surgery for treatment of selected lesions.

Serbinenko, in 1974, first described the use of detachable balloons for the treatment of aneurysms.[5] This technology has been refined and expanded in the United States by Hieshima and coworkers to treat aneurysms throughout the intracranial circulation.[44,45] The technique allows treatment by occlusion of the parent vessel from which the aneurysm originates, or preferably, with preservation of the parent vessel by direct aneurysm occlusion. A series of 84 patients in whom the aneurysm was treated while preserving the parent artery showed complete aneurysm obliteration in 77.4 percent with follow-up of 3 to 68 months (mean of 35.5 months), and subtotal occlusion in 22.6 percent.[45] All these cases were considered not amenable to surgical therapy or had been explored and found to be unclippable. The complication rate, including fatal hemorrhages and strokes, was 32 percent. The complications were much more frequent in large aneurysms that had presented with hemorrhage and for which no surgical therapy could be given. Among 87 cases of cavernous carotid artery aneurysms, which generally have a more benign course than other intracranial aneurysms, the parent vessels were spared in 22 percent and occluded in 78 percent.[44] Significant complications consisting of nonfatal stroke occurred in only 4.5 percent of these patients. Among a series of 21 vertebrobasilar artery aneurysms that could not be treated surgically, vertebral artery occlusion was performed.[46] In this group there were good outcomes consisting of complete obliteration in 62 percent, subtotal occlusion of the aneurysm in 28 percent, death in 5 percent, and failed treatment in 5 percent. In another series of 16 patients with surgically untreatable, high-risk aneurysms, 12 cases (75 percent) had excellent results without neurologic complications.[47] There were three deaths (18.8 percent) related to the treatment and one death from rupture of a second untreated aneurysm. The patients from these reports would all be considered high risk.

The technology of endovascular treatment of intracranial aneurysms is rapidly changing. While the complication rate has been high, it must be remembered that these lesions have no other treatment. Advances continue to be made in this form of therapy. The use of detachable platinum coils may markedly change the way aneurysms are treated in the future.[48,49] This new technology has many advantages over balloons, and while still experimental, initial results are promising.

Because arterial occlusion, aneurysm rupture, and intracranial hemorrhage may complicate endovascular treatment of aneurysms, most patients are initially observed in the ICU afterward. The neurologic examination is monitored for signs suggestive of hemorrhage or cerebral ischemia. New symptoms or signs are reevaluated with CT scanning of the brain. Blood pressure is carefully monitored and maintained at normal levels. Evidence of cerebral ischemia may be treated with volume expansion, induced hypertension, or use of Nimodipine,[47,54,72] using a Swan-Ganz or central venous catheter to monitor intravascular volume and cardiac output.

ANGIOPLASTY FOR VASOSPASM

Intracranial arterial spasm occurs in approximately 30 percent of patients with aneurysmal subarachnoid hemorrhage, usually within 5 to 12 days of the hemorrhagic event.[50–52] Recognized as a serious complication, it increases the risk of cerebral infarction and contributes to the high mortality and morbidity rates associated with aneurysmal bleeding: less than 50 percent of patients survive and only 36 percent of patients return to full employment.[53,54]

Cerebral vasospasm is a diffuse process, although there is a tendency for involvement of vessels in the circle of Willis.[50,55–58]

The involvement of a particular vessel may extend over a long distance or be focal. The mechanisms that result in vasospasm are not clearly understood but may include vasoconstriction from endogenous agents released from subarachnoid blood,[56,59] intimal hyperplasia,[60,61] and muscular contraction producing anoxia in the wall of the vessel.[62–66]

Many pharmacologic agents have been evaluated to treat this condition, but none are known that consistently reverse the clinical manifestations.[63,64,67–71] Medical therapies such as use of calcium channel blockers, induced arterial hypertension, or expanded intravascular volume have also been advocated. However, these therapies are associated with complications, and their effectiveness remains to be adequately demonstrated.[72]

The use of transluminal angioplasty to treat vasospasm associated with aneurysmal subarachnoid hemorrhage was first described in 1984 and shown to reverse arterial spasm and restore cerebral perfusion in patients with aneurysm subarachnoid bleeding.[73]

In the first report, 33 patients with symptomatic vasospasm benefited from this procedure. They demonstrated a marked improvement in their neurologic condition accompanied by angiographic evidence of arterial widening, although details of the neurologic exams were not given.[73] Since that first report, a new microballoon has been developed for dilation of intracranial arterial spasm resulting from subarachnoid hemorrhage.[74] The balloon is composed of a silicon shell attached to a 2.0 French catheter. It inflates symmetrically and from the proximal end to the distal end. It generates a very low pressure, less than 1 atm, so has less risk of rupturing the vessel.

Using this new balloon, angioplasty reversed the neurologic deficits in nine of thirteen patients with symptomatic vasospasm after subarachnoid hemorrhage, all of whom had failed medical therapy.[75] The four patients who had no improvement were in the Hunt and Hess grades 4 and 5 neurologic condition, which places them in a poor prognostic category.[76] In another series, eight of ten patients with symptomatic vasospasm improved after angioplasty.[77] Improvement in neurologic function has been documented to occur even when the deficits have been longstanding, over 36 h.[78]

The complications from angioplasty of intracranial vessels have been very low. Among the two largest series of 23 patients, there were three complications which included hemorrhage from an unclipped aneurysm, middle cerebral artery occlusion, and hemorrhagic infarction, possibly caused by reperfusion of an infarcted area of the brain.[75,77] Fatal rupture of a vessel has also been described.[79] These complications can be reduced by not dilating blood vessels associated with unclipped aneurysms, not treating vascular territories with known infarction, and not overinflating the balloon.

The use of angioplasty to treat vasospasm after subarachnoid hemorrhage is a new therapy with the results unproven but encouraging. There are many issues surrounding this therapy that are unresolved, particularly timing of therapy and the effect on small blood vessels and perfusion of the microcirculation.[75] However, in the acute stages of vasospasm it has been shown that spastic vessels can be dilated and distal circulation improved. Such patients should routinely be managed in the ICU to continue optimal control over hemodynamic status, ongoing hemodynamic therapy,[72] and careful monitoring.

CEREBRAL ARTERIOVENOUS MALFORMATIONS

The endovascular treatment of cerebral arteriovenous malformations began as an alternative to surgical therapy in the 1960s.[3] At the time this form of therapy began, the surgical treatment of cerebral arteriovenous malformations was only occasionally successful in completely removing the lesion and usually was only performed on small lesions in noneloquent areas of the brain.[3] In the setting of poor surgical results Luessenhop and Spence described the first endovascular approach to treating an arteriovenous malformation through an endovascular approach.[2] At first, embolic agents were delivered to the malformations utilizing flow patterns from proximal catheter locations. As catheter technology improved, it became possible to deliver embolic agents from catheters lodged in or adjacent to the malformation, thereby increasing safety and effectiveness.

The indications to treat an arteriovenous malformation are primarily related to prevention of hemorrhage. Hemorrhage is one of the most common presentations of a cerebral arteriovenous malformation, with the frequency ranging from 30 to 86 percent in large series.[80–82] The mortality from the first hemorrhage is around 10 percent, and morbidity is at least 30 percent.[83] Once a hemorrhage has occurred, the risk of another hemorrhage within the first year is about 6 percent, and for subsequent years the risk of hemorrhage is about 3 to 4 percent a year with an annual mortality rate of 1 percent.[84,85] Among one of the largest series with long-term follow-up, 23 percent of patients were dead as a result of hemorrhage from the malformation, and the presentation, by hemorrhage, headache, seizures or neurologic deficits, did not alter the ultimately poor prognosis for many of these lesions.[85]

The indications for therapy of a cerebral arteriovenous malformation include treatment of lesions that have bled to prevent rehemorrhage, uncontrolled headaches, progressive neurologic deficits, uncontrolled seizures, and as a preoperative or preradiosurgery adjunct. In addition, lesions with identified risk factors for hemorrhage, such as venous occlusive disease and aneurysms, should also be considered for treatment.

The methods used in treating an arteriovenous malformation are complex. Superselective angiography is used to define the vascular supply to the lesion and thereby avoid occluding normal vessels. Prior to occlusion of a vessel, functional testing can be performed with amobarbitol to evaluate whether or not any functional brain is supplied by the vessels, and to reposition the catheter as necessary to avoid those normal branches.[12-15] Generally embolizations are performed with the patient awake so that constant neurologic monitoring can be performed. A wide variety of embolic agents are available for producing vascular occlusion, including balloons, wire coils, liquid adhesives, and particles. The decision to use one agent over another is largely determined by the experience of the interventionalist.

The results of embolization of cerebral arteriovenous malformations have been the subject of 14 recent series, each reporting on at least 15 patients.[10,12,13,17-27] These reports are retrospective studies of the results of embolizations. The studies do not address a uniform set of questions, although they do give data concerning results of embolization.

The primary benefits of embolization is preoperative reduction in blood flow (Fig. 16-1). Embolization can change a very vascular lesion into an avascular tangle of thrombosed vessels. The surgical removal is significantly easier and faster, requiring less removal of normal brain adjacent to the lesion.

Prevention of hemorrhage has not been clearly shown to be a result of embolization. However, recognition of risk factors for hemorrhage, such as aneurysms within the nidus of an arteriovenous malformation and occlusion of that vessel, would appear to offer some protection against further hemorrhage. In four of these large series, there were no recurrent hemorrhages among 78 to 100 percent of patients treated who had originally presented with hemorrhage.[12,19,21,27] Resolution or significant improvement of headaches after embolization was noted in 50 to 71 percent of patients treated.[12,18,27] Neurologic dysfunction due to these lesions may improve after embolization. In three of these large series where neurologic deficits were evaluated, improvement occurred in 50 to 59 percent.[18,20,27] Reduction in seizure frequency is variable after embolization. Resolution or reduction was noted in 7 to 61 percent of treated patients.[12,18,27]

Complications from embolization may include transient neurologic deficits, strokes, and hemorrhage. Transient neurologic deficits occurred in 2.5 to 31 percent of patients.[20-22,24,25] The highest rates were seen when liquid adhesives were used as the embolic agent. Strokes occurred in 1.6 to 20 percent of patients, and again the highest risk was associated with use of liquid adhesives rather than particulate agents.[10,12,13,17-20,22-27] Among these reports including 503 patients, there were 22 hemorrhages, for an overall risk of 4.3 percent. When a hemorrhage did occur, 31.8 percent were fatal, underscoring the seriousness of this complication. This poor outcome from hemorrhage can probably be significantly reduced by early recognition and management, which has only recently been described.[86,87] As with patients with aneurysms, those undergoing embolization of AVM's should initially be managed in the ICU for early identification of complications and subsequent treatment.

ATHEROSCLEROTIC DISEASE

Percutaneous transluminal angioplasty of brachiocephalic vessels, including the innominate, subclavian, vertebral, and external and internal carotid arteries, is now being performed in selected cases. This technique appears to be safe and effective in treating hemodynamically significant lesions. Follow-up has included angiographic and clinical evaluation up to 4 years later and has shown generally stable clinical and angiographic results. Among 165 patients treated, there was a successful angiographic result in 162 patients.[88-93] Lesions most commonly treated were in the common carotid or internal carotid artery, although

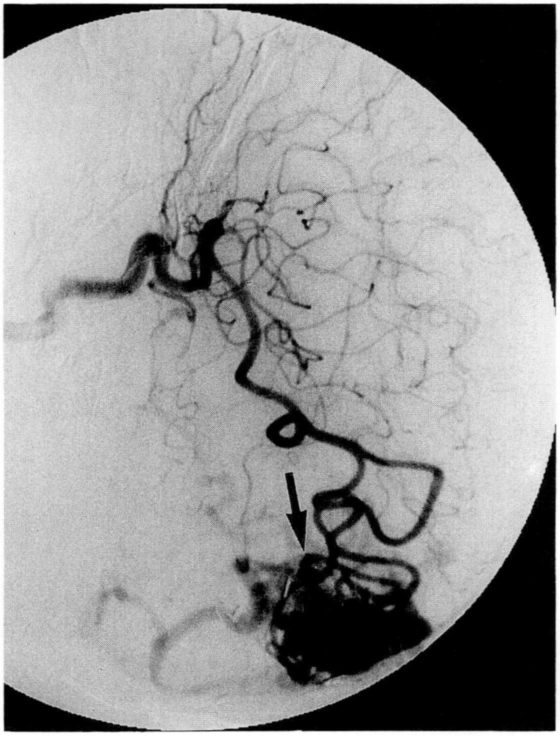

A

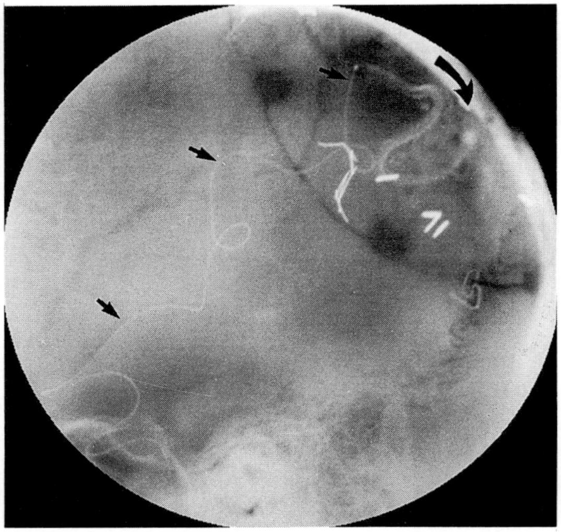

B

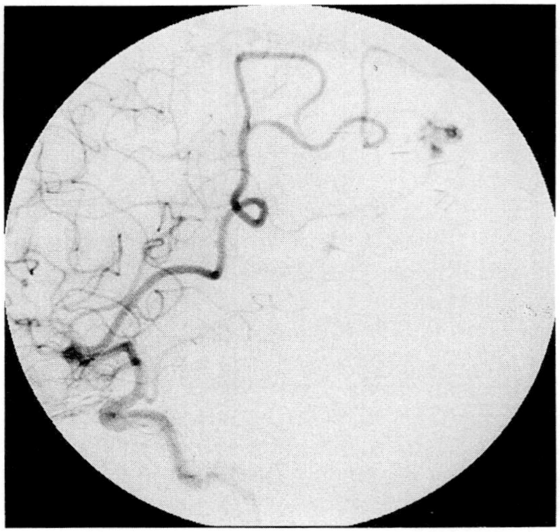

C

Figure 16-1 *A*. Left internal carotid artery injection, lateral view, shows a left occipital lobe arteriovenous malformation (arrow) in a 48-year-old man with seizures. An attempt to remove the malformation 10 years ago was stopped because of uncontrolled bleeding. *B*. Left middle cerebral artery distal branch injection, lateral view, shows supply to the malformation (curved arrow). The course of the catheter is shown (straight arrows). Three other arterial pedicles similar to this one were catheterized, tested with sodium amobarbitol, and embolized with platinum coils and polyvinyl alcohol particles. *C*. Left internal carotid artery injection, lateral view, shows minimal residual filling of the malformation. Surgical excision of the mass of mostly thrombosed vessels was performed without difficulty.

there is beginning to be extensive experience with all the vascular areas. Three of the 165 patients either had residual stenosis or the angioplasty catheter could not be advanced across the stenotic lesion.[88,89] Two patients had restenosis in follow-up.[90] Temporary ischemic complications occurred in five patients.[90,91] There was only one permanent stroke, in a patient with basilar artery atherosclerotic disease.[89]

Despite the promising results of this form of therapy, there is not widespread acceptance of this treatment. There is a valid concern of distal embolization of debris from the plaques subjected to angioplasty, and this problem has been shown to occur.[94] However, the clinical results would suggest distal embolization is infrequently significant. Recurrent stenosis from myointimal hyperplasia is another concern with this technique as with the surgical technique.[95] The initial reports with long-term follow-up do not show this problem to be especially prevalent.

CAROTID-CAVERNOUS ARTERIOVENOUS FISTULAS

Carotid-cavernous fistulas are of two types, direct or indirect. Direct types are usually solitary connections between the cavernous segment of the internal carotid artery and the cavernous sinus. Most of these direct types are the result of head trauma. Indirect, or dural type, carotid-cavernous fistulas are usually composed of multiple connections between branches of the internal and external carotid arteries in the cavernous sinus and veins in the cavernous sinus. These indirect fistulas are usually spontaneous in origin and characterized by slow flow and associated with a higher rate of spontaneous closure. Carotid-cavernous fistulas of either type may result in loss of vision, bruit, exophthalmos, glaucoma, ophthalmoplegia, or intracranial hemorrhage. These signs and symptoms may require urgent treatment.[96]

The treatment of choice of direct carotid-cavernous fistulas is transarterial embolization with preservation of flow through the internal carotid artery.[97] In a series of 206 patients with direct carotid-cavernous fistulas treated by transarterial balloon embolization, 88 percent had the fistula closed with preservation of flow through the carotid artery.[98] Occlusion of the internal carotid artery was required in 12 percent of patients to close the fistula. The complication rate for strokes was 2.4 percent.

Transarterial embolization may also be performed with platinum wires. This approach has been used successfully in cases where balloons were ineffective because of difficulty in navigating them into the fistula or because sharp spicules of bone break the balloon each time it is inflated. In a series of five patients, the fistula was closed in three with preservation of flow through the internal carotid artery.[99] One patient had a carotid occlusion when a coil was partly left in the internal carotid artery. The other patient's fistula could only be closed with a balloon in addition to the coils.

When transarterial embolization of direct carotid-cavernous fistulas is unsuccessful, alternative treatments are available. Transvenous embolization has been described as an effective approach to treating these lesions. In a series of 12 patients treated, 11 were completely cured and one had subtotal occlusion of the fistula with improved clinical symptoms.[100] A direct surgical exposure of the cavernous sinus can be performed for closure of these fistulas by packing the sinus with wires or balloons, although this procedure is seldom necessary.[101]

The treatment of choice of indirect, or dural, carotid-cavernous fistulas is through a transvenous route as clearly shown by Halbach and others.[102] The multiplicity of arterial feeders going into these fistulas makes the transarterial route less likely to succeed because if any arterial inflow remains, it will likely hypertrophy and the fistula will re-form. The inferior petrosal sinus is most commonly used to access the cavernous sinus fistula. Among 13 patients treated by this approach, the fistula was closed completely in 12 and partly in 1.[102]

The superior ophthalmic vein is another route used in the transvenous approach. This vein may be reached by either the femoral percutaneous approach or exposure of the angular vein in the face, which leads into the superior ophthalmic vein. This approach has been used in four patients with complete closure of the fistula in all cases.[103] Other reports of the superior ophthalmic vein approach have also been successful.[104,105]

Although some patients may be placed on the general ward after an uncomplicated fistula occlusion, many patients should have initial monitoring in the ICU because of the risk of carotid occlusion and cerebral ischemia, particularly after transarterial fistula closure.

DURAL ARTERIOVENOUS FISTULAS

Dural arteriovenous fistulas represent 10 to 15 percent of all arteriovenous malformations.[106] They occur most often in the region of the transverse and sigmoid sinus, although they may occur in any region of the head where dura is found, including the superior sagittal sinus, inferior petrosal sinus, anterior cranial fossa, and around the deep cerebral venous system or vein of Galen.[107-111] In adults, these lesions are thought to be acquired from small vessels that form in a thrombosed sinus or vein.[112] Although most dural sinuses develop spontaneously, trauma and hypercoagulable states have been suggested as predisposing factors to the development of some fistulas.[112]

The presentation of these fistulas includes pulse-synchronous tinnitus or bruit, headache, loss of vision, altered mental status, and neurologic deficits.[113] Dural fistulas may also cause intracranial hemorrhage. The pattern of venous drainage from these lesions accounts for most of the presentations. High-flow fistulas that drain into a large sinus usually have a bruit. Drainage of arterialized veins into the cavernous sinus region or orbital veins may produce deficits of ocular movement, proptosis, or loss of vision. Drainage into veins in the brain may result in headache, neurologic deficits from venous hypertension, or hemorrhage from rupture of thin-walled veins carrying blood under increased pressure.

Treatment of dural arteriovenous fistulas may be complex. Compression therapy and embolization through feeding arteries can ameliorate symptoms related to these fistulas, particularly those lesions in certain anatomical locations such as the cavernous sinus. If transarterial embolization is incomplete, and it usually is, collateral supply will develop and symptoms may recur. Surgical therapy is difficult because of the tremendous blood flow into many of these lesions. There is a 15 percent rate of major morbidity and mortality for surgical therapy of dural fistulas in the transverse and sigmoid sinuses, mostly related to massive blood loss.[114] In certain locations, however, such as the anterior cranial fossa, the surgical treatment is preferred and usually successful with little morbidity.[108,109]

The most recent developments in treating dural arteriovenous fistulas include treatment by approaching these lesions through the draining vein and a combined approach of transarterial embolization, transvenous embolization, and surgery.[109,115,116] This combination of techniques has led to improved outcomes in lesions that previously would have been very difficult to treat. In a series of 16 patients treated by this combined approach, all patients were either cured or improved, and there was no serious permanent morbidity.[115] This combination of treatments has also lead to improved results in lesions that heretofore were almost considered untreatable, as in the deep cerebral venous system around the vein of Galen.[111]

Such complex combined therapy can be augmented by posttreatment management in the ICU, with attention to maintaining normal systemic and cerebral hemodynamics. Children with vein of Galen aneurysms should particularly be monitored in the ICU (or pediatric ICU) after treatment in order to identify posttreatment cerebral edema, hydrocephalus, or hemorrhage.

DIRECT ENDOVASCULAR THROMBOLYTIC THERAPY FOR DURAL SINUS THROMBOSIS

Spontaneous thrombosis occasionally occurs in cerebral veins or dural sinuses. This type of thrombosis is different from that occurring as a result of an infectious process. Dural sinus thrombosis may exhibit a wide spectrum of clinical findings, ranging from asymptomatic incidental findings to catastrophic fatal courses.[117-126] Patients with symptomatic dural sinus occlusion commonly have headaches, papilledema, seizures, and focal neurologic deficits. The natural history of a dural sinus thrombosis that produces occlusion is also variable. The reported mortality rates range from 10 to 50 percent.[117,122] The lower mortality rates may be related in part to the diagnosis of asymptomatic sinus thrombosis. Factors thought to be of prognostic significance, such as the rate of evolution of thrombosis, coma, age, and involvement of cerebral veins[118,119,122,126] have not been substantiated in a larger series.[117] Therefore, outcomes seem to be unpredictable; some patients have a dramatic, spontaneous recovery, while others have a rapidly declining and often fatal clinical course. The natural history makes treatment regimens difficult to compare. For dural sinus thrombosis resulting from an infectious process, antibiotics are the mainstay of therapy. The therapy for spontaneous dural sinus thrombosis is more controversial. Surgical reconstruction of a thrombosed sinus has been described but has not gained widespread acceptance.[127] Systemic heparin is often used to prevent the additional spread of a thrombus, but this therapy is also controversial[117,118,128] and does not treat the involved, occluded sinus directly. The use of high-dose, peripheral urokinase therapy in conjunction with heparin was associated with the clinical and angiographic improvement in two series of five patients each.[126,128] Others, however, have reported poor results from this therapy that apparently were related to intracranial hemorrhage.[120,123]

Recent reports have shown the successful use of local fibrinolytic agents for the treatment of dural sinus thrombosis in four of five patients.[121,124,129] Local administration of urokinase obviates the need for high doses that result in systemic fibrinolytic effects. In two patients, urokinase was infused locally by a catheter placed directly into the superior sagittal sinus. The catheter was placed by performing a burr-hole craniotomy in one patient and by a percutaneous puncture of the superior sagittal sinus through the anterior fontanel in the other patient. More recently, catheterization of the superior sagittal sinus through the percutaneous jugular venous approach has been used with good results in two of three patients. There have been no significant complications from these approaches.

Tumors

Preoperative embolization of tumors is performed to reduce blood loss during surgery. Meningiomas, which account for 15 percent of intracranial tumors, are the most commonly treated intracranial tumor.[130] These tumors are benign, and complete surgical excision is the most effective form of therapy. The tumor derives most of its blood supply from the dura from which the tumor arises. Because of the tumor's origin from the dura, the blood supply often cannot be interrupted early in the resection, and bleeding remains a problem throughout the case. This problem is particularly apparent with tumors that arise from the sphenoid wing or base of the skull. Other tumors, such as schwannomas and glomus jugulare tumors may also be treated in a similar fashion.[131]

Embolization of meningiomas is usually performed 1 to 3 days prior to resection.[132–135] Delay beyond that time may allow revascularization of the tumor from collaterals. The embolization procedure should be performed at the time of the initial angiogram, as the procedure is straightforward enough to obviate the need for a separate control angiogram. The vessels which supply the tumor are usually branches of the external carotid artery, primarily the middle meningeal artery (Fig. 16-2). Other branches from either the vertebral artery or internal carotid artery may also provide routes for embolization, although the risks of causing a stroke are higher. Prior to embolization it is necessary to fully evaluate the functional and anatomical significance of the vessel to be embolized. The branches always have collaterals that connect with the intracranial circulation or ophthalmic artery, and there is the risk of sending embolic agents intracranially if these connections are unrecognized. High-resolution digital subtraction angiography is usually adequate in evaluating these connections. These branches also provide blood supply to cra-

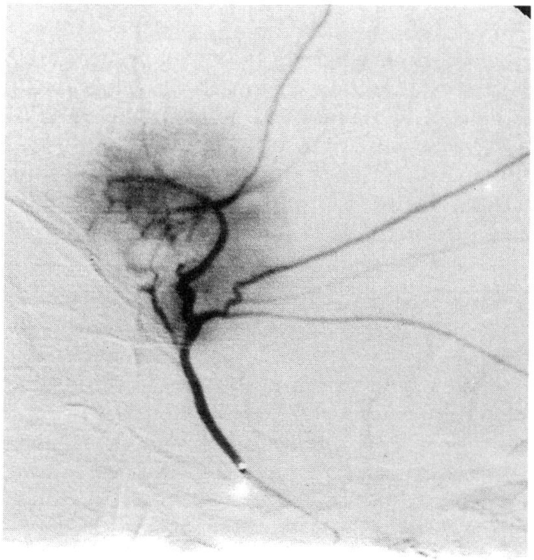

Figure 16-2 Middle meningeal artery injection, lateral view, shows the vascular blush of a medial sphenoid ridge meningioma. This pedicle, which is deep to the tumor and difficult to interrupt surgically, may be more superselectively catheterized, tested with lidocaine, and, if there are no cranial nerve deficits, embolized with particulate agents. The embolization results in nearly complete devascularization of the tumor.

nial nerves, and occlusion can result in cranial nerve palsies. The testing of a vessel prior to embolization with either lidocaine or amobarbital provides a degree of safety.[14,16]

The choice of embolic agent is usually restricted to particulate agents because of their safety and effectiveness.[131–135] While smaller particles, less than 300 μm in diameter, may penetrate into the lesion and cause more extensive thrombosis, there is the risk that particles of this small size may enter vessels that cannot be resolved on the usual angiographic equipment and flow into vessels supplying cranial nerves or the brain. Larger particles are usually sufficient to occlude the feeding pedicles and produce the expected devascularization of the tumor, with less risk of flowing through small collaterals.

The risk of embolization of tumors prior to surgical resection should be extremely low if collateral vessels are recognized and functional testing with lidocaine and amobarbitol is performed prior to vessel occlusion. Among larger series the rare complications were more often related to the angiogram rather than the embolization itself.[131–135] With such careful treatment planning it is unusual to need ICU management after tumor embolization unless the patient has a large tumor with probable increased intracranial pressure or the potential for hydrocephalus with tumor swelling or increased peritumoral edema.

SCALP ARTERIOVENOUS FISTULAS (CIRSOID ANEURYSMS)

Cirsoid aneurysms are abnormal arteriovenous communications that most often occur in the scalp or face.[136] The fistulous connections are associated with a large draining vein or varix. The clinical manifestations relate primarily to the size of the fistula. Clinically, the patients present with symptoms of loud bruits, hemorrhage, scalp necrosis, pain, throbbing headaches, and a cosmetic deformity. In the past, treatment relied on surgical excision or ligation of feeding arteries.[137] Surgery was necessarily extensive and often associated with excessive blood loss. If the surgery were incomplete, the fistula would re-form as collaterals developed.

Transarterial embolization of scalp arteriovenous fistulas has more recently been performed as definitive treatment or as an adjunct to treatment.[138] However, arterial embolization often occludes vessels proximal to the fistula, and recurrence commonly develops secondary to recruitment of collateral supply. Embolizing a scalp arteriovenous fistula through the draining vein was first described by Clarisse and others and may be a more effective therapy when embolization is used alone.[139]

An approach that uses a variety of techniques has been most successful in treating these lesions.[140–142] These procedures all rely on depositing the embolic agent directly in the fistulous site, rather than in proximal arteries or draining veins. These approaches may include superselective arterial embolization using glue, coils, balloons, or silk suture. The fistulas may also be reached through a retrograde approach through the draining vein. This approach is particularly useful when the feeding arteries are so tortuous the embolization catheters will not reach the fistula. Direct, percutaneous puncture of the fistula is also an effective therapy. Either absolute alcohol, glue, or wire coils can be placed in the fistula and produce thrombosis.

These combinations of techniques may lead to cure in 70 to 100 percent of patients treated.[140–142] Surgery may be necessary to remove the thrombosed mass or small residual fistula in some cases, although blood loss should be minimal. Complications rarely occur and are usually related to necrosis of the overlying skin, particularly if alcohol has been misdirected into the subcutaneous tissues or if there is a history of ishemia over the fistula. The surgical repair is typically a much easier procedure after the fistula has thrombosed.

EPISTAXIS

Epistaxis may originate either anteriorly or posteriorly in the nose. Anterior epistaxis is usually a self-limiting problem that needs no treatment, while posterior sources are less easily treated by direct pressure and may need nasal packing to stop. If bleeding cannot be controlled by packing, it is considered intractable and needs either surgical or endovascular therapy. The endovascular approach has the advantage of ease and effectiveness and may be repeated if necessary. This approach requires only light sedation, and the hospital stay is reduced compared to surgical ligation of the distal branches of the internal maxillary artery.[143] Epistaxis from any cause, including trauma, hypertension, vascular malformations, tumors, or bleeding disorders, may be treated with these techniques. In two series of 41 patients with intractable idiopathic epistaxis treated by endovascular therapies, control of bleeding was obtained in 95 percent with no significant complications.[143,144] There was only one complication described after treatment of epistaxis, a transient ischemic attack.[145] These methods may also be used successfully after surgical ligation of the internal maxillary artery has failed. In a series of 11 patients receiving endovascular therapy after failed surgery, all patients had control of bleeding.[146] One complication in this series was related to skin necrosis, a result of occlusion of multiple vessels providing collateral supply to an area of soft tissue. Only in a patient with significant hemorrhage and shock would ICU care seem necessary. In such patients, fluid resuscitation and transfusion (as outlined in Chap. 13) would be appropriate, while interventional therapy is used to control hemorrhage.

VENOUS SAMPLING FOR CUSHING'S DISEASE

The efficacy of petrosal sinus sampling for diagnosing Cushing's disease and providing lateralization of tumor has been documented.[1] Sampling of petrosal sinus blood in conjunction with corticotropin-releasing hormone stimulation is probably 100 percent sensitive and specific for differentiating Cushing's disease from ectopic adrenocorticotropic hormone syndrome. However, as Miller and Doppman note, the technique of petrosal sinus catheterization was abandoned for over a decade because the need for this type of diagnostic imaging was obviated by computed tomography and more recently magnetic resonance imaging.[147] As a result, few radiologists are able to perform the technique. Because of the recent emphasis on this technique and the experience neurointerventionalists have in using the inferior petrosal sinus as a conduit to treating carotid-cavernous fistulas, this technique is being performed more commonly.

The development of new catheters may lead to further improvements of the reliability and success of this technique, particularly for lateralizing tumors. Difficulties with petrosal sinus sampling may result from anatomical variants, and inaccurate sampling of peripheral blood will occur if the catheter is not positioned within the inferior petrosal sinus. Lateralization of tumors may be erroneous if there is crossover of blood from one cavernous sinus to the other side.[148] There are channels which connect the right and left cavernous sinuses in most people.[149] Superselective catheterization of the cavernous sinus can usually be performed with little difficulty, and the concentration of adrenocorticotropic hormone is higher in the cavernous sinus than inferior petrosal sinus near the jugular bulb (Fig. 16-3). With sampling taken directly from the cavernous sinus, false lateralization from crossover flow of blood from one cavernous sinus to the other may be prevented. Further evaluation of superselective catheterization of the cavernous sinuses for this test are ongoing.

INTRAARTERIAL FIBRINOLYSIS FOR STROKE

The use of fibrinolytic agents for the treatment of cerebral arterial occlusions was first clearly described by Fletcher and coworkers.[150] Enthusiasm was reduced by the high incidence of hemorrhagic complications which occurred in about 25 percent of the patients treated with systemic urokinase. Local intraarterial therapy has been tried and appears to be associated with a lower rate of hemorrhagic complications.[151] Using this selective delivery of urokinase, the posttreatment rate of hemorrhage has been reduced to 13 percent.[152] Theron and coworkers described the treatment of patients with acute internal carotid or middle cerebral occlusion.[153] They were able to classify this series of patients into three categories based on location of the occlusion. The patients who had a patent circle of Willis and lenticulostriate arteries and those with distal middle cerebral artery occlusions did better than those patients with occlusion

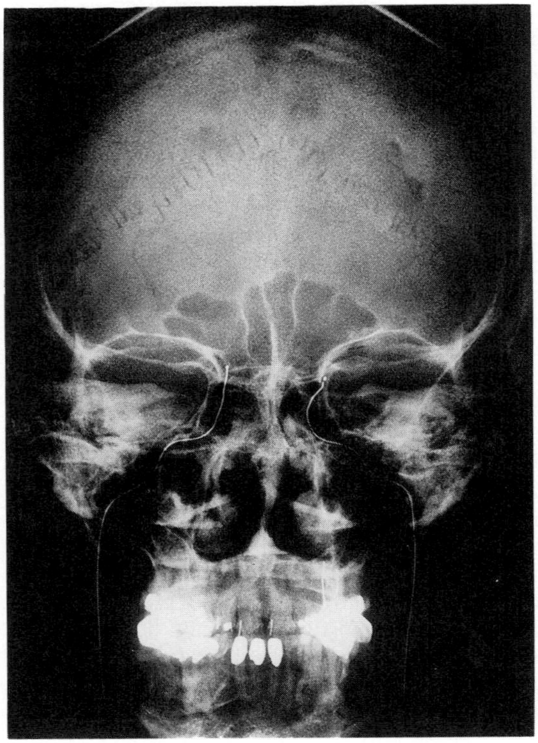

A

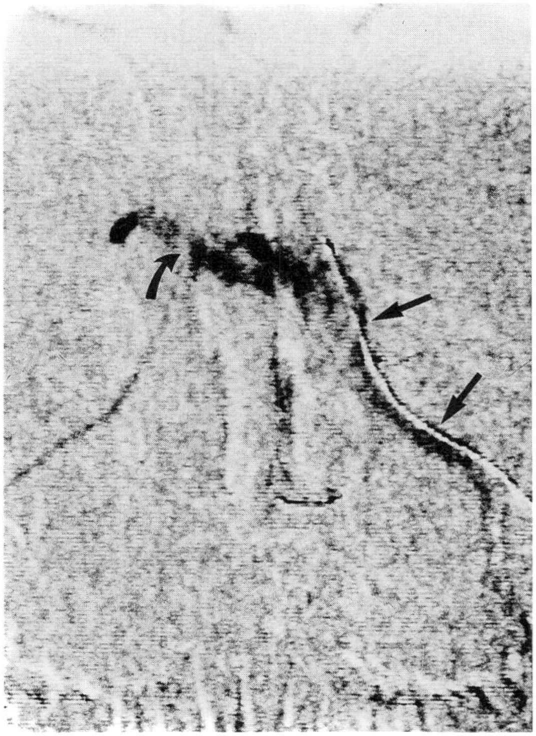

C

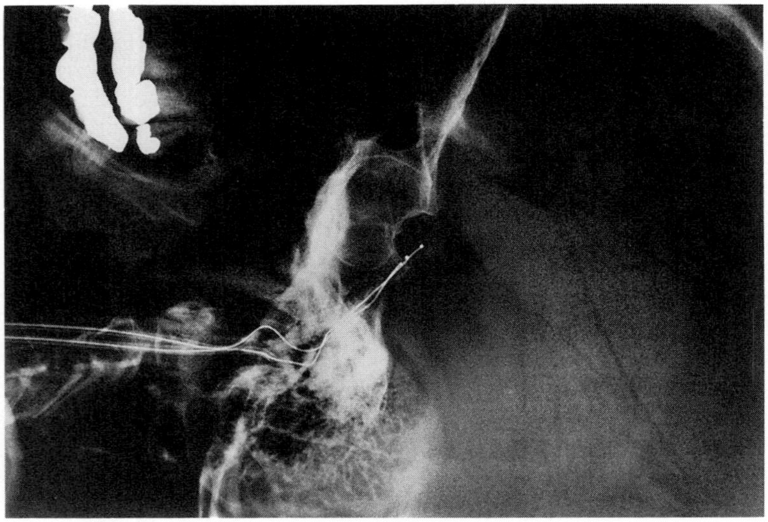

B

Figure 16-3 Frontal (*A*) and lateral (*B*) plain skull x-rays show Tracker catheters in the right and left cavernous sinuses. The position of these catheters allows venous sampling and accurate diagnosis and lateralization of tumors within the pituitary. *C*. Right cavernous sinus venogram, frontal view, shows flow of contrast from the right cavernous sinus (curved arrow) to the left inferior petrosal sinus (straight arrows). This crossover of flow may account for some false lateralizations that occur when venous sampling is obtained in the inferior petrosal sinus at the jugular bulb.

involving the circle of Willis or lenticulostriate arteries. Only the patients in this latter group had their treatment complicated by hemorrhage. Based on these findings, intraarterial fibrinolysis is probably safe in the first two groups, but unsafe in the group composed of patients with occlusion of the circle of Willis or lenticulostriate arteries if given 4 or 5 h after the event. The efficacy of this therapy is not yet known. Because of the risk of posttreatment intracerebral hemorrhage, initial management in the ICU with attention to neurologic monitoring, stability of blood pressure, and maintenance of normal intravascular volume is necessary.

REFERENCES

1. Brooks B: The treatment of traumatic arterio-venous fistula. *South Med J* 23:100, 1930.
2. Luessenhop AJ, Spence WT: Artificial embolization of the cerebral arteries for treatment of arteriovenous malformations. *JAMA* 172:1153, 1960.
3. Luessenhop AJ: Interventional neuroradiology: A neurosurgeon's perspective. *AJNR* 11:625, 1990.
4. Djindjian R, Cophegmonon J, Theron J, et al.: Embolization by supraselective arteriography from the femoral route in neuroradiology. Review of 60 cases. 1. Technique, indications and complications. *Neuroradiology* 6:20, 1973.
5. Serbinenko FA: Balloon catheterization and occlusion of major cerebral vessels. *J Neurosurg* 41:125, 1974.
6. Debrun G, Lacour P, Caron JP, et al.: Detachable balloon and calibrated-leak balloon techniques in the treatment of cerebrovascular lesions. *J Neurosurg* 49:635, 1978.
7. Romadanov AP, Scheglov VI: Intravascular occlusion of saccular aneurysms of the cerebral arteries by means of a detachable balloon catheter. In: Krayenbuhl H (ed): *Advances and Technical Standards in Neurosurgery*, vol 2. Berlin, Springer-Verlag, 1982, chap 3, pp 25–48.
8. Osborn AG: Technical aspects of cerebral angiography. In: *Introduction to Cerebral Angiography*. Hagerstown, Pennsylvania, Harper & Row, 1980, chap 1, pp 1–32.
9. Weinstein MA, Modic MT, Furlan AJ, et al.: Digital subtraction angiography. In: Wilkins RH, Rengachary SS (eds): *Neurosurgery*, vol 1. New York, McGraw-Hill, 1985, chap 25, pp 280–288.
10. Vinuela F, Fox AJ, Debrun G, Pelz D: Preembolization superselective angiography: Role in the treatment of brain arteriovenous malformations with isobutyl-2 cyanoacrylate. *AJNR* 5:765, 1984.
11. Spiegel SM, Vineula F, Goldwasser MJ, et al.: Adjusting polymerization time of isobutyl-2 cyanoacrylate. *AJNR* 7:109, 1986.
12. Fournier D, TerBrugge KG, Willinsky R, et al.: Endovascular treatment of intracerebral arteriovenous malformations: Experience in 49 cases. *J Neurosurg* 75:228, 1991.
13. Fox AJ, Pelz DM, Lee DH: Arteriovenous malformations of the brain: Recent results of endovascular therapy. *Radiology* 177:51, 1990.
14. Horton JA, Kerber CW: Lidocaine injection into external carotid branches: Provocative test to preserve cranial nerve function in therapeutic embolization. *AJNR* 7:105, 1986.
15. Wada J, Rasmussen T: Intracarotid injection of sodium amytal for the lateralization of cerebral speech dominence. *J Neurosurg* 17:266, 1960.
16. Horton JA, Dawson RC: Retinal Wada test. *AJNR* 9:1167, 1988.
17. Bank WO, Kerber CW, Cromwell LD: Treatment of intracranial arteriovenous malformations with isobutyl 2-cyanoacrylate: Initial clinical experience. *Radiology* 139:609, 1981.
18. Berthelsen B, Lofgren J, Svendson P: Embolization of cerebral arteriovenous malformations with bucrylate. Experience in a first series of 29 patients. *Acta Radiol* 31:13, 1990.
19. Cromwell LD, Harris AB: Treatment of cerebral arteriovenous malformations: Combined neurosurgical and neuroradiologic approach. *AJNR* 4:366, 1983.
20. Debrun G, Vinuela FV, Fox AJ, Drake CG: Embolization of cerebral arteriovenous malformations with bucrylate. Experience in 46 cases. *J Neurosurg* 56:615, 1982.
21. Deruty R, Lapras C, Patet JD, et al.: Intra-operative embolization of cerebral arteriovenous malformations by means of isobutylcyanoacrylate (experience in 20 cases). *Neurol Res* 8:109. 1986.
22. Halbach VV, Higashida RT, Yang P, et al.: Preoperative balloon occlusion of arteriovenous malformations. *Neurosurgery* 22:301, 1988.
23. Pelz DM, Fox AJ, Vinuela F, et al.: Preoperative embolization of brain AVMs with isobutyl-2 cyanoacrylate. *AJNR* 9:757, 1988.
24. Purdy PD, Samson D, Batjer HH, Risser RC: Preoperative embolization of cerebral arteriovenous malformations with polyvinyl alcohol particles: Experience in 51 adults. *AJNR* 11:501, 1990.
25. Ter Brugge KG, Lasjaunias P, Chiu MC: Surgical neuroangiography of intracranial vascular malformations. *Can J Neurol Sci* 14:70, 1987.
26. Vinuela FV, Debrun GM, Fox AJ, et al.: Dominant-hemisphere arteriovenous malformations: Therapeutic embolization with isobutyl-2-cyanoacrylate. *AJNR* 4:959, 1983.

27. Wolpert SM, Barnett FJ, Prager RJ: Benefits of embolization without surgery for cerebral arteriovenous malformations. *AJNR* 2:535, 1981.
28. O'Mahony BJ, Bolsin SNC: Anaesthesia for closed embolisation of cerebral arteriovenous malformations. *Anaesth Intensive Care* 16:318, 1988.
29. Hacke W, Zeumer H, Berg-Dammer E: Monitoring of hemispheric or brainstem functions with neurophysiologic methods during interventional neuroradiology. *AJNR* 4:382, 1983.
30. Cromwell LD, Kerber CW: Modification of cyanoacrylate for therapeutic embolization: Preliminary experience. *AJR* 132:799, 1979.
31. Brothers MF, Kaufmann JCE, Fox AJ, et al.: n-Butyl 2-cyanoacrylate—substitute for IBCA in interventional neuroradiology: Histopathologic and polymerization time studies. *AJNR* 10:777, 1989.
32. Vinters HV, Lundie MJ, Kaufmann JCE: Long-term pathological follow-up of cerebral arteriovenous malformations treated by embolization with bucrylate. *N Engl J Med* 314:477, 1986.
33. Rao VRK, Mandalam KR, Gupta AK, et al.: Dissolution of isobutyl 2-cyanoacrylate on long-term followup. *AJNR* 10:135, 1989.
34. Horton JA, Marano GD, Kerber CW, et al.: Polyvinyl alcohol foam-gelfoam for therapeutic embolization: A synergistic mixture. *AJNR* 4:143, 1983.
35. Jack CN Jr, Forbes G, Dewanjee MK, et al.: Polyvinyl alcohol sponge for embolotherapy: Particle size and morphology. *AJNR* 6:595, 1985.
36. Scialfa G, Scotti G: Superselective injection of polyvinyl alcohol microemboli for the treatment of cerebral arteriovenous malformations. *AJNR* 6:957, 1985.
37. Repa I, Moradian GP, Dehner LP, et al.: Mortalities associated with use of a commercial suspension of polyvinyl alcohol. *Radiology* 170:395, 1989.
38. Quisling RG, Mickle JP, Ballinger W: Small particle polyvinyl alcohol embolization of cranial lesions with minimal arteriolar-capillary barriers. *Surg Neurol* 25:243, 1986.
39. Lanman TH, Martin NA, Vinters HV: The pathology of encephalic arteriovenous malformations treated by prior embolotherapy. *Neuroradiology* 30:1, 1988.
40. Eskridge JM, Harling RP: Preoperative embolization of brain AVMs using surgical silk and polyvinyl alcohol (abstr). *AJNR* 10:882, 1989.
41. Pevsner PH, Klara P, Doppman J, et al.: Ethyl alcohol: Experimental agent for interventional therapy of neurovascular lesions. *AJNR* 4:388, 1983.
42. Strother CM, Laravuso R, Rappe A, et al.: Glutaraldehyde cross-linked collagen (GAX): A new material for therapeutic embolization. *AJNR* 8:509, 1987.
43. Taki W, Yonekawa Y, Iwata H, et al.: A new liquid material for embolization of arteriovenous malformations. *AJNR* 11:163, 1990.
44. Higashida RT, Halbach VV, Dowd C, et al.: Endovascular detachable balloon embolization therapy of cavernous carotid artery aneurysm: Results in 87 cases. *J Neurosurg* 72:857, 1990.
45. Higashida RT, Halbach VV, Barnwell SL, et al.: Treatment of intracranial aneurysms with preservation of the parent vessel: Results of percutaneous balloon embolization in 84 patients. *AJNR* 11:633, 1990.
46. Aymard A, Gobin YP, Hodes JE, et al.: Endovascular occlusion of vertebral arteries in the treatment of unclippable vertebrobasilar aneurysms. *J Neurosurg* 74:393, 1991.
47. Hodes JE, Aymard A, Gobin YP, et al.: Endovascular occlusion of intracranial vessels for curative treatment of unclippable aneurysms: Report of 16 cases. *J Neurosurg* 75:694, 1991.
48. Guglielmi G, Vinuela F, Sepetka I, Macellari V: Electrothrombosis of saccular aneurysms via endovascular approach. Part 1: Electrochemical basis, technique, and experimental results. *J Neurosurg* 75:1, 1991.
49. Guglielmi G, Vinuela F, Dion J, Duckwiler G: Electrothrombosis of saccular aneurysms via endovascular approach. Part 2: Preliminary clinical experience. *J Neurosurg* 75:8, 1991.
50. Allcock JM, Drake CG: Ruptured intracranial aneurysm—the role of arterial spasm. *J Neurosurg* 22:21, 1965.
51. Mullan S: Conservative management of the recently ruptured aneurysm. *Surg Neurol* 3:27, 1975.
52. Sahs AL, Nishioka H, Torner JC, et al.: Cooperative study of intracranial aneurysm and subarachnoid hemorrhage: A long term prognostic study. *Arch Neurol* 41:1140, 1984.
53. McKissock W, Paine KW, Walsh L: An analysis of the results of treatment of ruptured intracranial aneurysm: A report of 722 consecutive cases. *J Neurosurg* 17:762, 1960.
54. Smith RR, Yoshika J: Intracranial arterial spasm. In: Wilkins RH, Rengachary SS (eds): *Neurosurgery*. New York, McGraw-Hill, Inc., 1985, chap 162, pp 1355–1362.
55. Du Boulay G: Distribution of spasm in the intracranial arteries after subarachnoid haemorrhage. *Acta Radiol (Diagn)* 1:257, 1963.
56. Ecker A, Riemenschneider PA: Arteriographic demonstration of spasm of the intracranial arteries. With special reference to saccular arterial aneurysms. *J Neurosurg* 8:660, 1951.
57. Fisher CM, Kistler JP, Davis JM: Relation of cerebral vasospasm to subarachnoid hemorrhage visualized by

computerized tomographic scanning. *Neurosurgery* 6:1, 1980.
58. Graf CJ, Nibbelink DW: Cooperative study of intracranial aneurysms and subarachnoid hemorrhage: Report on a randomized treatment and study. *Stroke* 5:557, 1974.
59. Echlin F: Experimental vasospasm, acute and chronic, due to blood in the subarachnoid space. *J Neurosurg* 35:646, 1971.
60. Alksne JF, Greenhoot JH: Experimental catecholamine-induced chronic vasospasm. Myonecrosis in vessel wall. *J Neurosurg* 41:440, 1974.
61. Fein JM, Flor WJ, Cohan JL, Parkhurst J: Sequential changes of vascular ultrastructure in experimental cerebral vasospasm. Myonecrosis in subarachnoid arteries. *J Neurosurg* 41:49, 1974.
62. Conway LW, McDonald LW: Structural changes of the intradural arteries following subarachnoid hemorrhage. *J Neurosurg* 37:715, 1972.
63. Endo S, Suzuki J: Experimental cerebral vasospasm after subarachnoid hemorrhage. The participation of adrenergic nerves of cerebral vessel walls. *Stroke* 10:703, 1979.
64. Flamm ES, Yasargil MG, Ranssohoff J: Alteration of experimental cerebral vasospasm by adrenergic blockade. *J Neurosurg* 37:294, 1972.
65. Tanabe Y, Sakata K, Yamadad H, et al.: Cerebral vasospasm and ultrastructural changes in cerebral arterial wall. An experimental study. *J Neurosurg* 49:229, 1978.
66. Tanishima T: Cerebral vasospasm: Contractile activity of hemoglobin in isolated canine basilar arteries. *J Neurosurg* 53:787, 1980.
67. Ellis EF, Nies AS, Oates JA: Cerebral arterial smooth muscle contraction by thromboxane A2. *Stroke* 8:480, 1977.
68. Chyatte D, Rush N, Sundt TM: Prevention of chronic experimental cerebral vasospasm with ibuprofen and high dose methylprednisolone. *J Neurosurg* 59:925, 1981.
69. Sundt TM Jr: Chemical management of cerebral vasospasm. In: Whisnant JP, Sandok BA (eds): *Cerebral Vascular Disease. Proceedings of the 9th Princeton Conference, 1974.* New York, Grune & Stratton, 1975, chap 4, pp 77–81.
70. Tani E, Maeda Y, Fukumori T: Effect of selective inhibitor of thromboxane A2 synthetase on cerebral vasospasm after early surgery. *J Neurosurg* 61:24, 1984.
71. Wilkins RH: Attempted prevention or treatment of intracranial arterial spasm: A survey. In: Wilkins RH (ed): *Cerebral Arterial Spasm.* Baltimore, Williams & Wilkins, 1979, chap 89, pp 542–555.
72. Kassell NF, Peerless SJ, Durward QJ, et al.: Treatment of ischemic deficits from vasospasm with intravascular volume expansion and induced arterial hypertension. *Neurosurgery* 11:337, 1982.
73. Zubov YN, Nikiforov BM, Shustin VA: Balloon catheter technique for dilatation of constricted cerebral arteries after aneurysmal SAH. *Acta Neurochir (Wien)* 70:65, 1984.
74. Higashida RT, Halbach VV, Dormandy B, et al.: New microballoon device for transluminal angioplasty of intracranial arterial vasospasm. *AJNR* 11:233, 1990.
75. Higashida RT, Halbach VV, Cahan LD, et al.: Transluminal angioplasty of intracerebral vessels for treatment of intracranial arterial spasm. *J Neurosurg* 71:648, 1989.
76. Hunt WE, Hess RM: Surgical risk as related to time of intervention in the repair of intracranial aneurysms. *J Neurosurg* 28:14, 1968.
77. Newell DW, Eskridge JM, Mayberg MR, et al.: Angioplasty for the treatment of symptomatic vasospasm following subarachnoid hemorrhage. *J Neurosurg* 71:654, 1989.
78. Barnwell DL, Higashida RT, Halbach VV, et al.: Transluminal angioplasty of intracerebral vessels for cerebral arterial spasm: Reversal of neurological deficits after delayed treatment. *Neurosurgery* 25:424, 1989.
79. Linsky ME, Horton JA, Rao GR, Yonas H: Fatal rupture of the intracranial carotid artery during transluminal angioplasty for vasospasm induced by subarachnoid hemorrhage. *J Neurosurg* 74:985, 1991.
80. Amacher Al, Allcock JM, Drake CG: Cerebral angiomas: The sequelae of surgical treatment. *J Neurosurg* 37:571, 1972.
81. Aminoff MJ: Treatment of unruptured cerebral arteriovenous malformations. *Neurology* 37:815, 1987.
82. Mackenzie I: The clinical presentation of the cerebral angioma: A review of 50 cases. *Brain* 78:184, 1953.
83. Heros RC, Tu Y-K: Is surgical therapy needed for unruptured arteriovenous malformations? *Neurology* 37:279, 1987.
84. Graf CJ, Perret GE, Torner JC: Bleeding from cerebral arteriovenous malformations as part of their natural history. *J Neurosurg* 58:331, 1983.
85. Ondra SL, Troupp H, George ED, Schwab K: The natural history of symptomatic arteriovenous malformations of the brain: A 24-year follow-up assessment. *J Neurosurg* 73:387, 1990.
86. Halbach VV, Higashida RT, Dowd CF, et al.: Management of vascular perforations that occur during neurointerventional procedures. *AJNR* 12:319, 1991.
87. Purdy PD, Batjer HH, Samson D: Management of hemorrhagic complication from preoperative emboli-

zation of arteriovenous malformations. *J Neurosurg* 74:205, 1991.
88. Vitek JJ: Percutaneous transluminal angioplasty of the external carotid artery. *AJNR* 4:796, 1983.
89. Higashida RT, Hieshima GB, Tsai FY, et al.: Transluminal angioplasty of the vertebral and basilar artery. *AJNR* 8:745, 1987.
90. Kachel R, Basche St, Heerklotz I, et al.: Percutaneous transluminal angioplasty (PTA) of supra-aortic arteries especially the internal carotid artery. *Neuroradiology* 33:191, 1991.
91. Bockenheimer SAM, Mathias K: Percutaneous transluminal angioplasty in arteriosclerotic internal carotid artery stenosis. *AJNR*; 4:791, 1983.
92. Wiggli U, Gratzl O: Transluminal angioplasty of stenotic carotid arteries: Case reports and protocol. *AJNR* 4:793, 1983.
93. Tsai FY, Matovich V, Hieshima G, et al.: Percutaneous transluminal angioplasty of the carotid artery. *AJNR* 7:349, 1986.
94. DeMonte F, Peerless SJ, Rankin RN: Carotid transluminal angioplasty with evidence of distal embolization. Case report. *J Neurosurg* 70:138, 1989.
95. Culicchia F, Spetzler RF, Flom RA: Failure of transluminal angioplasty in the treatment of myointimal hyperplasia of the internal carotid artery: Case report. *Neurosurgery* 28:148, 1991.
96. Halbach VV, Hieshima GB, Higashida RT, Reicher M: Carotid cavernous fistulae: Indications for urgent treatment. *AJNR* 8:627, 1987.
97. Debrun GB, Lacour P, Fox AJ, et al.: Traumatic carotid cavernous sinus fistulas: Etiology, clinical presentation, diagnosis, treatment, results. *Semin Intervent Radiol* 4:242, 1987.
98. Higashida RT, Halbach VV, Tsai FY, et al.: Interventional neurovascular treatment of traumatic carotid and vertebral artery lesions: Results in 234 cases. *Am J Radiol* 153:577, 1989.
99. Halbach VV, Higashida RT, Barnwell SL, et al.: Transarterial platinum coil embolization of carotid-cavernous fistulas. *AJNR* 12:429, 1991.
100. Halbach VV, Higashida RT, Hieshima GB, et al.: Transvenous embolization of direct carotid cavernous fistulas. *AJNR* 9:741, 1988.
101. Hosobuchi T: Electrothrombosis of carotid cavernous fistulas. *J Neurosurg* 41:657, 1974.
102. Halbach VV, Higashida RT, Hieshima GB, et al.: Transvenous embolization of dural fistulas involving the cavernous sinus. *AJNR* 10:377, 1989.
103. Monsein LH, Debrun GM, Miller NR, et al.: Treatment of dural carotid-cavernous fistulas via the superior ophthalmic vein. *AJNR* 12:435, 1991.
104. Courtheoux P, Labbe D, Hamel C, et al.: Treatment of bilateral spontaneous dural carotid-cavernous fistulas by coils and sclerotherapy. *J Neurosurg* 66:468, 1987.
105. Teng MMH, Guo WY, Huang CI, et al.: Occlusion of arteriovenous malformations of the cavernous sinus via the superior ophthalmic vein. *AJNR* 9:539, 1988.
106. Newton TH, Cronqvist S: Involvement of the dural arteries in intracranial arteriovenous malformations. *Radiology* 93:1071, 1969.
107. Barnwell SL, Halbach VV, Dowd CF, et al.: Dural arteriovenous fistulas involving the inferior petrosal sinus: Angiographic findings in six patients. *AJNR* 11:511, 1990.
108. Martin NA, King WA, Wilson CB, et al.: Management of dural arteriovenous malformations of the anterior cranial fossa. *J Neurosurg* 72:692, 1990.
109. Barnwell SL, Halbach VV, Dowd CF, et al.: A variant of arteriovenous fistulas within the wall of dural sinuses. Results of combined surgical and endovascular therapy. *J Neurosurg* 74:199, 1991.
110. Halbach VV, Higashida RT, Hieshima GB, et al.: Treatment of dural arteriovenous malformations involving the superior sagittal sinus. *AJNR* 9:337, 1988.
111. Halbach VV, Higashida RT, Hieshima GB, et al.: Treatment of dural fistulas involving the deep cerebral venous system. *AJNR* 10:393, 1989.
112. Houser OW, Campbell RJ, Sundt TM: Arteriovenous malformations affecting the transverse dural venous sinus: An acquired lesion. *Mayo Clin Proc* 54:651, 1979.
113. Vinuela F, Fox AJ, Pelz DM: Unusual clinical manifestations of dural arteriovenous malformations. *J Neurosurg* 64:554, 1986.
114. Sundt TM Jr, Piepgras DG: The surgical approach to arteriovenous malformations of the lateral and sigmoid dural sinuses. *J Neurosurg* 59:32, 1983.
115. Barnwell SL, Halbach VV, Higashida RT, et al.: Complex dural arteriovenous fistulas. Results of combined endovascular and neurosurgical treatment in 16 patients. *J Neurosurg* 71:352, 1989.
116. Halbach VV, Higashida RT, Hieshima GB, et al.: Transvenous embolization of dural fistulas involving the transverse and sigmoid sinuses. *AJNR* 10:385, 1989.
117. Bousser GJ, Chiras J, Bories J, Castaigne P: Cerebral venous thrombosis—a review of 38 cases. *Stroke* 16:199, 1985.
118. Castaigne P, Laplane D, Bousser MG: Superior sagittal sinus thrombosis (Correspondence). *Arch Neurol* 34:788, 1977.
119. Ehlers H, Courville CB: Thrombosis of internal cerebral veins in infancy and childhood. Review of literature and report of five cases. *J Pediatr* 8:60, 1936.
120. Gettelfinger DM, Kokmen E: Superior sagittal sinus thrombosis. *Arch Neurol* 34:2, 1977.
121. Higashida RT, Helmer E, Halbach VV, Hieshima GB: Direct thrombolytic therapy for superior sagittal sinus thrombosis. *AJNR* 10:S4, 1989.

122. Krayenbuhl HA: Cerebral venous and sinus thrombosis. *Clin Neurosurg* 14:1, 1967.
123. Rousseaux P, Bernard MH, Scherpereel B, Guyot JF: Thrombose des sinus veineux intra-craniens. *Neurochirurgie* 24:197, 1978.
124. Scott JA, Pascuzzi RM, Hall PV, Becker GJ: Treatment of dural sinus thrombosis with local urokinase infusion. *J Neurosurg* 68:284, 1988.
125. Smith KR: Idiopathic bilateral sigmoid sinus occlusion in a child. *J Neurosurg* 29:427, 1968.
126. Vines FS, Davis DO: Clinical-radiological correlation in cerebral venous occlusive disease. *Radiology* 98:9, 1971.
127. Sindou M, Mercier P, Bokor J, Brunon J: Bilateral thrombosis of the transverse sinus: Microsurgical revascularization with venous bypass. *Surg Neurol* 13:215, 1980.
128. Di Rocco C, Iannelli A, Leone G, et al.: Heparin-urokinase treatment in aseptic dural sinus thrombosis. *Arch Neurol* 8:431, 1981.
129. Barnwell SL, Higashida RT, Halbach VV, et al.: Direct endovascular thrombolytic therapy for dural sinus thrombosis. *Neurosurgery* 28:135, 1991.
130. Guthrie BL, Ebersold MJ, Scheithauer BW: Neoplasms of the intracranial meninges. In: Youmans JR (ed): *Neurological Surgery*. Philadelphia, Saunders, 1990, chap 112, pp 3250–3315.
131. Abramowitz J, Dion JE, Jensen ME, et al.: Angiographic diagnosis and management of head and neck schwannomas. *AJNR* 12:977, 1991.
132. Macpherson P: The value of pre-operative embolisation of meningioma estimated subjectively and objectively. *Neuroradiology* 33:334, 1991.
133. Manelfe C, Lasjaunias P, Ruscalleda J: Preoperative embolization of intracranial meningiomas. *AJNR* 7:963, 1986.
134. Hieshima GB, Everhart FR, Mehringer CM, et al.: Preoperative embolization of meningiomas. *Surg Neurol* 14:119, 1980.
135. Richter H-P, Schachenmayr W: Preoperative embolization of intracranial meningiomas. *Neurosurgery* 13:261, 1983.
136. Watson WL, McCarthy WD: Blood and lymph vessel tumors: A report of 1056 cases. *Surg Gynecol Obstet* 71:569, 1940.
137. Khodadad G: Arteriovenous malformations of the scalp. *Ann Surg* 177:79, 1973.
138. Kasdon DL, Altemus LR, Stein BM: Embolization of a traumatic arteriovenous fistula of the scalp with radiopaque gelfoam pledgets: Case report and technical note. *J Neurosurg* 44:753, 1976.
139. Clarisse J, Gozet G, Cornil JP, et al.: The fluid plastic embolization: An experimental study—report of two cases of arteriovenous fistula. *J Neuroradiol* 2:29, 1975.
140. Barnwell SL, Halbach VV, Dowd CF, et al.: Endovascular treatment of scalp arteriovenous fistulas associated with a large varix. *Radiology* 173:533, 1989.
141. Mourao GS, Hodes JE, Gobin YP, et al.: Curative treatment of scalp arteriovenous fistulas by direct puncture and embolization with absolute alcohol. *J Neurosurg* 75:634, 1991.
142. Heilman CB, Kwan ES, Klucznik RP, Cohen AR: Elimination of a cirsoid aneurysm of the scalp by direct percutaneous embolization with thrombogenic coils. *J Neursurg* 73:296, 1990.
143. Vitek J: Idiopathic intractable epistaxis: Endovascular therapy. *Radiology* 181:113, 1991.
144. Strutz J, Schumacher M: Uncontrolled epistaxis. Angiographic localization and embolization. *Arch Otolaryngol Head Neck Surg* 116:697, 1990.
145. Merland JJ, Melki JP, Chiras K, et al.: Place of embolization in the treatment of severe epistaxis. *Laryngoscope* 90:1694, 1980.
146. Breda SD, Choi IS, Persky MS, Weiss M: Embolization in the treatment of epistaxis after failure of internal maxillary artery ligation. *Laryngoscope* 99:809, 1989.
147. Miller DL, Doppman JL: Petrosal sinus sampling: Technique and rationale. *Radiology* 178:37, 1991.
148. Miller DL, Doppman JL, Nieman LK, et al.: Petrosal sinus sampling: Discordant lateralization of ACTH-secreting pituitary microadenomas before and after stimulation with corticotropin-releasing hormone. *Radiology* 176:429, 1990.
149. Elster AD, Chen MYM, Richardson DN, Yeatts PR: Dilated intercavernous sinuses: An MR sign of carotid-cavernous and carotid dural fistulas. *AJNR* 12:641, 1991.
150. Fletcher AP, Alkjaersig N, Lewis M, et al.: A pilot study in urokinase therapy in cerebral infarction. *Stroke* 7:135, 1976.
151. Zeumer H, Hundgen R, Ferberta A, Rigelstein EB: Local intraarterial fibrinolytic therapy in inaccessible internal carotid occlusion. *Neuroradiology* 26:315, 1984.
152. Del Zoppo GJ, Zeumer H, Harker LA: Thrombolytic therapy in stroke: Possibilities and hazards. *Stroke* 17:595, 1986.
153. Theron J, Courtheoux P, Casasco A, et al.: Local intraarterial fibrinolysis in the carotid territory. *AJNR* 10:753, 1989.

CHAPTER 17

The Intensive Care Management of Patients with Epilepsy

Gregory D. Cascino

INTRODUCTION

The intensive care unit (ICU) management of the neurosurgical patient may include evaluation and treatment of epileptic seizures. Seizures may occur in patients with or without a presurgical history of epilepsy or a seizure disorder, i.e, recurrent unprovoked seizures. Generalized convulsive status epilepticus is a medical emergency and requires prompt attention and immediate termination of seizure activity to avoid neurologic morbidity. The diagnostic evaluation, treatment, and prognosis of seizure activity in the ICU depends on the type(s) of seizure and underlying precipitating factors. This chapter will review the treatment of the adult patient with seizures in the neurosurgical ICU.

I. PATIENTS WITH EPILEPSY

The patient with epilepsy often is receiving antiepileptic drug (AED) therapy prior to undergoing a neurosurgical procedure. The most common type of seizure disorder in the adult patient is partial epilepsy associated with an anatomically restricted or localized region of seizure onset.[1-3] Almost 45 percent of patients with partial epilepsy have a medically refractory seizure disorder.[1,4] Partial epilepsy may be associated with complex partial, simple partial, or secondarily generalized tonic-clonic seizures.[5,6] The distinction between complex and simple partial seizures depends on the presence of impaired consciousness during the seizure.[5,6] During the complex partial seizure the patient is often poorly responsive and postictally is amnestic for the details of the ictal behavior.[5,6] The majority of generalized tonic-clonic seizures, *grand mal attacks*, are partial in onset with secondary generalization.[5,6] Most complex partial seizures emanate from the anterior temporal lobe.[6] The term *temporal lobe epilepsy*, however, should be discouraged because approximately 20 percent of complex partial seizures are of extratemporal (mainly frontal lobe) origin.[6] Generalized epilepsy suggests a bihemispherical onset of seizure activity as determined by the ictal behavior and the electrophysiologic change. Types of generalized seizures include absence (*petit mal*), tonic-clonic, and myoclonic seizures.[5] Generalized epilepsy may be idiopathic or symptomatic in origin. The latter often occurs in patients with mental retardation and medically refractory seizures.[5]

The AEDs of choice for partial epilepsy are carbamazepine (CBZ) and phenytoin (PHT).[7–9] Other potentially effective AEDs include sodium valproate (VPA), phenobarbital (PB), and primidone (PM).[7,8] The barbiturates are limited in value because of neurotoxicity, i.e., sedation and cognitive alterations.[10] PHT and CBZ have been demonstrated to be similar in efficacy in patients with partial seizure disorders.[7] CBZ is available in a 200-mg scored tablet or a 100-mg chewable tablet. A suspension form of the drug also can be used. Unfortunately, CBZ is highly insoluble and is not available for parenteral administration. Initially, concerns regarding hematologic toxicity of CBZ were exaggerated, and this potential adverse reaction is not unique to CBZ. The metabolism of CBZ may be profoundly affected by combination therapy with other AEDs. The patient may tolerate high blood levels of CBZ when used in monotherapy; however, neurotoxicity commonly develops with polypharmacy.[11] Most patients should receive multiple CBZ doses per day, e.g., 3 or 4 times a day (tid or qid) depending on the total daily dose and the presence of side effects.

PHT can be administered with one or two daily doses in most patients because of the drug half-life (approximately 24 to 36 h). More frequent dosing, e.g., PHT 100 mg tid, is unnecessary and may be associated with AED noncompliance. The metabolism of PHT depends on the drug level. At higher plasma concentrations a small change in the drug dose may produce a significant change in the blood level. For example, a patient receiving a PHT dose of 300 mg per day with a blood level of 15 mg/mL may develop drug toxicity when the dose is increased to 400 mg/day and the blood level is raised to greater than 30 mg/mL. At doses of 200 mg/day or greater the dose should be increased or decreased by approximately 30 to 50 mg/day. CBZ and PHT are available in a suspension that can be taken orally or through a nasogastric tube. Importantly, PHT suspension should not be administered with tube feedings or antacids because of interference with drug absorption.

Several AEDs are effective in the management of generalized tonic-clonic seizures.[8] VPA is the preferred drug for the patient with generalized epilepsy who has multiple seizure types, e.g., tonic-clonic, myoclonic, and absence. VPA at present is only available for oral use, i.e., divalproex sodium 125 mg, 250 mg, 500 mg, and valproic acid 250 mg. A valproic acid syrup (250 mg/5 mL) can also be used. A sprinkle form of the drug has recently been introduced. Intravenous VPA is under investigation in the United States. The plasma concentration of the drug is not useful in deciding on the drug dose (even less than with CBZ and PHT). Most patients initially receive VPA 15 mg/kg, and the dose can be increased as needed and tolerated to 50 to 60 mg/kg. Common dose-related side effects include tremor, weight gain, and hair loss. The idiosyncratic hepatopathy associated with VPA appears to be restricted to young children and should not be a reason to exclude this drug in the adult population.[12]

One concern regarding the use of VPA in the operative patient is the potential for increased intracranial bleeding.[8] VPA may produce thrombocytopenia and inhibit the second phase of platelet aggregation.[8] The latter may only be recognized by checking a bleeding time. At our institution, if possible, VPA is usually discontinued at least 1 to 2 weeks prior to a neurosurgical procedure. An important drug interaction involving VPA is its effect on PB metabolism. Symptomatic PB toxicity may occur in patients receiving both drugs because of the inhibition of PB metabolism by VPA.

In the treatment of epilepsy, monotherapy is always preferred to polypharmacy because of the increase in neurocognitive problems associated with multiple medications.[11] The addition of a second drug in a patient with poorly controlled seizures is associated with complete seizure control in 11 percent of patients but produces AED toxicity in 90 percent of patients.[13] Combination therapy or polypharmacy should also be discouraged because of significant alterations in plasma concentrations.[10] Benzodiazepine drugs are not first-line because of neurotoxicity and the development of tachyphylaxis. Patients with partial epilepsy should not be considered medically refractory until they have received maximally tolerated monotherapy with CBZ or PHT. AED plasma concentrations are only a relative indicator of drug dosing. The most important parameters in assessing medication requirement are seizure activity and drug toxicity. Patients may tolerate high AED levels with monotherapy. Drug toxicity refers to clinical symptoms related to AED medication and not an elevation in the AED plasma concentration. The goals of treatment for the patient with epilepsy are to render the individual seizure-free and to avoid AED toxicity.

II. PRESURGICAL EVALUATION OF THE PATIENT WITH EPILEPSY

The presurgical evaluation of the patient with epilepsy (not restricted to surgical ablative procedures for intractable seizure epilepsy) begins with an ascertainment of seizure activity, i.e., the type and frequency of seizures, and AED dosages. Patients experiencing generalized tonic-clonic seizures may be more likely to develop generalized convulsive status epilepticus. The electroencephalogram (EEG) may be useful to indicate the type of seizure but should not be used to indicate medication requirements. The goals of treatment include prevention of consciousness-impairing seizures (especially generalized tonic-clonic seizures) and avoidance of AED toxicity. The latter may significantly complicate postoperative care, e.g., vomiting and drowsiness. The symptoms of AED-induced neurotoxicity may suggest a more sinister neurologic problem requiring neurosurgical care, e.g., hydrocephalus.

The potential causes for increased seizure activity in the patient with epilepsy in the perioperative period include a reduction in AED plasma concentration due to an inability to take medication, an increase in stress associated with surgery, sleep deprivation after surgery because of pain, and the use of potentially epileptogenic drugs, e.g., enflurane and thorazine. Patients may be unable to receive certain AEDs while in the operating room, e.g., CBZ, VPA, and PM. Substitution with other AEDs, e.g., PHT or PB, that can be administered intravenously may be considered (see below). If patients are in a seizure remission and tolerating the preoperative AED medication, then alteration in therapy may not be necessary. CBZ can often be administered the morning of surgery and continued when the patient is able to postoperatively take oral medications. Documentation of CBZ levels after surgery may be useful to indicate the appropriate drug dose (different than with the use of CBZ as maintenance therapy during outpatient care).

A problem that may occur with CBZ during the postoperative period is the development of AED toxicity. CBZ levels may be raised by propoxyphene (Darvon or Darvocet) and erythromycin because of an interference in CBZ metabolism.[8] Combination of AEDs should be discouraged because of AED toxicity and alteration in drug metabolism (see above). If patients are to be started on PHT prior to surgery, then an oral or intravenous loading dose may be necessary. The maintenance dose of PHT is 3 to 8 mg/kg.[8] Starting a patient on this dose will not achieve a therapeutic plasma concentration for 7 to 21 days. Oral loading of PHT can be performed by dividing the loading dose (18 mg/kg) into three oral doses of 6 mg/kg in a 24-h period.[14,15] A therapeutic level will be achieved in 14 to 24 h.[14,15] Intravenous PHT loading should be discouraged unless emergent because of the potential morbidity (see below).

Phenobarbitol also has significant toxicity when administered intravenously (see below). Another concern regarding the use of PB in the postoperative period is the sedative effect that may interfere with the neurologic examination. If PB must be started because of an inability to receive other AEDs, e.g., PHT and CBZ allergy, then the drug may be administered intravenously in the operating room and in the ICU as discussed below. Additional boluses of PB may be indicated depending on recurrent seizure activity. A maintenance dose of PB, e.g., 120 mg/day, begun prior to surgery may not produce a therapeutic blood level for several weeks! After surgery, patients can receive the preoperative AED medication if appropriate for their seizure disorder. Frequent plasma concentration monitoring postoperatively may be most helpful for the patient experiencing seizures and/or AED toxicity. Increasing the dose of a medication in a seizure-free patient because of a low serum level alone should be discouraged.

III. STATUS EPILEPTICUS[16]

Status epilepticus (SE) is "a condition characterized by an epileptic seizure that is so frequently repeated or so prolonged as to create a fixed and lasting condition."[17] A more substantive definition is continuous seizure activity lasting for 30 min or longer, or recurrent seizures occurring with impairment of consciousness that are not associated with return of consciousness between seizure activity. There are as many different types of SE as there are types of seizures. The term SE should not only refer to generalized tonic-clonic status (GTCS) which is the most frequently occurring form.[14] GTCS and nonconvulsive SE of the partial type, complex partial status (CPS), require emergent treatment to avoid neurologic morbidity.[18]

The incidence of GTCS is approximately 60,000 to 160,000 patients per year in the United States.[19] Recent estimates of the mortality rate have suggested a figure of 1 to 2 percent.[20] The morbidity associated with GTCS includes memory and intellectual changes.[21] GTCS is a medical emergency and requires prompt attention and immediate termination of seizure activity.[10] GTCS in experimental models of epilepsy can produce neuronal death related to ongoing seizure activity, even when metabolic abnormalities are corrected and the animals are ventilated and paralyzed.[22] Paralyzing agents should be avoided in the management of SE because of the inability to monitor seizure activity. SE occurs more commonly in patients with partial seizure disorders and remote symptomatic epilepsy, e.g., head trauma.[20] In approximately 75 percent of patients with GTCS the seizures are partial at onset with secondary generalization.[18,19] The majority of patients with generalized convulsive status have an identifiable etiology of the seizure activity.[20,23] The common causes are neurologic disorders, e.g., stroke or cerebral neoplasm, and drug-related and metabolic alterations.[20,23] Inadequate AED levels is one of the most common causes of SE in patients with epilepsy.[14]

The initial management of the patient with suspected generalized convulsive status may include observation of the patient to make certain of the diagnosis. The treatment of SE has significant potential morbidity; therefore, the diagnosis should be confirmed clinically.[14] Common clinical disorders that may emulate SE include toxic-metabolic encephalopathies, postictal states, medication-related tremor, nonepileptic myoclonus, shivering related to anesthetic withdrawal, and decerebrate and decorticate posturing. Patients who are postictal after a single seizure should also not be considered to be in status. The treatment of simple partial SE, e.g., repetitive focal motor seizures, is different than GTCS because of the potential for neurologic morbidity.[14] Patients in simple partial SE may be aggressively treated with oral AEDs and should not receive the treatment outlined below for intractable GTCS.[14]

When a patient is diagnosed as experiencing GTCS, the EEG technologist should be contacted to arrange for an emergent EEG study. Treatment of the patient in GTCS should not be deferred until EEG confirmation. The EEG becomes critical in a patient who has received a paralyzing agent, to confirm the diagnosis of nonconvulsive SE, and when certain medications are used in the treatment of intractable SE (see below). Appropriate life support should of course be rendered to the patient.[14,18,19] A soft plastic airway should be inserted in the patient's mouth if possible. Personnel capable of endotracheal intubation will need to be contacted. No object should be forced in the patient's mouth, e.g., tongue blade to protect the patient from "swallowing the tongue." Monitoring the blood pressure, respiratory rate, and ECG is critical (especially when intravenous AEDs are used). Two large intravenous catheters should be inserted (preferably in the forearm and not in the hand). Initial blood studies should include a determination of AED levels, and routine laboratory studies. A neurologist should be contacted for assistance in selecting and administering AED medication.

The goals of treatment in the patient with GTCS include (1) stopping seizure activity, (2) avoiding neurologic morbidity related to the seizures and/or the treatment, and (3) identifying and treating the underlying factors. The medicine of choice to treat SE is a drug that works promptly, is highly effective and safe, and can be administered orally when the patient recovers. This ideal drug unfortunately does not exist, and less satisfactory AEDs must be considered. Only several AEDs are commonly used in the management of GTCS, and these include diazepam (DZP), lorazepam (LZP), PHT, and PB (Table 17-1).[14,18,19] Thiamine 100 mg and 50 mL of 50% glucose can be administered intravenously prior to the AEDs. If the patient is actively seizing when evaluated, then a benzodiazepine medication should be used initially. DZP is the only benzodiazepine drug approved by the Food and Drug Administration for treatment of SE. DZP should be administered no faster than 5 mg/min, with a total dose not to exceed 0.25 mg/kg.[14,24] LZP can be administered at 2 mg/min, with the total dose not to exceed 0.1 mg/kg.[14,24] LZP and DZP may be equivalent in efficacy; however, LZP has an important advantage, which is the prolonged duration of action relative to DZP.[25,26] The benzodiazepines when administered intravenously may produce cardiac and respiratory failure.[14,24] Both drugs have a rapid onset of action, e.g., 1 to 2 min after administration. All

Table 17-1 Management of Generalized Convulsive Status Epilepticus[16]

Appropriate life support
Thiamine 100 mg IV, 50% glucose 50 mL IV
Diazepam 5 mg/min (maximal dose 0.25 mg/kg) IV or lorazepam 2 mg/min (maximal dose 0.1 mg/kg) IV
and
Phenytoin 50 mg/min (loading dose 18 mg/kg) IV
if seizure activity is stopped
Initiate phenytoin maintenance therapy (3 to 8 mg/kg per day)
if seizure activity continues
Phenobarbital 100 mg/min (loading dose 20 mg/kg) IV
if seizure activity continues
Phenytoin 50 mg/mL (10-mg/kg dose) IV
if seizure activity continues
Pentobarbital 5 mg/kg IV followed by 1 to 3 mg/kg per h
or
Phenobarbital 100 mg/min IV (10 mg/kg every 30 min until clinical and electrographic seizure activity is terminated)
or
Isoflurane anesthesia

patients with GTCS should receive a long-acting AED in addition to benzodiazepine therapy.

PHT is the preferred long-acting drug because of its minimal sedative and respiratory depressant effect compared to PB.[27] The loading dose of PHT (18 mg/kg) should be administered to the patient intravenously no faster than 50 mg/min.[28] PHT can precipitate in glucose solutions and should only be given in a saline solution.[14,28] Intravenous PHT contains propylene glycol and alcohol and may be associated with significant morbidity, e.g., cardiac arrhythmias, hypotension, and cardiac arrest.[14,24,28] PHT may also cause a chemical phlebitis and tissue damage related to extravasation of the drug, "the purple glove syndrome."[14,28] The latter complication with intravenous PHT may be the most common and most underrecognized. The skin changes can lead to significant tissue loss and rarely may require amputation of a limb. Most patients at our institution who have developed the purple glove syndrome have been elderly patients with impaired levels of consciousness. Presumbly they were unable to communicate effectively the pain associated with extravasation of the drug to stop PHT administration. A new preparation of PHT under investigation, fosphenytoin, may have less toxicity when used intravenously. Importantly, the patient after receiving a loading dose of PHT will require maintenance therapy within 24 h. The onset of action of intravenous PHT is approximately 30 min (although in some patients it may be effective within minutes of administration).[29] If the patient had been receiving PHT prior to developing SE, the loading dose should not change unless the plasma concentration is known. The treating physician should assume that the patient does not have an adequate AED level. PHT should not be given to patients with SE if they have a known history of hypersensitivity to the drug, cardiac failure, or greater than second-degree atrioventricular block.[14] PHT may still be used in patients with a history of PHT refractory complex partial seizures who develop GTCS. In the majority of patients the combination of the benzodiazepine drugs and PHT will prove effective in the treatment of SE.

Phenobarbital is the second most commonly used long-acting AED in the management of SE.[14,18,19,24] The loading dose of PB is 20 mg/kg, and the drug is administered at 100 mg/min. Intubation will be necessary during PB administration because of respiratory depression that occurs with PB levels greater than 35 μg/mL.[30] PB is contraindicated in patients with a known hypersensitivity to the drug and porphyria.[14,24] The maintenance dose of PB should be started within 24 h of the loading dose. The peak concentration of PB may be achieved 60 min after infusion; however, seizure control may occur within several minutes because of the increased uptake in the brain of PB during SE.[24,29]

The patients who have not responded to the above treatment would be considered to have intractable SE. A neurologist with a special interest in SE should be contacted. Continuous EEG monitoring should be performed to evaluate the patient's response to therapy. While considering other options an additional bolus of PHT, e.g., 10 mg/kg, can be administered.[25] The patient should not leave the ICU until the clinical and/or electrical SE has ceased. Neuroimaging studies need to be deferred until effective seizure control has been obtained. The options that remain include (1) high-dose PB therapy; (2) short-acting anesthetic drugs, e.g, pentobarbital or thiopental; or (3) inhalation anesthetic drugs, e.g., isoflurane (Table 17-1).[14,24,31-34] Other potential AEDs that are rarely used include (1) paraldehyde, (2) rectal valproate, or (3) lidocaine.[14,24] Potential reasons for patients to continue in status are inadequate doses of PHT and PB, intramuscular administration of AEDs, an uncorrected metabolic abnormality, or the presence of a cerebral mass lesion. Nearly all patients with idiopathic generalized epilepsy will have been effectively treated with conventional medications. Approximately 65 percent of patients with partial epilepsy will stop seizing with PHT and the benzodiazepine drugs.[18]

High-dose PB therapy has been used successfully in patients with medically refractory SE.[33] There is no maximum level of PB beyond which additional medication is ineffective. The drug can be given at 10-mg/kg increments every 30 min (regardless of the total dose) until generalized seizure activity has ceased. This form of therapy for SE should only be used in the ICU. Hypotension is less likely to occur with PB than with pentobarbital, obviating the need for vasopressor therapy. The recent experience at the Mayo Clinic has indicated the efficacy and safety of high-dose phenobarbital therapy in the adult and pediatric patient.

Short-acting anesthetic agents are the most commonly used drugs in the management of intractable GTCS.[31] The advantages of these drugs include the rapid onset of action, predictable EEG alterations, reduction in cerebral metabolic rates, and short half-life. Patients will require continuous blood pressure and central venous pressure monitoring. Pentobarbital (half-life of 21 to 41 h) is administered at 5 mg/kg and then continued at 1 to 3 mg/kg per h.[14,24] Continuous EEG monitoring is utilized to make certain that the seizure activity has ceased and to produce a burst-suppression pattern or an isoelectric EEG. The pentobarbital dose can be lowered every 2 to 4 h to see if the electrical SE will reoccur.[24] The efficacy of pentobarbital and thiopental has been demonstrated in patients with medically refractory GTCS.[14,24,31,32] Patients should only receive these agents in an appropriately staffed ICU and after adequate initial therapy, i.e, benzodiazepine drugs, PHT, and PB. Thiopental has the disadvantage of being stored in fat; therefore, the anesthetic effect may be quite prolonged. Pentobarbital is the preferred short-acting anesthetic drug.[31]

The final approach for refractory GTCS is the use of inhalation anesthetics.[33] Isoflurane has been demonstrated to be effective in the treatment of intractable SE.[33] These agents require the presence of an anesthesiologist for administration and are not preferred in the management of these patients.

A diagnostic evaluation is performed concomitant with treatment of the electrical and clinical seizure activity in patients with GTCS. Potential reasons for SE have already been mentioned. Certain metabolic abnormalities, e.g., hypocalcemia and hyponatremia, may increase seizure tendency. Patients with metabolic disturbances may have ictal features suggesting focal seizure activity, e.g., hyperglycemic-induced epilepsia partialis continua.[35] The EEG is used to confirm the diagnosis of GTCS and may reveal localization-related changes to indicate partial seizure onset. Neuroimaging studies, computed tomography, and magnetic resonance imaging may identify an epileptogenic lesion and the need for surgical treatment.[36] A spinal fluid examination in select patients may be necessary to exclude a central nervous system infection.

IV. EPILEPSY SURGERY

Surgery for focal epilepsy is the most effective alternative treatment for the patient with medically refractory seizures.[37] The most common and safest procedure performed is an anterior temporal lobectomy. Most patients with seizures emanating from the temporal lobe have pathologically verified mesial temporal sclerosis.[38] Foreign-tissue pathology, tumor, or vascular malformation is identified in nearly 30 percent of these patients.[38]

Prior to considering a patient a candidate for epilepsy surgery the individual must have been demonstrated to be refractory to maximally tolerated AED therapy.[39] Patients should be considered for surgery within 1 to 2 years of diagnosis if successful seizure control cannot be attained.[1,39] Most patients who fail to respond well to CBZ and PHT are not rendered seizure-free with other AEDs. Therefore, surgery should not be considered a procedure of last resort after all possible combinations of AEDs have been used.

The most frequently performed procedure for intractable epilepsy is resection of the epileptogenic brain tissue.[40] Other procedures that have been shown to be effective in some patients include lesionectomy, hemispherectomy, corpus callosotomy, and amygadalohippocampectomy.

Prior to surgery the patients will have received a comprehensive epilepsy evaluation.[39] This will have included neuroimaging studies, neuropsychometry, speech-language testing, visual perimetry and long-term EEG monitoring.[39] The latter procedure is critical to localize the epileptogenic zone, i.e., the site of seizure onset.[41] Invasive EEG recordings, e.g., using subdural grid and/or depth electrodes, may be necessary in select patients.[41] Functional neuroimaging studies, e.g., positron emission tomography, may identify a localization-related abnormality associated with partial epilepsy that may assist in identification of potential surgical candidates.[42] The goals of epilepsy surgery are similar to the goals of AED therapy: (1) render the individual seizure-free, (2) avoid neurologic morbidity, and (3) allow the patient to become a participating and productive member of society, i.e., pursue educational and employment opportunities.[1]

Patients admitted for epilepsy surgery are often receiving multiple AEDs in the toxic range. Preoperatively at the Mayo Clinic the patients are loaded orally on PHT if possible (if they are not receiving PHT already). An additional intravenous bolus, e.g., PHT 500 mg, is administered in the operating room. VPA had been discontinued prior to surgery because of the alleged bleeding complications (see above). A PHT level is checked shortly after surgery, and the patient is given a maintenance dose of the drug. CBZ is restarted in patients who have been receiving maintenance CBZ prior to surgery.

Shortly after surgery the second AED is withdrawn, and if possible, the patient receives only one AED. For patients who are unable to take PHT (see above), PB may be used in the operating room and immediately after surgery. The PB may be slowly tapered later if the patient prefers another AED. Usually the patient stays in the ICU overnight and then is transferred to the neurosurgical floor. The AED levels are monitored prior to and after surgery. If seizure activity occurs in the immediate postoperative period, the patient is often kept intubated and in the ICU. The patient will receive intravenous PHT or PB if parenteral AED therapy is necessary.

Postoperative generalized tonic-clonic seizures at our institution have been most common in patients undergoing extratemporal surgery (mainly frontal lobe). GTCS that develops is treated as outlined above. Most patients (even if seizure-free) receive AED therapy (preferably monotherapy) for approximately 2 years after surgery. Select patients may be gradually withdrawn from AED medication at that time if they have a successful surgical outcome. The rationale for this delay in withdrawing therapy is that the effect of the surgery on seizure tendency cannot be determined for 1 to 2 years.

REFERENCES

1. Dreifuss FE: Goals of surgery for epilepsy. In: Engel J Jr (ed): *Surgical Treatment of the Epilepsies.* New York, Raven, 1987, pp 31–49.

2. Rayport M: Role of neurosurgery in management of medication—resistant epilepsy. In: *Plan for Nationwide Action in Epilepsy.* Washington D.C., DHEW Publications, 1977, pp 314–324.
3. Hauser WA, Kurland LT: The epidemiology of epilepsy in Rochester, Minnesota 1936–1967. *Epilepsia* 16:1, 1967.
4. Ward AA Jr: Perspectives for surgical treatment of epilepsy. In: Ward AA Jr, Penry JK, Purpura D (eds): *Epilepsy.* New York, Raven, 1983, pp 371–390.
5. Engel J Jr: Epileptic seizures. In: Engel J Jr (ed): *Seizures and Epilepsy.* Philadelphia, FA Davis, 1989, pp 137–178.
6. Williamson PD, Wieser HG, Delgado-Escueta AV: Clinical characteristics of partial seizures. In: Engel J Jr (ed): *Surgical Treatment of the Epilepsies.* New York, Raven, 1987, pp 101–120.
7. Mattson RH, Cramer JA, Collins JF, et al.: Comparison of carbamazepine, phenobarbital, phenytoin and primidone in partial and secondarily generalized tonic-clonic seizures. *N Engl J Med* 313:145, 1985.
8. Engel J Jr: Antiepileptic drugs. In: Engel J Jr (ed): *Seizures and Epilepsy.* Philadelphia, FA Davis, 1989, pp 410–474.
9. Schmidt D: Drug-resistant partial epilepsy: Clinical and pharmacological criteria. In: Wieser HG, Elger CE (eds): *Presurgical Evaluation of Epileptics.* New York, Springer-Verlag, 1987, pp 321–324.
10. Thompson PJ, Trimble MR: Anticonvulsant drugs and cognitive function. *Epilepsia* 12:531, 1982.
11. Lesser RP, Pippenger CE, Luders H, et al.: High-dose monotherapy in treatment of intractable seizures. *Neurology* 34:707, 1984.
12. Dreifuss FE, Santilli N, Langer DH, et al.: Valproic acid hepatic fatalities: A retrospective review. *Neurology* 37:379, 1987.
13. Schmidt D: Two anti-epileptic drugs for intractable epilepsy with complex partial seizures. *J Neuro Neurosurg Psychiatry* 45:1119, 1982.
14. Browne TR, Mikati M: Status epilepticus. In: Ropper AH, Kennedy SF (eds): *Neurological and Neurosurgical Intensive Care,* 2d ed. Rockville, MD, Aspen Publishers, 1988, pp 269–288.
15. Wilder BJ, Ramsay ER, Wilmore LJ, et al.: Efficacy of intravenous phenytoin and treatment of status epilepticus: Kinetics of central nervous system penetration. *Ann Neurol* 1:511, 1977.
16. Cascino GD: Status epilepticus. In: Gress DR (ed): *Clinicians Guide to Neurological Emergencies.* New York, Marcel Dekker. In press.
17. Gastaut H: Classification of status epilepticus. *Adv Neurol* 34:15, 1977.
18. Delgado-Escueta AV, Treiman DM: Focal status epilepticus: Modern concepts. In: Luders H, Lesser RP (eds): *Epilepsy: Electroclinical Syndromes.* New York, Springer-Verlag, 1987, pp 347–391.
19. Delgado-Escueta AV, Wasterlain C, Treiman DM, Porter RJ: Status epilepticus: Summary. *Adv Neurol* 34:537, 1983.
20. Hauser WA: Status epilepticus: Epidemiologic considerations. *Neurology* 40(suppl 2):9, 1990.
21. Dodrill CB, Wilensky AJ: Intellectual impairment as an outcome of status epilepticus. *Neurology* 40(suppl 2):23, 1990.
22. Meldrum BJ, Vigouroux RA, Brierly JB: Systemic and epileptic brain damage: Prolonged seizures in paralyzed, artificially ventilated baboons. *Arch Neurol* 28:82, 1973.
23. Janz D: Etiology of convulsive status epilepticus. *Adv Neurol* 34:47, 1983.
24. Engel J Jr: Status epilepticus. In: Engel J Jr (ed): *Seizures and Epilepsy.* Philadelphia, FA Davis, 1989, pp 256–280.
25. Treiman DM: The role of benzodiazepines in the management of status epilepticus. *Neurology* 40(suppl 2):32, 1990.
26. Leppik IE, Derivan AT, Holman RW, et al.: Double-blind study of lorazepam and diazepam in status epilepticus. *JAMA* 249:1452, 1983.
27. Wilder BJ: Efficacy of phenytoin in treatment of status epilepticus. *Adv Neurol* 34:441, 1983.
28. Albani M: How to use phenytoin. In: Moreselli PL, Penry JK, Pippenger CE (eds): *Antiepileptic Drug Therapy.* New York, Raven, 1982, pp 253–262.
29. Leppik IE, Hauser WA, Lothman E, et al.: Status epilepticus: Questions and answers. *Neurology* 40(suppl 2):47, 1990.
30. Gabor AJ: Lorazepam versus phenobarbital: Candidates for drug of choice for treatment of status epilepticus. *Journal of Epilepsy* 3:3, 1990.
31. Van Ness PC: Pentobarbital and EEG burst suppression in treatment of status epilepticus refractory to benzodiazepines and phenytoin. *Epilepsia* 31:61, 1990.
32. Young GB, Blume WT, Bolton CF, Warren KG: Anesthetic barbiturates in refractory status epilepticus. *Can J Neurol Sci* 7:291, 1980.
33. Ropper AH, Kofke WA, Bromfield EB, et al.: Comparison of isoflurane, halothane, and nitrous oxide in status epilepticus. *Neurology* 19:98, 1986.
34. Crawford TO, Mitchell WG, Fishman LS, Snodgrass S: Very-high-dose phenobarbital for refractory status epilepticus in children. *Neurology* 38:1035, 1988.
35. Singh BM, Strobos RJ: Epilepsia partialis continua associated with nonketotic hyperglycemia: Clinical and biochemical profile of 21 patients. *Ann Neurol* 8:155, 1980.

36. Sperling MR, Wilson G, Engel J Jr, et al.: Magnetic resonance imaging in intractable partial epilepsies: Correlative studies. *Ann Neurol* 20:57, 1986.
37. Cascino GD: Intractable partial epilepsy: Evaluation and management. *Mayo Clin Proc* 65:1578, 1990.
38. Babb TL, Brown WJ: Pathological findings in epilepsy. In: Engel J Jr (ed): *Surgical Treatment of the Epilepsies.* New York, Raven, 1987, pp 511–540.
39. Andermann F: Identification of candidates for surgical treatment of epilepsy. In: Engel J Jr (ed): *Surgical Treatment of the Epilepsies.* New York, Raven Press, 1987, pp 51–70.
40. Engel J Jr: Alternative therapy. In: Engel J Jr (ed): *Seizures and Epilepsy.* Philadelphia, FA Davis, 1989, pp 443–474.
41. Quesney LF, Gloor P: Localization of epileptic foci. In: Gotman J, Ives JR, Gloor P (eds): Long-term monitoring in epilepsy. *Electroencephalogr Clin Neurophysiol Suppl* Amsterdam, Elsevier, 37:165, 1985.
42. Chugani HT, Shewmon DA, Peacock WJ, et al.: Surgical treatment of intractable neonatal seizures: The role of positron emission tomography. *Neurology* 38:1178, 1988.

CHAPTER 18

The Intensive Care Management of Patients with Brain Tumors

Michon Morita
Brian T. Andrews
Philip H. Gutin

INTRODUCTION

Modern neurosurgical techniques and improved diagnostic imaging now permit the routine performance of neurosurgical operations that were rarely attempted only a generation ago. Neurosurgeons can now reasonably expect to operate successfully on brain tumors with minimal morbidity and mortality. The routine care of neurosurgical patients with brain tumors has increasingly come to include preoperative and postoperative intensive care involving closer and more sophisticated monitoring and management. This chapter will discuss the indications for intensive care management, types of monitoring and interventions, and prophylaxis for adverse events that may be encountered in the preoperative and postoperative management of patients with brain tumors.

PREOPERATIVE INTENSIVE CARE

Patients with brain tumors may present in extremis and require intensive medical management before surgery. In such cases, admission to the intensive care unit (ICU) allows the clinical condition to be stabilized and a complete preoperative evaluation to be performed. The immediate cause may not be discovered until further tests can be performed or after surgical intervention. The reasons for deterioration include status epilepticus, intratumoral hemorrhage, and increased intracranial pressure (ICP) due to cerebral swelling or hydrocephalus.

Status Epilepticus

Occasionally, patients with brain tumors present with status epilepticus requiring admission to the ICU. Up to 26 percent of patients with status epilepticus have brain tumors.[1,2] In such cases, the clinician's immediate concern is to control the seizures; the underlying brain tumor may not be diagnosed until the seizures have been controlled. In patients with a seizure disorder caused by a previously diagnosed tumor, seizures may be precipitated by tumor progression, worsening edema, electrolyte disorders, or a low anticonvulsant level. The acute pharmacologic management of status epilepticus caused by brain tumors is similar to that of idiopathic status epilepticus (see Chap. 17).[3]

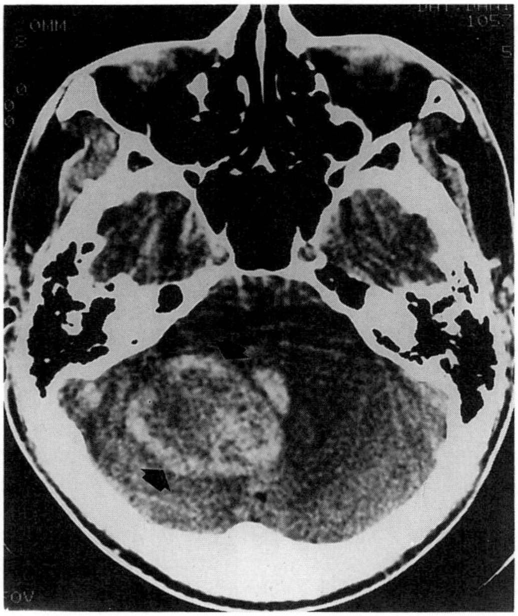
A

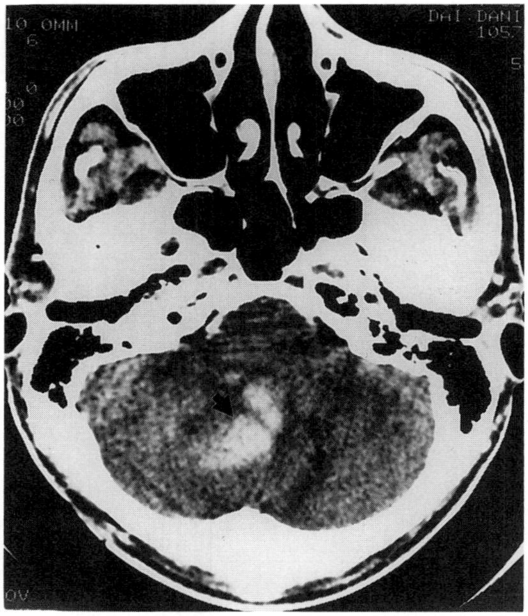
B

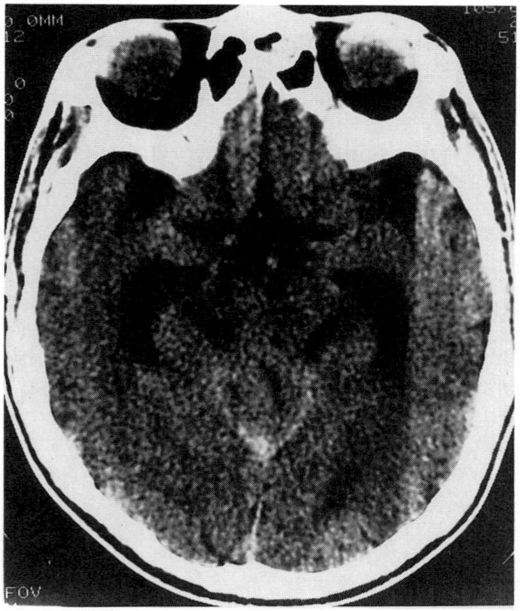
C

Figure 18-1 Unenhanced axial CT scans from a 65-year-old man with gastric carcinoma who came to the emergency room with vomiting, somnolence, and truncal ataxia show a right cerebellar hemispheric tumor (A, large arrows), hemorrhage (B, small arrows), and obstructive hydrocephalus (C).

Spontaneous Intracranial Hemorrhage

Spontaneous intracranial hemorrhage due to a brain tumor can also cause sudden deterioration requiring intensive care. Retrospective reviews have shown intratumoral hemorrhage in 1.3 to 9.6 percent of patients with brain tumors[4-10]; in recent series, acute hemorrhage was the initial manifestation of the tumor in 0.6 percent of cases. Overall 1.4 to 2.3 percent of patients with brain tumors have acute neurologic deterioration caused by an intratumoral hemorrhage.[11,12] Among glial tumors, mixed oligodendroglioma-astrocytomas and glioblastomas are most likely to hemorrhage (29.2 and 20 percent, respectively); of all intracranial tumors, metastatic melanomas have the highest hemorrhage rate (50 percent).[12] Metastatic carcinoma (Fig. 18-1), atrial myxoma, and choriocarcinoma may also bleed. Pituitary adenomas[10-14] may hemorrhage into the sella and suprasellar region, causing so-called pituitary apoplexy, with abrupt loss of vision; these tumors may also cause acute subarachnoid hemorrhage and symptoms of a ruptured aneurysm. Other factors associated with an acute tumoral hemorrhage are neoplastic aneurysms,[13-16] anticoagulation therapy,[17] minor trauma,[18,19] and placement of intraventricular catheters.[20,21]

In cases of intracranial hemorrhage due to tumor, emergent measures should be taken to stabilize the patient by intubation and mechanical ventilation, hyperosmolar agents, controlling seizures, or treating hydrocephalus, followed by further diagnostic evaluation. Intratumoral hemorrhage is suggested by hematoma surrounded by edema or unenhanced computed tomography (CT) scans followed by additional tumor enhancement on contrast-enhanced scans (Fig. 18-1). The definitive diagnosis of tumor is based on surgical evacuation of the clot and biopsy of the cavity wall or suspected tumor mass.

Acute Deterioration without Hemorrhage

Sudden deterioration without hemorrhage or seizure can also result from focal brain swelling or acutely increased ICP. This may occur after an initially insidious or progressive course that may not have prompted medical attention, as with a slowly growing and finally massive meningioma. In such cases, unenhanced CT scans frequently show hypodense regions suggesting brain swelling, mass effect, and compressed ventricles, often associated with an enhancing intra- or extra-axial mass (Fig. 18-2).

Acute Deterioration due to Hydrocephalus

Abrupt neurologic deterioration due to obstructive hydrocephalus is most common with third-ventricular and infratentorial tumors and may also occur with tumor hemorrhage or hemispheric compression of ventricular outflow (Fig. 18-3). The appropriateness of routine preoperative external ventricular drainage (EVD) in third-ventricular and infratentorial tumors is a controversial issue. It is clearly necessary in stuporous or comatose patients with acutely enlarged ventricles. Bilateral EVD may be necessary in patients with

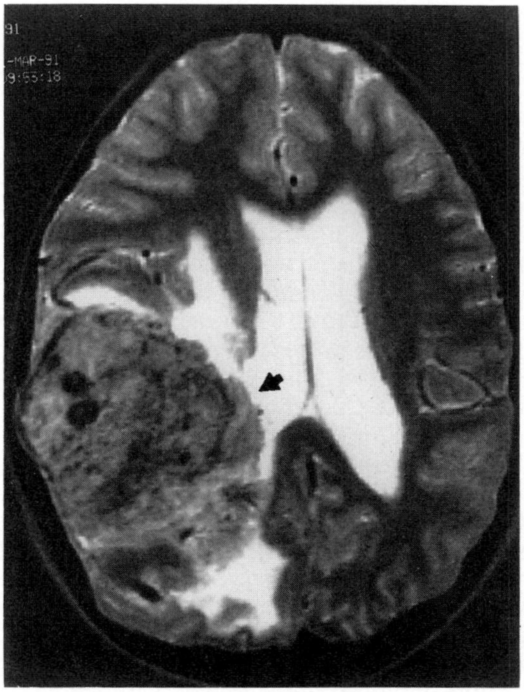

Figure 18-2 Axial MR images from a 12-year-old girl with progressive headaches show a right convexity tumor, later confirmed as a meningioma, that caused a mass effect and a midline shift.

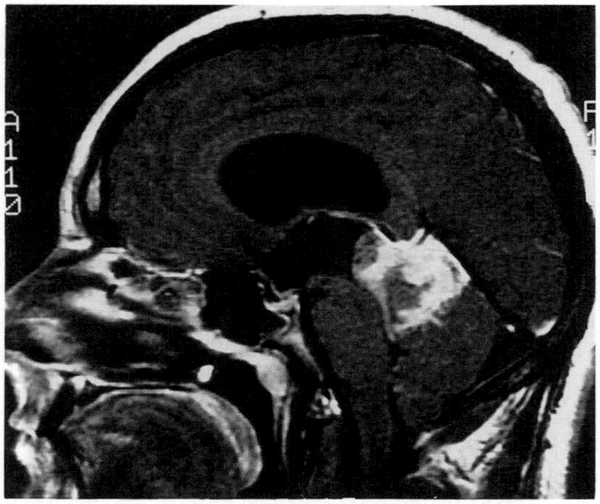

Figure 18-3 Sagittal MR images from a 35-year-old man who presented with headache and depressed level of consciousness show hemorrhage into a pineal tumor and associated hydrocephalus.

third-ventricular tumors or colloid cysts that cause bilateral obstruction of ventricular outflow.

Arguments in favor of preoperative EVD include the improvement in the patient's neurologic condition by relief of hydrocephalus, the possibility of avoiding a postoperative shunt, the prevention of sudden rapid deterioration due to a further increase in ICP in an unshunted patient, and the creation of a *slack brain* during subsequent surgery. EVD also allows ICP monitoring and direct treatment of the hydrocephalus through drainage of cerebral spinal fluid (CSF) as needed. Arguments against preoperative EVD, except in the severest cases, include the risk of infection, hemorrhage,[20,21] parenchymal injury, and upward herniation if the tumor is in the posterior fossa,[22] and the possibility of managing the hydrocephalus with corticosteroids alone. Some neurosurgeons routinely place a shunt preoperatively in patients with hydrocephalus, many of whom ultimately require shunting,[23–27] even though this exposes the patient to many of the same risks as EVD and to possible tumor seeding to the peritoneum as well.[28] Others attempt to minimize the risk of infection associated with external drainage by placing a ventricular catheter connected to a subcutaneous reservoir; this allows telemetric ICP monitoring and intermittent ventricular drainage and can be converted to shunt if necessary.[29,30]

POSTOPERATIVE INTENSIVE CARE

Early detection and prompt treatment of clinical deterioration are the primary reasons for admitting patients with brain tumors to the ICU postoperatively. Thus, careful neurologic and, at times, ICP monitoring are key elements of ICU care. Patients who remain intubated after surgery may also require ventilatory support and respiratory care. The causes of postoperative clinical deterioration are quite varied and include delayed emergence from anesthesia, intracranial hemorrhage, hydrocephalus, focal brain swelling, increased ICP, electrolyte disturbances, seizures, vasospasm, cerebral infarcts, and aspiration. General postoperative care, such as pain control and monitoring of systemic vital signs and functions, can also be improved in the ICU. In addition, delayed invasive therapeutic interventions, including reintubation, mechanical ventilation, ventriculostomy, and other forms of monitoring can be performed more quickly and easily if the patient is already in the ICU. The disadvantages of ICU admission are the greater cost, the monopolization of resources, and decreased patient privacy and family contact. Generally, we monitor all patients in the ICU for at least 24 h after uneventful tumor surgery, and longer if the operation was lengthy and complex, if the patient remains intubated, if specific monitoring is needed, or if complications arise.

INTRACRANIAL PRESSURE MONITORING

The purpose of monitoring ICP in patients with brain tumors is to detect and treat excessive elevation in ICP, which may be elevated postoperatively as a result of intracranial hematoma, cerebral edema, and hydrocephalus. These causes are all potentially remediable but require prompt identification and early intervention to achieve an optimal outcome. Postoperative ICP monitoring is safe and helpful in the early detection of elevated ICP as a cause of clinical deterioration.[31] ICP monitoring after surgery is not always performed routinely but is generally indicated when the likelihood of brain swelling or need for ventricular drainage is suggested at the time of surgery or when neurologic function is not expected to recover immediately after anesthesia.

Types of Monitoring

Many types of ICP monitors are available for monitoring the ventricular, intraparenchymal, subarachnoid, subdural, and epidural spaces. They range from simple fluid-filled catheters to screws, bolts, and fiber-optic systems (see Chap. 3). No single device is ideal for all cases of ICP monitoring in the brain tumor patient, but each system has advantages and drawbacks.

Ventricular Monitors Ventriculostomy is the most widely used method of recording ICP and is generally considered the most accurate. It has been reliably used in a wide variety of clinical situations as a method of ICP monitoring[32] and is the only method that permits treatment of increased pressure through drainage of ventricular fluid. A ventriculostomy can be placed during the craniotomy and left for subsequent monitoring and CSF drainage, or it may be placed in the ICU under local anesthesia. The principal disadvantages of a ventriculostomy are a higher rate of central nervous system infection (estimated at 4 to 5 percent[33,34]), the risk of parenchymal injury, and the occurrence of parenchymal hematomas (as high as 4 percent in one series[35]) with catheter placement. Another disadvantage is the difficulty of cannulating the ventricle in some patients with severely increased ICP and slit ventricles or shifted intracranial contents. Ventriculostomy is the best method to use in patients with hydrocephalus in whom drainage of CSF may be useful or in patients requiring intraoperative ventricular cannulation and postoperative ICP monitoring.

Recently, a new experimental telemetric ventricular ICP monitoring system has been tried in a small series of patients after surgery for posterior fossa and third-ventricular tumors.[29] This system was used in conjunction with conventional shunt systems and by itself with a subcutaneous reservoir and can be used for long-term monitoring in patients who may be expected to develop hydrocephalus. There are no elements exiting through the skin, and pressure can be measured intermittently or continuously. This system seems to be a good alternative for monitoring children with hydrocephalus, but further studies are needed to evaluate its safety and efficacy.

Subdural Monitors A subdural monitor can easily be placed at the time of surgery and left for subsequent monitoring. A fluid-filled catheter with multiple side holes can be used to transduce ICP readings with an accuracy comparable to that of ventriculostomy.[32] This method may have a lower infection rate (1 percent in a series of 110 patients[35]) than vetriculostomy and does not require cortical puncture. The drawbacks are the difficulty of placing the subdural catheter through a burr hole alone[36] and the tendency of the system to dampen out, resulting in a loss of accuracy, in patients with severely elevated ICP. This is probably the best system to place at the time of a craniotomy when there is no particular need to cannulate the ventricle, or it may be used at the bedside in a patient with small or shifted ventricles, albeit with more difficulty than a fiber-optic transducer or subarachnoid screw.

Fiber-optic Monitors The fiber-optic probe with the transducer in the tip, initially developed by Camino Laboratories, has been used for intracranial monitoring.[37] Fiber-optic monitors are extremely simple to place through a small twist-drill hole and function in almost any intracranial compartment, including parenchyma, ventricles, and the posterior fossa.[38] They do not require a patient to remain in constant position in relation to an external transducer. The major drawbacks appear to be the fragility and expense of the system.

Subarachnoid Screws Like fiber-optic monitors, subarachnoid screw monitors (Richmond bolts) are easy to insert; they may be placed through a twist-drill hole under local anesthesia in the ICU and can be used preoperatively or after accidental or routine removal of an existing ICP monitor. Unlike fiber-optic monitors, however, a subarachnoid screw must be positioned in the subarachnoid space for optimal efficacy. In a series of 650 patients monitored with subarachnoid screws, 49 of whom were perioperative brain tumor patients, the central nervous system infection rate during an average monitoring time of 5 days was only 0.7 percent.[38] The major problem was the difficulty of placing the screw in the subarachnoid space, which resulted in an 8 percent failure rate for attempted recordings. There is also evidence that subarachnoid screws may be less accurate than subdural and ventricular monitors,[32] but overall they appear to provide adequate information to detect abnormal ICP elevations after resection of brain tumors. These monitors are best suited for placement in the ICU or to replace an existing ICP monitor. However, we prefer to use the fiber-optic monitor if it is available.

Direct Posterior Fossa Monitoring Direct recording from the posterior fossa has occasionally been used to monitor ICP after resection of posterior fossa tumors.[39,40] Under normal physiologic conditions, ICP is completely equilibrated between the infratentorial and supratentorial compartments through free flow of CSF. After removal of a posterior fossa tumor, however, focal blockage of the basal cisterns or fourth-ventricular outflow may compromise CSF flow, which may result in large intercompartmental pressure gradients and eventually lead to transtentorial or tonsillar herniation. The possibility that measurement of supratentorial ICPs may inadequately reflect the status of the infratentorial compartment suggests an advantage of monitoring posterior fossa ICP directly.

Neurosurgeons have been reluctant to place ICP monitors in the posterior fossa for fear of causing CSF leakage, cranial nerve dysfunction, and brainstem irritation. Recently, the safety and efficacy of subdural[39] and intraparenchymal[40] monitoring in the posterior fossa after resection of infratentorial tumor were assessed in two series of 20 and 7 patients, respectively. Most patients underwent simultaneous posterior fossa and supratentorial monitoring for up to 5 days without adverse effects. A distinct pattern of transtentorial intercompartmental pressure gradients was reported: Infratentorial pressure rose 50 percent immediately after surgery and then gradually declined. However, only three patients had pressure elevations that required intervention, and in two of them, the increase would have been immediately detected with a supratentorial monitor; the third patient lacked a simultaneous supratentorial monitor. Thus, convincing evidence does not yet exist to show that posterior fossa monitors provide otherwise unavailable information that can prompt intervention earlier and more efficaciously than conventional supratentorial monitors.

Duration of Monitoring

When to discontinue monitoring is largely an empirical decision. We discontinue monitoring after ICP has remained normal for 24 h without ventricular drainage, mannitol infusion, or hyperventilation and after the patient's clinical condition has improved to the point where the neurologic examination will suffice for monitoring intracranial events. Because the infection rate increases sharply after about 7 days, the monitor site should be changed if further monitoring is required. In such cases, the fiber-optic system has the advantage that it can be moved easily and safely to a different site. Patients undergoing EVD because of hydrocephalus will either need a new drain or conversion to a permanent ventricular shunt.

OTHER TYPES OF MONITORING

In most patients undergoing craniotomy at our institution, arterial catheters are placed at surgery. This facilitates blood drawing and allows continuous and accurate blood pressure monitoring for the first 24 h after surgery or until the patient is discharged from the ICU. Other invasive intravascular monitoring, including central venous catheters and pulmonary artery catheters, may be necessary in hemodynamically unstable patients (see Chap. 1) but are rarely used for patients with brain tumors. Central venous catheters may also be used for volume expansion in the rare postoperative brain tumor patient with symptomatic cerebral vasospasm. Patients in the ICU routinely undergo electrocardiography and pulse oximetry, and fluid intake and output via Foley catheter are monitored hourly.

Brainstem Auditory Evoked-Potential Monitoring

Brainstem auditory evoked-potential monitoring has been suggested as an alternative to direct posterior fossa pressure monitoring after surgery for tumors of the posterior fossa.[41,42] This method appears to be quite sensitive for detecting increased posterior fossa pressure but requires the continuous presence of a trained observer and has not been evaluated in adequate numbers of patients.

INTRACRANIAL PRESSURE CONTROL

Vasogenic Edema in Brain Tumor Patients

The predominant form of cerebral edema associated with brain tumors is peritumoral vasogenic edema.[43] Peritumoral edema is a prominent finding both before and after surgery and often accounts for more clinical neurologic deficits than the tumor mass itself; if severe, it can depress the level of consciousness and cause life-threatening increases in ICP. Furthermore, intraoperative manipulation of brain tissue and focal brain ischemia may exacerbate vasogenic edema, leading to a potentially explosive degree of brain swelling and devastating brain injury.

The commonly accepted mechanism of vasogenic edema is that it results from increased capillary permeability and a breakdown of the blood-brain barrier, which allows macromolecules to leak into the extracellular space.[44] These macromolecules then exert an osmotic gradient for free water to enter the perivascular space and are eventually deposited in the extracellular space, predominantly in white matter, but also in gray matter. Abnormal vascular permeability is responsible for the contrast enhancement seen on CT scans and magnetic resonance images of brain tumors. Possible mediators of this abnormal vascular permeability include histamine, serotonin, glutamate, polyamines, lymphokines, leukotrienes,[45] tumor plasminogen activators,[46] and a protein vascular permeability factor.[47] No single mechanism appears to explain all cases.

Meningiomas and Cerebral Edema

Certain meningiomas are the only histologically benign tumors that cause severe cerebral edema. The brain swelling can be severe enough to cause significant morbidity beyond that from compression by the tumor itself. It has been seen with both large and small meningiomas and frequently complicates the postoperative management. Several recent studies have attempted to identify factors associated with this phenomenon.[48-51] It is possible that the mechanisms of edema formation around meningiomas and primary glial neoplasms are different. Meningiomas with meningiotheliomatous[51] or hemangiopericytic features,[49] higher cellularity, increased vascularity, larger size, and higher mitotic activity are all associated with more severe edema.[48] At the cellular level, it remains unclear whether the edema is caused by a leaky blood-tumor barrier, which lacks tight junctions, or by active secretion of fluid, as suggested by some electron microscopic studies.[51]

Management of Vasogenic Peritumoral Edema (Table 18-1)

Glucocorticoids Glucocorticoids have long been known to reduce the edema associated with brain tumors.[52] The possible mechanisms of this action include reduced capillary and blood-brain barrier permeability[53,54]; increased sodium, potassium, and water flux across the capillary-tissue interface[55]; and direct inhibition of tumor growth.[56] At the cellular level, glucocorticoids bind to specific steroid receptors on target cells, forming a steroid-receptor complex, but subsequent cellular events have not yet been elucidated. Glucocorticoids have been shown to decrease the extracellular fluid content,[57] which reduces brain swelling. This decrease is manifested clinically by lower ICP and fewer neurologic deficits in patients receiving glucocorticoids.

Glucocorticoids act fairly quickly; decreased capillary permeability is detectable as early as 1 h after a single dose of dexamethasone and lasts about 12 h.[58] Perioperative glucocorticoids are recommended whenever significant postoperative brain swelling is expected because of severe preoperative brain swelling or intraoperative manipulation of brain. We routinely administer dexameth-

Table 18-1 Treatment of Edema or Mass Effect Related to Brain Tumors

Head of bed elevation 20–30°
Glucocorticoids (dexamethasone 8–32 mg/day)
Volume restriction (usually 1200–1800 mL/day)
Furosemide (10–20 mg every 6–12 h)
Mannitol (0.25–1.0 g/kg intravenously every 6–12 h)
Hyperventilation (to achieve P_{CO_2} of 25–30 mmHg)

asone, 4 mg orally every 6 h, for several days before elective tumor surgery; if significant edema or mass effect is present or if clinical deterioration has occurred, higher doses are given intravenously. Postoperatively, intravenous dexamethasone is continued in the ICU and tapered as the clinical condition of the patient permits.

The overall clinical response to glucocorticoids for cerebral ischemia is best in patients with cerebral metastases, intermediate in those with glioblastomas and astrocytomas, and worst in those with meningiomas.[59] Studies of human tumor and peritumoral specimens have shown increased concentrations of glucocorticoid receptors in metastatic tumors and meningiomas,[60] which may contribute to the variable clinical response to glucocorticoids.

Glucocorticoids may cause a variety of adverse effects, including exacerbation of hyperglycemia, occasional frank diabetes mellitus, and euphoria. Less frequent but more serious risks include gastrointestinal hemorrhage, psychosis, osteonecrosis, impaired wound healing, and impaired immune function, leading to an increased risk of infection. The benefits in the perioperative management of brain tumors usually outweigh the untoward effects, which can usually be treated without immediately discontinuing the corticosteroids. Hyperglycemia may require administration of oral hypoglycemic drugs or insulin and discontinuation of steroid therapy. Patients receiving glucocorticoids should also take an H_2 inhibitor, such as cimetidine, or famotidine, or sucralfate, as prophylaxis against gastrointestinal irritation. Sedatives are prescribed as necessary for the psychiatric side effects of glucocorticoids. Osteonecrosis appears to be only a sporadic risk, which may be minimized by reducing the dose and duration of steroid therapy to the minimum needed to treat the edema.[61]

Diuretics for Increased ICP Diuretics and hyperosmolar agents decrease brain swelling by increasing serum osmolarity, which leads to an osmolar gradient that forces free water from the extracellular compartment. The agents most commonly used for this purpose are mannitol, furosemide, and concentrated albumin (see previous chapters). Because renal function must be adequate for these agents to have a lasting effect, they should not be used in patients with renal impairment. Serum sodium and osmolarity should also be monitored, and further administration of diuretics should be avoided if serum sodium rises above 150 mEq/L or osmolarity above 320 mOsm/L.

One limitation of diuretic and hyperosmolar therapy for increased ICP is gradual insensitivity to these agents after the osmolarity of the extracellular space has equilibrated with that of the serum. Another limitation is hemodynamic: hyperosmolar agents may cause volume overload in the short-term, and diuretics cause volume depletion in the long-term.

Hyperventilation Hyperventilation may be used to reduce ICP in patients with progressive focal deficits or depressed consciousness due to severe brain swelling in whom diuretics and fluid restriction do not control ICP (see earlier chapters). As in head trauma patients, P_{CO_2} should be maintained at 25 to 30 mmHg.

Barbiturate Coma Although it is rarely needed in patients with brain tumors, barbiturate coma is used to treat refractory elevations in ICP. Sodium thiopental is often used; the dose should be adjusted to suppress EEG bursts without causing an excessive decrease in blood pressure. Barbiturates exert a protective effect by slowing cerebral metabolism, which reduces cerebral blood volume and pressure (see earlier chapters).

Other Treatments for Increased ICP The usual nonpharmacologic measures for decreasing ICP are head elevation and maintenance of adequate jugular venous outflow if uncontrolled. A pharmacologic measure is adequate control of seizures, which greatly increases cerebral metabolism and blood flow.

Lazaroids Lazaroids are experimental steroid-like compounds without a glucocorticoid effect that appear to protect the brain and alleviate vasospasm. There are two classes of these compounds, the 21-amino steroids and the 2-methylaminochromans. Both have antioxidant and antilipolytic functions in vitro and have been shown to decrease angiographic vasospasm in experimental subarachnoid hemorrhage[62] and to enhance neurologic recovery after experimental head injury.[63]

The effectiveness of U-74006F, a 21-amino steroid, in the treatment of experimental peritumoral edema has been evaluated in two studies. In one study, it did not prevent tumor growth or edema formation.[64] The other study showed decreased tumor size and less neurologic dysfunction in treated animals than in controls[65]; however, there was no difference in peritumoral edema formation, which suggests that neurologic dysfunction was prevented by a mechanism unrelated to edema formation.

The safety of lazaroids in the treatment of head injury is being tested in humans. It remains to be seen what role, if any, these compounds will have in the clinical treatment of vasogenic edema due to brain tumors.

Nonsteroidal Anti-Inflammatory Drugs Nonsteroidal anti-inflammatory drugs are used extensively to treat nonneural inflammation but have never been evaluated in the treatment of vasogenic edema in patients with brain tumors. A recent study in a rat glioma model showed that ibuprofen and indomethacin significantly decreased extravasation of protein.[66] These drugs may prove useful as adjunct therapies for peritumoral brain edema.

ROUTINE PERIOPERATIVE INTENSIVE CARE

Fluid Management

If serious postoperative brain swelling is expected, fluid intake should routinely be limited to 1200 to 1500 mL/day, or even less in patients with hyponatremia. Further dehydration can be obtained with alternating doses of mannitol and furosemide to attain serum osmolarities greater than 300 mOsm/dL in patients with symptomatic brain swelling or prophylactically in patients with apparent brain swelling at surgery.

Several studies have shown that hyperglycemia increases the risk of cerebral infarction due to ischemic injury.[67,68] Therefore, we generally use normal saline as our intravenous fluid, withhold solutions that contain dextrose, and monitor serum glucose, especially in patients receiving high-dose steroids. If the serum glucose level is greater than 200 mg/dL, treatment with short-acting insulin preparations and continued glucose monitoring should be considered.

Feeding and Nutrition

Feeding can be started as soon as patients are alert and demonstrate intact cough, swallow, and gag reflexes. A barium swallow can be performed to assess the swallowing function, and fiber-optic laryngoscopy can be used to assess vocal cord apposition; this may be particularly important in patients with tumors of the posterior fossa, foramen magnum, and cranial base, which may affect the lower cranial nerves (IX, X, XI). If there is a prolonged decrease in alertness or neurologic swallowing or coughing difficulty, a small-caliber, soft nasoduodenal feeding tube should be placed so that feedings can begin without delay. A dietary consultation, calorie count, and assessment of nitrogen balance should be considered to optimize nutrition (see Chap. 7).

Management of Deep Venous Thrombosis and Pulmonary Embolism

As the perioperative morbidity and mortality rates for brain tumor surgery have declined, deep venous thrombosis (DVT) and pulmonary embolism (PE) have emerged as significant causes of morbidity and mortality after elective procedures for brain tumors. Postoperative venous thrombosis of the calf is estimated to occur in 29 to 43 percent of neurosurgical patients[69,70]; in one series, 3 percent of all perioperative deaths among patients undergoing elective intracranial surgery were attributable to PE.[71] The importance of DVT and PE as causes of morbidity and mortality in hospitalized patients has led to a staggering array of clinical publications and recommendations for management; the literature on DVT and PE in neurosurgical patients has been reviewed by Swann and Black.[72] Decisions regarding the prophylaxis, diagnosis, and treatment of thromboembolic disease in patients with brain tumors are frequently made in the ICU.

Risk Factors The risk factors for DVT and PE in general medical and surgical patient populations include increased age of the patient, the type and duration of surgery, a history of DVT, leg trauma, immobility, malignancy, hypercoagulable states, dehydration, varicose veins, heart failure, pregnancy, gram-negative sepsis, obesity, oral contraceptive use, and inflammatory bowel disease. Many of these factors, particularly limb paresis, prolonged operations, iatrogenic dehydration, and malignant disease, are frequently present in perioperative patients with brain tumors.

Surgery causes systemic changes in platelet and coagulation function that favor thrombosis, and longer operations carry a greater risk of thrombosis. In one study of patients undergoing cranial or spinal operations, the incidence of DVT determined by ^{125}I-fibrinogen uptake was 50 percent in patients whose operations lasted 4 h or more, but was only 24 percent in those who underwent shorter procedures.[70]

The question of whether a brain tumor increases the risk of DVT remains largely unanswered. The original studies that identified malignancy as a risk factor did not attempt to distinguish among various types of malignancies, except to note that pancreatic cancer appeared to be more frequently associated with DVT.[73] Patients with primary brain tumors may lack some of the systemic pathologic changes of malignant disease that predispose to thromboembolism, such as a hypercoagulable state. Not surprisingly, no major study has identified primary brain neoplasms as an independent risk factor for DVT. Indeed, a review of 100 neurosurgical patients found no significant difference in the incidence of DVT in patients who had a craniotomy and those who had a laminectomy.[70] On the other hand, Brisman and Mendell noted an increased incidence of DVT in patients with suprasellar tumors versus all other brain tumors, which they related to hypothalamic derangements causing dehydration.[74]

Diagnosis of DVT The diagnosis of DVT and PE in patients with brain tumors is no different from that in other hospitalized patients. Both invasive and noninvasive tests can be used. For DVT, noninvasive tests include ^{125}I-fibrinogen scanning, impedance plethysmography, and Doppler ultrasound; however, all these techniques lack sensitivity and specificity. Venography, an invasive test, is much more accurate but carries its own morbidity. For PE, noninvasive tests include ventilation-perfusion scanning and pulmonary angiography, which is the most definitive test. Up to 83 percent of DVTs in brain tumor patients are asymptomatic.[70] Therefore, if PE is suspected clinically, the diagnosis and treatment should be aggressively pursued irrespective of evidence of DVT.

The value of screening asymptomatic patients for DVT has not yet been evaluated in neurosurgical patients. Although the expense of screening would be high, the potential benefit in prevented cases of PE could also be great. In one study, preoperative ^{125}I-fibrinogen scanning showed DVT in 9 percent of patients undergoing elective intracranial procedures.[75]

Prophylaxis Against Deep Venous Thrombosis

Mechanical Measures Several mechanical measures to prevent DVT in brain tumor patients are often endorsed, including leg elevation during surgery, early ambulation, physiotherapy, and elastic stockings, but they have never been shown to reduce the risk of DVT or PE. The only mechanical measure proven to reduce the risk of DVT is external pneumatic compression boots. Two randomized, prospective studies have shown unequivocally that intermittent external pneumatic compression reduces the risk of DVT in neurosurgical patients[76,77] and should be recommended for all patients undergoing major intracranial surgery. At our institution, elastic stockings and external pneumatic compression boots are placed routinely in the operating room and are not removed until the patient is ambulatory and has been discharged from the ICU.

Mini-dose Heparin The efficacy of mini-dose heparin (5000 U subcutaneously every 12 h) as perioperative prophylaxis for DVT has been demonstrated, but its use in perioperative neurosurgical patients is not universally accepted. Cerrato and associates[75] showed that perioperative mini-dose heparin decreased the incidence of DVT from 34 to 6 percent. However, even though the safety of this prophylactic measure was demonstrated in two series,[75,78] considerable concern remains about exacerbating problems with intraoperative hemostasis and perioperative intracranial hemorrhage in patients undergoing neurosurgical operations. The effectiveness of mini-dose heparin in the prophylaxis of PE has not been evaluated.

Dextran Intravenous dextran prophylaxis reduces the risk of fatal PE[79] but is probably contraindicated in patients with intracranial tumors, as defects in the blood-brain barrier could allow dextran to leak into the interstitial space and cause cerebral edema.[80]

Treatment of Deep Venous Thrombosis

Anticoagulation The objectives of treatment of DVT in patients with brain tumors are to prevent PE, to minimize clot progression, to prevent clot recurrence, and to provide local extremity care. The standard therapy has been full anticoagulation with heparin, followed by oral anticoagulation with warfarin for approximately 6 months. This regimen reduces the risk of subsequent PE, minimizes clot progression, and decreases the risk of clot recurrence, but it does have risks. Heparin can cause osteopenia, thrombocytopenia, and hemorrhage, while warfarin is associated with adverse drug interactions, birth defects, and hemorrhage. Current therapies for DVT still have high rates of complications, including leg swelling, venous stasis, ulceration, gangrene, and gastrointestinal bleeding. The safety of anticoagulation in patients with brain tumors has never been evaluated, but cases of hemorrhage from unsuspected brain tumors have been reported after administration of anticoagulants.[17] Recent intracranial surgery also increases the risk of hemorrhage due to anticoagulants; in one series, 9 of 21 neurosurgical patients suffered hemorrhagic complications.[81] To reduce the risk of hemorrhage, systemic anticoagulants should not be administered for at least 2 weeks after intracranial surgery.[80] If DVT or PE develops during this time, placement of a Greenfield filter or other form of inferior vena cava interruption should be considered. After 2 or 3 weeks, systemic anticoagulation may be started, and the patient's coagulation status should be carefully monitored by laboratory studies.

Inferior Vena Cava Interruption Because of the high risk of hemorrhagic complications with anticoagulation for the first several weeks after surgery and because of the danger of untreated DVT, an inferior vena cava interrupting device is probably the best means of preventing PE. A recent study demonstrated the safety and efficacy of the Greenfield filter without anticoagulation as primary therapy for DVT.[82] The filter,[83] which can be placed under local anesthesia alone, was used in 42 patients who did not receive anticoagulants; there were no permanent complications related to filter placement, and no patient had a PE. Even though no treatment was directed to the clot itself, ulceration of the lower extremity due to venous stasis was less common than has been reported in patients with DVT treated with anticoagulants alone (5 versus 17 percent).[84]

Treatment of PE Patients with a documented PE after surgery for brain tumors receive supportive care, supplemental oxygen, intravenous hydration, vasopressors, and invasive intravascular monitoring, if needed, as well as presumptive treatment for DVT. Anticoagulation and/or inferior vena cava interruption are used to prevent further embolism. Fibrinolytics, which are used to lyse the pulmonary clot in cases of PE, are contraindicated in postoperative neurosurgical patients; they should be used with extreme caution before surgery for brain tumors, especially vascular tumors, which are most likely to hemorrhage.[85] Since pulmonary emboli frequently occur in the perioperative period, transvenous inferior vena cava interruption using a Greenfield filter, without anticoagulation, is often the only treatment recommended.

Gastritis and Ulcer Prophylaxis

The incidence of gastritis and peptic ulcer disease is increased by a number of risk factors found in patients with brain tumors in the ICU. Intracranial pathology by itself is a risk factor for gastritis, and the incidence of hemorrhagic ulceration of the upper gastrointestinal tract as autopsy is 2 times higher (12.5 versus 6.0 percent) in patients who died of intracranial causes than in those who died of other causes.[86] Furthermore, many patients are taking glucocorticoids, which further increases the risk. Therefore, prophylaxis for gastritis is recommended for all ICU patients with brain tumors. At our institution, intravenous H_2 inhibitors, such as famotidine or cimetidine, or sucralfate are used routinely in all ICU patients with brain tumors.

Postoperative Airway Management

As with other patients undergoing intracranial surgery, patients with brain tumors are extubated as soon as they can manage their airway and hyperventilation is no longer necessary. Occasionally, patients with brainstem and lower cranial nerve deficits may have new postoperative neurologic deficits requiring longer intubation. These are seen frequently with lower cranial nerve schwannomas, foramen magnum and posterior fossa meningiomas, brainstem gliomas, and glomus jugulare tumors. In such patients the gag reflex and lower cranial nerve functions should be carefully assessed before extubation. Prolonged or permanent loss of lower cranial nerve function should prompt consideration of placing a tracheostomy for long-term airway management.

Routine Diagnostic Studies

Few routine studies are really needed in the perioperative management of patients with brain tumors. Daily monitoring of electrolytes and urine specific gravity is sufficient to detect hypothalamic disturbances of fluid balance, and daily glucose and urine glucose measurements will detect hyperglycemia and glycosuria in patients taking corticosteroids. More frequent measurements may be necessary after operations in the region of the hypothalamus and third ventricle and in patients with severe brain edema in whom dehydration therapy or diuretics are being used. Glucose intolerance warrants more frequent blood glucose measurements and treatment as already noted. Periodic checking of arterial blood gases is necessary while patients are being managed on or weaned from the respirator.

Anticonvulsants

Perioperative administration of anticonvulsants is recommended in most patients with brain tumors, including those undergoing supratentorial operations and those with preexisting seizure disorders. Routine use of anticonvulsants is not recommended for patients with tumors confined to the infratentorial space and those undergoing transsphenoidal operations, or placement of a ventricular shunt only. Anticonvulsant therapy, usually phenytoin, may be started preoperatively and supplemented intraoperatively with intravenous doses, or an intraoperative intravenous loading dose may be given, followed by daily intravenous dosing until the patient can tolerate oral doses. If the patient has never taken anticonvulsants, the dose may be adjusted empirically to attain standard therapeutic levels. Otherwise, the occurrence of seizure activity or anticonvulsant toxicity should be used to guide adjustment to the patient's own therapeutic level. We routinely use phenytoin as first-line intravenous therapy, followed by carbamazepine, and then phenobarbital if necessary. Routine loading and maintenance dosing are shown in Table 18-2.

In general, critically ill patients with brain tumors of the cerebral hemispheres should probably be given some form of anticonvulsant prophylaxis because seizures could greatly complicate the course of their illness. Overall, 50 percent of all brain tumors have been reported to be associated with seizures,[87] and fever, electrolyte disturbances, and other drugs are known to lower the threshold for seizures.

CONCLUSION

The indications for ICU care of patients with brain tumors include uncontrolled seizures, sudden deterioration due to hemorrhage into a tumor, focal brain swelling, hydrocephalus, increased ICP, as well as routine postoperative observation. The types of monitoring used include ICP monitoring, evoked-potential monitoring, and invasive intra-

Table 18-2 Routine Loading and Maintenance Doses of Commonly Used Anticonvulsants for Perioperative Seizure Prophylaxis

Drug	Route*	Loading dose, g	Maintenance dose, mg/day	Empiric serum level, μg/mL
Phenytoin	IV or PO	1	300	10–20
Phenobarbital	IV or PO	Up to 1.4	180–200	10–30
Carbamazepine	PO	None	Start at 400, adjust to 800–1200	4–12

*IV = intravenous; PO = per os (by mouth).

vascular monitoring, while types of interventions include hyperventilation, glucocorticoids, diuretics and hyperosmolar therapy, direct removal of cerebrospinal fluid, barbiturate coma, and several experimental approaches including nonsteroidal anti-inflammatory drugs and lazaroids. Prophylactic measures should include attention to a variety of common complications including thromboembolism, seizures, aspiration, gastrointestinal irritation, and fluid and electrolyte imbalances. Future developments in these areas will undoubtedly yield greater opportunities to improve the care of patients with brain tumors.

REFERENCES

1. Janz D: Conditions and causes of status epilepticus. *Epilepsia* 2:170, 1961.
2. Rowan AJ, Scott DF: Major status epilepticus: A series of 42 patients. *Acta Neurol Scand* 46:573, 1970.
3. Brodie M: Status epilepticus in adults. *Lancet* 336:551, 1990.
4. Drake CG, McGee D: Apoplexy associated with brain tumours. *Can Med Assoc J* 84:303, 1961.
5. Globus JH, Sapirstein M: Massive hemorrhage into brain tumor. *JAMA* 120:348, 1942.
6. Jellinger K: Pathology and aetiology of ICH. In: Pia HW, Langmaid C, Zierski J (eds): *Spontaneous Intracerebral Haematomas: Advances in Diagnosis and Treatment.* Berlin, Springer-Verlag, 1980, pp 13–29.
7. Oldberg E: Hemorrhage into gliomas: A review of eight hundred and thirty-two consecutive verified cases of glioma. *Arch Neurol Psychiatry* 30:1061, 1933.
8. Padt JP, De Reuck J, vander Eecken H: Intracerebral hemorrhage as initial symptom of a brain tumor. *Acta Neurol Belg* 73:241, 1973.
9. Pia HW: The surgical treatment of intracerebral and intraventricular haematomas. *Acta Neurochir (Wien)* 27:149, 1972.
10. Scott M: Spontaneous intracerebral hematoma caused by cerebral neoplasms: Report of eight verified cases. *J Neurosurg* 42:338, 1975.
11. Wakai S, Yamakawa K, Manaka S, et al.: Spontaneous intracranial hemorrhage caused by brain tumor: Its incidence and clinical significance. *Neurosurgery* 10:437, 1982.
12. Kondziolka D, Bernstein M, Resch L, et al.: Significance of hemorrhage into brain tumors: Clinicopathological study. *J Neurosurg* 67:852, 1987.
13. Andrews BT, Raffel C, Rosegay H: Subarachnoid hemorrhage from a peripheral intracranial aneurysm associated with a malignant glioma: Report of a case. *Neurosurgery* 17:645, 1985.
14. Ho KL: Neoplastic aneurysm and intracranial hemorrhage. *Cancer* 50:2935, 1982.
15. Momma F, Beck H, Miyamoto T, et al.: Intracranial aneurysm due to metastatic choriocarcinoma. *Surg Neurol* 25:74, 1986.
16. Pullar M, Blumbergs PC, Phillips GE, et al.: Neoplastic cerebral aneurysm from metastatic gestational choriocarcinoma. *J Neurosurg* 63:644, 1985.
17. Everett BA, Kusske JA, Pribram HW: Anticoagulants and intracerebral hemorrhage from an unsuspected meningioma. *Surg Neurol* 11:233, 1979.
18. Mandybur TI: Intracranial hemorrhage caused by metastatic tumors. *Neurology* 27:650, 1977.
19. Mangianiello LOJ: Massive spontaneous hemorrhage in gliomas. A report of seven verified cases. *J Nerv Ment Dis* 110:277, 1949.
20. Vaquero J, Cabezudo JM, de Sola RG, et al.: Intratumoral hemorrhage in posterior fossa tumors after ventricular drainage. *J Neurosurg* 54:406, 1981.
21. Zuccarello M, Dollo C, Carollo C: Spontaneous intratumoral hemorrhage after ventriculoperitoneal shunting. *Neurosurgery* 16:245, 1985.
22. Epstein F, Murali R: Pediatric posterior fossa tumors: Hazards of the "preoperative" shunt. *Neurosurgery* 3:348, 1978.
23. Abraham J, Chandy J: Ventriculo-atrial shunt in the management of posterior fossa tumors: Preliminary report. *J Neurosurg* 20:252, 1963.
24. Albright L, Reigel DH: Management of hydrocephalus secondary to posterior fossa tumors. *J Neurosurg* 46:52, 1977.
25. Bohm B, Mohadjer M, Hemmer R: Preoperative continuous measurements of ventricular pressure in hydrocephalus occlusus with tumors of the posterior fossa: The value of ventriculoauricular shunt. *Adv Neurosurg* 5:194, 1978.
26. Gruss P, Gaab M, Knoblich OE: Disorders of CSF circulation after interventions in the area of the posterior cranial fossa with prior shunt operation. *Adv Neurosurg* 5:199, 1978.
27. Hekmatpanah J, Mullan S: Ventriculo-caval shunt in the management of posterior fossa tumors. *J Neurosurg* 26:609, 1967.
28. Hoffman HJ, Hendrick EB, Humphries RP: Metastasis via ventriculoperitoneal shunt in patients with medulloblastoma. *J Neurosurg* 44:562, 1976.
29. Chapman PH, Cosman E, Arnold M: Telemetric ICP monitoring after surgery for posterior fossa and third ventricular tumors. *J Neurosurg* 60:649, 1984.
30. Schmid UD, Seiler RW: Management of obstructive hydrocephalus secondary to posterior fossa tumors by steroids and subcutaneous ventricular catheter reservoir. *J Neurosurg* 65:649, 1986.

31. Constantini S, Cotev S, Rappaport ZH, et al.: Intracranial pressure monitoring after elective intracranial surgery. *J Neurosurg* 69:540, 1988.
32. Mollman HD, Rockswold GL, Ford SE: A clinical comparison of subarachnoid catheters to ventriculostomy and subarachnoid bolts: A prospective study. *J Neurosurg* 68:737, 1988.
33. Smith RW, Alksne JF: Infections complicating the use of external ventriculostomy. *J Neurosurg* 44:567, 1976.
34. Wyler AR, Kelly W: Use of antibiotics with external ventriculostomies. *J Neurosurg* 37:185, 1972.
35. North B, Reilly P: Comparison among three methods of intracranial pressure recording. *Neurosurgery* 18:730, 1986.
36. Wilkinson HA: Comment. *Neurosurgery* 18:732, 1986.
37. Ostrup RC, Luerssen TG, Marshall LF, et al.: Continuous monitoring of intracranial pressure with a miniaturized fiberoptic device. *J Neurosurg* 67:206, 1987.
38. Winn HR, Dacey RG, Jane JA: Intracranial subarachnoid pressure recording: Experience with 650 patients. *Surg Neurol* 8:41, 1977.
39. Rosenwasser RH, Kleiner LI, Krzeminski JU, et al.: Intracranial pressure monitoring in the posterior fossa: A preliminary report. *J Neurosurg* 71:503, 1989.
40. Piek J, Bock WJ: Continuous monitoring of cerebral tissue pressure in neurosurgical practice—experiences with 100 patients. *Intensive Care Med* 16:184, 1990.
41. Park CK: Accuracy of ICP monitoring in posterior fossa lesions. *J Neurosurg* 72:832, 1990. Letter.
42. Rosenwasser RH: Response. *J Neurosurg* 72:832, 1990.
43. Klatzo I: Neuropathological aspects of brain edema. *J Neuropathol Exp Neurol* 26:1, 1967.
44. Hossman KA, Wechsler W, Wilmes F: Experimental peritumorous edema. Morphological and pathophysiological observations. *Acta Neuropathol* 45:195, 1979.
45. Black KL, Hoff JT, McGillicuddy JE, et al.: Increased leukotriene C4 and vasogenic edema surrounding brain tumors in humans. *Ann Neurol* 19:592, 1986.
46. Quindlen EA, Bucher AP: Correlation of tumor plasminogen activator with peritumoral cerebral edema. *J Neurosurg* 66:729, 1987.
47. Criscuolo GR, Merrill MJ, Oldfield EH: Further characterization of malignant glioma-derived vascular permeability factor. *J Neurosurg* 69:254, 1988.
48. Challa VR, Moody DM, Marshall RB, et al.: The vascular component in meningiomas associated with severe cerebral edema. *Neurosurgery* 7:363, 1980.
49. Smith HP, Challa VR, Moody DM, et al.: Biological features of meningiomas that determine the production of cerebral edema. *Neurosurgery* 8:428, 1981.
50. Gilbert JJ, Paulseth JE, Coates RK, et al.: Cerebral edema associated with meningiomas. *Neurosurgery* 12:599, 1983.
51. Phillippon J, Foncin JF, Grob R, et al.: Cerebral edema associated with meningiomas: Possible role of a secretory-excretory phenomenon. *Neurosurgery* 14:295, 1984.
52. Galicich JH, French LA: Use of dexamethasone in the treatment of cerebral edema resulting from brain tumors and brain surgery. *Am Pract* 12:169, 1961.
53. Pappius HM, McCann WP: Effects of steroids on cerebral edema in cats. *Arch Neurol* 20:207, 1969.
54. Shapiro WR, Posner JB: Corticosteroid hormones. Effects in an experimental brain tumor. *Arch Neurol* 30:217, 1974.
55. Long DM, Hartmann JF, French LA: The response of human cerebral edema to glucosteroid administration. An electron microscopic study. *Neurology* 16:521, 1966.
56. Gurcay O, Wilson C, Barker M, et al.: Corticosteroid effect on transplantable rat glioma. *Arch Neurol* 24:266, 1971.
57. Yamada K, Ushio Y, Hayakawa T, et al.: Effects of methylprednisolone on peritumoral brain edema. *J Neurosurg* 59:612, 1983.
58. Shapiro WR, Hiesiger EM, Cooney GA, et al.: Temporal effects of dexamethasone on blood-to-brain and blood-to-tumor transport of ^{14}C-alpha-aminoiso-butyric acid in rat C_6 glioma. *J Neurooncol* 8:197, 1990.
59. Reulen HJ, Hajidimos A, Hase U: Steroids in the treatment of brain edema. In: Schurmann K, Brock M, Reulen HJ, et al. (eds): *Cerebello-Pontine Angle Tumors. Advances in Neurosurgery, vol 1.* New York, Springer-Verlag, 1973, pp 92–99.
60. Yu Z-Y, Wrange Ö, Boëthius J, et al.: A study of glucocorticoid receptors in intracranial tumors. *J Neurosurg* 55:757, 1981.
61. Fast A, Alon M, Weiss S, et al.: Avascular necrosis of bone following short-term dexamethasone therapy for brain edema. *J Neurosurg* 61:983, 1984.
62. Zuccarello M, Marsch JT, Schmitt G, et al.: Effect of the 21-aminosteroid U-74006F on cerebral vasospasm following subarachnoid hemorrhage. *J Neurosurg* 71:98, 1989.
63. Hall ED, Yonkers PA, McCall JM, et al.: Effects of the 21-aminosteroid U74006F on experimental head injury in mice. *J Neurosurg* 68:456, 1988.
64. Megyesi JF, Farrell CL, Del Maestro RF: Investigation of an inhibitor of lipid peroxidation U74006F on tumor growth and protein extravasation in the C6 astrocytoma spheroid implantation glioma model. *J Neurooncol* 8:133, 1990.
65. King WA, Black KL, Ikezaki K, et al.: Tumor-associated neurological dysfunction prevented by lazaroids in rats. *J Neurosurg* 74:112, 1991.
66. Reichman HR, Farrell CL, Del Maestro RF: Effects of steroid and nonsteroid anti-inflammatory agents on vascular permeability in a rat glioma model. *J Neurosurg* 65:233, 1986.
67. Rehncrona S, Rosen C, Siesjo B: Excessive cellular aci-

dosis: An important mediator of neuronal damage in the brain. *Acta Physiol Scand* 110:435, 1980.
68. Rehncrona S, Rosen C, Siesjo B: Brain lactic acidosis and ischemic cell damage. 1. Biochemistry and neurophysiology. *J Cereb Blood Flow Metab* 1:297, 1981.
69. Joffe SN: Incidence of postoperative deep vein thrombosis in neurosurgical patients. *J Neurosurg* 42:201, 1975.
70. Valladares JB, Hankinson J: Incidence of lower extremity deep vein thrombosis in neurosurgical patients. *Neurosurg* 6:138, 1980.
71. Wetzel N, Anderson MC, Shields TW: Pulmonary embolism as a cause of death in the neurosurgical patient. *J Neurosurg* 17:664, 1960.
72. Swann KW, Black PM: Deep vein thrombosis and pulmonary emboli in neurosurgical patients: A review. *J Neurosurg* 61:1055, 1984.
73. Coon WW: Epidemiology of venous thromboembolism. *Surg Gynecol Obstet* 143:149, 1977.
74. Brisman R, Mendell J. Thromboembolism and brain tumors. *J Neurosurg* 38:337, 1973.
75. Cerrato D, Ariano C, Fiacchino F: Deep vein thrombosis and low-dose heparin prophylaxis in neurosurgical patients. *J Neurosurg* 48:378, 1978.
76. Skillman JJ, Collins RED, Coe NP, et al.: Prevention of deep vein thrombosis in neurosurgical patients: A controlled, randomized trial of external pneumatic compression boots. *Surgery* 83:354, 1978.
77. Turpie AGG, Gallus AS, Beattie WS, et al.: Prevention of venous thrombosis in patients with intracranial disease by intermittent pneumatic compression of the calf. *Neurology* 27:435, 1977.
78. Barnett HG, Clifford JR, Llewellyn RC: Safety of minidose heparin administration in neurosurgical patients. *J Neurosurg* 47:27, 1977.
79. Gruber UF, Saldeen T, Brokop T, et al.: Incidences of fatal postoperative pulmonary embolism after prophylaxis with dextran 70 and low-dose heparin: An international multicentre study. *Br Med J* 280:69, 1980.
80. Powers SK, Edwards MSB: Prophylaxis of thromboembolism in the neurosurgical patient: A review. *Neurosurgery* 10:509, 1982.
81. DiRicco G, Marini C, Rindi M, et al.: Pulmonary embolism in neurosurgical patients: Diagnosis and treatment. *J Neurosurg* 60:972, 1984.
82. Fink JA, Jones BT: The Greenfield filter as the primary means of therapy in venous thromboembolic disease. *Surg Gynecol Obstet* 172:253, 1991.
83. Greenfield L, McCurdy J, Brown P, Elkins R: A new intracaval filter permitting continued flow and resolution of embolic complications. *Surgery* 73:599, 1973.
84. Kakkar VV, Lawrence D: Hemodynamic and clinical assessment after therapy for deep venous thrombosis. *Am J Surg* 150:54, 1985.
85. National Institutes of Health Consensus Development Conference: Thrombolytic therapy in thrombosis. *Stroke* 12:17, 1981.
86. Karch SB: Upper gastrointestinal bleeding as a complication of intracranial disease. *J Neurosurg* 37:27, 1972.
87. Rasmussen T: Surgery of epilepsy associated with brain tumors. In: Purpura DP, Penry JK, Walter RD (eds): *Neurosurgical Management of the Epilepsies. Advances in Neurology, vol 8.* New York, Raven, 1975, pp 227–239.

CHAPTER 19

The Neurosurgical Pediatric Patient

Gregory Hammer
James N. Lindsay

INTRODUCTION

Since the development of specialized pediatric intensive care units (ICUs) in the 1970s, the field of pediatric intensive care has matured into a distinct specialty. It is now standard practice for hospitals in which significant numbers of critically ill children are managed to have a multidisciplinary pediatric ICU. Such a unit offers care provided by a variety of pediatric surgeons and other specialists in conjunction with pediatric physicians who have subspecialty training in pediatric critical care. In addition, care is provided by specially trained pediatric nurses, respiratory therapists, pharmacists, and social workers in a highly coordinated effort. Critically ill infants and children may at times be cared for, however, in adult ICUs owing to trauma center designation or limited access to a pediatric facility. The purpose of this chapter is to provide guidance regarding the care of the neurosurgical pediatric patient who may not necessarily be located in a pediatric ICU.

Management of the pediatric neurosurgical patient demands a broad-based knowledge of general neurologic intensive care as well as an understanding of pediatric anatomy and physiology. Principles of adult neurologic intensive care are covered extensively in other chapters of this text. The focus of this chapter, therefore, will be to review pediatric anatomy and physiology pertinent to neurologic intensive care, followed by discussion of important differences between adult and pediatric pathophysiology and management.

The newborn, infant, and young child are not merely small adults. There are numerous important anatomic and physiologic differences between patients in these age groups and their adult counterparts. Indeed, there are many developmental changes which occur following birth and throughout childhood which produce dramatic anatomic and physiologic consequences. For example, morphologic development of the airway from birth to young adulthood produces changes with which the practitioner must be familiar to facilitate safe and effective management. Maturational changes in pediatric circulatory, respiratory, and central nervous system (CNS) physiology have profound impact on the diagnosis and treatment of the neurologically injured child. This chapter will review normal anatomy and physiology of the pediatric respiratory, circulatory, and central nervous systems; principles of renal physiology and fluid and electrolyte balance in children; and essential nutritional considerations. We will then review the pathophysiology of these systems while providing an overview of care of the critically ill child.

Closed head injury is the most common diagnosis that results in admission of a pediatric patient to an adult ICU.[1A] For that reason, as developmental and physiologic differences are presented, attention will be drawn to these differences and their importance in the head-injured child.

THE RESPIRATORY SYSTEM

The purpose of the respiratory system is to exchange oxygen and carbon dioxide across the alveolar-capillary membrane. Respiratory failure is the inability of the respiratory system to perform this function, leading to inadequate delivery of oxygen to tissues to meet their metabolic demands (hypoxia) and/or the accumulation of carbon dioxide in the tissues and bloodstream (hypercarbia). Both hypoxia and hypercarbia are associated with untoward physiologic consequences. The causes of respiratory failure in children, as in adults, include impaired control of ventilation, neuromuscular disorders, structural impairment of the thorax (both extrathoracic and intrathoracic), airway obstruction, and alveolar disease states. Many of these conditions may be seen in the pediatric neurosurgical patient. Impaired control of ventilation may be secondary to head trauma, intracranial hemorrhage, elevated intracranial pressure, CNS infection, status epilepticus, or drug intoxication. Trauma to the cervical cord or phrenic nerve may precipitate neuromuscular failure. Trauma to the chest may produce pneumothorax, hemothorax, or flail chest, causing structural impairment and consequent respiratory failure. Extrathoracic airway obstruction may be caused by trauma from a previously indwelling tracheal tube, resulting in edema, hemorrhage, stenosis, or vocal cord injury. Intrathoracic airway obstruction may be concomitant with neurologic injury, such as with pulmonary edema due to near-drowning or "neurogenic" pulmonary edema, aspiration of gastric contents, or pulmonary contusion or hemorrhage. Many features of the anatomy and physiology of the pediatric patient may result in predisposition to respiratory failure from these causes.

From the naris to the terminal bronchiole, the calibers of the airways in infants and children are anatomically small. Because the resistance to gas flow through airways is inversely proportional to the fourth power of their radius (Poiseuille's law), there is an inherently elevated resistance to gas flow in the airways of infants and children. Any lesion which causes further airways narrowing may raise gas-flow resistance to a critical level. This may limit gas flow such that adequate alveolar gas exchange cannot occur, thereby causing respiratory failure. Patients with normal CNS function will increase their effort of breathing in response to airway obstruction in an attempt to overcome elevated resistance to gas flow. Patients with CNS impairment may have limited ability to increase their respiratory effort and may be especially predisposed to respiratory failure. Resulting hypoxia and hypercarbia may exacerbate existing CNS damage. Infants are also predisposed to respiratory failure because of their increased metabolic requirements as compared with adults. Infants normally consume approximately 6 to 8 mL O_2/kg body weight per min and produce about an equal amount of CO_2, compared with a normal minute O_2 consumption and CO_2 production of approximately 3 mL/kilogram of body weight per minute in an adult.[18] Conditions which cause reduced alveolar gas exchange in infants, therefore, produce a more precipitous drop in arterial O_2 saturation and elevation of arterial CO_2 tension. Infants may, therefore, be predisposed to the "secondary injury" of hypoxia and/or hypercarbia and the associated adverse outcome following recovery from a primary CNS injury.

Examples of extrathoracic airway lesions which

may cause elevated resistance to gas flow in pediatric patients include edema and hemorrhage of the nose, tongue, posterior pharynx, and supra- or subglottic tissues. These may be produced by trauma, such as facial injuries incurred in a fall or motor vehicle accident, or by infections of the extrathoracic respiratory tract, including laryngotracheobronchitis and supraglottitis. Infants are often obligate nasal breathers, so otherwise minor inflammation and swelling of the nasal mucosa may cause intermittent extrathoracic airway obstruction. Patients with CNS injury may have diminished tone of the hypopharynx due to brainstem or lower cranial nerve dysfunction or coma, contributing to inspiratory obstruction. In children up to the age of about 7 or 8 years, the subglottic trachea is the narrowest segment of the extrathoracic respiratory tract, as opposed to the vocal cord or glottic opening in the adult. Therefore, further narrowing of the subglottic trachea in infants and children may cause a critical stenosis, diminished gas flow, and respiratory failure. Such narrowing may be produced by infection, such as laryngotracheobronchitis, or by trauma due to a previously indwelling tracheal tube.

In the neurologically impaired pediatric patient, the diagnosis of respiratory failure must be made promptly and treated rapidly in order to avoid secondary neurologic injury. The appearance of tachypnea, nasal flaring, exhalatory grunting, and intercostal retractions signal the need for immediate intervention in the infant or child with CNS injury. Alternatively, signs of respiratory depression, including decreased respiratory rate for age with somnolence, also merit urgent treatment. Respiratory failure may be accompanied by tachycardia or bradycardia, hypertension or hypotension, depending upon the underlying condition and age of the patient. In the neonate and infant, for example, limited sympathetic neural tone may predispose to bradycardia secondary to hypoxia.

Monitoring of the neurologically impaired patient with respiratory compromise should include continuous ECG, respiratory rate, and pulse oximetry, as well as frequent blood pressure measurements by automated cuff or continuous intraarterial monitoring. Arterial CO_2 tension may be estimated with transcutaneous CO_2 monitoring or nasal capnometry.[2,3] Except in the preterm infant at risk for retinopathy of prematurity, supplemental oxygen should be continuously administered to achieve oxygen saturation by pulse oximetry of 98 to 100 percent. If the oxygen saturation cannot be maintained in this range (or $Pa_{O_2} > 80$ to 100 mmHg) despite an FI_{O_2} of > 0.60, if respiratory acidemia exists, or if heart rate and/or blood pressure are adversely affected in the presence of respiratory distress, tracheal intubation should be performed and mechanical ventilation should be instituted. These modalities should also be utilized in the presence of impending or existing unconsciousness, absent protective airway reflexes, intracranial hypertension, or severe neuromuscular weakness.

Tracheal Intubation

Important considerations or goals for tracheal intubation in infants and children include maintenance of alveolar gas exchange and oxygenation, prevention of pulmonary aspiration of gastric contents, and control of intracranial pressure. In achieving these goals, optimal use of special equipment is mandatory, and pharmacologic therapy may be essential.

Prior to tracheal intubation, bag-and-mask ventilation should be performed with 100 percent oxygen. A continuous oxygen source and bag-and-mask system with the appropriately sized face mask for positive-pressure ventilation should be maintained for this purpose at each patient's bedside. Circuits employing self-inflating bags or anesthesia bags may be utilized safely and effectively, as long as the operator is familiar with the specifications of the system in use. A range of oropharyngeal and nasopharyngeal airways should be readily available to maintain extrathoracic airway patency during bag-and-mask ventilation. As with adult patients, nasopharyngeal airways should not be employed in the presence of basilar skull fracture with possible discontinuity of the nasopharyngeal mucosa, nor in patients with bleeding diatheses.

All patients with CNS injury and respiratory failure should be considered as having a "full stomach." CNS injury and respiratory failure alone may be associated with increased gastric acidity and volume. Therefore, patients with both disorders might logically be assumed to be at especially high risk for gastric regurgitation and pulmonary aspiration. Bag-and-mask ventilation may result in gaseous distension of the stomach, increasing this risk. The appropriate application of cricoid pressure during bag-and-mask ventilation and laryngoscopy reduces the likelihood of this potentially catastrophic event by occluding the esophagus. Cricoid pressure should be maintained until correct placement of the tracheal tube has been confirmed by auscultation.

Special equipment for performing tracheal intubation in infants and children includes appropriately sized laryngoscope blades and tracheal tubes. Anatomic features of the infant's airway may render tracheal intubation more difficult than in the adult patient. These features include large head size relative to neck, shoulders, and thorax; small mandibular size; relatively large tongue; and a glottis which is displaced cephalad and anteriorly (see Fig. 19-1). In neonates and infants, a straight laryngoscope blade (e.g., Miller, Wis-Hipple) may be most efficacious. Such a blade is designed to directly elevate the epiglottis, which is typically soft and floppy in the first 12 to 18 months of life. After this age, a curved blade (e.g., MacIntosh), designed to indirectly elevate the epiglottis by displacing the vallecula anteriorly, is preferred by some operators. Suggested blade styles and sizes are listed in Table 19-1. The range of suggested tracheal tube sizes by age is also listed in Table 19-1. Because the subglottic trachea is the narrowest lumen of the extrathoracic airway in children younger than 7 or 8 years of age, *uncuffed tracheal tubes* are generally employed in this age group. It should be noted that for an individual patient these tube sizes are cho-

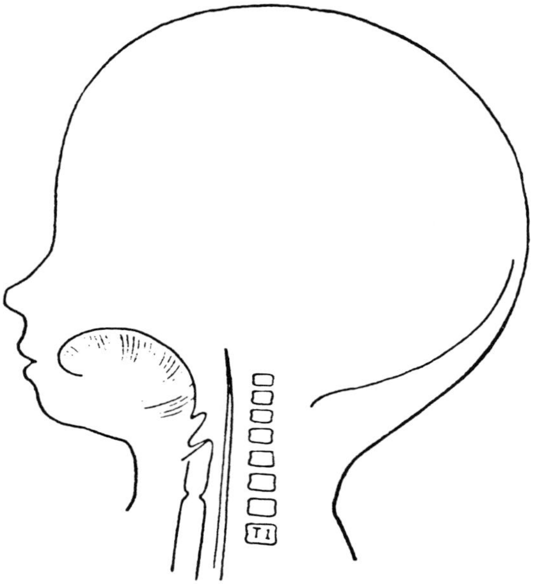

Figure 19-1 Infant airway; large head; small lumens; large tongue; larynx cephalad (C3-C4 versus C5-C6); larynx anterior; airway narrowest at level of cricoid (versus vocal cords).

Table 19-1 Endotracheal Tube and Laryngoscope Blade Sizes by Age

Age	Tube size (I.D., mm)	Laryngoscope blade
Preterm infant		
Weight < 1500 g	2.5	Miller 0
Weight > 1500 g	3.0	Miller 0 or 1
Term newborn	3.0–3.5	Miller 1
3–9 months	3.5	Miller 1
9–15 months	4.0	Miller 1 or Wis-Hipple 1.5
15–24 months	4.5	Wis-Hipple 1.5 or MacIntosh 2
3–4 years	4.5–5.0	Wis-Hipple 1.5 or MacIntosh 2
5–6 years	5.0–5.5	Miller 2* or MacIntosh 3
7–8 years	5.5–6.0	Miller 2* or MacIntosh 3
9–10 years	6.0 cuffed	Miller 2* or MacIntosh 3
11–14 years	6.5 cuffed	Miller 2* or MacIntosh 3
15–18 years	7.0 cuffed	Miller 2* or MacIntosh 3
>18 years (male)	8.0 cuffed	Miller 2* or MacIntosh 3

*May substitute Wisconsin or other straight blade.

sen empirically. If the indwelling tracheal tube is too small, leakage of inspired gas around the tube may preclude maintenance of adequate lung volumes and alveolar ventilation. If the tracheal tube is too large, pressure exerted against the tracheal mucosa may cause ischemic injury leading to subglottic scarring and stenosis. Therefore, after confirmation of correct positioning of the tracheal tube, appropriate size must also be confirmed. During slow positive-pressure inspiration, the anterior neck overlying the trachea is auscultated. The inflating pressure at which a gas leak around the tracheal tube is first auscultated is noted. The tracheal tube size is generally appropriate if this initial leak occurs at between 10 and 35 cmH_2O. If the initial leak is auscultated at a pressure of 0 to 10 cmH_2O, the indwelling tube should be replaced with the next larger size (e.g., a no. 4.0 tube is replaced with a no. 4.5 tube). If no leak is auscultated at an inflating pressure of 35 cmH_2O, a smaller tube should be inserted if the patient's clinical status permits. Tracheal tubes may be secured with or without the use of suture material. The use of benzoin and waterproof tape is recommended.

Pharmacologic Therapy

Therapy to control intracranial pressure (ICP) during laryngoscopy and tracheal intubation in the pediatric patient is similar to that applicable to adult patients. When bag-and-mask ventilation is begun, hyperventilation should be instituted and 100 percent oxygen administered. Pharmacologic therapy is often essential in order to provide the best possible conditions for tracheal intubation and to prevent or minimize elevation of ICP during laryngoscopy and tracheal intubation. Agents which are recommended include barbiturates, narcotics, muscle relaxants, and local anesthetics.

Barbiturates produce sedation and/or hypnosis, a decrease in cerebral oxygen consumption, and a diminution in cerebral blood flow. Barbiturates also may cause hypotension, a decrease in cardiac output, and inadequate cerebral perfusion. These circulatory effects are caused by increased venous capacitance, myocardial depression, and a decrease in systemic arteriolar tone. These effects may be especially pronounced in patients with diminished intravascular volumes and/or myocardial dysfunction. Thiopental is the barbiturate most commonly used prior to tracheal intubation. The dose in pediatric patients is 4 to 7 mg/kg IV. This dose should be reduced in patients with diminished intravascular volumes and/or myocardial dysfunction. Thiopental should not be given to patients with low cardiac output, as further depression of myocardial function can be anticipated. The circulatory and neurologic effects of this dose of thiopental generally dissipate after 10 to 20 min.

Narcotics cause a diminution in sympathetic neural response to such stimuli as laryngoscopy, tracheal intubation, and pharyngeal or tracheal suctioning. Narcotics, when administered in appropriate doses, may therefore prevent or decrease the tachycardia and hypertension which often results from these procedures. Many narcotics, including morphine and meperidine, may cause histamine-mediated vascular dilatation and consequent increase in cerebral blood flow.[4] These drugs, therefore, should be avoided if possible. Fentanyl does not produce histamine release and causes minimal circulatory depression in most patients. All narcotics, however, may cause decreased cardiac output and hypotension in patients with diminished intravascular volumes and/or severe myocardial dysfunction and should be used in reduced doses or avoided in this setting. The administration of fentanyl in a dose of 8 to 10 μg/kg IV, in combination with thiopental, usually results in minimal sympathetic neural response to laryngoscopy and tracheal intubation.[5] This dose rarely produces chest wall rigidity, which more commonly results from higher doses. Pupillary constriction, slowing of the heart rate, and decreased response to voice and other stimuli may persist for 2 to 3 h following this dose of fentanyl.

Muscle relaxants facilitate tracheal intubation by causing increased mandibular mobility and vocal cord paralysis. These drugs also facilitate efficient mechanical ventilation and control of intracranial pressure by reducing muscular tone of the chest wall and diaphragm. This reduces impedance to gas flow and prevents coughing and its associated increase in cerebral blood flow. Agents commonly used in pediatric and adult patients include succinylcholine, vecuronium, pancuronium, and atracurium. Succinylcholine has a rapid onset, producing profound neuromuscular blockade within 60 s following a dose of 1 to 1.5

mg/kg IV. Its offset is also usually rapid due to metabolism by pseudocholinesterase, with dissipation of paralysis generally within 5 to 7 min following administration. Succinylcholine produces muscle relaxation by causing disorganized muscle depolarization. Resultant muscle activity may result in hyperkalemia and release of myoglobin in some patients. This may occur in patients following burn or crush injuries, denervation (upper motor neuron) injuries, or renal failure. Rarely, succinylcholine may trigger malignant hyperthermia. In patients with pseudocholinesterase deficiency, muscle relaxation may persist for several hours. Alteration of heart rate may also occur, including tachycardia or bradycardia. Because of these adverse effects, the use of succinylcholine should be limited. The use of succinylcholine is most appropriate when rapid onset *and offset* of neuromuscular blockade are imperative.

Vecuronium is a nondepolarizing muscle relaxant with a duration of action intermediate between that of succinylcholine and pancuronium. While the usual "intubating" dose is 0.1 mg/kg IV, onset is hastened by the administration of doses 2 to 4 times this amount. The onset of profound muscle relaxation after the administration of 0.3 to 0.4 mg/kg of vecuronium IV is approximately 90 s, and in most cases tracheal intubation can be facilitated after approximately 60 s.[6] The duration of paralysis after a dose of 0.1 mg/kg IV is approximately 40 to 45 min, and increases to approximately 115 min after 0.4 mg/kg IV is administered.[6] Duration of action is prolonged in patients with impaired biliary excretion and severe renal insufficiency. Vecuronium is not associated with alteration of heart rate or blood pressure, or with the other adverse effects associated with succinylcholine.

Pancuronium is a longer-acting muscle relaxant commonly used in the management of neurosurgical patients both in the operating room and the ICU. Because of its vagolytic effect, pancuronium frequently causes undesired tachycardia and may cause hypertension. As with vecuronium, the usual intubating dose of pancuronium is 0.1 mg/kg IV. Newer, long-acting, nondepolarizing muscle relaxants not yet widely used in pediatric patients include doxacurium and pipecuronium. Because these agents do not produce the tachycardia associated with pancuronium, they may become more commonly utilized in the future.

Atracurium is another intermediate-acting, nondepolarizing muscle relaxant, with onset and duration of action similar to vecuronium. An advantage of atracurium is its metabolism by Hofmann degradation and, to a lesser extent, by ester hydrolysis, both of which are minimally affected by hepatic and/or renal dysfunction. Atracurium may, however, produce histamine-mediated hypotension and increased cerebral blood flow when given in the usual intubating doses, so it has limited use in neurosurgical patients.

Sympathetic neural stimulation produced by laryngoscopy and tracheal intubation may be modulated by the use of local anesthetics. Lidocaine may be delivered via aerosol as a 4% solution in order to topically anesthetize the tongue, pharynx, vocal cords, and trachea. Intravenous lidocaine administered 60 to 90 s prior to laryngoscopy diminishes untoward sympathetic response. The dose is 1 to 1.5 mg/kg IV.[7] This dose is not likely to produce myocardial depression except in the presence of preexisting, severe myocardial dysfunction.

Mechanical Ventilation

The goal of mechanical ventilation in the neurosurgical pediatric patient is to assure optimal exchange of oxygen and carbon dioxide across the alveolar capillary membrane while causing minimal adverse effects on cerebral perfusion. Mechanical ventilation of the adult patient has been described in Chap. 1. Considerations pertaining to infants and children will be briefly described below.

Several important developmental aspects of respiratory mechanics impact upon the practice of mechanical ventilation of the pediatric patient. The normal respiratory rate of the newborn is 20 to 60 breaths per minute, as opposed to 12 to 16 in the adult. Inspiratory time in the infant is normally 0.4 to 0.5 s,[8] compared to about 1.25 s in the adult. Tidal volume, on the other hand, remains relatively constant throughout childhood development at approximately 6 to 8 mL/kg.[9,10] Maximum inspiratory flow in the infant is about 20 L/min,[11] compared with 300 to 600 L/min in the adult. The static and dynamic differences in the developing respiratory system dictate the technical requirements of respiratory support in infants and children.

In the neonate and infant, ventilators which are pressure-limited and/or time-limited are most commonly employed. These ventilators offer the advantages of avoiding excessive inflating pressures and, presumably, decreased risk of barotrauma. However, a decrease in the compliance (or conductance) of the patient's respiratory system (or ventilator circuit) will cause a reduction in delivered tidal volume. An increase in either parameter, conversely, will result in an increased tidal volume. Examples of these types of ventilators include the Babybird, Bear Cub, Sechrist, and Infant Star ventilators.

Volume-limited ventilators, on the other hand, deliver a relatively constant volume of gas despite changes in the patient's chest compliance. The presence of high inflating pressures signal decreased compliance or conductance of the breathing circuit (e.g., occluded tracheal tube) or the patient (e.g., offset of neuromuscular blockade, bronchospasm). Disadvantages of these ventilators include the potential generation of very high inflating pressures and the possibly increased risk of barotrauma. With proper monitoring of inspiratory pressure, including the use of alarms, however, changes in the patient's pulmonary mechanics can be observed and the risk of excessive barotrauma minimized. Because of technical difficulties in accurately delivering very small tidal volumes (e.g., under 100 mL), volume-limited ventilators are primarily used in patients weighing over 10 kg. In addition, gas leaks around uncuffed tracheal tubes represent an important source of "volume loss." The magnitude of such gas leaks commonly varies with the patient's head position. As a result, there may be a variable discrepancy between inspiratory and exhalatory tidal volumes related to head position. It is important, then, to monitor both inspired and exhaled tidal volumes closely in pediatric patients with indwelling uncuffed tracheal tubes in order to facilitate appropriate alveolar ventilation. The Siemans 900C is an example of a volume-limited ventilator. The Puritan-Bennett 7200 and Bear 2 ventilators may be used in either a volume- or pressure-limited mode.

There are many other variations in features offered by different types of pediatric mechanical ventilators, including mechanisms for power drive, modes of initiating inspiration, and patterns of inspiratory flow. Of primary importance is that the practitioners be familiar with the various types of mechanical ventilators available at their institutions, including associated features, benefits, and hazards. There is no substitution for bedside observation of the patient. When mechanical ventilation is utilized, for example, the physician should monitor thoracic excursion and ventilatory pattern to ensure that the desired parameters are achieved. The patient should be continuously observed for signs of respiratory distress, indicating the need for ruling out occlusion of the tracheal tube, ventilator malfunction, or a change in chest compliance. Vigilance is essential in order to obviate secondary CNS injury due to mishap associated with mechanical ventilation. Elevation of mean airway pressure, for example, due to inadvertent positive end-expiratory pressure (PEEP) or high inflating pressures, can cause untoward elevation of intracranial pressure. Monitors such as ventilator alarms, pulse oximetry, and capnography should be maintained at all times.

THE CIRCULATORY SYSTEM

An understanding of basic cardiovascular dynamics in the developing child is essential for the care of the neurosurgical pediatric patient. The fundamentals of circulatory physiology in the neonate, infant, and child will be reviewed. In addition, basic considerations of the physical examination and monitoring of the circulatory system will be discussed. Finally, therapies for low cardiac output and hypertension, both of which may exacerbate brain injury, will be presented.

During the transition from normal fetal to neonatal life, there are many changes in the circulation. Immediately after birth, there is a large decrease in pulmonary vascular resistance and an increase in pulmonary blood flow concomitant with oxygenation and inflation of the lungs. As the placental circulation is removed from the circulation, the right and left ventricles, having operated in parallel during fetal life, begin to function in series. Systemic vascular resistance increases, and there is functional closure of the foramen ovale followed by anatomic closure of the ductus arteriosus. Within a few days after birth, the normal infant circulation is similar to the adult circulation. The pulmonary vascular resistance, having dropped dramatically shortly after birth, remains somewhat higher than in the adult and continues to decrease over the first few months of life. The systemic arterial blood pressure is lower in the infant and increases to adult values by the time of adolescence. In the infant, stroke volume is relatively limited, so increased cardiac output is largely mediated by increased heart rate. The stroke volume and cardiac output increase with age, while the heart rate decreases with age. Other differences between the developing pediatric heart and that of the adult include oxygen consumption, response to hypoxemia, and autonomic innervation.

Following birth, oxygen consumption in the term neonate rises from approximately 4.5 mL O_2/kg body weight per min to 8 mL O_2/kg body weight per min at the age of 1 month.[1] Oxygen consumption increases further with exposure to a cold environment and as body temperature deviates either above or below normal. The infant has a diminished ability to maintain neutral body temperature in the presence of variations in environmental temperature. This may precipitate systemic lactic acidemia as oxygen consumption exceeds the ability of the heart to generate sufficient cardiac output to meet such demands. It is therefore of critical importance that infants be maintained in a thermoneutral environment at all times, with appropriate use of warming devices such as radiant heating lamps.

Acute hypoxia, like hypo- or hyperthermia, is a potent stimulus for a reactive increase in cardiac output (although, paradoxically, hypoxia may cause bradycardia in the neonate). This increase in cardiac output is mediated in part by increased sympathetic efferent stimulation.[12] The developing heart is better able to tolerate acute severe hypoxia than the adult heart. This is, at least in part, related to the increased capacity of the immature myocardium to maintain anaerobic metabolism due to improved glycolytic activity.[13] The infant's myocardium allows it to survive more prolonged exposure to acute severe hypoxia than the adult. Unfortunately, the infant brain does not appear to be similarly protected against hypoxic-ischemic injury. Therefore, among infants there is a predisposition toward brain-injured survival following severe hypoxia as compared with adults.

Autonomic control of the heart and circulation is less well developed in the infant than the adult. The infant appears to have a relative predominance of parasympathetic neural tone, with a diminution of generalized sympathetic innervation. The infant may, for example, exhibit an exaggerated vagotonic response to hypoxemia, laryngoscopy, or gastroesophageal reflux, leading to bradycardia. Conversely, the infant may demonstrate increased sensitivity to exogenous catechols. For example, norepinephrine dose-response curves in fetal, newborn, and adult lambs show that fetal heart muscle is 3 times more sensitive to norepinephrine than the adult myocardium.[14] Physicians caring for critically ill pediatric patients should be aware that, because of developmental differences, pharmacologic manipulation of the circulation may differ from that of the adult patient.

As with adult patients, recognition of impending or existing circulatory failure in children is largely dependent on the physical examination. Dyspnea, tachycardia, cardiomegaly, and hepatomegaly are the hallmarks of congestive heart failure in infants and children. Because of the infant's relatively soft, incompletely calcified thoracic cage, dyspnea is often accompanied by suprasternal, intercostal, and subcostal retractions. Tachycardia may be seen relatively early in the course of cardiac failure in the infant, because cardiac output is more dependent on heart rate than increased stroke volume. Hepatomegaly may also appear early because of the increased distensibility of the liver. Distension of neck veins, however, is relatively difficult to appreciate in infants and young children. Chest radiography may be useful in differentiating cardiac from pulmonary disease and to aid in assessment of cardiomegaly. The presence of thymic tissue, especially during the first 3 years of life, may give the false impression of cardiomegaly. The ratio of the true transverse cardiac to transverse thoracic diameter, or cardiothoracic index, should be less than 0.65 during the first year of life, less than 0.60 during the second year of life, and less than about 0.50 after the age of 6 years.[15] Interpretation of other diagnostic studies in pediatric patients also demands familiarity with age- and size-related differences between these and adult patients. Correct noninvasive measurement of blood pressure requires appropriate selection of cuff size, as too small a cuff may overestimate the pressure. During the first months to years of life, significant electrocardiographic changes occur with which the interpreter must be familiar. Descriptions of techniques for vascular access to facilitate placement of central venous, pulmonary artery, and systemic arterial catheters is beyond the scope of this chapter and are described elsewhere.[16]

Therapies to ameliorate low cardiac output and hypertension in pediatric patients are, in principle, similar to those utilized in adults. Because of the above-mentioned differences in autonomic regulation of the pediatric circulation, certain differences in pharmacologic strategies may obtain. Inotropic drugs should be very carefully titrated in infants, as infants may demonstrate pronounced sensitivity to these agents for reasons described above. Primary hypertension is uncommon in infancy and early childhood. In infants with secondary hypertension as a manifestation of brain injury, the primary cause of blood pressure elevation, such as elevated intracranial pressure, should be aggressively treated before antihypertensive agents are invoked. Beta blockers should be used with extreme caution in infants. These agents may cause a precipitous fall in cardiac output owing to its relative dependency upon heart rate in the first year of life.

THE NERVOUS SYSTEM

The child's nervous system is poorly developed at birth. An understanding of the neurologic examination, and postnatal development of the skull, cervical spine, and brain is helpful in treating the pediatric neurosurgical patient.

The Pediatric Neurologic Examination

The normal child's neurologic examination changes over time as a reflection of the maturation of the child's brain. The neurologic examination is different for the newborn, the infant, the toddler, and the older child. Detailed descriptions of the normal child's neurologic examination are readily available.[38, 39]

Practitioners may be challenged initially when performing a neurologic examination on a child. They will be aided by patience and knowledge of normal developmental milestones as listed in Table 19-2.

Much of the younger child's neurologic examination may be accomplished by simple observation with attention to the child's general appearance, level of alertness, and spontaneous motor activity. This may be followed by noting the child's response to the stimuli of light, sound, and gentle touch. An examination of the tone is performed when the child is relaxed. Assessment of tone and muscle strength is obtained with attention to symmetry in the exam. Cranial nerves are myelinated at birth and can be examined at all ages. A formal sensory exam requires cooperation and is difficult in the child less than 5 years of age.

Certain cranial nerve findings that are abnormal in adults may be normal in children. Young infants may have an asymmetric blink. Dysconjugate gaze occurs occasionally in infancy. Strabismus is not uncommon in 3- to 6-year-old children. Infants may have irregular movements of the tongue both on protrusion and at rest. The infant's optic disc margins are often indistinct and slightly elevated.[40]

Infants have normal reflexes that disappear with age. The newborn Moro or startle reflex disappears after 6 months. Bilateral extensor plantar reflex

Table 19-2 Motor Developmental Milestones

1 week	Extends head in prone position
3–4 months	Has head control
5–6 months	Rolls prone to supine
6–7 months	Rolls supine to prone
7–8 months	Sits alone and transfers objects hand to hand
9–11 months	Stands holding on
11–12 months	Walks with assistance
13–15 months	Walks by self
18 months	Climbs stairs with assistance
24 months	Runs

Source: Adapted from Swaiman[39] and Venes et al.[40]

can be normal up to 1 year of age. The normal infant's deep tendon reflexes may be absent. More commonly, the normal infant's deep tendon reflexes are brisk and ankle clonus can be elicited.

Peripheral nerves are not myelinated at birth, so evaluation of both gross and fine motor activity is dependent on the child's age. The motor developmental milestones provide a reference against which to evaluate an individual infant or child. Regardless of developmental stage, the motor examination should be symmetric. Hand preference is rare in the first 18 months[40] and may suggest an abnormality when present. Raimondi and Hirschauer describe an unusual syndrome of asymmetry in head-injured patients under 3 years consisting of unilateral Babinski reflex, hemiparesis, and ocular deviation that was benign in 97 percent of the cases but may represent a state of subclinical seizures.[19]

When evaluating muscle tone, it is important to remember that the infant usually has dominance of flexor muscles and that extremities may be normally flexed even during sleep. Hypotonia or flaccidity is abnormal at all ages.

The newborn may have a massive injury to the cerebrum yet preserve limb movement. If there is flaccidity or lack of movement of one or more limbs, the lesion involves the spinal cord or peripheral nerve rather than the cerebrum.

Examination of the head with attention to head trauma may reveal abnormalities peculiar to infants. The anterior fontanel is usually flat when the infant is upright and is normally pulsatile with increasing size during crying. A tense fontanel suggests increased ICP. While a unilateral retinal hemorrhage may have no significance, *bilateral retinal hemorrhages* suggest a dramatic rapid increase in ICP and are often associated with a subdural hemorrhage.[19] Combined subdural and retinal hemorrhages are associated with nonaccidental trauma that occurs with a shaking injury.

The child's head circumference should be measured to assess enlargement from increasing ICP. Otherwise, assessment of increased ICP is similar in children and adults. Vomiting as a sign of increased pressure is seen more commonly in children than in adults. Papilledema is not an acute sign of increased ICP in children and indicates a longer period of increased pressure than in adults.

The pediatric neurosurgical patient may have an abnormal level of consciousness for a variety of reasons including increased ICP, metabolic abnormalities, and the presence of medications. The physicians and nurses must, in a consistent and objective manner, document this exam at hourly intervals. Rather than relying on subjective descriptions such as "lethargic" or "stuporous," the adult Glasgow coma scale (GCS) is often used for this purpose (see Table 12-1). However, it is difficult to use the GCS even on a completely normal preverbal child who, at best, would only score 2 on the verbal score (for *nonspecific sounds*) and 5 on the motor score (for *localizes pain*) for a total of 11 out of 15.

There is no consensus on how to score the younger pediatric patient. Some authors prefer to adapt the GCS by making a modified children's scale, giving, for example, a verbal score of 5 if the infant coos or babbles (Table 19-3). Another alternative is to use the children's coma scale (Table 19-4). This scale is for infants, has a range of scores from 3 to 11, and is designed to evaluate subcortical and brainstem function. The proponents of

Table 19-3 Modified Coma Scale for Infants*

Response	Score
Eye opening	
Spontaneous	4
To speech	3
To pain	2
None	1
Verbal	
Coos, babbles	5
Irritable cries	4
Cries to pain	3
Moans to pain	2
None	1
Motor	
Normal spontaneous movements	6
Withdraws to touch	5
Withdraws to pain	4
Abnormal flexion	3
Abnormal extension	2
None	1

*Range of score is from 3 to 15. Although this score is similar to the adult Glasgow coma scale, it has not been validated as a predictor of outcome after closed head injury in infants. *Source:* James and Trauner.[56]

Table 19-4 Children's Coma Scale*

Response	Score
Ocular	
Pursuit	4
Extraocular muscles (EOM) intact and reactive pupils	3
Fixed pupils or EOM impaired	2
Fixed pupils and EOM paralyzed	1
Verbal	
Cries	3
Spontaneous respirations	2
Apneic	1
Motor	
Flexes and extends	4
Withdraws from painful stimuli	3
Hypertonic	2
Flaccid	1

*Range of scores is from 3 to 11. *Source:* Raimondi and Hirschauer.[18]

this scoring system feel that it offers prognostic outcome value for the head-injured patient under 36 months old.[19]

Regardless of what system is used, physicians and nurses need to assess pupillary function, verbal response, and motor response in a frequent, consistent manner. Any deterioration in the exam demands attention and an explanation.

The Skull

A diagram of the newborn skull is seen in Fig. 19-2. The frontal, parietal, squamous-temporal, and squamous-occipital bones grow radially until the sites of the sutures are reached. The anterior fontanel closes at about 1 year of age. A review showed that the anterior fontanel closed between 7 and 19

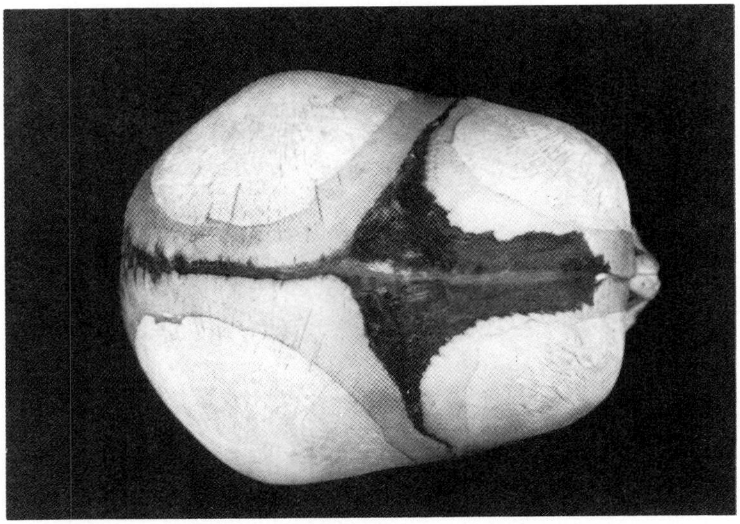

Figure 19-2 Typical suture alignment of the newborn skull with large anterior fontanel. (*Source:* Hollinger and Goodrich.[20])

months of age in 90 percent of the cases studied.[17] By this time the cranial sutures are closed as well.

The infant skull with an open fontanel, soft calvaria, and open, moveable sutures is different from the adult's skull. One advantage to the open fontanel is that it allows a visual and tactile assessment of the infant's intracranial pressure. Also the infant's skull can continue to expand somewhat and partially compensate for the slowly developing increases in pressure that accompany hydrocephalus, hematomas, or other intracranial mass lesions.

However, the open fontanel does not fully protect the child against elevated intracranial pressure (ICP). It may add some small extra compensatory volume, but the presence of split sutures and a bulging fontanel denotes elevated ICP and suggests that compensatory mechanisms have become exhausted.[18]

Because the skull is elastic, it can absorb some of the energy associated with trauma instead of transmitting the energy to the brain. However, rather than protecting the brain, the soft skull may also allow more brain compression and distortion than in the adult in the setting of head trauma. The compliant skull may allow more to-and-fro motion of the brain with a shaking injury that can lead to a tearing of the bridging veins between the cortex and the venous sinuses, leading to the formation of subdural hematomas. Additionally, the floor of the anterior and middle fossa is smooth with few convolutional markings providing less resistance to brain movement. The infantile skull may therefore predispose a child to a higher possibility of subdural hematoma.[19]

The infant's skull may be fractured in a different manner than the adult's skull. A depressed skull fracture may occur without an associated scalp laceration.[20] Skull fractures in infants tend to have a larger separation than in the adult or occur with diastasis of the sutures.[21A] Occasionally, an infant with a skull fracture and underlying laceration of the dura may develop a "delayed growing skull fracture" due to the entrapment of an arachnoid cyst.[21B]

The Cervical Spine

There are important anatomic and biomechanic differences between the adult and pediatric spine. These differences result in a different pattern of injury and different radiologic findings.

The newborn spine is elastic, and the laxity of ligaments allows longitudinal distraction of up to 2 in.[22] However, since the newborn spinal cord can only stretch a quarter of an inch, injuries to the spinal cord can occur during traction on the head at the time of delivery.

Developmental differences in children under 8 years of age predispose them to upper cervical injuries. More horizontal orientation of the facet joints of the upper cervical vertebrae, and anterior wedging of the vertebral bodies, allow increased forward movement of the upper cervical spine with flexion. The child with a large, heavy head and less well-developed neck musculature can develop increased angular momentum, with flexion and extension resulting in cervical spine injury.

Radiographic diagnosis of cervical spine injuries in children is complicated by a number of pediatric normal variants. The distance between the anterior arch of C1 and the dens can be up to 5 mm in children, whereas in adults it is never more than 3 mm. Pseudosubluxation of C2 on C3 occurs in up to 40 percent of children, with more than 50 percent of these children having a 3-mm or greater degree of shift.[23] Pseudosubluxation of C3 on C4 is a less common normal variant, occurring 15 percent of the time. Epiphyseal plates in the spine close between 2 and 10 years and can resemble fractures. Unless the physician is aware of these normal variants, an incorrect diagnosis can easily be made.

Of more concern are the false-negative cervical spine films. Although the "syndrome of spinal cord injury without radiologic abnormality" (SCIWORA) is reported in adults, it is much more common in children.[24] It is thought that either transient dislocation of the spine occurs followed by spontaneous reduction or that a flexion-extension injury results in a vascular insult to the cord. In a series of pediatric cervical spine injuries reported by Pang and Wilberger,[24] two-thirds of the children had normal cervical spine films. Half of the patients in this series presented with delayed symptoms up to 96 h after injury. Some of the injuries were severe, including cases of complete quadriplegia due to spinal cord transection.

Finally, while only 1 to 3 percent of all cervical

spine injuries occur in children, the pattern of injury is different in young children. When cervical spine injuries do occur, they are more likely to be at the occipitocervical junction or upper cervical segments. They may vary from rotary subluxation of the atlas on the axis after mild trauma to more severe and catastrophic injury to C1 and C2.[25]

The Brain

The newborn's brain is poorly developed and functions mainly at a subcortical level. Brainstem reflexes are present, but the cortical functions of fine motor movement and cognitive functions are less well-developed. The autonomic nervous system exists in an immature form and is more responsive to parasympathetic stimuli that can cause bradycardia than to sympathetic stimuli.

The newborn has a relatively large head since the brain has already reached 25 percent of the weight of the adult brain. Intrauterine growth resulted in rapid cell division with most neuronal cell division complete by 20 weeks' gestation.[17] Rapid growth of the brain continues postnatally, with a doubling in size in the first 6 months of age. The brain reaches 75 percent of adult size by 2 years of age, as shown in Fig. 19-3. This postnatal growth consists of proliferation of glial cells, dendritic arborization, and myelination (Fig. 19-4). The postnatal growth of the brain results in increases in its volume, weight, and complexity.

Because of its rapid growth and differentiation, the brain is particularly vulnerable to injury during the first few months of life. While neurons do not regenerate, they do respond to injury by forming new synaptic connections. Additional connections may either decrease the amount of permanent neurologic damage or may result in increasing disability and spasticity. Myelination of motor roots, sensory roots, and pyramidal tracts is complete by about 2 years of age.[17]

The type and pattern of traumatic injuries to the

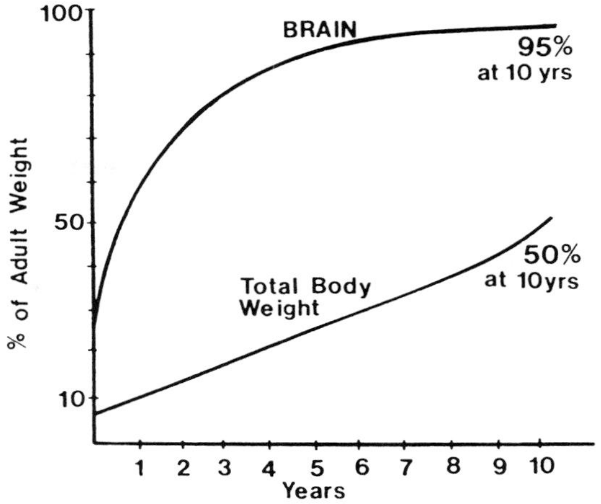

Figure 19-3 There is early accelerated growth of the brain compared to that of the whole body. (*Source:* Peacock.[17])

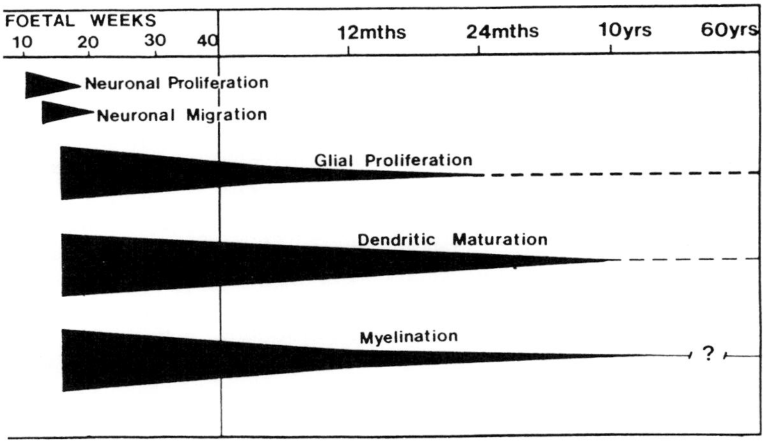

Figure 19-4 Significant brain development occurs postnatally. (*Source:* Peacock.[17])

brain reflects the structural development of the brain and skull at different ages.

Epidural hematomas provide one example of the relationship between brain development and pattern of injury. Epidural hematomas are uncommon in children, especially in those under 2 years of age. The close and strong attachment between the skull and dura may make bleeding into the epidural space less likely.[26]

While epidural hematomas are uncommon, subdural hematomas are more common following severe head injury in infancy. Mechanical factors within the skull, the meninges, and the brain predispose the infant to this injury. The infant's brain has more mobility within the skull, resulting in stretching and tearing of cortical veins. The absence of arachnoidal adhesions to the dura may also result in venous bleeding.[20] With slow venous bleeding and no documented history of trauma, these infants may present many hours after their injury with seizures, decreased level of consciousness, and elevated ICP.

Some common adult injuries are uncommon in infancy. The contrecoup lesion seen in nearly 90 percent of fatal adult brain injuries is extremely rare in infancy.[27] Other injuries are more common in infants than in older children and adults. Brain lacerations occur in young infants more commonly than in older children. This might be explained by the thin and mobile skull, which may be fractured or depressed into the brain, or by the lack of myelination resulting in a gelatinous consistency of the brain that increases its risk of shearing. Injuries to the basal ganglia after blunt trauma are more common in infants and may be the only injury present. This may be explained as a vascular injury with stretching of the lenticular perforating vessels of the middle cerebral artery leading to infarction.[28]

Not only do children with trauma have a different pattern of injury than do adults, but they have a different response to traumatic brain injury. The usual adult findings of decreased cerebral blood flow and decreased cerebral metabolism are seen in children with severe subarachnoid hemorrhage or diffuse axonal injury. An alternative response consisting of increases in cerebral blood flow and possibly increases in metabolism is also seen in children but is relatively uncommon in adults. This second pediatric response has been described by Bruce and coworkers as diffuse cerebral swelling.[29] Part of the evidence for this is radiographic. In fatal pediatric closed head injury, the most common findings on computed tomography are absence of significant hemorrhage, a diffusely swollen brain, small ventricles, and loss of the perimesencephalic cisterns and subarachnoid space.[26,30]

It is possible that increases in cerebral blood flow and resultant increases in cerebral blood volume account for this diffuse brain swelling.[30] Bruce and associates suggest that brain swelling caused by increased cerebral blood flow is more likely than cerebral edema caused by increased brain water because the swelling occurs rapidly and because radiographically the computed tomography scan resembles hyperemia more than edema.[29] Possible explanations for this diffuse brain swelling include (1) increased cerebral blood flow caused by decreased vascular resistance with loss of autoregulation and (2) increased brain metabolism resulting in increased cerebral blood flow. More recently it has been argued that diffuse traumatic edema, rather than cerebral congestion, is the cause of the cerebral swelling.[31]

Whatever the explanation, it appears that the head-injured child with diffuse brain swelling may have a different injury than the adult.

Cerebral Blood Flow and Cerebral Hemodynamics

There are differences in cerebral blood flow between children and adults. Control of cerebral blood flow may also be different in the child, but this is difficult to document.

The distribution of the arterial cerebral vessels is complete at birth, and the cerebral venous vessels are completely developed soon after birth.

The infant's cerebral blood flow of 90 to 100 mL/min per 100 g of brain weight is nearly twice the adult's rate of 53 mL/min per 100 g of brain weight. In contrast, the newborn's cerebral blood flow is only 40 mL/min per 100 g of brain.[32–34] Cerebral function is compromised at a cerebral blood flow of 15 to 20 mL/min per 100 g. Infarction in the infant's brain does not occur until cerebral blood flow is less than 10 mL/min per 100 g, a lower level than in the adult.[20]

Control of Cerebral Blood Flow It is also likely that the control of cerebral blood flow is different in the child. The response of cerebral blood flow to Pa_{CO_2} may be different in children. While hyperventilation below a Pa_{CO_2} of 20 mmHg does not decrease cerebral blood flow in adults, it can be effective in children. Studies have shown decreasing cerebral blood flow in head-injured children continued until Pa_{CO_2} was 15 mmHg.[35] In newborn animal models, cerebral blood flow continued to decrease until the Pa_{CO_2} was 12 to 15 mmHg.[33] Some have used jugular venous catheterization to measure arterial-jugular oxygen differences ($AJDO_2$) as a means of comparing cerebral blood flow to cerebral metabolism. A rise in $AJDO_2$ suggests a relative uncoupling of blood flow to metabolic needs and the potential onset of cerebral ischemia. Monitoring of $AJDO_2$ and maintenance of jugular venous oxygen tension above 20 mmHg is recommended for prolonged hyperventilation below a Pa_{CO_2} of 20 mmHg.[35]

The relationship between P_{O_2} and cerebral blood flow is also different in the infant. The neonate is adapted to a lower intrauterine oxygen tension, and the newborn's hemoglobin F has an increased affinity for oxygen. Cerebral blood flow in the older child increases in response to hypoxia with a P_{O_2} of under 50 mmHg, but this doesn't occur in infants until the P_{O_2} is under 25 mmHg.[20]

Autoregulation of cerebral blood flow is also different in infants in that autoregulation occurs at much lower systemic arterial blood pressures. The normal mean arterial blood pressure of the newborn of 40 mmHg is much less than the normal adult cerebral perfusion pressure. Cerebral blood flow is decreased and autoregulation may be lost in the sick infant with respiratory distress syndrome or asphyxia. In these cases cerebral blood flow is pressure-dependent, resulting in ischemia or hemorrhage.[20]

Control of Intracranial Pressure The control of ICP is perhaps the principal task in the neurosurgical care of infants.[36] There are a wide variety of pediatric neurosurgical conditions which may be accompanied by increased ICP, including congenital lesions, tumors, infections, and head trauma.

While the basic mechanisms that result in increased ICP in the adult apply in the child, the previously noted differences in control of cerebral blood flow and differences in control of systemic arterial blood pressure mean that caution must be used when applying adult management algorithms to the child.

The normal values for ICP are different in children. The neonate has an ICP of 2 mmHg or less, the 1-year-old infant has an ICP of 2 to 6, and the older child has a ICP of 3 to 13.[36,37] Technical problems may make it very difficult to measure the ICP in infants.

There is also data suggesting that cerebral compliance may be different in infants than in older children and adults. The slope of the infant's pressure-volume curve is steeper, reflecting that while the addition of a 10-mL volume may be well tolerated in the adolescent, that same volume change may be lethal in an infant (Fig. 19-5).[36] However, once suture separation has occurred as a result of slowly increasing pressure, the infant brain can tolerate larger increases in intracranial volume than can the adult brain.

Control of elevated ICP in the child follows similar guidelines as in the adult and is fully reviewed in Chap. 3. General measures of head elevation, sedation, and avoidance of noxious stimuli are observed. Hyperventilation to a Pa_{O_2} of 20 to 30 mmHg may be sufficient. Extremes of hyperventilation, down to a Pa_{CO_2} of 12 to 15 mmHg may be effective in lowering ICP in the infant or young child, but there is a risk of ischemia unless $AJDO_2$ is monitored and jugular venous oxygen tension is kept over 20 mmHg.[35] High-dose barbiturate therapy and osmotherapy entail the same risks in the pediatric patient as in the adult patient. These risks can be minimized by a balanced approach including initial use of isovolemic dehydration, hyperventilation, and, lastly, judicious use of barbiturates.

Central Nervous System Monitoring

Computed tomography (CT) scans of the head are often obtained electively to provide prognostic information and are obtained emergently for diagnostic purposes when a deterioration of the neurologic exam occurs. In infants with an open fontanel, imaging by ultrasound (Fig. 19-6) provides the advantage of portability, although cer-

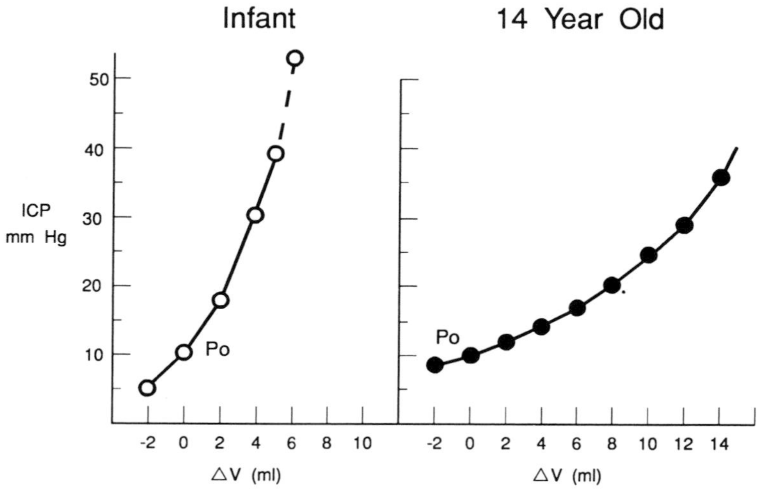

Figure 19-5 These two pressure-volume curves were generated in a normal infant and in a normal teenager by injecting and withdrawing cerebral spinal fluid. The infant's curve is steeper indicating less compliance, and the infant is less able to buffer additional volume compared with the teenager. (*Source:* Shapiro and Marmarou.[36])

tain areas of the brain are not accessible and the resolution of the scan is inferior to CT. Continuous EEG monitoring is useful in detecting seizures in children when the exam is obscured by neuromuscular blockade. Fourier transformation of the EEG signal by compressed spectral array processing (Fig. 19-7) provides a three-dimensional display of the EEG, preserving information about frequency, amplitude, and symmetry of the signal over an extended period of time.

Electrophysiologic monitoring is becoming more common in the pediatric patient to help assess outcome following head trauma or hypoxic-ischemic encephalopathy. Auditory evoked potentials (EPs) provide a means of assessing the brainstem function in a comatose child. The EP is

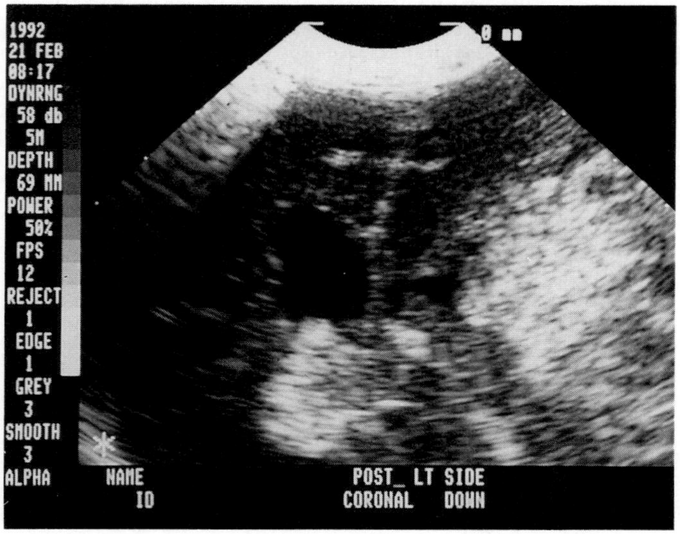

Figure 19-6 This coronal ultrasound of a neonate with a large intraparenchymal hematoma shows a midline shift from left to right with enlargement of the right lateral ventricle.

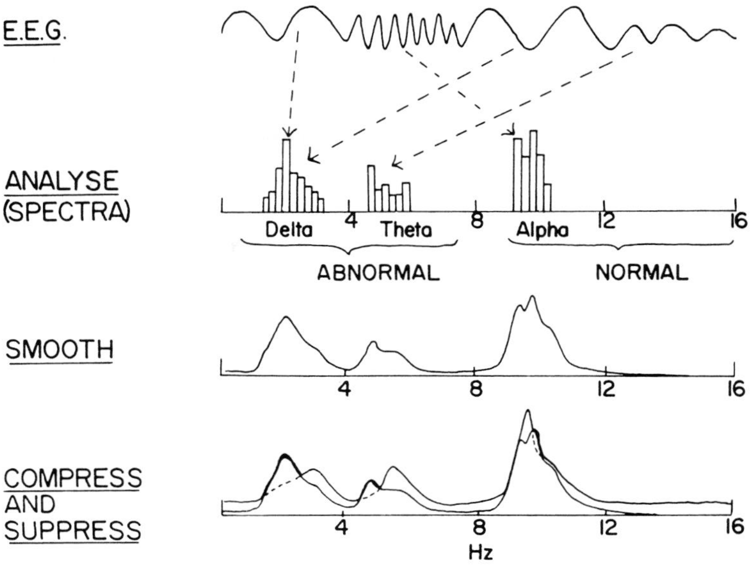

Figure 19-7 Fast Fourier transformation of conventional EEG data results in the spectra shown above. This data is smoothed and compressed. (*Source:* Bickford et al.[57])

virtually unaffected by medications, including high-dose barbiturate therapy, that otherwise result in an isoelectric EEG.[41] Lütschg and coworkers studied 43 comatose children after head trauma or asphyxia and found that a loss of auditory EP components was associated with a poor outcome.[42] Fisher and coworkers studied 89 children after cardiac arrest from a submersion accident and found that auditory EPs had a prognostic value for predicting outcome.[43]

FLUID AND ELECTROLYTE REQUIREMENTS

Fluid and electrolyte therapy in children can be challenging for a number of reasons. First, although the fluid requirements per kilogram of weight are higher in children than in adults, the total amount of fluid administered is small, necessitating that all fluid sources be totaled to avoid overhydration. Second, the body fluid compartments vary with age. Third, maintenance fluid and electrolyte requirements change with weight. Finally, infants have a limited ability to self-regulate intravascular volume because of diminished renal concentrating ability.

The relationship of fluid compartments with age is shown graphically in Fig. 19-8. Intravascular volume as a percentage of weight also decreases with age, as shown in Table 19-5.

Maintenance Fluid Requirements

The child's maintenance fluid requirement is approximately 1500 mL per square meter of surface area per day. However, rather than using a surface area formula, this requirement is usually expressed on the basis of weight. Note the relationship between fluid requirement and caloric requirements in Table 19-6.

As an example, for the 10-kg infant who requires 100 mL/kg per day of maintenance fluid, urinary losses will be 50 to 55 mL/kg, stool losses will be 0 to 5 mL/kg, skin losses will be 30 mL/kg, and pulmonary losses will be 15 mL/kg.

Table 19-5 Blood Volume Related to Age

Age	Intravascular volume, mL/kg
Premature	100
Newborn	90
3–24 mo	80
>24 mo	70

Source: From Hollinger.[20]

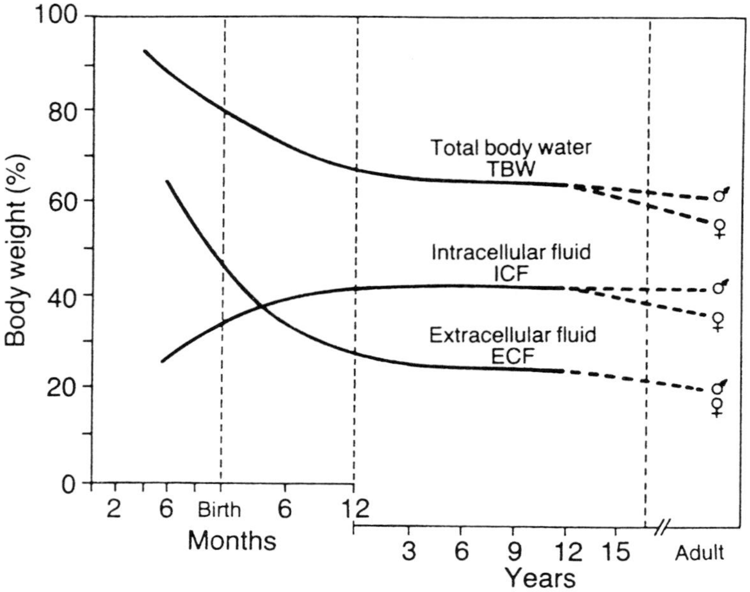

Figure 19-8 Distribution of body water as a percent of body weight approaches adult values by 1 year of age. (*Source:* Fris-Hansen, et al.[58] and Weinberg and Hickman.[59])

Assessment of hydration status is similar in children as in adults. Additional signs of dehydration in the infant include a sunken anterior fontanel, decrease or absence of tears when crying, and decreased skin turgor with tenting of the skin. With overhydration, hepatomegaly may be noted and eyelid edema is often present. A dehydrated infant should receive an initial bolus of 20 mL/kg of isotonic crystalloid such as lactated Ringer's solution and then be reevaluated.

Maintenance fluid requirements per kilogram weight are increased in all infants because of the increased heat loss from the higher ratio of skin surface area to body mass in infants compared to adults. Excessive losses from hyperthermia, diarrhea, nasogastric suction, or indwelling drains will rapidly lead to dehydration if these losses are not measured and replaced.

Table 19-6 Fluid and Caloric Requirements on Basis of Weight

Weight, kg	Fluid requirement	Caloric requirement
0–10	100 mL/kg	100 cal/kg
10–20	1000 mL plus 50 mL/kg for weight over 10 kg	1000 cal plus 50 cal/kg for weight over 10 kg
>20	1500 mL plus 20 mL/kg for weight over 20 kg	1500 cal plus 20 cal/kg for weight over 20 kg

While overhydration is undesirable for the pediatric neurosurgical patient, there is no advantage to dehydration with resultant hypovolemia. Normovolemia should be maintained at all times. If osmotherapy to control elevated ICP is desired, the goal should be a *euvolemic dehydration* with elevation of serum osmolality to 300 to 320 mOsm/L while maintaining normal intravascular volume. If diuresis from mannitol or furosemide results in hypovolemia, physiologic blood volume can be maintained by replacing urinary losses with packed cells, fresh frozen plasma, or other isotonic fluids such as lactated Ringer's solution or normal saline.[44]

Electrolyte Requirements

Maintenance fluid should contain 3 mEq of sodium per 100 mL water and 2 mEq of potassium per 100 mL water. Adjustments will be needed based on the patient's serum electrolyte values and the need to replace electrolytes lost in diarrhea or gastric secretions.

Regulation of serum calcium, phosphorous, and magnesium in children is similar to this regulation in adults as reviewed in Chap. 7. Serum phosphorous levels are maintained higher in infants (4.5 to 8.5 mg/dL) and in children (3.7 to 5.9 mg/dL), possibly because of increased growth hormone level and decreased gonadal hormones.[45] Hypocalcemia is not uncommon in stressed newborns and may be suspected in the neonate with jitters or seizures.

Hyponatremia

As is the case with adults, the pediatric patient may become hyponatremic from (1) receiving excessive free water, (2) by the mechanism of inappropriate secretion of antidiuretic hormone, or (3) by cerebral salt-wasting,[46] as described in previous chapters. Serum sodium needs to be measured frequently to detect and correct hyponatremia. Hyponatremic seizures may occur with a sodium below 125 mEq/L and are difficult to control without partial correction of the serum sodium. This may be achieved by the administration of a 3% saline infusion. Unappreciated hyponatremia may result in significant morbidity in the pediatric neurosurgical patient. A number of reports have described fatal cerebral edema caused by excessive hyponatremia in the pediatric patient recovering from head injury.[47,48] For that reason, it is reasonable to begin maintenance fluid in the head-injured patient as lactated Ringer's with 5% dextrose rather than using hypotonic quarter normal saline.

Renal Maturity

The kidneys continue to mature after birth. The newborn's glomerular filtration rate is only 2.5 mL/min, increases to 15 mL/min at 6 months of age, to 50 mL/min in the preschooler, and finally reaches the adult value of 130 mL/min.[49] The newborn has limited renal concentrating ability and is able to concentrate urine to only 700 mOsm/kg in comparison to the adult value of 1400 mOsm/kg.

NUTRITIONAL REQUIREMENTS

Nutritional requirements vary tremendously from the needs of the 3-kg newborn to the needs of the 60-kg adolescent. There are a number of differences between pediatric and adult requirements that will be discussed.

Table 19-7 outlines how protein and caloric requirements are related to age. Infants have the highest caloric requirement in calories per kilogram per day because of their rapid growth, increased activity, and larger heat losses resulting from a proportionately higher body surface area.

Earlier nutritional support is needed in infants than in adults because infants have decreased energy stores and have an increased basal metabolic rate (BMR). The BMR of infants is 40 to 50 kcal/kg per day, and the BMR of adults is 25 to 30 kcal/kg per day.[50] An estimated 50 percent of children in a pediatric ICU have protein-calorie malnutrition.[51] Excessive periods of catabolism will lead to breakdown of protein stores to provide substrate for gluconeogenesis. This will result in loss of muscle mass. Caloric requirements are increased in children and adults by the same factors, such as fever, trauma, increased respiratory rate, and sepsis.

Infants and neonates are considered to have the additional essential amino acid requirements of cysteine and tyrosine. Children do have a requirement for the four fat-soluble vitamins (A, D, E,

Table 19-7 Fluid, Caloric, and Protein Requirements by Age

	Requirements per day		
	Fluid	Calories	Protein
Infant (0–1 year, 0–10 kg)	100 mL/kg	100–110 per kg	2 g/kg
Child (1–5 year, 10–20 kg)	1000 mL + 50 mL/kg over 10 kg	80 per kg	1.5 g/kg
Child (5–10 year, 20–40 kg)	1500 mL + 20 mL/kg over 20 kg	55 per kg	1 g/kg
Adolescent (>10 years, >40 kg)	1900 mL + 20 mL/kg over 40 kg	2000–2500	1 g/kg

Source: Adapted from Snyderman.[55]

and K) and nine water-soluble vitamins. A special pediatric multivitamin preparation for children under 12 years is given by intravenous infusion.

A pediatric dietician may assist in the assessment of baseline nutritional status by anthropometry of height, weight, and head circumference as well as in calculating caloric and protein requirements.

Enteral Feedings

Enteral feedings are preferred when possible to preserve the integrity of the gut, to stimulate gastrointestinal hormone secretion, to decrease the risk of bacterial translocation, and to avoid the risks associated with central hyperalimentation. The risk of pulmonary aspiration can be decreased by placing a soft, pliable, weighted feeding tube that is advanced beyond the pylorus. Continuous administration of feedings further decreases the incidence of diarrhea. Gastric residual volumes of less than 5 mL/kg or less than 1 h of feeding are usually tolerated. A variety of standard pediatric formulas are available. If these are not tolerated, an elemental formula can be used. Feedings should be started slowly and advanced every 12 h until nutritional goals are met. Metoclopramide can be given to increase gastrointestinal motility if gastric residual volumes are excessive. However, poor tolerance to enteral feeds following head injury is common, necessitating parenteral nutrition.[52]

Parenteral Nutrition

Peripheral parenteral nutrition (PPN) may supplement enteral feedings. The maximum nutrient concentrations administered through a peripheral vein are 2% amino acids and 12.5% glucose. PPN alone can promote positive nitrogen balance but cannot provide adequate caloric needs for the stressed child without the concomitant administration of excessive amounts of fluid.

If adequate nutrition cannot be provided enterally or by peripheral vein, central parenteral hyperalimentation should be started within 5 to 7 days of hospitalization. With central parenteral nutrition, glucose, amino acids, and fats are increased gradually until nutritional goals are met. Glucose is increased daily by 2.5 percent increments in infants and 5 percent increments in children. Careful monitoring of glucose is needed to prevent hypergylcemia, since in experimental models, hyperglycemia increases cerebral ischemic injury.[52] Protein is begun at 1 g/kg per day and increased by 0.5 g/kg per day until protein goals are met. Fats, provided as 10 or 20% intralipids, are started at 1 g/kg per day given over 20 to 24 h. Fats are increased by 0.5 to 1.0 g/kg per day to a usual maximum of 2 to 3 g/kg per day as tolerated avoiding hyperlipemia. Fat calories are usually limited to 40 percent of total calories but can be increased to 60 percent of total calories if additional carbohydrate is not tolerated.

HEMATOLOGIC SYSTEM

There are several areas in which the child's hematologic system differs from that of the adult.

First, children have a larger intravascular volume per weight than do adults. A premature infant's intravascular volume is nearly 100 mL/kg. This decreases to 90 mL/kg in the newborn, 80 mL/kg in the 3- to 24-month-old, and 70 mL/kg in the older child.[20] While infants have a larger blood volume per kilogram weight, they have a much smaller absolute blood volume than an older child. This is relevant since a 60-mL hemorrhage in an 8-kg infant represents a loss of nearly 10 percent of the total blood volume. An infant may have sufficient scalp and/or intracranial hemorrhage to cause anemia, decreased cardiac output, and hypotension.[44]

Second, the "normal" laboratory values for the complete blood count vary with age. The average hemoglobin concentration is 13 mg/dL at birth, falls to 11 mg/dL at 3 months of age, and returns to 13 mg/dL at 6 months of age.[53] Infants have higher white blood cell counts than do adults. There is no difference in platelet count between infants and adults. However, clotting factors don't reach adult levels until 1 to 12 months of age resulting in a great variation in the infant's prothrombin time and partial thromboplastin time.[54]

Third, the newborn's hemoglobin is different. The newborn has 75 percent of the hemoglobin as hemoglobin F and only 25 percent as the adult hemoglobin A. Fetal hemoglobin decreases to 20 percent by 4 months and to less than 2 percent by

12 months of age. Hemoglobin F binds oxygen more tightly than does hemoglobin A, resulting in a left shift of the oxygen-hemoglobin dissociation curve in the newborn.[53]

Blood Transfusion Therapy

Transfusion of blood or blood products in children is based on the child's weight. A transfusion of 10 mL/kg of packed cells will increase the hematocrit by about 10 percent. The usual dose of platelets, 1 unit per 5 kg, should increase the platelet count by about 50,000. Since platelets are usually suspended in 50 to 60 mL plasma, this is a platelet transfusion of about 10 mL/kg. Finally, fresh frozen plasma is also given in a volume of 10 to 15 mL/kg for initial treatment of coagulopathy.

Hypocalcemia resulting in hypotension may accompany transfusions with citrate-containing blood products. This is most likely with transfusions of large volumes of fresh frozen plasma, which has the greatest amount of citrate per volume of any blood product. Hypocalcemia and, occasionally, hypotension have been seen in infants receiving 1 to 2.5 mL/kg per min of fresh frozen plasma. Infants are at higher risk both because of their smaller calcium reserves and because a larger portion of their blood volume may be replaced more rapidly. This may be treated with 10 mg/kg of 10% calcium chloride injected slowly via a central venous catheter or by 20 to 30 mg/kg of 10% calcium gluconate administered via a peripheral vein.

SUMMARY

Care of infants and children with neurosurgical diseases remains one of the greatest challenges in intensive care medicine. Anatomic and physiologic changes in these patients occur during maturation and impact profoundly upon their medical and surgical management. An understanding of such developmental changes in addition to an indepth knowledge of general neurologic intensive care is essential to the appropriate care of critically ill pediatric patients.

In this chapter, we have outlined fundamentals of pediatric anatomy and physiology which pertain to care of the neurosurgical pediatric patient. The principles described in this chapter should be integrated with essential information contained within the other chapters in this text. As a result, an improved understanding of the problems of infants and children with neurosurgical diseases may facilitate optimal care of these challenging patients.

ACKNOWLEDGMENTS

The authors thank Betisha Allen for assistance with this manuscript.

REFERENCES

1A. Pettigrew AH, Singer JS, Falade E, Friedman H: The pediatric intensive care network of northern and central California: A regional approach. DHHS Grant #MCJ-063336, Santa Cruz, 1986.

1B. Dawes GS: *Fetal and Neonatal Physiology*, Chicago, Yearbook Medical, 1973, p 191.

2. Bucher HU, Fanconi S, Fallenstein F, Duc G: Transcutaneous carbon dioxide tension in newborn infants: Reliability and safety of continuous 24-hour measurement at 42°C. *Pediatrics* 78:631, 1986.
3. Hess D: Capnometry and capnography: Technical aspects, physiologic aspects, and clinical applications. *Resp Care* 35:557, 1990.
4. Flacke JW, Flacke WE, Bloor BC, et al.: Histamine release by four narcotics: A double-blind study in humans. *Anesth Analg* 66:723, 1987.
5. Martin DE, Rosenberg H, Aukburg SJ, et al.: Low-dose fentanyl blunts circulatory responses to tracheal intubation. *Anesth Analg* 61:680, 1982.
6. Tullock WC, Diana P, Cook DR, et al.: High-dose vecuronium: Onset and duration. *Anesth Analg* 67:S235, 1988.
7. Stoelting RK: Circulatory changes during direct laryngoscopy and tracheal intubation: Influence of duration of laryngoscopy with or without prior lidocaine. *Anesthesiology* 47:381, 1977.
8. Mushin WW, Rendell-Baker L, Thomspon PW, Mapleson WW (eds): Clinical aspects of controlled respiration. In: *Automatic Ventilation of the Lungs*, Oxford, Blackwell Scientific, 1980, p 33.
9. Nelson NM: Neonatal pulmonary function. *Pediatr Clin North Am* 13:769, 1966.
10. Doershuk CF, Fisher BJ, Matthews LW: Pulmonary physiology of the young child. In: Scarpelli EM (ed): *Pulmonary Physiology of the Fetus, Newborn, and Child.* Philadelphia, Lea and Febiger, 1975, p 166.
11. Auld PAM: Pulmonary physiology of the newborn infant. In: Scarpelli EM (ed): *Pulmonary Physiology of*

the Fetus and Newborn Child. Philadelphia, Lea and Febiger, 1975, p 140.

12. Downing SE: Neural regulation of circulation during hypoxia and acidosis with special reference to the newborn. *Fed Proc* 31:1209, 1972.
13. Dawes GS, Mott JC, Shelley HJ: The importance of cardiac glycogen for the maintenance of life in foetal lambs and newborn animals during anoxia. *J Physiol* 146:516, 1959.
14. Friedman WF: The intrinsic physiologic properties of the developing heart. In: Friedman WF, Lesch M, Sonnenblick E (eds): *Neonatal Heart Disease*. New York, Grune and Stratton, 1973, p 21.
15. Schieber RA: Noninvasive recognition and assessment of the failing circulation. In: Swedlow DB, Raphaely RC (eds): *Cardiovascular Problems in Pediatric Critical Care*. New York, Churchill Livingstone, 1986, p 90.
16. Tabata BK, Kirsh JR, Rogers MC: Diagnostic tests and technology for pediatric intensive care. In: Rogers MC (ed): *Textbook of Pediatric Intensive Care*. Baltimore, Williams and Wilkins, 1987, pp 1406–1413.
17. Peacock WJ: The postnatal development of the brain and its coverings. In: Raimondi AJ, Choux M, Rocco CD (eds): *Head Injuries in the Newborn and Infant*. New York, Springer Verlag, 1986, chap 4, pp 53–66.
18. Bruce DA: Concepts of intracranial volume and pressure. In: James HE, Anas NG, Perkin RM (eds): *Brain Insults in Infants and Children: Pathophysiology and Management*. Orlando, Grune & Stratton, 1985, chap 2, pp 19.
19. Raimondi AJ, Hirschauer J: Clinical criteria—children's coma score and outcome scale for decision making in managing head injured infants and toddlers. In Raimondi AJ, Choux M, Rocco CD (eds): *Head Injuries in the Newborn and Infant*. New York, Springer Verlag, 1986, chap 10, pp 141–150.
20. Hollinger IB, Goodrich JT: Pediatric neuroanesthesia. In: Frost EAM (ed): *Clinical Anesthesia in Neurosurgery*, 2d ed. Boston, Butterworth, 1991, chap 13, pp 287–333.

21A. Mealey J: Skull fractures. In: McLaurin RL, Schut L, Venes JL, Epstein F (eds): *Pediatric Neurosurgery*, 2d ed. Philadelphia, Saunders, 1989, chap 20, pp 263.

21B. Stein B, Tenner ST: Enlargement of skull fracture in childhood due to cerebral herniation. *Arch Neurol* 26:137, 1972.

22. Menezes AH, Godersky JC, Smoker WRK: Spinal cord injury. In: McLaurin RL, Schut L, Venes JL, Epstein F (eds): *Pediatric Neurosurgery*, 2d ed. Philadelphia, Saunders, 1989, chap. 24, pp 298.
23. Wilberger JE: Anatomy and biomechanics of the immature spine. In: Wilberger JE (ed): *Spinal Cord Injuries in Children*. New York, Futura, 1986, chap 1, pp 1.
24. Pang D, Wilberger JE: Spinal cord injury without radiographic abnormalities in children. *J Neurosurg* 57:114, 1982.
25. Wilberger JE: Clinical aspects of specific spinal injuries. In: Wilberger JE (ed): *Spinal Cord Injuries in Children*. New York, Futura, 1986, chap 4, pp 69.
26. James HE: Head injury in infants, children, and adolescents. In: Nussbaum E (ed): *Pediatric Intensive Care*, 2d ed. New York, Futura, 1989, chap 4, pp 39–54.
27. McLaurin RL, Towbin R: Diagnosis and treatment of head injury in infants and children. In: Youmans JR (ed): *Neurological Surgery*, 3d ed. Philadelphia, Saunders, 1990, chap 68, pp 2149.
28. McLaurin RL, Towbin R: Cerebral damage. In: Raimondi AJ, Choux M, Rocco CD (eds): *Head injuries in the Newborn and Infant*. New York, Springer Verlag, 1986, chap 13, pp 183–202.
29. Bruce DA, Alavi A, Bilaniuk L: Diffuse cerebral swelling following head injuries in children. *J Neurosurg* 54:170, 1981.
30. Rockoff MA, Kennedy SK: Physiology and clinical aspects of raised intracranial pressure. In: Ropper AH, Kennedy SF (eds): *Neurological and Neurosurgical Intensive Care*, 2d ed. Rockville, Aspen, 1988, chap 2, pp 9–22.
31. Clasen RA, Penn RD: Traumatic swelling and edema. In: Cooper PR (ed): *Head Injury*, 2d ed. Baltimore, Williams and Wilkins, 1987, chap 5, pp 285–312.
32. Tabaddor K: Intracranial pressure. In: Frost EAM (ed): *Clinical Anesthesia in Neurosurgery*, 2d ed. Boston, Butterworth, 1991, chap 3, pp 45–62.
33. Bruce DA: Cerebrovascular dynamics. In: James HE, Anas NG, Perkin RM (eds): *Brain Insults in Infants and Children: Pathophysiology and Management*. Orlando, Grune & Stratton, 1985, chap 5, pp 53–60.
34. Bruce DA: Cerebrovascular dynamics following brain insults. In: James HE, Anas NG, Perkin RM (eds): *Brain Insults in Infants and Children: Pathophysiology and Management*. Orlando, Grune & Stratton, 1985, chap 8, pp 83–90.
35. Bruce DA: Ventilation, hyperventilation, megaventilation, and cerebral blood flow. In: James HE, Anas NG, Perkin RM (eds): *Brain Insults in Infants and Children: Pathophysiology and Management*. Orlando, Grune & Stratton, 1985, chap 25, pp 257–262.
36. Shapiro K, Marmarou A: Mechanisms of intracranial hypertension in children. In: McLaurin RL, Schut L, Venes JL, Epstein F (eds): *Pediatric Neurosurgery*, 2d ed. Philadelphia, Saunders, 1989, chap 17, pp 238.
37. Trauner DA: Increased intracranial pressure. In: Swaiman KF (ed): *Pediatric Neurology: Principles and Practice*. St Louis, Mosby, 1989, chap 13, pp 169–176.
38. Swaiman KF: Neurologic examination of the older child. In: Swaiman KF (ed): *Pediatric Neurology: Prin-*

ciples and Practice. St Louis, Mosby, 1989, chap 2, pp 15–34.

39. Swaiman KF: Neurologic examination after the newborn period until 2 years of age. In: Swaiman KF (ed): *Pediatric Neurology: Principles and Practice*. St Louis, Mosby, 1989, chap 3, pp 35–44.
40. Venes JL, Linder SL, Elterman RD: Neurological examination of infants and children. In: Youmans JR (ed): *Neurological Surgery*, 3d ed. Philadelphia, Saunders, 1990, chap 2, pp 37.
41. Chiappa KH: Electrophysiologic monitoring. In: Ropper AH, Kennedy SK: *Neurological and Neurosurgical Intensive Care*. Rockville, Aspen, 1988, chap 10, pp 129–156.
42. Lütschg J, Pfenninger J, Ludin HP: Brain-stem auditory evoked potentials and early somatosensory evoked potentials in neurointensively treated comatose children: *Am J Dis Child* 137:421, 1983.
43. Fisher B, Hicks G, Peterson B: The use of brainstem auditory evoked response testing to assess neurologic outcome following near drowning in children: *Crit Care Med*, 20:578, 1992.
44. Walker ML, Storrs BB: Medical management of head injuries in neonates and infants. In: Raimondi AJ, Choux M, Rocco CD (eds): *Head Injuries in the Newborn and Infant*. New York, Springer Verlag, 1986, chap 11, pp 151–162.
45. Dabbagh S, Ellis D: Regulations of fluids and electrolytes in infants and children. In: Motoyama EK, Davis PJ (eds): *Smith's Anesthesia for Infants and Children*. St Louis, Mosby, 1990, chap 4, pp 105–142.
46. Nelson PB, Seif SM, Maroon JC: Hyponatremia in intracranial disease: *J Neurosurg* 55:938, 1981.
47. Berger MS, Pitts LH, Lovely M: Outcome from severe head injury in children and adolescents. *J Neurosurg*, 62:194, 1985.
48. Humphreys RP, Hendrick EB, Hoffman HJ: The head-injured child who "talks and dies." *Child's Nervous System* 6:139, 1990.
49. Hazinski MF, van Stralen D: Physiologic and anatomic differences between children and adults. In: Levin DL, Morriss FC (eds): *Essentials of Pediatric Intensive Care*. St Louis, Quality Medical, 1989, chap 2, pp 5–17.
50. Reed MD: Principles of total parenteral nutrition. In: Blumer JL (ed): *A Practical Guide to Pediatric Intensive Care*. St Louis, Mosby, 1990, chap 92, pp 582–591.
51. Smith BC, Hickman RO, Morray JP: Nutritional support. In: Morray JP (ed): *Pediatric Intensive Care*. 1989, chap 3, pp 21–42.
52. Kirvela O, Kvetan V, Askanazi J: Parenteral nutrition. In: Frost EAM (ed): *Clinical Anesthesia in Neurosurgery*, 2d ed. Boston, Butterworth, 1991, chap 23, pp 533.
53. Rudolph AM, Hoffman JIE, Rudolph CD: *Rudolph's Pediatrics*, Norwalk, CT, Appleton & Lange 1991, p 1094.
54. Cook DR, McLaurin RL, Schut L, et al. (eds): Pediatric neuroanesthesia and intensive care. In: McLaurin RL, Schut L, Venes JL, Epstein F (eds): *Pediatric Neurosurgery*. Philadelphia, Saunders, 1989, chap 54, pp 565.
55. Snyderman SE: Total parenteral alimentation. In: Zimmerman SS (ed): *Critical Care Pediatrics*. Philadelphia, Saunders, 1985, chap 9, pp 65–69.
56. James HE, Trauner DA: The Glasgow coma scale. In: James HE, Anas NG, Perkin RM (eds): *Brain Insults in Infants and Children*. Orlando, Grune & Stratton, 1985, chap 16, pp 179–182.
57. Bickford RG, Billinger TW, Fleming NI, Steward L: The compressed spectral array. *Proc San Diego Biomed Sym*, 11:365, 1975.
58. Fris-Hansen BJ, Holiday MA, Stapleton T: Total body water in children. *Pediatrics*, 7:321, 1951.
59. Weinberg MG, Hickman RO: Fluid and electrolyte management. In: Morray JP (ed): *Pediatric Intensive Care*. Norwalk, CT, Appleton and Lange, 1989, chap 1, p 3.

CHAPTER 20

Ethical Issues of Care Withdrawal in the Intensive Care Unit

John M. Luce

THE COMPLEXITY OF WITHHOLDING AND WITHDRAWING LIFE SUPPORT

Definition

The withholding and withdrawal of life support are processes by which various medical interventions either are not given to or are taken away from patients with the expectation that they will die as a result.[1,2] These processes are carried out in many medical settings but are especially common in the intensive care unit (ICU), where an array of therapies capable of sustaining life are employed. An example of *withholding* life support is not providing mechanical ventilation to a patient who if not placed on a ventilator will probably die. An example of *withdrawing* life support is removing mechanical ventilation from a patient, with the provision that the patient will neither be ventilated again nor resuscitated if he or she decompensates. This second patient is different from a third patient who is being weaned from mechanical ventilation and will be ventilated again or resuscitated if he or she deteriorates during the weaning process.

Strictly speaking, all patients who die while receiving close medical attention in an ICU or elsewhere do so as a direct result of the withholding or withdrawal of life support. This is either because a decision has been made in advance of decompensation not to resuscitate the patient, or because vigorous resuscitation will not be provided indefinitely if decompensation occurs. For example, the third patient described earlier would receive cardiopulmonary resuscitation (CPR), if he or she were to suffer an unexpected cardiopulmonary arrest during weaning, but CPR would be discontinued if a viable cardiac rhythm could not be restored in a reasonable amount of time. The withdrawal of life support from this third patient is comparable to the withholding of CPR from the second patient, except for the fact that with the second patient deliberate planning has taken place before cardiopulmonary arrest. It is this more deliberate form of withholding and withdrawal that will be focused on in this chapter.

Brain Dead Patients

The only patients who die in the ICU prior to withholding and withdrawal of life support are those who have been declared brain dead, with complete and irreversible loss of function of the cerebral hemispheres and brainstem. These patients frequently receive mechanical ventilation and other forms of life support either because the diagnosis of brain death has not yet been confirmed by apnea testing (after which the ventilator will be removed), or because vital organs such as the heart and kidneys are being preserved for organ donation and transplantation. Indeed, if transplantation is accomplished, withholding or withdrawal of mechanical ventilation and other therapies usually takes place in the operating room, where the patient's organs are harvested. Because interventions such as mechanical ventilation are removed after death, instead of before death, in brain dead patients these interventions are better thought of as organ support rather than life support.

What Form of Life Is Supported?

Biological Life

The mention of brain death raises the question of what form of life is being supported. One form is *biological* life, which requires not only functional organs but also a functional organism. Brain dead patients are considered biologically dead because they have lost the integrative functions of the brainstem, without which individual organs cannot survive for a prolonged period.

Sentient Life

Brain dead patients are distinguished from biologically alive patients in a persistent vegetative state who maintain brainstem and hence integrative function but have lost the sentient functions of the cerebral hemispheres. Without *sentient* life, patients in a persistent vegetative state are incapable of self-awareness or social interaction; however, they may successfully tolerate weaning from mechanical ventilation and be capable of breathing on their own.

Worthwhile Life

A third form of life is *worthwhile* life, a life that is considered worth living by the patient, by other persons, or by society. This form of life does not lend itself to medical diagnosis, and it is open to many interpretations. For example, some might consider life worthwhile only if it contained less pain than pleasure, whereas others might see pain as a necessary part of living or even take pleasure in it. Similarly, one patient who cannot ventilate and oxygenate adequately without the ventilator may prefer to have mechanical ventilation withdrawn because he or she considers life no longer worth living, but another patient in the same condition might prefer to remain on the ventilator because he or she still wants to live. In our society, which values freedom of choice and has adequate critical care resources at present, a patient is allowed to refuse treatment or to accept or request it based upon his or her perception of whether life is worthwhile.

JUDICIAL DECISIONS

The Quinlan Case

Perhaps the best-known judicial decision regarding the withholding and withdrawal of life support occurred in the case of *In Re Karen Ann Quinlan* (1976), in which the father of a girl who was in a persistent vegetative state petitioned the court to be appointed guardian with the power to remove her from mechanical ventilation. The lower court denied the petition, but the New Jersey Supreme Court reversed the decision. In doing so, the court reasoned that patients generally would accept or refuse medical treatment on the basis of its ability to support sentient life rather than mere biological existence. Having concluded that Ms. Quinlan, if she had been capable of making decisions herself, would have forgone therapy that could only prolong biological life but not sentient life, the court decided that her right to privacy would be abrogated if she were prevented the exercise of this right on her behalf. The court therefore granted the father's petition, allowing him to exercise "substituted judgment" for his daughter, and stated that life support could be withdrawn if physicians and a hospital ethics committee agreed that such support did not alter Ms. Quinlan's underlying condition.[3]

The Barber Case

The case of *Barber v. Superior Court* (1983) confirmed the utility of substituted judgment and also answered the question of physician liability in withholding or withdrawing life support. This case involved two California physicians who performed surgical closure of an ileostomy on a Mr. Herbert, who subsequently suffered cardiopulmonary arrest. Five days later they determined that his coma was irreversible; with the consent of his family, the physicians withdrew not only mechanical ventilation but also intravenous fluids and nutrition. Although the family found no fault with this at the time, the physicians were accused of murder by a district attorney.

After the case was heard by several courts, the California Court of Appeals ruled that because the physicians had considered it medically futile to continue life support because sentient life could not be restored, the physicians had not failed to perform their duty. The court did not distinguish between removing mechanical ventilation or removing fluids and nutrition because all were interventions that could either help or hurt the patient. The court thereby discarded the traditional dichotomy between ordinary and extraordinary forms of treatment in favor of a distinction between measures that benefit and burden. Finally, the court held that, without evidence of malevolence, family members are the proper surrogates for an incompetent patient, and that prior judicial approval is not necessary if families and physicians decide to withhold or withdraw support.[3]

The Cruzan Case

The most recent case to wrestle with the issue of withholding and withdrawing life support is that of *Cruzan vs. Missouri*, which was heard by the U.S. Supreme Court in 1990. This case involved Nancy Cruzan, a young woman in a persistent vegetative state who required tube feeding rather than mechanical ventilation. Believing that she would not want to live in such a state, her parents asked to have tube feeding discontinued and were authorized to do so by a trial judge in Missouri. However, the Missouri Supreme Court reversed this decision, arguing that no one could exercise Ms. Cruzan's right to refuse treatment on her behalf. The court also said that because the state had an interest in preserving life regardless of its quality, support could be terminated only if it could be shown by "clear and convincing evidence" that Ms. Cruzan had rejected such treatment.

The U.S. Supreme Court, while acknowledging that patients had a constitutional right to refuse lifesaving hydration and nutrition, also concluded that the Constitution did not prohibit Missouri or other states from requiring evidence of a patient's wishes regarding life support. The reasons for this decision, given by Chief Justice Rehnquist for the five-justice majority, were that states have a legitimate interest in "the protection and preservation of human life," that "the choice between life and death is a deeply personal decision," and that abuses can occur in the case of incompetent patients who do not have "loved ones available to serve as surrogate decision makers."[4]

The minority dissent to the *Cruzan* decision, which was written by Justice Brennan for three of the four dissenting justices, was based on the position that the right of patients to refuse treatment was greater than the state's interest in supporting life. Even if the preservation of life was a legitimate state interest, Justice Brennan argued, the Missouri decision probably would lead to more deaths by discouraging health professionals from initiating medical interventions because of fear that later the interventions could not be withdrawn. By requiring strong evidence of a patient's wishes, Missouri was accused of depriving Ms. Cruzan of the best judgment of those who loved her and of forcing her loved ones to suffer due to the protraction of her persistent vegetative state. Finally, Justice Brennan argued that Missouri was out of touch with reality in expecting patients to write elaborate documents about all the ways in which their lives could or could not be supported. By ignoring the insights of family and friends, the Missouri statute "transforms [incompetent] human beings into passive subjects of medical technology."[4]

Although the *Cruzan* decision stated that the Missouri law, requiring clear and convincing evidence of a formally competent patient's wishes, is constitutional and may be used in Missouri, it did not require that other states follow Missouri's lead, nor did it prevent Missouri from changing its statute. The decision also did not alter the laws, ethical principles, or clinical practices permitting the withholding or withdrawal of life support that have evolved in the United States since the *Quinlan* case 14 years earlier. Additionally, in the *Cruzan* decision the Supreme Court affirmed the right of competent patients to refuse life-sustaining treatment and did not treat the withholding or withdrawal of hydration and nutrition differently from the withholding and withdrawal of other medical interventions. And finally, the Supreme Court highlighted the desirability of all persons filling out advance directives to facilitate medical decision making if and when they become critically ill.[5]

ADVANCE DIRECTIVES

Advance directives are of two types: (1) instructional directives, such as living wills, in which patients specify the conditions under which they would accept or not accept various kinds of life support; and (2) proxy directives, such as the durable power of attorney for health care, in which patients indicate other persons who are authorized to make medical decisions for them in the event that they become unable to do so themselves. Under the terms of the Patient Self Determination Act of 1990, medical facilities that admit patients sponsored by Medicare or Medicaid are required as of December 1, 1991 to inquire whether patients have advance directives, to inform them or their surrogates of what form of advanced directives are available in their state, and to assist them in filling out directives. It is hoped that this legislation will obviate the need for controversial decisions such as that involving Nancy Cruzan.

CARDIOPULMONARY RESUSCITATION

If Missouri's position in the *Cruzan* case was out of touch with reality, as Justice Brennan argued, it may have been because of the fact that relatively little information regarding the reality of withholding or withdrawing life support is available in the medical or lay literature. Most writings on the subject have dealt with issues such as CPR and do-not-resuscitate (DNR) orders. Regarding CPR, it has been noted that most institutions adopted universal CPR policies when this technology was first introduced in 1960. However, recent studies have shown that many patients do not want CPR and that it is rarely effective in hospitalized patients[6] or in those over 70 years of age.[7] This has led the American Heart Association[8] and other groups to state that CPR is not required in terminally, irreversibly ill patients. At the same time, New York and other states have drafted statutes stipulating that patient preferences regarding CPR be solicited on or shortly after hospital admission. Although seeking input from patients and families seems appropriate in most situations, some investigators have argued that patient autonomy is irrelevant when CPR has no potential medical benefit and that this information should not be even offered to the terminally, irreversibly ill.[9]

DO-NOT-RESUSCITATE ORDERS

Despite emerging policies in New York State and elsewhere, most studies[10–13] have demonstrated that DNR orders are written relatively late in a patient's admission, even when the patient is hospitalized in an ICU. Justification for the orders frequently is lacking, as are treatment goals after the order is written. The brief interval between writing an order and death or ICU discharge suggests that the DNR order often represents a decision point for placing broader limits on therapy. Indeed, although many hospital policies consider DNR status compatible with aggressive medical management, in actual practice the writing of a DNR order usually leads to less aggressive care.

HOW LIFE SUPPORT IS WITHHELD OR WITHDRAWN FROM THE CRITICALLY ILL

The fact that the writing of a DNR order often results in less aggressive care was borne out in a study of the withholding and withdrawal of life support from critically ill patients we conducted in two hospitals affiliated with the University of California, San Francisco.[1] This study took place in the medical-surgical ICUs of Moffitt-Long Hospital and San Francisco General Hospital. Moffitt-Long Hospital is a 560-bed tertiary care facility with an 18-bed medical-surgical ICU, a 5-bed neurosurgical ICU, and an 8-bed coronary care unit. San Francisco General Hospital is a 430-bed facility containing a level 1 trauma center that has a 14-bed medical-surgical ICU, and an 8-bed coronary care unit.

The medical-surgical ICUs at the two hospitals are the setting for a multidisciplinary training program in critical care medicine that involves attending faculty, fellows, and residents from the departments of anesthesia, medicine, and surgery. These intensive care teams are consulted about all admissions to the ICU, and they assist the primary services (such as surgery, medicine, and pediatrics) with patient care. The medical-surgical ICU did not provide care for all the critically ill patients treated at either hospital during the study period; in fact, they provided care for a disproportionate number of surgical patients. Nevertheless, because the study investigators were part of the medical-surgical intensive care teams, and because the two units functioned in a similar fashion, only patients admitted to these two ICUs were included in the study.

All patients over 1 year of age who were admitted to one of the two-medical surgical ICUs from July 1987 through June 1988, and from whom life support was subsequently withheld or withdrawn, were identified by the attending critical-care physicians for inclusion in the study. Patients who were included were expected to die after the withholding or withdrawal of life support, either in the ICUs or shortly after transfer to other areas of the hospital. The latter were transferred with the provision that they would not be resuscitated or readmitted to the ICUs if their conditions deteriorated. Also included were organ donors who were brain dead and from whom cardiopulmonary support was withdrawn in the operating room rather than the ICU, because the process leading to organ donation is similar to the process leading to the withholding or withdrawal of support in other patients.

A three-part, detailed, standardized questionnaire was used to collect information about the patients, their families, and the physicians and nurses who cared for them. This questionnaire had a closed format, according to which most questions required choosing among a limited number of responses. The first part of the questionnaire was completed by the critical care fellows, who reviewed the patients' medical records to determine age, sex, diagnoses on admission and discharge, outcome, length of stay in the ICU, DNR status, any previously expressed wish to limit care, and the sequence in which life support was withheld or withdrawn. The fellows also interviewed the attending physicians and chief residents on the primary services to determine why life support had been withheld or withdrawn. The second and third parts of the questionnaire were completed by a research nurse and the family counselors in the ICUs. It focused on the intensive care nurses' and the families' understanding of and involvement in the withdrawal process.

A total of 1719 patients were admitted to the medical-surgical ICUs during the 1-year study period; 968 patients were admitted to Moffitt-Long Hospital and 751 to San Francisco General Hospital. Life support was withheld or withdrawn from 115 of the 1719 patients admitted (7 percent)—36 of those admitted to the ICU at Moffitt-Long Hospital (4 percent), and 79 of those at San Francisco General Hospital (11 percent). Of the total of 115, support was withheld from 22 (19 percent) and withdrawn from 93 (81 percent).

Of the 1719 patients admitted to the two ICUs, 198 died there (12 percent)—127 (13 percent) of those admitted to the ICU at Moffitt-Long Hospital and 71 (9 percent) of those at San Francisco General Hospital. Eighty-nine (45 percent) of the 198 patients who died in the ICUs died after support was withheld or withdrawn. The remaining 26 of the 115 patients from whom support was withheld or withdrawn were transferred from the ICUs with the expectation that they would die. Only 1 of these 26 patients was discharged from the hospital; the remainder died on the ward within 2 weeks of discharge from the ICU.

The median stay in the ICU for all patients was 2 days (3 days at Moffitt-Long Hospital and 2 days at San Francisco General Hospital). The median stay of the patients who died in the ICUs as a result of the withholding or withdrawal of life support was 8 days at Moffitt-Long Hospital and 4 days at San Francisco General Hospital. These stays were considerably longer than those of patients who survived after treatment in the ICU and patients who died there but did not have life support withheld or withdrawn.

Neurosurgical disorders were present in 66 patients from whom support was withheld or withdrawn; this included 6 (17 percent) of the patients from whom support was withheld or withdrawn at Moffitt-Long Hospital and 60 (76 percent) at San Francisco General Hospital. The corresponding median stays in the ICU were 4 and 3 days, respectively. Eighteen patients were considered brain dead, 17 of whom were at San Francisco General Hospital. Head trauma accounted for 10 (56 percent) of the cases of brain death; intracerebral and subarachnoid hemorrhage and anoxic injury were responsible for five (28 percent) and three (17 percent) of the cases of brain death, respectively. Five patients were organ donors. Seventeen neurosurgical patients from whom support was withheld or withdrawn were admitted postoperatively. Twelve of the 17 had had emergency surgery. The median stay in the ICU was 9 days at Moffitt-Long Hospital and 14 days at San Francisco General Hospital.

Respiratory failure was present in 30 patients from whom support was withheld or withdrawn (excluding those with postoperative multiple-organ failure) during their admission to the ICU. The median duration of intensive care was 7 days at both hospitals. Four patients had severe underlying lung disease and were admitted because of a decline in pulmonary function. Six patients, three at each hospital, had the acquired immunodeficiency syndrome (AIDS); five of the six had *Pneumocystis carinii* pneumonia, and one had diffuse pulmonary lymphoma. The remainder of the patients had severe acute lung injury due to sepsis, aspiration, or multiple trauma.

Fourteen patients from whom support was withheld or withdrawn were admitted with known underlying cancers. All but two of these patients were admitted to the ICU at Moffitt-Long Hospital. Eleven of the 14 patients had solid tumors. Eight of the 14 had respiratory failure, three were postoperative, one had a brain tumor, one was bleeding from an upper gastrointestinal hemorrhage, and one had intra-abdominal sepsis. The median stay in the ICU was 3 days. Only three patients had hematologic cancers, and two of these had previously undergone bone marrow transplantation. Their numbers were too small to permit definitive conclusions, but the patients with hematologic cancers tended to stay in the ICU longer (9, 21, and 27 days) than the patients with solid tumors.

The issue of withholding or withdrawing life support usually first came up during the work rounds of the primary and intensive care teams. The primary attending physicians and the attending physicians in the ICU then began to discuss the issue with the patients (if they were sufficiently competent to make medical decisions) or their families (if family members were available).

Five (4 percent) of the 115 patients from whom support was withheld or withdrawn, were competent in the judgment of their physicians. Three of these patients had severe underlying lung disease and either elected not to be intubated during an exacerbation (one patient) or declined reintubation after repeatedly unsuccessful attempts to wean them from mechanical ventilation (two patients). The other two patients had AIDS with respiratory failure; one declined to receive ventilatory support for *Pneumocystis* pneumonia, and the other had previously expressed a desire to limit the duration of mechanical ventilation.

The great majority of the patients—110 of the 115 from whom support was withheld or withdrawn (96 percent)—were not competent to make the decisions themselves. Family members were involved in the decisions to withhold or withdraw support from 102 (93 percent) of these 110 patients. For the remaining eight patients (7 percent), all at San Francisco General Hospital, no family members could be found. Seven of these eight patients were admitted after severe traumatic injuries, three of which were neurosurgical. The decisions to withhold or withdraw support from these eight incompetent patients who had no accessible family members were the result of the deliberations of the primary attending physician and the attending physician in the ICU, after consultation with other physicians about the prognosis.

Once a consensus was reached among the attending physicians and the patients or family members, DNR orders were written for 107 (93 percent) of the 115 patients before support was withheld or withdrawn. These orders were always written by the primary attending physicians. Orders were not written for the five patients who were organ donors or for three patients whose attending physicians were present at the bedside during the process of withdrawing life support. Of the 107 for whom DNR orders were written, 105 (98 percent) died or were discharged from the unit within 48 h of the DNR order.

Thirteen patients had previously expressed a wish to limit terminal care through a living will or in discussions with families or friends. None had signed a durable power of attorney for health care, which is sanctioned by California law. The median length of stay in the ICU for these patients was 7 days, which was not different from the group as a whole. However, four patients with solid tumors who had expressed such a wish had a median stay of 2 days.

The presence of brain death was cited by the primary attending physician as the sole reason for withholding or withdrawal of support from the 18 patients who were brain dead. A poor prognosis was given as the reason for withholding or withdrawing support from the other 97 patients. Additional reasons given for withholding or withdrawing support from specific patients were the futility of continued intervention in 29 (30 percent), extreme suffering in 8 (8 percent), and a request by the patient or a family member in 6 (6 percent). There were no family members who requested the withholding or withdrawal of life support while the patient was competent; in the past, such requests at the two institutions have not been honored and would not be viewed today as violating the patient's autonomy. Although the allocation of resources was discussed frequently among the physicians caring for the patients, concern about resources was never cited as a reason for withholding or withdrawing support, nor was the lack of availability of ICU beds cited (although the units were frequently full).

Family members were available for 106 (92 percent) of the 115 patients, and all those available were involved in the process of deciding whether life support should be withheld or withdrawn. As noted earlier, relatives of 102 of the incompetent patients and 4 of the competent patients were available. Ninety-six (91 percent) of the 106 families either agreed with the course of withholding or withdrawing support suggested by the physicians or had asked beforehand that support be withheld or withdrawn; 10 (9 percent) of the families disagreed at first with the suggested course, but 8 of these 10 accepted the recommendations within 2 to 3 days; and 2 families continued to insist on intensive care against the advice of physicians, and in these cases care was administered until the time of the patients' deaths.

Twenty-six (60 percent) of the 43 families who were interviewed with regard to their attitudes toward the process of withholding and withdrawal said they believed that the patients or their families should make such decisions jointly with the physicians; 12 (28 percent) thought that the physicians should make these decisions on their own; and 4 (9 percent) thought these decisions should be the exclusive responsibility of patients or their families.

Support was withheld from 22 patients and withdrawn from 93; as noted earlier, 5 patients were organ donors. At both institutions mechanical ventilation was the intervention most commonly withdrawn, and the use of vasopressors was the intervention most frequently withheld. The initial step in withdrawing mechanical ventilatory support usually consisted of discontinuing supplemental oxygen and positive end-expiratory pressure. If these actions did not result in death, patients were then placed on a T-piece. Sedatives and analgesic agents were administered during the process of withholding or withdrawing support to 68 (70 percent) of the 97 patients who were not brain dead. Antibiotics, blood transfusions, intravenous fluids, and dialysis were withheld from 8 patients and withdrawn from 13. In the patients from whom these interventions were withdrawn, mechanical ventilation or vasopressors were withdrawn either simultaneously or within a few hours.

The applicability of the findings of this study are uncertain because no one has extensively studied the withholding and withdrawal process in ICUs before. Nevertheless, the 7 percent incidence of withholding or withdrawing life support in the study was comparable to the 0.4 to 13.5 percent range of frequency of DNR orders in medical-surgical ICUs[13] and the 14 percent incidence of such orders in a medical ICU,[12] assuming that support was withheld or withdrawn after DNR orders were written, as was the case in this study.

The most important finding of the study was that brain death and poor prognosis were the major reasons for withholding or withdrawing life support. Other findings were that patients were most often unable to participate in decision making, but that family members were willing to take an active part; advance directives were rarely available and did not significantly shorten time in the ICU; DNR orders were almost always written and were crucial turning points in patient care; and allocation of resources was never cited as a reason for withholding or withdrawing life support, even though it was an issue discussed frequently in the ICUs.

WITHHOLDING AND WITHDRAWAL OF LIFE SUPPORT FROM PATIENTS WITH SEVERE HEAD INJURY

After completing this previous study, my colleagues and I concluded that head trauma was the most common underlying condition in critically ill patients from whom life support was withheld or withdrawn at San Francisco General Hospital. We also reasoned that severe head injury might provide a model of how physicians and patient families use prognostic information to make decisions regarding the foregoing of life-sustaining therapy. Nevertheless, we could not determine how frequently life support was withheld or withdrawn from patients with head injuries at our institution because we did not follow all patients with this condition who were admitted to the medical-surgical ICU, only those from whom life support was withheld or withdrawn. We also had limited information regarding the accuracy of physician prognostication, how physicians communicate their prognoses to families, how families arrive at their own assessment of prognosis, and how families act upon this assessment.

Because of these limitations, we performed a second study to better characterize how life support was withheld or withdrawn from all patients admitted by the neurosurgery service to the medical-surgical ICU at San Francisco General Hospital from January 1990 through December 1990 with head injuries and a Glasgow coma scale score of 7 or less.[14] Once again we included patients who were brain dead because the processes of foregoing life-sustaining care in patients who are brain dead is similar to that in patients who are not brain dead but are severely neurologically impaired. The second study was conducted not only in the medical-surgical ICU but also in a nearby 4-bed constant-observation room and an adjacent 30-bed ward for neurosurgical patients. Although intubated patients are cared for in both the observation room and the ward, patients requiring mechanical ventilation must be cared for in the ICU.

The neurosurgery service at San Francisco General Hospital is supervised by three attending physicians who are full-time faculty of the University of California, San Francisco. The service also contains chief residents and general surgery residents and interns who rotate among various teaching hospitals in the university. The neurosurgery chief residents rotate through San Francisco General Hospital on a 6-month basis. During that time, they have consistent responsibility for the service in the ICU, the constant-observation room, and the neurosurgery ward. Among these responsibilities are regular communication with patients and their families regarding therapy and its possible limitation. Because the chief residents are primarily responsible for such communication, they and not their attendings were interviewed during the course of this study.

A detailed, standardized questionnaire was used by the ICU family counselor to collect demographic information and outcome data and to interview the patients' physicians and families at specific intervals in the hospital course. This questionnaire had a closed format, according to which most questions required choosing between a limited number of options, although open comments were solicited when appropriate. Demographic information and outcome data were collected, and interviews of physicians and families were conducted at the time patients were admitted to the ICU, later during the ICU stay if the patient's condition changed, upon transfer to the constant-observation room or the ward, and at discharge from the hospital if discharge occurred. Outcome data were also collected, and family interviews were conducted by telephone 6 months after patient admission.

At the various time intervals, the physicians were asked to predict the patients' likely outcome using five categories of functioning: good recovery, moderate disability, severe disability, vegetative, and death. The physicians also were asked what functional prognosis they communicated to families and how well the families appeared to understand this communication using a 10-point scale. In addition, the physicians were asked to indicate on a scale of 10 which reasons were important to them in recommending the withholding or withdrawal of life support if such recommendations were made; a score of 5 or more was interpreted as being an affirmative response. These reasons include brain death, poor prognosis, futility, patient suffering, unacceptable quality of life if patients survived, patient or family wish, further care too costly, and limited bed or nurse availability. Finally, the physicians were asked to choose from a number of scenarios that occurred after the withholding or withdrawal of life support was recommended and to describe how life support was withheld or withdrawn.

At the same time intervals, the families were asked what they believed would be the patient's outcome, using the same five categories, and how important patient eye opening and body movement were in reaching this prognosis. In addition, the families were asked what functional prognosis was communicated by the physicians and how well the families understood this information, using a 10-point scale. During their first interview, the families were asked to discuss their emotional closeness to the patients, whether another family member or close friend had experienced a severe neurosurgical or neurologic illness, and the outcome of that illness. If the withholding or withdrawal of life support was recommended by physicians, the families were asked to indicate what reasons were important to them in considering withholding or withdrawing life support, choosing from the same list used by the physicians and using the same 10-point scale. Six months after patient admission, the families were asked in retrospect how well they considered physician communication, what strategies might be used to improve communication, what factors were important in their own assessment of prognosis, and how they felt in general about the process of withholding or withdrawal of life support if it occurred.

A total of 47 patients were included in the study during the 12-month period. These patients were from 18 to 83 years of age, with a mean age of 44 years. Thirty-six of the 47 patients (77 percent) were men, and 11 (23 percent) were women. Twenty-five of the 47 patients (53 percent) were Caucasian, 5 (11 percent) were African-American, 9 (19 percent) were Hispanic, 6 (13 percent) were Asian, and 2 (4 percent) had other ethnic heritage. Motor vehicle accidents accounted for 18 (38 percent) of the patients' head injuries, falls for 8 (17 percent), assault with blunt objects for 7 (15 percent), gunshot wounds for 5 (11 percent), other forms of penetrating trauma for 2 (4 percent), and other causes for 7 (15 percent). The mean Glasgow coma scale score for all patients was 5.0

Twenty-two of the 47 patients (46 percent) in this study died. Twenty patients died during hospitalization and two died following discharge. Eleven of the patients who died were determined to be brain dead; seven of these were organ donors. All seven patients who were organ donors were declared dead in the ICU and therefore were said to have died there, although their organs were harvested in the operating room and support was withdrawn from them there. Three other patients who were not brain dead also died in the ICU. Thus, a total of 14 patients died in the ICU. The two patients who died following discharge did so at rehabilitation centers. All patients who died were hospitalized at San Francisco General Hospital from 1 to 18 days, with a mean stay of 5 days.

Of the 25 patients who survived, 5 were transferred to other acute care facilities under the requirements of their health insurance plans. Fourteen patients were transferred to rehabilitation centers after completing acute hospitalization at San Francisco General Hospital. The patients who were discharged had stays at San Francisco General Hospital of 5 to 60 days, with a mean stay of 25 days.

Life support was withheld or withdrawn from 24 of the 47 patients (51 percent) with severe head injury. Twenty-two of the patients from whom life support was withheld or withdrawn died and two were discharged alive. All 22 patients who died did so during the withholding or withdrawal of life support; they included all 14 patients who died in the ICU. The hospital stay for those patients who had life support withheld or withdrawn and died was from 1 to 40 days, with a mean of 5 days ($p < 0.05$ compared to patients who did not have life support withheld or withdrawn). The hospital stay for those patients who had life support withheld or withdrawn but were discharged ranged from 44 to 62 days, with a mean of 54 days.

Families were available to participate in medical decisions for 45 of the 47 patients (96 percent). Families were available to participate in medical decisions for 23 of the 24 patients (96 percent) from whom life support was withheld or withdrawn. Of the family members of patients from whom life support was withheld or withdrawn, 9 (38 percent) were parents, 5 (17 percent) were spouses or significant others, 4 (25 percent) were children of legal age, and 3 (13 percent) were siblings.

Of the 45 available families, only 5 (11 percent) had another family member who had experienced a serious neurosurgical or neurologic illness, and none said that the experience had an impact on decision making during the present study. Thirty-one of the 47 families, 15 of whom were families of patients from whom life support was withheld or withdrawn, answered the question regarding the importance of patient eye opening and body movement in their own prognostication. Fifteen of the 31 (48 percent) attributed no importance to eye opening and body movement; 4 said that the presence of eye opening and body movement had led them to expect a good outcome; 12 said that the absence of eye opening and body movement led them to expect a poor outcome. Only four family members were aware of patients having previously expressed wishes regarding intensive care. Only a single patient had prepared a living will, and none had durable powers of attorney for health care.

Complete data regarding the prognosis given patients by their physicians on admission to the ICU, at the time of transfer to the ward, and on hospital discharge were available for 35 patients. Life support was withheld or withdrawn from 23 of these 35 patients. A higher functional class generally was predicted at every interval for patients from whom life support was not withheld or withdrawn.

A change in prognosis by physicians was defined as any change from one functional class to another at any interval of the study. Only 5 of the 23 patients from whom life support was withheld or withdrawn manifested a change in prognosis, and this change was for the worse in three of the five patients. The two patients who had life support withheld and withdrawn and improved both survived. One of these patients was initially predicted to be vegetative, but the prognosis was changed to brain death; life support was withheld or withdrawn at this point but was reinstituted at the family's request when the patient remained vegetative instead. The other patient was initially expected to have a full recovery but deteriorated so much that brain death was predicted; when the patient appeared to be vegetative and brain death was unlikely, supportive care was resumed at the family's request. Both of these patients remained vegetative through the end of the study.

Prognosis became more favorable for five patients, most of whom initially were in higher functional categories; four of the five were initially considered moderately or severely disabled and then improved. None of these patients were even considered for withholding or withdrawal of life support. Prognosis became less favorable for six patients, three of whom had life support withheld or withdrawn, as noted earlier, and three of whom did not. Another four patients deteriorated but then improved such that the prognosis of three of the patients was the same as originally indicated.

Data regarding the prognosis given patients by their families at the various time intervals were available for 42 patients, including all those from whom life support was withheld or withdrawn. These prognoses and those made by physicians were completely congruent for 31 patients (73 percent). In the case of two patients, the physicians' prognosis reflected a higher functional category than the family noted. In the case of nine patients, the families' prognosis reflected a higher functional category than the physicians noted. The physician and family prognosis became congruent later in the hospital course for one patient.

Data regarding what prognosis the physicians believed they communicated to the family and what prognosis the family believed was being communicated were available for 43 patients. In these 43 cases, only 7 families (16 percent) differed in their understanding of the prognosis communicated by physicians; in 6 of the 7 situations, there was a difference of a single functional category. Also in 6 of 7 instances, the families believed a more favorable prognosis had been communicated than the physicians believed.

The reasons that physicians recommended withholding or withdrawal of life support and that families decided to accept these recommendations were similar in this study. Both groups cited brain death in 11 patients, poor prognosis in 9, futility in 8, and an unacceptable quality of life in 7. Family requests anticipated physician recommendations to forego life-sustaining therapy in four cases, and in another four cases the families' expression of prior requests on the part of patients were followed. In no cases were the cost or availability of care cited.

Three scenarios emerged after physicians recommended foregoing of life-sustaining therapy. In 11 cases (50 percent), patients were declared brain dead and no option for care existed. For another 10 patients (41 percent), families agreed to withhold or withdraw life support after physician recommendations. Another family (6 percent) initially disagreed with this recommendation but agreed to it after the patient was transferred to another acute care hospital. Two families (12 percent) refused and earlier disagreed with the recommendation, and care was continued at San Francisco General Hospital. In all cases in which the family disagreed with physician recommendations, their wishes to continue life-sustaining therapy were acted on.

Life support was withheld or withdrawn for 14 patients in the ICU; included were 11 brain dead patients who were counted as dying in the ICU but actually had therapy removed in the operating room after their organs were harvested. Life support was withheld or withdrawn from an additional six patients in the observations room or on the ward, from two patients in rehabilitation centers, from one patient in another acute care facility, and from one patient in a chronic care facility. Do-not-resuscitate orders were written for all 24 patients before the withholding or withdrawing of life support began.

As in the first study, therapy was more often withdrawn than withheld. Mechanical ventilation was withdrawn from a total of 10 patients (41 percent); three other patients (13 percent) had oxygen and three (13 percent) had endotracheal tubes withdrawn. Medications, including antibiotics, were withheld from three patients (13 percent), all of whom were in the constant-observation room or on the ward and were not ventilator-dependent. Because DNR orders were written for all 24 patients, CPR was by definition withheld from all patients as well. It was the only therapy withdrawn from one patient.

Information was available from only 29 families 6 months after patient admission because only 33 families could be located and 4 did not offer comments. Of those families that were interviewed in depth, six stated that frequent and clear communication was of great value to them during their family members' hospitalization, although one family felt that the information provided them was inadequate. Four families commented that they valued joint decision making involving them and physicians, whereas one family said that decision making was entirely a family perogative. Three families appreciated the availability of interpreters to assist in communication, and two families cited the usefulness of clergy in this process. The fact that patients were organ donors was seen as helpful by three families. Belief in miracles was a paramount concern for an additional three families. One family said that more time was needed to come to grips with critical illness. Another family noted that physicians did not mention potential psychiatric sequellae in their discussions of prognosis. Still another commented on the difficulty of caring for a head-injured patient with severe disabilities.

The results of this study demonstrate that life support was frequently withheld or withdraw from patients with severe head injury at San Francisco General Hospital, and that most patients died when life support was withheld or withdrawn. The functional prognosis of patients from whom life support was withheld or withdrawn was poorer than that of patients who continued to receive life support, and it never improved beyond the vegetative state. Physician recommendations to forego life-sustaining therapy was based almost entirely on poor prognosis, which was expressed either in those terms or in terms of brain death, futility, and an unacceptable quality of life if the patient survived. Families usually agreed with physician recommendations, although some asked for and received further life support for patients. Agreement presumably occurred because families shared the physicians' interpretation of prognosis, perhaps because the families expected the same functional outcome for patients due to their own assessment or because physician communication of prognosis was generally clear.

DEATH MANAGEMENT

The two studies described in detail above are the first to document how and why life support is withheld or withdrawn from critically ill patients, including those with severe head injury and other neurosurgical disorders. Many of the aspects of foregoing life-sustaining therapy explored in the studies are supported by consensus statements and a growing literature on ethical issues in critical care practice.[2,3,15–18] Such issues are likely to become even more important in the future as clinicians focus on how to better manage patients during death and as society faces the challenge of allocating scarce resources in and outside of the ICU.

REFERENCES

1. Smedira NG, Evans BH, Grais LS, et al.: Withholding and withdrawal of life support from the critically ill. *N Engl J Med* 322:309, 1990.
2. Luce JM: Ethical principles in critical care. *JAMA* 263:696, 1990.
3. Luce JM, Raffin TA: Withholding and withdrawal of life support from critically ill patients. *Chest* 94:621, 1988.
4. Annas GJ: Sounding board: Nancy Cruzan and the right to die. *N Engl J Med* 323:670, 1990.
5. Annas GJ, Arnold B, Aroskar M, et al.: Occasional notes: Bioethicists' statement on the U.S. Supreme Court's *Cruzan* decision. *N Engl J Med* 323:686, 1990.
6. Beddell SE, Delbanco TL, Cook EF, Epstein FH: Survival after cardiopulmonary resuscitation in the hospital. *N Engl J Med* 309:569, 1983.
7. Murphy DJ, Murray AM, Robinson BE, Campion EW: Outcomes of cardiopulmonary resuscitation in the elderly. *Ann Intern Med* 111:199, 1989.
8. American Heart Association: Standards and guidelines for cardiopulmonary resuscitation and emergency cardiac care. *JAMA* 255:2841, 1986.
9. Blackhall LJ: Must we always use CPR? *N Engl J Med* 317:1281, 1987.
10. Lo B, Saika G, Strull W, et al.: "Do-not-resuscitate" decisions—a prospective study at three teaching hospitals. *Ann Intern Med* 145:1115, 1985.
11. Bedell SE, Pelli D, Maher P, Cleary PD: Do-not-resuscitate orders for critically ill patients in the hospital—how are they used and what is their impact? *JAMA* 256:233, 1986.
12. Younger SJ, Lewandowski W, McClish DK, et al.: "Do-not-resuscitate" orders—incidence and complications in a medical intensive care unit. *JAMA* 253:54, 1985.
13. Zimmerman JE, Knaus WA, Sharpe JM, et al.: The use and implications of do-not-resuscitate orders in intensive care units. *JAMA* 255:351, 1986.
14. Luce JM, O'Callahan J, Fink C, Pitts LH: Withholding and withdrawal of life support from patients with severe head injury. *Am Rev Respir Dis*. Abstract. In press.
15. Schneiderman LJ, Spragg RG: Ethical decisions in discontinuing mechanical ventilation. *N Engl J Med* 318:984, 1988.
16. NIH Workshop Summary: Withholding and withdrawing mechanical ventilation. *Am Rev Respir Dis* 134:1327, 1986.
17. Jonsen AR, Siegler M, Winslade WJ: *Clinical Ethics*, 2d ed. New York, Macmillan, 1986.
18. American Thoracic Society Bioethics Task Force: Withholding and withdrawing life-sustaining therapy. *Am Rev Respir Dis* 144:726, 1991.

CHAPTER 21
Brain Death and Organ Donation

Grant E. Gauger

Despite long-standing recognition of a human being's dependence for survival on cardiac and respiratory function, it is the activity of the brain that progressively has come to define the life of the individual and its limits.

Two practical concerns have benefited from such definition: the focus of resources on the care of patients who might recover from illness or injury, and organ donation on behalf of others with advanced disease of any of several organ systems. Intelligent response to these concerns requires some understanding of the concept of brain death, including its neurologic and laboratory features. The clinical applications of such understanding are still evolving.

CONCEPT OF BRAIN DEATH

In a recent discussion, C. Miller Fisher has noted that ". . . human life is best defined in terms of preservation of the brain and mind. Brain function is the final determinant of life, not the beat of the heart. The brain and mind are the essence of mankind; they constitute meaningful life and their absence defines human death."[1] These comments reflect the fact that the heart can continue to act, for a time, when brain activity has been irretrievably lost. Although cardiac death produces brain death, the reverse may not be true over the short term. The same scientific progress that has made modern technological support of critically ill or injured patients so successful has also elicited more careful thought concerning the definition of death.

As Fisher states, "It is one matter to speak of the death of the brain but quite another to use brain death determined clinically and electrically as the determinant of death of a person, officially for legal purposes."[1] This recognizes not only the now-accepted identity of death of the brain with the death of the person, but the litigious "climate of general public unease about brain death . . . , partly engendered by sensational fiction," noted by Sweet.[2]

The unease may also be shared by physicians, since published criteria of brain death have provoked controversy and disagreement, and the proliferation of terminology has produced very serious semantic confusion.

The terms *whole brain death, brain death, brainstem death, cerebral death,* and *irreversible coma* have varying implications, as delineated by Pallis.[3] Confusion of the last term[4] with *persistent vegetative state*,[5] clearly not synonymous with brain death, limits its usefulness. Whole brain death implies a presently nonexistent capacity to assess activity in every brain area. Cerebral death suggests loss of hemispheric activity underlying higher functions. (However, where defined as *total destruction of the brain*, it may be synonymous with brain death.) Brain death was defined in the Report of the President's Commission (1981) as "the irreversible cessation of all functions of the entire brain, including the brainstem."[6]

These definitions and their implications are not trivial, since they determine what conditions, findings, and test results establish brain death. It cannot be declared if it is not defined.

The use of irreversible loss of brain function as the major criterion of death is a modern phenomenon that follows several individual and organizational investigations of the subject. The widely known 1968 Harvard study considered that the comatose patient was dead when responsiveness to external stimuli and inner need was absent.[4] Two clinical examinations performed by a competent physician, with an interval of 24 h or more between them, were recommended, with supplementation by electroencephalography (EEG) when possible.

In 1981 the President's Commission for the Study of Bioethics and Medicine suggested criteria for brain death which included time between examinations of 6 h in those patients in whom irreversible damage was obvious, or where the mechanism of injury was known.[6] In the case of anoxic injury, a waiting period of 24 h was recommended. Ancillary tests were advised in the case of children under 5 and when less than 12 h had elapsed before the repeat examination.

Although no single set of guidelines for the determination of brain death has been legally adopted by all states, the National Conference of Commissioners on Uniform State Laws was among several organizations endorsing the 1981 Report of the President's Commission. This included the statement that "An individual who has sustained either (1) irreversible cessation of circulatory and respiratory function, or (2) irreversible cessation of all functions of the entire brain, including the brainstem, is dead. A determination of death must be made in accordance with accepted medical standards."[6]

Thus, the concept of total and irreversible loss of functioning of the whole brain as the determinant of death has received the endorsement of a presidential commission and progressive acceptance by students of the law. The complex sequence of studies of the factors associated with the declaration of brain death has been summarized in a comprehensive review by Black.[7]

Pallis's observation that brainstem death is the "physiological core of brain death" is highly useful in eliminating confusion. It is internally consistent and physiologically sound. As he notes, it ". . . implies an irreversibly unconscious patient with irreversible apnoea and irreversible loss of brainstem reflexes." Further, ". . . the crucial attribute of irreversibility can only be established by due attention to context. There must be a known and sufficient "primary diagnosis" to account for the patient's condition, and all reversible causes of brainstem dysfunction must have been excluded. The passage of sufficient time and resort to all relevant therapeutic measures are also essential components of irreversibility."[3]

This emphasis on the brainstem can inform a practical assessment of neurologic findings and the selection of supplementary tests. It is also consistent with the conclusion that "Death of the brain occurs when the organ irreversibly loses its capacity to maintain the vital integrative functions regulated by the vegetative and consciousness-mediating centers of the brainstem."[8]

CLINICAL CRITERIA

Criteria for the determination of brain death are concisely outlined in Table 21-1[9] and are more fully developed in the President's Commission study.[6] They refer to the findings on the clinical examination and to the results of confirmatory tests

Table 21-1 Criteria for Determination of Brain Death

Absent cerebral and brainstem function
Well-defined, irreversible etiology
Persistent absence of all brain function after observation and/or treatment
Hypothermia, drug intoxication, metabolic encephalopathy, and shock excluded

(Table 21-1). A recent outline of clinical tests of brain death is presented in modified form (Table 21-2).[9]

The patient must demonstrate unresponsive coma. Spontaneous movements are usually absent, although rare complex movement of spinal origin has been described.[10] Seizures, shivering (revealing hypothalamic activity), or decerebrate or decorticate posturing indicating brainstem function are not consistent with brain death.[11] By contrast, spinal activity, including muscle-stretch reflexes, plantar flexion, plantar withdrawal (triple flexion), or tonic neck and abdominal reflexes, may be present and does not exclude brain death.[12]

The pupils need not be dilated,[13] but they must be unreactive to light in the absence of major cataract, primary ocular trauma, or agents compromising the light response, including neuromuscular blocking compounds, glutethimide, opiates, scopolamine, dopamine, or atropine.

Absence of the corneal reflex may reflect facial paresis. There is a suggestion that its threshold is influenced by the duration of lid closure.[14]

The oculocephalic (doll's eye) reflex is tested by rotating the patient's head. Movement of the eye within the orbit indicates retention of some brainstem function.

Table 21-2 Clinical Tests of Brain Death

Cerebral unresponsiveness
No spontaneous motor activity
Absent pupillary, corneal, and oculocephalic/oculovestibular reflexes
Absent cough reflex with deep tracheal suctioning
No increase in heart rate in response to intravenous administration of atropine
No respiratory efforts on apnea testing ($PA_{CO_2} > 60$ mmHg)

The oculovestibular (caloric) reflex may persist despite loss of the doll's eye response. It is tested by the infusion of cold water into each ear canal, bathing the tympanic membrane for 20 to 30 s, with the head elevated 30°. Ocular motion as a response to this powerful labyrinthine stimulus is inconsistent with complete brainstem failure. Barbiturate or other intoxication and severe disease of the inner ear may compromise this test.

Presence of coughing or the gag reflex reveals function of glossopharyngeal and vagal mechanisms. The latter may also be assessed by the administration of 1.0 mg of atropine sulfate intravenously. Absence of an acceleration of heart rate indicates that the vagus was not moderating that rate before its pharmacological suppression.

The significance of respiratory action in the setting of hypercarbia has made the apnea test a widely discussed component of the diagnosis of brain death. Careless performance of the test may render it both invalid and a form of "self-fulfilling prophecy." Preoxygenation with 100 percent oxygen during mechanical ventilation and introduction of a 4- to 6-L/min oxygen flow by intratracheal catheter will permit the development of a hypercarbic state (P_{CO_2} of 60 torr) without accompanying hypoxia.[15] The time required is a function of a P_{CO_2} increase of approximately 3 to 6 torr/min. The total interval of apneic oxygenation may be minimized by an adjustment of ventilation which permits a pretest rise to high normal levels. Monitoring and documentation of oxygen and carbon dioxide levels are important in assuring that organs are not placed at risk of hypoxia, leading to compromise of later transplantation where appropriate.

Several conditions may undermine, or even fully invalidate, both clinical and confirmatory testing in the determination of brain death. These include hypothermia, shock, drug intoxication, metabolic coma, and hypophosphatemia.[16] A body temperature lower than 32°C, especially in association with ingestion of alcohol, makes either ancillary testing or an extended period of observation desirable. Similarly, barbiturate intoxication or the presence of diazepam, methaqualone, mecloqualone, trichlorethylene, meprobamate, narcotics, or other agents may make study of brain blood flow advisable in certification of brain death.[6] A brain death simulation by succinylcholine sensitivity, with full recovery, has also been described.[17]

The value of a skillful neurologic examination in diagnosing brain death can scarcely be overstated. Accomplished in the context of full historical and general physical findings, it forms the basis of this process. It may be performed in any setting, independent of the availability of one or more supplementary tests. These may be helpful, but they do not supplant the clinical assessment of brain function which remains the cornerstone of the diagnosis.

CONFIRMATORY TESTS

Powner has suggested an outline of confirmatory brain death tests (Table 21-3).[18] The absence of electrical activity on EEG study continues to be the most frequently cited ancillary observation in the establishment of brain death. A single EEG examination conducted with 2 μV/mm or higher sensitivity which shows absence of waveform activity during a period of 30 min is highly supportive of brain death. However, this conclusion is not justified if any of the compromising factors of shock, hypothermia, or drug intoxication is present.[19]

The American EEG Society has specified that "electrocerebral silence (ECS) or electrocerebral inactivity is defined as no electrical activity over 2 μV when recording from scalp or referential pairs 10 or more centimeters apart with interelectrode resistances under 10,000 ohms (or impedances under 6,000 ohms) but over 100 ohms."[20] Related technical requirements are important. These include identification of sources of artifact as influenced by the ICU environment and by amplification settings.

A repeat study should be considered when doubt about the character or significance of the recording exists. There is no uniform acceptance of the interval between examinations. When the criteria of brain death have been met on clinical grounds, repeated testing may not contribute any further "objective" information and may compromise the success of organ transplantation through further time passage.

Clinicians should recall that the EEG reflects the activity of a small proportion of cortical neurons and is not a measure of activity in all centers. It does not indicate brainstem processes and cannot exclude the activity of scattered cellular clusters. Residual EEG activity in the presence of a nonfunctioning brainstem has been described.[21] It appears that the EEG infrequently contributes predictive information not already derived from a thorough neurologic examination.[22]

The presence of electrical activity elicited by visual, auditory, or somatosensory stimulation excludes the diagnosis of brain death.[18] Such evoked-potential study may provide helpful supplementary data.

The measurement of intracranial blood flow may be the most certain available means of documentation of the presence of brain death. The absence of flow on four-vessel angiography has been considered diagnostic of brain death. The usefulness of this test may be greatest in patients whose assessment is complicated by metabolic or pharmacologic factors, or hypothermia. Transcranial Doppler study permits detection of cerebral blood flow. A pattern suggesting an alternating intraluminal motion has been described in brain dead patients.[23]

Radionuclide imaging can be a valuable indicator of cerebral blood flow. Activity confined to the sagittal sinus has been described in patients with angiographically demonstrated loss of the cerebral circulation.[24] The less invasive and portable nature of the radionuclide method contributes to its usefulness.[25]

Table 21-3 Confirmatory Brain Death Tests

Dependent upon neuronal function
Clinical examination
EEG and cerebral function monitor
Evoked potentials
Biochemical correlates
Dependent upon intracranial blood flow
Angiography (contrast)
Radioisotope angiography
Ultrasonography
Digital subtraction angiography/venography
Computed tomography
Intracranial pressure
Echoencephalography
Ophthalmic artery blood flow

Other confirmatory tests which are directly or indirectly reflective of intracranial blood flow include digital subtraction angiography, ultrasonography, ophthalmic artery flow, echoencephalography, and ICP measurement. ICP monitoring may be useful in patients under treatment with large doses of barbiturates which invalidate EEG findings. Cerebral perfusion pressure approaches zero as ICP reaches or exceeds mean systemic pressure. Loss of the pulsatile character of the ICP tracing usually follows. It has occasionally persisted even when angiography has documented absence of cerebral blood flow.[26]

Although data concerning the cerebral circulation may provide highly significant ancillary support, they are nevertheless inferential with respect to neuronal activity. Two modern approaches more directly address the location and extent of cerebral metabolism.

Positron emission tomography monitors chemical reactions of the brain on-line, providing kinetic, and not simply structural, information. Its use is limited by radiopharmaceutical and equipment constraints. Magnetic resonance spectroscopy may become a readily available means of demonstrating the absence of high-energy phosphates and thus the loss of the engine of cellular life within the brain.[27]

DIAGNOSIS OF BRAIN DEATH IN CHILDREN

The determination of brain death in pediatric patients is not fundamentally different from that in adults. It should, however, reflect recognition of the possibility of greater potential for recovery of the child's brain, especially in infancy. The use of a method of blood flow determination in supplementing the clinical examination is advised where any question exists regarding cerebral function. A task force has specifically addressed these and other related aspects, including recommended observation periods.[28]

For infants of age 7 days to 2 months, two examinations and EEGs separated by at least 48 h are advised. For ages 2 months to 1 year, two examinations and EEGs with a 24-h interval, or an examination, EEG, and radionuclide angiographic study demonstrating no visualization of cerebral arteries are recommended. For patients over 1 year with an "irreversible cause," an observation period of at least 24 h, without a requirement for laboratory testing, is specified.

The task force noted the difficulty in interpretation of clinical and laboratory findings in infants, and, especially, in premature newborns. The prognosis associated with hypoxic-ischemic encephalopathy may be obscure in any pediatric age category. A longer observation period, with supplementary blood flow information, may be essential in some of these cases.

DISCUSSION

A clear understanding of the definition and identification of brain death serves both the patient's family and the health professionals interacting with it. Relatives and friends are able to recognize the reality of their loss, and they are spared the prolonged anguish that uncertainty promotes. They can see and understand the fact and its permanence, and can begin sooner to move past the first shock of death. They can be helped by nurses, social workers, and physicians in the process of acceptance and in handling decisions which cannot be deferred.

The health care team, including intensive care workers, can direct its energies to the care of patients who may benefit from therapy, thereby focusing and conserving human and material resources. Critical care beds and equipment such as ventilators can be made available to patients who urgently need them.

The potential sense of psychological abandonment of the brain dead patient can be countered by explicit recognition and communication of the equivalence of brain death with the death of the individual.

As important as these benefits are, another may transcend them: the potential availability of organs and tissues on behalf of a large and growing number of patients whose lives depend on successful transplantation.

Many of these persons are otherwise in the prime of their lives, and they can be returned to vigorous productivity by highly effective pharmacologically supported surgical measures. Marginally satisfactory survival can be replaced by independence and a lasting high quality of life.

Unfortunately, the number of patients awaiting organ transplantation far exceeds the number of donors. These, in turn, represent a fraction of the potential donor pool.[29] Several factors have been shown to influence organ availability. They include the early identification of brain death, its communication to the family in clear and unequivocal terms, and the nature of the request for consideration of organ donation. Such a request should be made after brain death has been explained to family members, with an interval permitting them to begin the process of acceptance. The request need not be made by those most directly involved in the patient's care to that point. What appears most important in determining the success of the process of organ donation is the skill and experience of the person who raises this question with the family. A representative of the appropriate organ procurement organization who is sensitive to the range of personal, cultural, and ethical issues involved in each specific patient's circumstances may most effectively conduct this crucial discussion.

Thus it could be said that two processes of uncoupling are important in the intensive care setting of brain death and its consequences. The first is the dissociation between the function of the brain and that of other systems including circulation, making preparation for organ donation possible. The second uncoupling, that between the announcement of brain death and the request for organ donation, has been shown to be highly significant in the successful outcome of such requests.

Early identification of brain death can preserve both time and effort. Communication with families by persons best suited through training and temperament can further reduce stress and promote the efficiency of the process. Nevertheless, the application of concepts of brain death to the subject of organ and tissue donation and transplantation is unavoidably associated with several demands on physicians, nurses, and allied health workers. These include the continuing physiologic support of the organ donor following declaration of death.[30]

The clinical, psychological, and administrative difficulties can only be minimized and not eliminated. But, the final result can be the creation of new hope, often from tragedy, through the return to normal health of another person. And every such creation is, as Albert Camus expressed it, "a gift to the future."[31]

REFERENCES

1. Fisher CM: Brain death—a review of the concept. *J Neurosci Nurs* 23:330, 1991.
2. Sweet WH: Brain death (editorial). *N Engl J Med* 299:410, 1978.
3. Pallis C: Brainstem death. In: Vinken PJ, Bruyn GW, Klawans HL, Braakman R (eds): *Head Injury. Handbook of Clinical Neurology*, vol. 57. Amsterdam, Elsevier, 1990, pp 441–496.
4. A definition of irreversible coma. Report of the Ad Hoc Committee of the Harvard Medical School to examine the definition of brain death. *JAMA* 205:337, 1968.
5. Jennett B, Plum F: Persistent vegetative state after brain damage: A syndrome in search of a name. *Lancet* 1:734, 1972.
6. Guidelines for the determination of death. Report of the medical consultants on the diagnosis of death to the president's commission for the study of ethical problems in medicine and biomedical and behavioral research. *JAMA* 246:2184, 1981.
7. Black PMcL: Brain death (Parts 1 & 2). *N Engl J Med* 299:338, 393, 1978.
8. Plum F, Posner JB: *The Diagnosis of Stupor and Coma*, 3d ed. Philadelphia, FA Davis, 1982, p 322.
9. Darby JM, Stein K, Grenvik A, Stuart SA: Approach to management of the heartbeating "brain dead" organ donor. *JAMA* 261:2224, 1989.
10. Mandel S, Arenas A, Scasta D: Spinal automatism in cerebral death. *N Engl J Med* 307:501, 1982.
11. Polacek DJ, Grenvik A: Brain death. In: Parrillo JE (ed): *Current Therapy in Critical Care Medicine*, Philadelphia, B.C. Decker, 1987, p 236.
12. Caronna JJ: The neurological intensive care unit. In: Parrillo JE, Ayres SM (eds): *Major Issues in Critical Care Medicine*, Baltimore, Williams & Wilkins, 1984, p 202.
13. An appraisal of the criteria of cerebral death: A summary statement: A collaborative study. *JAMA* 237:982, 1976.
14. O'Leary DJ, Millodot M: Brain death and the corneal reflex. *Lancet* 2:1379, 1980.
15. Pitts LH, Kaktis J, Caronna J, et al.: Brain death, apneic diffusion oxygenation, and organ transplantation. *J Trauma* 18:180, 1978.
16. Young GB, Amaker AL, Paulseth JE, et al.: Hypophosphatemia versus brain death. *Lancet* 1:617, 1982.

17. Tyson RN: Simulation of cerebral death by succinylcholine sensitivity. *Arch Neurol* 30:409, 1974.
18. Powner DJ: The diagnosis of brain death in the adult patient. *J Intensive Care Med* 2:184, 1987.
19. Powner DJ: Drug-associated isoelectric EEGs: A hazard in brain-death certification. *JAMA* 236:1123, 1976.
20. Cohen RJ, Henry CE: The electroencephalogram in head injury. In: Becker DP, Gudeman SK, (eds): *Textbook of Head Injury*, Philadelphia, Saunders, 1989, p 273.
21. Jennett B, Gleave J, Wilson P: Brain death in three neurosurgical units. *Br Med J* 282:533, 1981.
22. Powner DJ, Fromm GH: The electroencephalogram in the determination of brain death. *N Engl J Med* 300:502, 1979.
23. Ropper AH, Kehne SM, Wechsler L: Transcranial Doppler in brain death. *Neurology* 37:1733, 1987.
24. Schwartz JA, Baxter J, Brill D, Burns JR: Radionuclide cerebral imaging confirming brain death. *JAMA* 249:246, 1983.
25. Goodman JM, Heck LL, Moore BD: Confirmation of brain death with portable isotope angiography: A review of 204 consecutive cases. *Neurosurgery* 16:492, 1985.
26. Wilkinson HA: Intracranial pressure monitoring: Techniques and pitfalls. In: Cooper, PR (ed): *Head Injury*, 2d ed. Baltimore, Williams & Wilkins, 1987, chap 12, pp 220–222.
27. Nakada T: Magnetic resonance spectroscopy in the study of brain metabolism. *Hospimedica* 7:51, 1990.
28. Guidelines for the determination of brain death in children. *Ann Neurol* 21:616, 1987.
29. Garrison RN, Bentley FR, Raque GH, et al.: There is an answer to the shortage of organ donors. SG&O 173:391, 1991.
30. Darby JM, Powner DJ, Stein KL, Grenvik A: Management of the organ donor. In: Rippe JM, Irwin RS, Alpert JS, Fink MP (eds): *Intensive Care Medicine*, Boston, Little, Brown, 1991, pp 1657–1659.
31. Camus A: *The Myth of Sisyphus*. New York, Vintage Books, 1959, p 151.

Index